Molecular Neuropharmacology

A Foundation for Clinical Neuroscience

NOTICE

Medicine is an ever-changing science. As new research and clinical experience broaden our knowledge, changes in treatment and drug therapy are required. The editors and the publisher of this work have checked with sources believed to be reliable in their efforts to provide information that is complete and generally in accord with the standards accepted at the time of publication. However, in view of the possibility of human error or changes in medical sciences, neither the editors, authors, nor the publisher nor any other party who has been involved in the preparation or publication of this work warrants that the information contained herein is in every respect accurate or complete, and they disclaim all responsibility for any errors or omissions or for the results obtained from use of the information contained in this work. Readers are encouraged to confirm the information contained herein with other sources. For example and in particular, readers are advised to check the product information sheet included in the package of each drug they plan to administer to be certain that the information contained in this book is accurate and that changes have not been made in the recommended dose or in the contraindications for administration. This recommendation is of particular importance in connection with new or infrequently used drugs.

Molecular
Neuropharmacology
A Foundation for
Clinical Neuroscience
SECOND EDITION

Eric J. Nestler, MD, PhD

Nash Family Professor of Neuroscience
Chairman, Department of Neuroscience and
Director of the Mount Sinai Brain Institute
Mount Sinai School of Medicine
New York, New York

Steven E. Hyman, MD

Professor of Neurobiology
Harvard Medical School
Provost
Harvard University
Cambridge, Massachusetts

Robert C. Malenka, MD, PhD

Nancy Friend Pritzker Professor of Psychiatry
and Behavioral Sciences
Director, Nancy Friend Pritzker Laboratory
Stanford University School of Medicine
Palo Alto, California

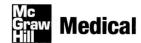

New York   Chicago   San Francisco   Lisbon   London   Madrid   Mexico City
Milan   New Delhi   San Juan   Seoul   Singapore   Sydney   Toronto

The McGraw·Hill Companies

Molecular Neuropharmacology: A Foundation for Clinical Neuroscience, Second Edition

2 3 4 5 6 7 8 9 0   CTP/CTP   12 11 10 9

ISBN 978-0-07-148127-4
MHID 0-07-148127-3

This book was set in Minion by International Typesetting and Composition.
The editors were Anne Sydor and Regina Y. Brown.
The production supervisor was Sherri Souffrance.
Project management was provided by Madhu Bhardwaj, International Typesetting and Composition.
The text was designed by Alan Barnett.
The cover was designed by Kelly Parr.
The illustration manager was Armen Ovsepyan.
China Printing & Translation Services, Ltd. was printer and binder.

This book is printed on acid-free paper.

Catalog-in-Publication Data is on file for this title at the Library of Congress.

This book is dedicated to our families:
Susan, David, Matt, and Jane
Barbara, Emily, Julia, and Charlie
Nick and Ben

CONTENTS

CONTRIBUTING AUTHORS TO THE SECOND EDITION

Olivia Carter, PhD
Harvard University
Boston, Massachusetts

Michael Donovan, PhD
University of Texas Southwestern Medical Center at
*   Dallas*
Dallas, Texas

Matthew Goldberg, PhD
University of Texas Southwestern Medical Center at
*   Dallas*
Dallas, Texas

Max Kelz, MD, PhD
University of Pennsylvania School of Medicine
Philadelphia, Pennsylvania

Anatol Kreitzer, PhD
University of California, San Francisco
San Francisco, California

Michael Lutter, MD, PhD
University of Texas Southwestern Medical Center at
*   Dallas*
Dallas, Texas

Michelle Monje, MD, PhD
Harvard Medical School
Boston, Massachusetts

Tarek K. Rajji, MD
University of Toronto
Canada

Erik Roberson, MD, PhD
University of California, San Francisco
San Francisco, California

David Stellwagen, PhD
McGill University
Montreal, Quebec

Steve Vernino, MD, PhD
University of Texas Southwestern Medical Center at
*   Dallas*
Dallas, Texas

Weifeng Xu, PhD
Stanford University
Palo Alto, Califonia

CONTRIBUTING AUTHORS
TO THE FIRST EDITION

John Alvaro, PhD
Yale University School of Medicine
New Haven, Connecticut

Jennifer A. Cummings, MD
University of California, San Francisco
San Francisco, California

Catharine Duman, PhD
Yale University School of Medicine
New Haven, Connecticut

Charles Glatt, MD, PhD
Cornell University Weill School of Medicine
New York, New York

Kelly Van Koughnet, PhD
Canadian Institutes of Health Research,
*   Ottawa, Ontario*

David Krantz, MD, PhD
University of California, Los Angeles
Los Angeles, California

Chris McBain, PhD
National Institute of Child Health & Development
Bethesda, Maryland

Thomas Neylan, MD
University of California, San Francisco
San Francisco, California

Heather Rieff, PhD
University of Virginia Medical Center
Charlottesville, Virginia

Nicole Ullrich, MD, PhD
Children's Hospital Boston and Harvard Medical
*   School*
Boston, Massachusetts

Dan Wolf, MD, PhD
University of Pennsylvania School of Medicine
Philadelphia, Pennsylvania

PREFACE

Neuropharmacology, the study of drug actions on the nervous system, comprises several areas of investigation of critical importance to science and medicine. Neuropharmacology involves studies aimed at understanding the mechanisms by which drugs alter brain function. These include medications used to treat a wide range of neurologic and psychiatric disorders as well as drugs of abuse. A primary goal of neuropharmacology is to use this information to develop new medications with ever-improving efficacy and safety for diseases of the nervous system. In addition, neuropharmacologic agents are valuable tools with which to probe the molecular and cellular basis of nervous system functioning. For example, drugs such as antidepressants, that produce their clinically relevant effects only after repeated administration, provide a means of learning about neural plasticity. Overall, much of what we now know about the nervous system—how individual neurons work, how neurons communicate with one another, and how neurons adapt over time to external stimuli—has come from studies using pharmacologic probes.

To comprehend the actions of a drug on the nervous system, a great deal more is needed than simply identifying the drug's initial target in the nervous system. Rather, one must understand the entire sequence of events that commences with the binding of a drug to an initial molecular target. The resulting alteration in the functioning of that target, the influence of that occurrence on the complex biochemical networks that exist within neurons, the subsequent changes in the output of the neuron, and their consequences for the functioning of circuits within which the targeted neuron exists are all important for gaining a real understanding of drug action. Only with an awareness of the many steps in the process can we grasp how a drug changes complex nervous system functions such as movement, cognition, pain, or mood. Thus, the action of a drug on the nervous system must be comprehended at many levels under both normal and pathologic conditions.

The organization of this textbook represents an attempt to build an understanding of drug action by adding the different levels of explanation layer by layer. As a result this book differs significantly from many other pharmacology texts, which are usually organized by drug class or by neurotransmitter. In this book, information on fundamental molecular and cellular building blocks is provided first so that it can serve as the basis for the material associated with neural functions. This permits the reader to relate fundamental neuropharmacology to neural systems and ultimately to clinical neuroscience.

The book is divided into three parts. Part 1 includes a brief discussion of general principles of neuropharmacology (Chapter 1), followed by a detailed presentation of nervous system function (Chapters 2–4), from electrical excitability to signal transduction to gene expression. Drugs that act on these basic components of neuronal function are mentioned in these early chapters.

In Part 2 information about the major neurotransmitter systems in the brain and spinal cord is presented (Chapters 5–8). Highlighted in these chapters are the molecular details of neurotransmitter synthetic and degradative enzymes, receptors, and transporter proteins. These proteins represent the initial targets for the large majority of known psychotropic drugs. Also included in Part 2 is a discussion of several types of atypical neurotransmitters, eg, neurotrophic factors, adenosine, endocannabinoids, and nitric oxide, among others (Chapter 8), which in recent years have been shown to profoundly influence the adult nervous system and to be potentially important in therapeutics.

Part 3 uses the basic information contained in Parts 1 and 2 to build a systems-level description of the major domains of complex nervous system function. Chapter 9 focuses on the autonomic nervous system; Chapter 10 on neuroendocrine function, Chapter 11 on pain and analgesia, Chapter 12 on sleep and arousal, Chapter 13 on cognition and behavioral control, Chapter 14 on emotion and mood, Chapter 15 on reinforcement and addiction, Chapter 16 on schizophrenia and other forms of psychosis, Chapter 17 on neurodegenerative diseases, in particular, Alzheimer disease and Parkinson disease, Chapter 18 on seizure disorders, and Chapter 19 on cerebrovascular illnesses such as stroke and migraine. Each chapter begins with a description of the normal neural mechanisms underlying a particular domain of nervous system functioning, followed by a discussion of the diseases that affect that domain. Drugs are discussed within the context of their influence on the neural circuits involved in both normal function and specific disease states.

The organization of *Molecular Neuropharmacology: A Foundation for Clinical Neuroscience* allows individual drugs to be discussed in several contexts. A drug is first mentioned when its initial target is described in Part 1 or 2. The drug is mentioned again in Part 3 in the context of its effect on complex neural functions. Many drugs are discussed in several chapters of Part 3 because they affect more than one domain; for example, first generation antipsychotic drugs not only reduce psychosis (Chapter 16), but also affect motor function (Chapter 17), sleep (Chapter 12), and neuroendocrine function (Chapter 10).

The book's structure also permits the incorporation of a great deal of clinical information, much of it representing the integration of modern molecular genetics with neuropharmacology. New insights on the molecular mechanisms underlying such disorders as Parkinson disease, Huntington disease, depression, schizophrenia, Alzheimer disease, stroke, and epilepsy, to name a few, are provided. Our knowledge of the molecular underpinnings of normal brain function and disease, particularly in cases that have been successfully investigated by genetics, may be in advance of developments in pharmacology. Consequently, the book includes many molecular insights, even though drugs may not yet exist that exploit such molecular knowledge. In this regard the book can be seen as presenting a template for the future in identifying molecular mechanisms for novel therapeutic approaches. We anticipate that subsequent editions of this book will describe the development of such novel medications and thereby gradually fill in these gaps in pharmacology.

The scientific and clinical explanations in *Molecular Neuropharmacology: A Foundation for Clinical Neuroscience* are written in a style that makes them accessible to a wide audience: undergraduate and graduate students as well as students in the medical and allied health professions. This book is also an excellent resource for residents in psychiatry, neurology, neurosurgery, rehabilitation medicine, and anesthesiology, and practicing clinicians and scientists in these areas. As a concise treatise of clinical information that provides descriptions of basic mechanisms and their clinical relevance, this book is suitable for both scientists and clinicians.

We would like to acknowledge the contributing authors who were instrumental in the initial phases of the preparation of this book, both the first and second editions. We also would like to thank Anne Sydor, Regina Brown, and their colleagues at McGraw-Hill, and Madhu Bhardwaj and her team at International Typesetting and Composition, for their crucial role in production of this second edition.

Eric J. Nestler
Steven E. Hyman
Robert C. Malenka
September, 2008

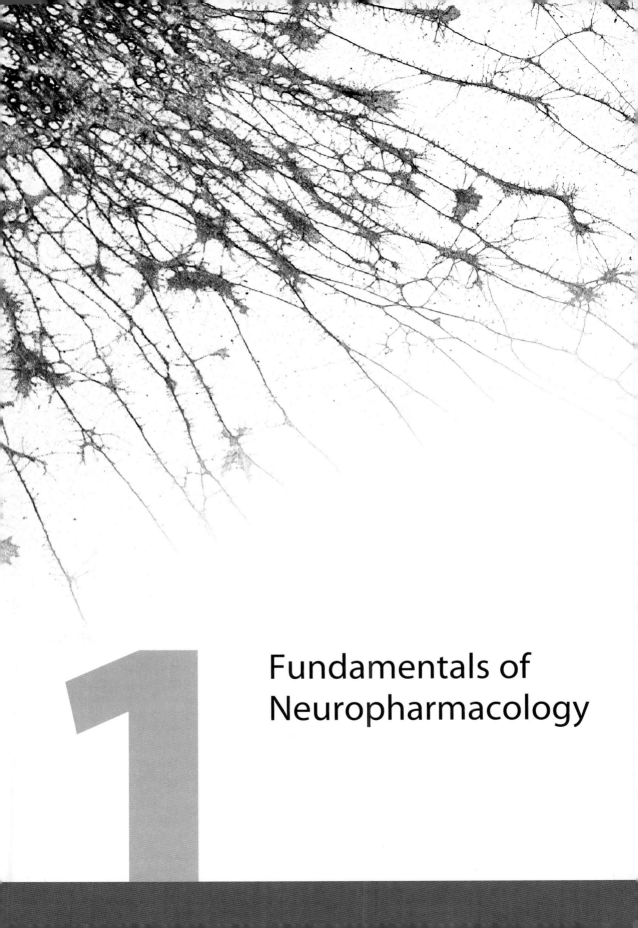

Fundamentals of Neuropharmacology

1

Basic Principles of Neuropharmacology

KEY CONCEPTS

- An understanding of drug action in the brain must integrate knowledge of the molecular and cellular actions of a drug with their effects on brain circuitry.

- The clinical actions of a drug in the brain often are due to neural plasticity—the long-term adaptations of neurons to the sustained short-term actions of a drug.

- The binding of a drug to its specific target(s) normally is saturable and stereoselective.

- The specific binding of a drug to its target is quantified according to its affinity for the target, expressed as a dissociation constant (K_d), and the total amount of binding (B_{max}).

- Potency of a drug describes the strength of binding between the drug and its target; efficacy describes the maximal biologic effects that the drug exerts by binding to its target.

- Drugs can be classified as agonists, partial agonists, inverse agonists, partial inverse agonists, or antagonists.

- Modern neuropharmacology takes advantage of the tools of molecular biology, genetics, and cell biology as well as combinatorial chemistry, which is used to generate novel molecules that may function as new drugs.

- Functional genomics and proteomics will help identify novel drug targets.

Neuropharmacology is the scientific study of the effects of drugs on the nervous system. Its primary focus is the actions of medications for psychiatric and neurologic disorders as well as those of drugs of abuse. Neuropharmacology also uses drugs as tools to form a better understanding of normal nervous system functioning. The goal of neuropharmacology is to apply information about drugs and their mechanisms of action to develop safer, more effective treatments and eventually curative and preventive measures for a host of nervous system abnormalities. The importance of neuropharmacology to medical practice, and to society at large, is difficult to overstate. Drugs that act on the nervous system, including antidepressant, antianxiety, anticonvulsant, and antipsychotic agents, are among the most widely prescribed medications. Moreover, commonly prescribed medications that act on other organ systems often are associated with side effects that involve the nervous system and in turn may limit their clinical utility. In addition, a substantial number of individuals use common substances, such as caffeine, alcohol, and nicotine, that are included in the domain of neuropharmacology because of their effects on the central nervous system (CNS). In a much smaller fraction of the population, these and other drugs are used compulsively, in a manner that constitutes an addiction. Drug abuse and addiction exact an astoundingly high financial and human toll on society through direct adverse effects, such as lung cancer and hepatic cirrhosis, and indirect adverse effects—for example, accidents and AIDS—on health and productivity. Still other common afflictions of the nervous system, such as Alzheimer disease as just one example, are awaiting effective medications, further emphasizing the importance of neuropharmacology.

Neuropsychopharmacology is an all-encompassing term that typically is applied to all types of drug effects that influence nervous system functioning. The term *psychopharmacology* is often used to describe the effect of drugs on psychologic parameters such as emotions and cognition. Drugs that influence behavior are known as *psychotropic* agents. In this book we use the term *neuropharmacology* to describe the study of all drugs that affect the nervous system, whether they affect sensory perception, motor function, seizure activity, mood, higher cognitive function, or other forms of nervous system functioning.

HOW DRUGS WORK

The actions of drugs that affect the nervous system are considerably more complicated than those of drugs that act on other organ systems. To understand how drugs act on the nervous system, it is critical to integrate information about the molecular and cellular actions of a drug with knowledge of how these actions affect brain circuitry—a circuitry that is constantly changing in structure and function in response to both pharmacologic and nonpharmacologic input from the environment. The complexity that underlies such actions can be illustrated by consideration of **fluoxetine,** a widely prescribed antidepressant, and **furosemide,** a widely prescribed diuretic. The chemical actions of these drugs are fairly simple. Both drugs initially bind to their specific protein target: fluoxetine binds to and inhibits serotonin transporters, which normally inactivate the actions of the neurotransmitter serotonin (Chapter 6), and furosemide binds to and inhibits Cl^- channels located in the ascending loop of Henle in nephrons of the kidney. However, the relation between the chemical and clinical actions of these drugs—particularly those of fluoxetine—requires a more elaborate explanation.

The association between furosemide's chemical and clinical activity is relatively straightforward. By inhibiting Cl^- transport in Henle's loop, furosemide causes more Cl^- to remain in the lumen of the nephron tubule, which in turn requires more H_2O to remain in the tubule. Furosemide exerts this same effect on all nephrons in the kidney, and the increase in H_2O in individual nephron tubules combines to cause diuresis at the level of the kidney. Diuresis is achieved as soon as effective concentrations of the drug reach the kidney's extracellular fluid, and is maintained with repeated use of the drug—for example, in the treatment of chronic congestive heart failure.

The relationship between the chemical and clinical actions of fluoxetine is more intricate and also more speculative. Most drugs that act on the nervous system interact with only the minute subset of the brain's neurons that express the initial protein target of the drug. Fluoxetine directly affects only those neurons that use serotonin as a neurotransmitter—a few 100 000 out of approximately 100 billion neurons in the brain. By inhibiting serotonin reuptake by these neurons, fluoxetine enhances serotonergic transmission throughout the brain, but little is known about where in the brain enhanced serotonin function causes an antidepressant effect. Similarly, little is known about which of serotonin's 14 known receptors must be activated to achieve an antidepressant response. Moreover, the mood-elevating effects of fluoxetine are not evident after initial exposure to the drug but require its continued use for several weeks. This delayed effect suggests that it is not the inhibition of serotonin transporters per se, but some adaptation to sustained increases in serotonin function that mediates the clinical actions of fluoxetine. However, where these adaptations occur in the brain, and the nature of the adaptations at the molecular level, have yet to be identified with certainty.

The clinical actions of fluoxetine, like those of many neuropharmacologic agents, reflect drug-induced *neural plasticity,* which is the process by which neurons adapt over time in response to chronic disturbance. Consequently, to understand fully the effects of a neuropharmacologic drug, we must determine not only the initial effects of the drug, but also the intraneuronal signals that control a neuron's adaptations over time, the interneuronal signals through which neurons communicate with one another, and the ways in which large groups of neurons operate in circuits to produce complex brain functions.

Parts I and II of this book explore the intraneuronal and interneuronal signals that enable communication among neurons, which are fairly well understood. Part III addresses the relationships between circuits of neurons and complex brain functions, about which much remains to be discovered.

DRUGS AS TOOLS TO PROBE BRAIN FUNCTION

Neuropharmacology has contributed to many important advances in the neurosciences during the past several decades. Drugs have been used as tools to dissect the functions of the brain and of individual nerve cells under normal and pathophysiologic conditions. Historically, neuropharmacology has involved the delineation of diverse molecules that function as neurotransmitters in the nervous system, including monoamines, amino acids, purines, and peptides. The identification of many of these neurotransmitters and the elucidation of their synthesis, degradation, and receptors occurred in conjunction with studies of synthetic and plant substances that were known to exert profound effects on behavior. The neuropharmacology of **ergot** alkaloids, **cocaine,** and **reserpine,** for example, led to the discovery and characterization of monoamine neurotransmitter systems; **opiate** alkaloids such as **morphine** led to endogenous opioid systems; **nicotine, muscarine,** and **cholinesterase inhibitors** led to cholinergic systems; and **caffeine** and related substances led to purinergic systems.

Neuropharmacology also played a fundamental role in the delineation of the numerous receptor subtypes through which neurotransmitters elicit biologic responses. The early idea that one neurotransmitter acts on only one receptor was replaced decades ago with the recognition that for each neurotransmitter there are multiple receptors. This discovery led to the development of synthetic drugs with increasing selectivity for individual types of receptors, and the evolution of these neuropharmacologic agents has represented important advances in clinical medicine. These advances include the use of selective β_1-**adrenergic antagonists** for cardiovascular disease, selective β_2-**adrenergic agonists** for asthma, μ-**opioid antagonists** for opiate overdose, and $5HT_{1d}$-**serotonin agonists** for migraine, to name just a few examples.

As well, the identification of multiple receptor subtypes for neurotransmitters contributed to the recognition of complex postreceptor signal transduction cascades through which receptors ultimately produce their biologic responses. From G proteins to second messengers to protein phosphorylation pathways to regulation of gene expression, studies of the effects of drugs on the nervous system have provided crucial windows onto the functioning of intracellular signaling. For instance, investigation of the mechanisms by which **organic nitrates** cause vasodilation in the treatment of angina led to the discovery of nitric oxide as a critical signaling molecule, and studies of **aspirin** and related nonsteroidal anti-inflammatory drugs (**NSAIDs**) led to the discovery of a host of signaling molecules derived from arachidonic acid, including prostaglandins and leukotrienes.

Drugs serve as prototypical external or environmental factors in determining how the brain adapts or maladapts over time in response to repeated perturbations. Many adaptations that occur in response to repeated drug exposure are models for adaptations to other external exposures, including stress and experience.

PRINCIPLES OF GENERAL PHARMACOLOGY

The ability of a drug to produce an effect on an organism is dependent on many of its properties, from its absorption to its stability to its elimination. To briefly summarize these processes, the first factor to be considered is the *route of administration,* which can determine how rapidly a drug reaches its target organ and which organs it affects. *Oral* administration typically results in a relatively slow onset of action. *Parenteral* describes all other routes of administration, including *subcutaneous* (under the skin), *intraperitoneal* (into the peritoneal–abdominal cavity), *intravenous* (into the venous system), *intracerebroventricular* (into the cerebral ventricular system), and *intracerebral* (into the brain parenchyma) delivery. The *bioavailability* of a drug determines how much of the drug that is administered actually reaches its target. Bioavailability can be influenced by *absorption* of the drug from the gut if administered orally. It also can be affected by *binding* of the drug to plasma proteins, which makes the drug unavailable to bind to its target. Moreover, it can be influenced by a drug's ability to penetrate the *blood–brain barrier* if the drug acts on the brain (Chapter 2), or its ability to permeate cell membranes if the drug acts on intracellular proteins.

Drug action also depends on the *stability* of the drug once it is absorbed, that is, how rapidly it is metabolized to inactive congeners or eliminated from the body through urine, bile, or exhaled air. Some drugs (*prodrugs*) must be converted into active metabolites before they can exert their biologic effects.

Each of these factors, which can be categorized as *pharmacokinetic* considerations, is a critical determinant of drug action and influences both the clinical use of drugs and the process of developing new agents. However, these pharmacokinetic properties are not discussed in detail in this book because they are not, strictly speaking, related to the underlying mechanisms of drug action—the *pharmacodynamic* features that are the primary concern of these chapters. As an introduction to this topic, a brief description of the process by which a drug interacts with its initial protein target follows. *Pharmacogenetics*, which describes the influence of an individual's genes in determining the response to a given drug, is also critical, but still in the earliest phases of understanding (see below).

Drug Binding

Neuropharmacology is changing rapidly in response to the molecular revolution. In previous decades, neuropharmacology focused on the role of the synapse and, more particularly, on the effects of drugs on neurotransmitters or neurotransmitter receptors. The action of drugs on synaptic targets remains an important field of investigation. The initial target of a drug generally determines the particular cells and neural circuits on which the drug acts and at the same time the potential efficacy and side effects of the pharmacologic agent. However, the molecular revolution has made it clear that the initial binding of a drug to its target—for example, the binding of a drug to a neurotransmitter receptor—is only the beginning of a signaling cascade that affects the behavior of cells and ultimately complex circuits.

When a drug binds to a protein, it affects the functioning of that protein, thereby establishing a form of *allosteric* regulation. A drug can conceivably bind to any site on a protein. A simple site may involve just a few contiguous amino acid residues in a protein's primary structure, while a relatively complex site may involve discontinuous residues from the protein's primary structure that are brought near each other by the protein's secondary and tertiary structures. Ultimately, the three-dimensional shape, or conformation, of a binding site and the electrostatic charges distributed across the site must complement the shape and charge of the drug. The interaction of a drug with its binding site can influence the intrinsic activity of the target protein, for example, the catalytic activity of an enzyme or the conductance of an ion channel, or it can influence the ability of the protein to interact with some other molecule, such as the ability of a receptor to bind to its neurotransmitter.

In classic studies of drug mechanisms of action, a mechanism is defined by a drug's ability to bind to an unknown receptor in tissue homogenates or on tissue sections. In these studies the drug, termed the *ligand,* is radiolabeled and incubated with a tissue preparation, which is washed extensively to remove loosely bound drug. A radioactive atom, typically ^{3}H, ^{14}C, or ^{125}I, must be added to the drug without altering its ligand-binding properties, a process that can be exceedingly difficult. Three major criteria are used to assess the resulting ligand binding. First, the binding should be *specific;* that is, the ligand must bind to its specific target protein. Specific binding must be distinguished from binding to other proteins or even to the wall of a plastic test tube. In many cases, binding is *stereoselective,* or specific for only one stereoisomer of a drug. Second, binding should be *saturable.* A limited amount of ligand binding occurs in the preparation because the amount of the specific target is limited. (A tissue preparation contains a finite amount of an individual receptor protein compared with a test tube wall, which is theoretically infinite.) Third, binding should attain a *steady state.* Time and other conditions, such as temperature, associated with incubation should enable the ligand binding to achieve a state of equilibrium.

The extent to which a ligand binds to a tissue preparation is a function of the concentration of the ligand **1-1**. The total binding of a ligand to the tissue preparation comprises two components: (1) specific binding, which is saturable, and (2) nonspecific binding, which is not saturable. In the ideal situation, in which binding to a specific receptor site is competitive and fully reversible in the steady state, specific binding can be defined as the fraction of total binding that can be displaced by incubating the radiolabeled ligand-tissue mixture with a large excess of unlabeled ligand. Conversely, the nondisplaceable radioactive portion of the preparation is considered nonspecific binding.

There are several discrepancies, however, between ideal and actual conditions. Not all binding to target proteins is truly reversible; the affinity of some ligand–receptor interactions is so high that resulting complexes

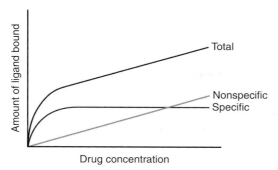

1-1 **Radioligand binding assay.** In this theoretical representation the amount of radioligand bound to a tissue preparation (eg, homogenate, brain slice) is a function of the concentration of the radioligand. Total binding is the total amount of binding observed. Nonspecific binding represents the nonsaturable portion of binding that is presumably not associated with the specific binding site under investigation; it is often calculated as the binding of radioligand that persists in the presence of a large excess of nonradiolabeled ligand. Specific binding is calculated as the difference between total and nonspecific binding and reflects the amount of radioligand bound to the specific binding site.

are not readily dissociable. Moreover, artifactual sites may be present and may show striking apparent specificity. While the ideal situation assumes that the tissue preparation contains just one specific target, in actuality many drugs can bind specifically to many related subtypes of a protein target; for example, serotonin binds to numerous subtypes of serotonin receptors. Consequently, the resulting binding curves can be quite complicated and difficult to interpret.

The specific binding of a ligand to a tissue preparation is quantified according to two properties: the *affinity* of the binding, which is expressed as a dissociation constant (K_d), and the *total amount* of the binding (B_{max}) **1-2**. These terms are analogous to those used in studies of enzyme kinetics—for example, the Michaelis–Menten equation—in which K_a is the activation constant for an enzyme and its cofactor, and V_{max} is the maximum catalytic activity of the enzyme. The K_d is defined as the concentration of ligand at which half of the specific binding sites are occupied; larger K_d values (eg, 100 nM versus 1 nM) reflect lower affinities of the drug. When ligand binding is plotted as a function of the log of drug concentration, a sigmoidal curve is obtained **1-2B**. Ligand binding data are often transformed mathematically to yield a

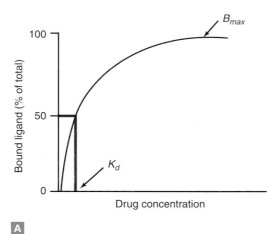

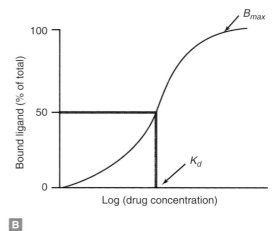

1-2 **Determination of K_d and B_{max} from radioligand binding assays.** The amount of specific radioligand binding to a specific site in a tissue preparation (determined in **1-1**) is plotted as a function of radioligand concentration, using a normal **A.** or semilogarithmic **B.** plot. The K_d is calculated as the concentration of radioligand that results in 50% of maximal binding (B_{max}). The semilogarithmic plot, which better illustrates the effects of low radioligand concentrations, places the K_d near the middle of the graph.

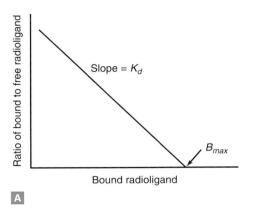

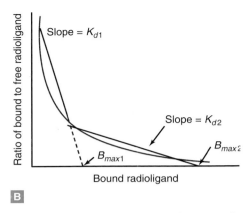

A   **B**

1-3   The Scatchard plot. Specific binding data are mathematically transformed to plot the ratio of bound to free radioligand as a function of bound radioligand. **A.** When one binding site is involved, the data follow a straight line. The slope of the line is the K_d and the x-intercept is the B_{max}. **B.** When more than one binding site is involved, the data follow convex curves, which can be converted into multiple straight lines. The slope of each line and its x-intercept represent the K_d and B_{max}, respectively, of each binding site.

Scatchard plot, in which the ratio of bound ligand to free ligand is plotted as a function of bound ligand **1-3** . Because it is difficult to measure the amount of free (unbound) ligand, total ligand minus bound ligand is used. The shape of Scatchard plots provides an indication of the number of binding sites in a tissue preparation, as well as the K_d and B_{max} values for each site.

Another method for studying ligand–target interactions makes use of *competition curves.* These curves describe the ability of a drug to compete with a radioligand in binding to a tissue preparation **1-4** . The drug concentration at which half of the radioligand binding is displaced (K_i) is a measure of the affinity of the drug for a binding site in the context of a specific radioligand. Historically, such competition studies have played an important role in defining many subtypes of neurotransmitter receptors. In general, such pharmacologic distinctions of receptors accurately predicted broad categories of receptor proteins, which subsequently were identified with greater precision by means of molecular cloning techniques, as discussed later in this chapter. In ideal situations, the competing drug and the radioligand bind to the same site of the target protein; such binding is termed *competitive.* In more complicated situations, the drug and radioligand bind to different sites on the same protein; in such cases, the binding is *noncompetitive* and results in far more complicated competition curves.

These assessments of ligand binding can be performed in several different types of tissue preparation. The traditional preparation is a tissue homogenate or membrane fraction, although extracts of solubilized

receptor or even samples of purified receptor may be used. An alternative approach, which provides critical data on the anatomic localization of a drug target, involves drug binding to tissue sections, a process termed *receptor autoradiography.*

As with any technique, the limitations of ligand binding assays must be appreciated. One of the most critical

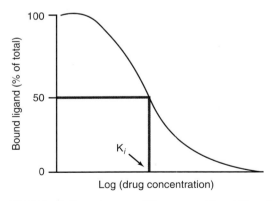

1-4   Radioligand competition curve. The ability of compounds to bind to a particular site in a tissue preparation can be compared by studying the ability of each to compete with a radioligand for a particular binding site. When the binding data are plotted on a semi-logarithmic graph, a sigmoidal curve results. The K_i represents the concentration of drug that results in a reduction of radioligand binding to 50% of maximal values.

limitations is that binding assays, and the determination of K_d, K_p and B_{max} values, are highly dependent on experimental conditions and therefore must be interpreted with considerable caution. The specific radioligand, the temperature of incubation, the salt and ionic content of the buffer, and the presence of different guanine nucleotides (Chapter 4) are among the factors that can exert dramatic effects on ligand binding. The cloning of receptors and other target proteins and the ability to express them on cells without confounding background—for example, without endogenous expression of the target—have made at least some aspects of characterizing the binding properties of drugs more straightforward.

Drug Efficacy

Binding studies describe the physical relationship between a drug and its target but do not directly assess the biologic consequences of this association. Although drug binding and biologic effect are intricately related, they help define two distinct aspects of drug action: *potency* and *efficacy*. Potency (affinity, or K_d) describes the strength of the binding between a drug and its target. Efficacy describes the biologic effect exerted on the target by virtue of the drug binding. These properties can be understood by considering the effect of a drug on a neurotransmitter receptor. As previously explained, the drug must physically bind to the receptor, which requires a physical attraction between the two. Subsequently, that binding must elicit a change in the receptor that leads to a biologic response. For a G protein–coupled receptor, drug binding must trigger a conformational change in the receptor that alters its interactions with its G protein α subunit. For a ligand-gated channel (receptor ionophore), drug binding must trigger a conformational change that opens or closes the pore that is intrinsic to the receptor.

Drugs differ dramatically with respect to their potency and efficacy. Traditionally, two categories of drug have been described: *agonist* and *antagonist*. When an agonist binds to a receptor, it mimics the endogenous neurotransmitter by producing the same conformational change and hence the same biologic response. According to this definition, all neurotransmitters are receptor agonists. When an antagonist binds to a receptor, it elicits no such change; thus, an antagonist is inherently inert and exerts a biologic effect only by interfering with an endogenous ligand. For opioid receptors, which are receptors for the endogenous opioid peptides such as the enkephalins, **morphine** and **naloxone** are classic examples of an agonist and antagonist, respectively. The differences in efficacy associated with agonists and antagonists are

independent of the affinity with which each binds to its receptor; both can exhibit high or low affinities. How can two molecules that bind to the same receptor site exert such different effects on the receptor? There are two possible explanations. An antagonist may share one moiety that is required for binding to the receptor with an agonist, but may lack a moiety required for efficacy. Alternatively, the antagonist and agonist may bind to overlapping but distinct sites on the receptor.

In addition to the actions of classic agonists and antagonists, an intermediate category of drug efficacy is exemplified by *partial agonists*. When a drug binds to a receptor and elicits only a partial biologic response, the drug presumably lacks a portion of the molecule required for full biologic effect or binds to a slightly different site on the receptor 1-5. An interesting situation arises when partial agonists possess high potency. At low drug doses, a mild agonist effect is obtained. At high doses, a similarly mild agonist effect is obtained because of limits in the intrinsic efficacy of the molecule. However, at high doses, the drug can antagonize the ability of a full agonist, including the endogenous neurotransmitter, to activate the receptor because its affinity is greater than that of the full agonist. For this reason, partial agonists are sometimes referred to as mixed agonists–antagonists. Partial agonists can be quite useful clinically; for example, **buprenorphine** is a partial agonist at opioid receptors

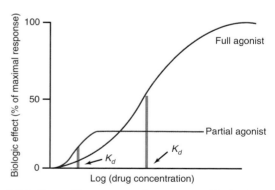

1-5 **Drug efficacy versus drug potency.** The biologic responses elicited by two drugs that bind to the same site are presented in this representation as a function of drug concentration. Efficacy refers to the maximal biologic response elicited by each drug. In this theoretical representation the partial agonist elicits a smaller maximal response than the full agonist. However, efficacy is independent of the potency (K_d) of the drug; the partial agonist shown is in fact more potent (possesses a higher affinity for the binding site) than the full agonist.

and is used in the treatment of chronic pain and opiate addiction. At low doses, buprenorphine elicits a mild analgesic and rewarding effect. Higher doses not only fail to yield a stronger effect, which limits the abuse liability of this drug, but also antagonize the action of full opioid agonists and thereby discourage abuse of opiates such as **morphine.**

Inverse agonists achieve efficacy in still another way. When an inverse agonist binds to a receptor, it elicits the biologic response that is the opposite of that associated with an agonist. If an agonist opens an ion channel, an inverse agonist closes the channel. If an agonist facilitates receptor-to-G protein coupling, an inverse agonist attenuates such coupling. The action of an inverse agonist requires some basal activity on the part of the receptor, which means that the receptor is not quiescent in the absence of ligand but instead possesses some level of intrinsic biologic activity, such as channel conductance or G protein coupling. Indeed, most receptors do exhibit such baseline activity.

Very few drugs can be placed in discrete categories—agonist, antagonist, and inverse agonist. Many drugs that are classically described as agonists, such as **morphine,** are not full agonists but strong partial agonists. Conversely, many drugs that are classically categorized as antagonists—for example, **naloxone**—are not completely inert and thus can be very weak partial agonists. Moreover, some neurotransmitters show less efficacy than synthetic drugs, which indicates that they also are partial agonists. Consequently, drugs should be thought of as existing on a continuum ranging from full agonist to inert antagonist to full inverse agonist 1-6 .

The complex nature of the interactions between drugs and their target receptors can be illustrated by a discussion of the γ-aminobutyric acid receptor (GABA$_A$)—an important receptor for the neurotransmitter GABA (Chapter 5). This receptor is a heteropentamer that has two main types of subunits, α and β. GABA binds to a site on the β subunit and triggers the opening of a Cl$^-$ channel that is intrinsic to the receptor complex. **Muscimol** (an agonist) and **bicuculline** (an antagonist) also bind at this site and thus compete with GABA. The α subunit of the GABA$_A$ receptor contains a binding site for a class of synthetic molecules known as **benzodiazepines.** Agonists that bind at this site, such as **diazepam,** are antianxiety agents that, when bound to the site, allosterically facilitate the ability of GABA to bind to and activate the GABA$_A$ receptor (Chapters 5 and 14). Antagonists at this site, such as **flumazenil,** bind to the site but do not affect receptor function. Because this site lacks endogenous ligands, flumazenil is clinically inactive

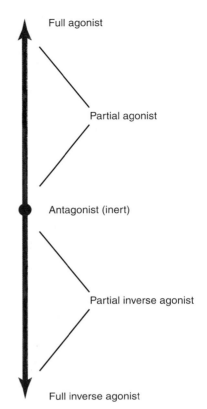

1-6 **Drug efficacy as a continuum.** Ligands for a receptor can be described as agonists (agents that activate the receptor), antagonists (agents that have no intrinsic effect on the receptor but can block the ability of agonists and inverse agonists to regulate the receptor), or inverse agonists (agents that regulate the receptor but produce effects opposite to those produced by agonists). However, ligands rarely can be placed into these discrete categories; instead they are distributed across a continuum. In strict pharmacologic terms, there are very few true antagonists, most being very weak partial agonists or inverse agonists, and very few full agonists or inverse agonists, most being strong partial agonists or inverse agonists.

when bound to the GABA$_A$ receptor; however, it can be used to treat diazepam overdose because it displaces diazepam from the binding site. Inverse agonists, such as **β-carboline,** which intensify anxiety, bind very near the benzodiazepine agonist site and allosterically inhibit the ability of GABA to bind to and activate the receptor. Diazepam and β-carboline are a noncompetitive agonist and inverse agonist, respectively, of the GABA$_A$ receptor, in that they interact with a binding site distinct from the GABA site.

Although this type of complex receptor pharmacology was first described for the GABA$_A$ receptor, a similar level of complexity can characterize drug interaction at virtually any type of receptor. This knowledge is contributing to the development of drugs with novel pharmacologic and hence clinical activity.

It must be emphasized that binding sites with a high affinity for drugs do not necessarily have an endogenous ligand. No evidence, for example, supports the existence of an endogenous ligand for the benzodiazepine binding site on the GABA$_A$ receptor. Rather, the discovery of this class of drugs and their binding site is testimony to the power and promise of medicinal chemistry to target distinctive features of proteins that are not exploited by nature.

Dose-Dependent Drug Response

That the effect of a drug on a target protein is dependent on the concentration of a drug is implicit in the discussions of drug binding and efficacy presented in the preceding sections. This dose dependency of drug action is one of the principal tenets of neuropharmacology and illustrates the importance of studying the effects of a wide range of drug doses.

One application of dose-response curves is in determining whether a form of treatment—for example, chronic exposure to an antidepressant—increases or decreases the responsiveness of a particular receptor system. Hypothetical cases are illustrated in **1-7**,

which shows that a reduction in receptor sensitivity in response to treatment is characterized by a rightward or downward shift in the dose-response curve, whereas an increase in receptor sensitivity is characterized by a leftward or upward shift in the dose-response curve.

Dose-response curves also can reveal that the biologic effects of a specific drug may not be a simple (monotonic) function of drug dose. The effects of some drugs vary in complex ways with respect to drug dose. When the effects of a drug are nonmonotonic, for example, they are represented by an inverted U-shaped curve **1-8**. Such drugs elicit a progressively greater biologic response with greater drug dose up to a point, after which higher drug doses begin to produce smaller effects. This shift in effect most likely occurs because the drug begins to act on a different target protein at higher drug doses, and action on the second target opposes the effects of the first. Alternatively, high doses may cause receptor desensitization.

The analysis of full dose-response curves is necessary to determine reliably whether a particular treatment causes an increase or decrease in drug responsiveness. **1-9** shows a leftward shift in the dose-response curve for a drug whose biologic effects are an inverted U-shaped function of drug concentration. Without an analysis of the full dose-response

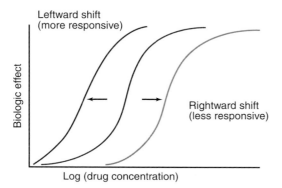

1-7 **Rightward and leftward shifts in dose-response curves.** A rightward, or downward, shift indicates a reduction in drug sensitivity: more drug is needed at all concentrations to elicit the same level of biologic response. A leftward, or upward, shift indicates an increase in drug sensitivity: less drug is needed at all concentrations to elicit the same level of biologic response.

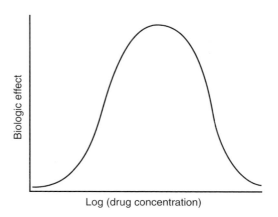

1-8 **Inverted U-shaped dose-response curve.** Dose-response curves that are placed on a semilogarithmic plot often are not sigmoidal, such as those in previous figures, but instead form an inverted U shape. Such curves contain an ascending limb at lower drug doses and a descending limb at higher drug doses. These curves indicate that the biologic response elicited by a drug progressively increases as the drug dose increases and subsequently peaks at a moderate dose; higher doses elicit progressively smaller responses.

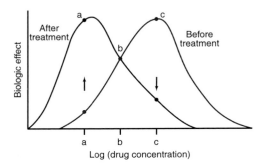

1-9 **Analysis of a full dose-response curve.** Because the biologic effects of many drugs are described by an inverted U-shaped dose-response curve, the effects of a drug should be analyzed over a wide range of doses. The graph shows a leftward shift in an inverted U-shaped dose-response curve occurring after an experimental treatment. With analysis of a single drug dose, it might be determined that the treatment causes (1) an increase in drug sensitivity (dose **a**); (2) no change in drug sensitivity (dose **b**); or (3) a decrease in drug sensitivity (dose **c**). The leftward shift in the dose-response curve becomes apparent only after a wide range of doses are analyzed.

curve, an investigator may incorrectly interpret effects of the drug; for example, depending on the concentration of drug used to activate the receptor, a shift in the curve may indicate a reduction, an increase, or a lack of change in drug response.

Drug Interaction With Nonreceptor Proteins

Although most principles of drug action have been ascertained from studies of neurotransmitter and hormone receptors, the same general principles apply to interactions between drugs and nonreceptor proteins. A drug binds to a specific site on a protein, which can be determined by means of ligand binding assays. Drug binding influences the function of a protein by either facilitating or inhibiting that protein's normal functioning, including its interactions with other macromolecules. Some drugs create a new function for the protein to which they bind; examples include **FK506** and related drugs that bind immunophilins (Chapter 4). When such drugs bind to immunophilin proteins, the proteins become potent inhibitors of calcineurin, a protein phosphatase.

The conditions under which two proteins interact are conceptually similar to those for drug–target interactions. Protein–protein interactions have emerged as a central theme of cell regulation (Chapter 4). The binding of proteins such as transcription factors to specific sequences of DNA, which is a key mechanism of gene regulation in development and in neural plasticity in the adult, also operates according to principles like those of drug-target interactions.

NEUROPHARMACOLOGY IN THE MOLECULAR ERA

Neuropharmacology originally was a phenomenologic science. An investigator administered a drug to an animal or a cell preparation and examined the response. There were two major drawbacks to this black box approach **1-10**. First, it did not elucidate the mechanisms of drug action and thus did not enable investigators to relate the initial action of a drug on its protein target to the clinical effects of the drug. Earlier in this chapter, it was pointed out that the actions of fluoxetine extend beyond inhibiting serotonin transporters or increasing serotonin function. To understand fully how fluoxetine works it is necessary to determine its action on the overall workings of the brain, from its effects on molecules and cells to its effects on neural systems and ultimately on behavior.

Second, traditional neuropharmacology depended on ligand binding studies to identify the protein targets of a drug and to understand its actions on brain function. Such protein targets were typically defined by potency series, which compared the ability of ligands to interact with different binding sites. However, many of the neurotransmitter receptors that were originally identified by ligand binding studies proved to be misleading once it became possible to identify individual proteins by molecular means with near-perfect precision. Whereas pharmacologic studies identified three major subtypes of serotonin receptors, we now know that 14 subtypes exist, with some subtypes misclassified by ligand binding experiments (Chapter 6).

Neuropharmacologists are currently using the penetrating tools of molecular biology and cellular physiology to extend their experimental repertoire. New research is aimed at defining the action of a drug on its cloned protein target in precise molecular terms and analyzing the protein target in various functional states, for example, in phosphorylated versus dephosphorylated states. Ultimately, investigators hope to delineate the crystal structure of these proteins before and after they are bound to a drug to better understand the ways in which a drug alters the shape and surface charges of a protein.

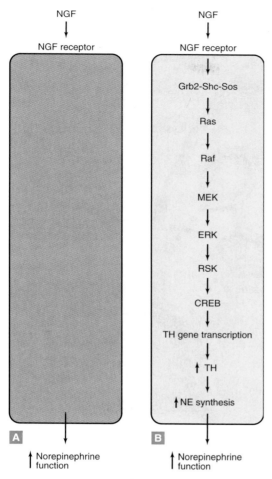

1-10 **A comparison of black box and mechanistic approaches to neuropharmacology.** The increased norepinephrine function in a sympathetic neuron caused by nerve growth factor (NGF) can be described in different ways. **A.** In classic studies, the effect of NGF was described in narrow, superficial terms—for example, NGF activates an NGF receptor—and insufficient attention was given to the detailed mechanisms by which drug-receptor interactions lead to a biologic response. **B.** In contrast, the tools of molecular and cell biology enable a detailed mechanistic description of NGF action, encompassing the delineation of the precise molecular steps by which activation of the NGF receptor leads to increased transcription of tyrosine hydroxylase (TH), the rate-limiting enzyme in norepinephrine synthesis. (Chapters 4 and 8 for definitions of the various proteins shown in this figure.)

Neuropharmacologists are also using new approaches to identify and validate novel targets for drug development, so that novel drugs can be synthesized to interact with those targets. *Combinatorial chemistry* is enabling the development of a large number of drugs with unique and diverse chemical structures. It incorporates knowledge of drug–target interactions at the molecular level, or *structure–activity relationships,* to determine what types of chemical moieties can be added to a drug to alter its actions on a protein target. Much of this initial characterization can now be carried out virtually, by exploring theoretical interactions between chemical structures of small molecules and three-dimensional structures of protein targets **1-11**. *High throughput screening* then allows the testing of a large number of chemical agents, which are promising by such chemi-informatic analyses, to discover their actual abilities to influence cloned proteins of interest. Finally, exploratory research is under way to use higher throughput behavioral analyses to facilitate the discovery of novel classes of compound that exert interesting, and potentially clinically useful, behavioral effects in laboratory animals. Together, these tools may enable researchers to develop any desired types of drugs–for example, agonists, antagonists, weak partial agonists, or inverse agonists–for any targeted proteins or behavioral endpoint.

An interesting question in the field is whether a specific drug is more desirable than a less specific one. The initial era of modern neuropharmacology focused on the search for ever more specific medicinal agents, for instance, moving from **antipsychotic drugs** which antagonize numerous receptors to more specific agents that antagonize just one receptor type. The expectation was that such "cleaner" drugs would show similar or even greater efficacy without the unwanted side effects of the "dirty" drugs. To date, however, such specific agents have been disappointing clinically, which has led to the realization that drugs with multiple targets may offer some advantages for complex brain diseases. The focus on specific agents is also somewhat semantic: fluoxetine is quite specific in that to a first approximation it antagonizes serotonin transporters only, but in doing so it promotes serotonin action at 14 receptors which are expressed by a large fraction of all of the brain's 100 billion nerve cells.

Molecular Diversity of the Brain

Traditional neuropharmacology focused on a very narrow subset of cellular proteins, which included neurotransmitter receptors and transporters and proteins involved in the synthesis or degradation of

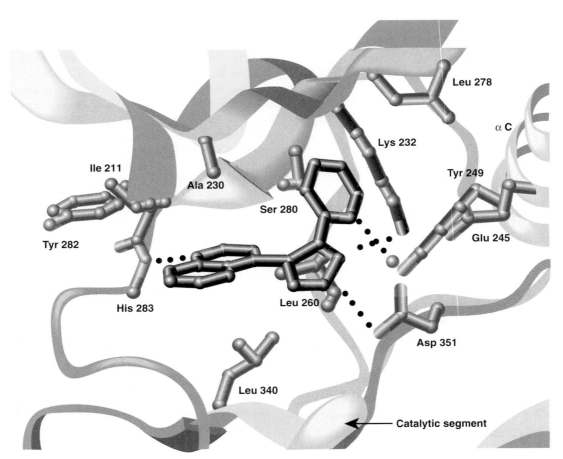

1-11 Three-dimensional representation of a drug binding to a protein target. The figure shows a small molecule (dark purple and red) interacting with specific amino acid residues in a 3D image of the transforming growth factor-β (TGF-β) type 1 receptor. This approach is being used to help investigators synthesize small-molecule antagonists of TGF and other growth factor receptors, which has been a major challenge in the field (Chapter 8). (From J Singh, Avila Therapeutics, Waltham, MA, with permission.)

neurotransmitters. Such proteins account for only a few thousand of perhaps hundreds of thousands of distinct gene products that are expressed in the brain once alternative splicing and protein processing are taken into account (Chapter 4).

The concentration on neurotransmitter-based drugs excessively narrowed the scope of neuropharmacology and interfered with the development of drugs based on new mechanisms of action. Focusing on the 100 000 or more proteins expressed in the brain but not based on neurotransmitters is likely to lead to the identification of fundamentally novel classes of neuropharmacologic agents. Over the next decade, *functional genomics* and *proteomics*—the processes of sequencing, identifying, and characterizing individual

gene products—will provide a template for exploring this vast array of proteins. Large numbers of proteins that regulate receptor sensitivity already have been identified, as have large numbers of modulatory proteins that govern these regulatory proteins. Indeed, it is an exciting prospect that the completion of the various genome projects will allow us to know the full set of receptors and regulatory proteins expressed by nerve cells. Neuropharmacology in the postgenomics era will be involved with the development of drugs aimed at a new set of proteins and the clarification of the mechanisms by which these drugs regulate brain function and behavior. This potential transformation of current treatment of psychiatric and neurologic disorders holds great promise for the future.

Pharmacogenetics

Pharmacogenetics represents the ultimate application of the molecular era to neuropharmacology. It holds the promise of *personalized medicine,* where an individual's particular genetic makeup predicts his or her response to a given medication. For instance, it should be possible one day to identify distinct etiologic subtypes of genetically heterogeneous disorders, such as **autism, schizophrenia,** and **epilepsy,** to name just a few examples, based on genetic testing. These findings could be combined with brain imaging or other technologies to define pathophysiologic subtypes of the illnesses and to thereby permit treatment with drugs aimed specifically at the underlying biologic abnormalities.

Pharmacogenetics is in the earliest stages of development, particularly for diseases of the nervous system, but a few examples are currently in clinical practice. *Cytochrome P450 enzymes,* which are encoded by the CYP gene superfamily, are involved in the metabolism of a large majority of all drugs. We now know that individuals with particular CYP gene variants metabolize certain drugs much more or less effectively than most people. Such genotypes account for some of the differences in drug responsiveness observed clinically, and have been used to approximate the unusually high or low drug doses required in these individuals.

To date, pharmacogenetics is being applied most widely to the treatment of cancer. **Monoclonal antibodies** directed against a particular type of cancer, or even specific for an individual's cancer, are in clinical use. The use of **tamoxifen,** an estrogen receptor antagonist, in the treatment of breast cancer is reserved for those individuals whose tumors express the estrogen receptor. Likewise, the use of epidermal growth factor (EGF) receptor antagonists, such as **gefitinib** or **erlotinib,** for treatment of several types of cancers is increasingly being targeted to individuals whose tumors express mutant forms of the receptor or its signaling proteins. This has recently been applied to **glioblastomas,** a particularly severe form of brain cancer: only 20% of glioblastomas respond to EGF receptor antagonists and recent work has shown that it is possible to predict those individuals who respond based on EGF receptor function in the tumors.

As large scale genetic studies of nervous system diseases progress, and specific causative or vulnerability genes are discovered, it should be possible to increasingly match a particular treatment with a particular patient. While this is many years on the horizon, it will truly usher in the molecular era of pharmacotherapeutics.

SELECTED READING

Brunton LL, Lazo JS, Parker KL. *Goodman and Gilman's The Pharmacological Basis of Therapeutics,* 11th ed. New York: McGraw-Hill; 2005.

Chung WK. Implementation of genetics to personalize medicine. *Gender Med.* 2007;4:248–265.

Daeffler L, Landry Y. Inverse agonism at heptahelical receptors: concept, experimental approach and therapeutic potential. *Fundam Clin Pharmacol.* 2000;14:73–87.

Guo Y, Shafer S, Weller P. et al. Pharmacogenomics and drug development. *Pharmacogenomics.* 2005;6: 857–864.

Gura T. A chemistry set for life. *Nature.* 2000;407: 282–284.

Mellinghoff IK, Wang MY, Vivanco I, et al. Molecular determinants of the response of glioblastomas to EGFR kinase inhibitors. *N Engl J Med.* 2005;353: 2012–2024.

Tecott LH, Nestler EJ. Neurobehavioral assessment in the information age. *Nature Neurosci.* 2004;7:462–466.

CHAPTER 2

Cellular Basis of Communication

- Neurons are the principal cells in the brain that process information. There is a great diversity of neuronal cell types based on morphology, chemistry, location, and connections.

- The nucleus and major cytoplasmic organelles in the cell body of neurons synthesize and process proteins, which are subsequently transported to their appropriate locations within the neuron.

- The axon transports molecules and conducts action potentials to presynaptic terminals to initiate communication with other neurons, which occurs at synapses.

- Dendrites, multiple fine processes that extend from the neuronal cell body, together with the cell body, serve as the primary structure for the reception of synaptic contacts from other neurons.

- The cytoskeleton—the inner scaffold of a neuron formed by a system of interconnected protein filaments called microtubules, intermediate filaments, and actin filaments—plays a key role in the structure of neurons and in the transport of various proteins and organelles from the cell body to axonal and dendritic processes.

- Three major classes of glia—astrocytes, oligodendrocytes, and microglia—play important supporting roles in brain function.

- The blood-brain barrier, formed by tight junctions between endothelial cells of capillaries in cerebral vascular beds, allows only small lipophilic substances to enter the brain from the general circulation.

- In their resting state, neurons maintain a negative electrical potential in relation to the extracellular environment. This results from differences between the intracellular and extracellular concentrations of K^+, Na^+, and Cl^- and the relative permeability of the cell membrane to these and other ions. The energy consuming Na^+/K^+ pump helps to maintain appropriate ionic gradients across the membrane.

- The generation of all-or-none action potentials relies on the activities of voltage-dependent ion channels, highly specialized proteins that allow the flow of a specific ion (K^+, Na^+, or Ca^{2+}) across neuronal membranes in response to changes in neuronal membrane potential.

- Sodium channels are the targets of many important drugs including local anesthetics and some antiseizure medications.

- The three general classes of potassium channels include voltage-gated potassium channels, calcium-activated potassium channels, and inward rectifiers.

- Entry of calcium into neurons through voltage-dependent calcium channels, of which there are five major classes—L-type, N-type, T-type, P/Q-type and R-type—is important for neurotransmitter release and activation of intracellular signaling cascades. L-type calcium channel blockers are used to treat ischemic heart disease and hypertension.

- Mutations in ion channels are the cause of several neurologic disorders, including certain inherited neuromuscular disorders.

It has been estimated that there are at least 100 billion neurons in the human brain, although this number in itself reveals little of the brain's complexity. Unlike other organs, the brain contains an enormous diversity of cell types. Depending on the definition of a neuronal cell type, there may be thousands in the brain—each with their own structural, biochemical, and functional properties. Yet, the complexity of the brain as an information processing organ extends beyond its cellular diversity. Neurons in the brain form diverse circuits that can range in scale from small local neuronal groups to long-distance projections. Any given neuron might function in more than one circuit and might commmunicate with thousands of other neurons.

Neuronal communication depends on both electrical and chemical carriers of information. The electrical mechanisms rely on the ability of each neuron to control the flow of ions across its membrane and thus to process and store information. Chemical signals are the means by which the vast majority of neurons communicate with each other. Neurons are not physically connected but are separated by a minute space, as small as 20 to 40 nm, called a *synapse* (the Greek word for clasp; **2-1**). The simplest synaptic arrangement involves an electrical impulse in one neuron, the presynaptic neuron, that triggers the release of a chemical substance, or neurotransmitter, which diffuses across the synaptic cleft and binds to specific receptors on another, the postsynaptic neuron. The binding of a neurotransmitter to its appropriate receptors precipitates changes in the electrical activity of the postsynaptic neuron, which in turn leads to the release of a neurotransmitter and further interneuronal communication. In a small fraction of cases, neurons physically connect with one another so that direct electrical transmission between the neurons can occur.

Neurons in the brain can form thousands of synapses with other neurons; extreme examples are a Purkinje cell in the cerebellum or a monoamine-containing cell in the brainstem that may form more than 100 000 synapses. Overall, in a single human brain, there are likely to be more than 100 trillion synapses. Complex processes of brain development that are not fully understood result in connections among neurons—some local, some over long distances—that are both highly specific and highly plastic.

The overall patterns of neural connectivity in the mammalian central nervous system (CNS) are dictated

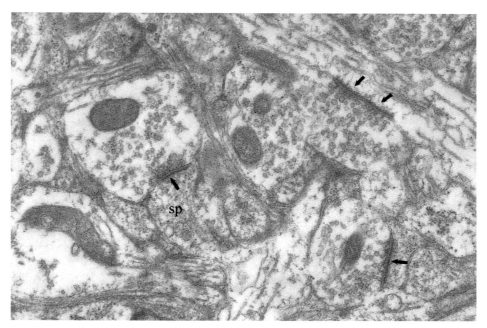

2-1 **Electron micrograph of excitatory synapses.** Each excitatory synapse forms an asymmetric junction, which exhibits a prominent postsynaptic thickening called the postsynaptic density (arrows). Axon terminals opposite the postsynaptic density contain small, spherical vesicles. One terminal can be seen making contact with a dendritic spine (sp). (Micrograph borrowed with permission from J. Buchanan, Stanford University School of Medicine.)

by a complicated set of genetically programmed interactions. Nevertheless, both spontaneous neural activity and neural activity that occurs in response to stimulation during gestation and throughout life have profound influences on the fine-tuning of an individual's pattern of synaptic connections. Although there are finite critical periods of early postnatal development during which the pattern of neural connectivity in some circuits is markedly influenced by experience, the adult brain is far more plastic than previously thought and synaptic connectivity is modified throughout life. Thus, unlike computers, which are sometimes represented as artificial brains, the neural circuitry of the mammalian brain is not hard-wired but instead constantly reacts and adapts to an ever-changing environment.

Although the neuron is the critical cell type for communication in neural networks, essential supporting roles are played by glial cells. The brain contains three major classes of glia: *astrocytes*, *oligodendrocytes*, and *microglia*. Astrocytes have the most diverse functions, which include maintenance of the extracellular milieu (the composition, including ion concentrations, of extracellular fluid in the brain) for healthy neuronal function, metabolism of certain neurotransmitters, and formation of the blood-brain barrier. Astrocytes also are critical in the CNS response to injury. Oligodendrocytes produce myelin sheaths that encase axons and facilitate the conduction of action potentials. Microglia, together with lymphocytes and macrophages that migrate to the CNS from the periphery, are the cellular components of the brain's immune system. All types of glia elaborate soluble factors, including neurotrophic factors and cytokines, which are involved in the maintenance of the nervous system and in its adaptation to changes in the environment (Chapter 8). Indeed, astrocytes are important in modulating the process of synaptic transmission. Glia also are key components in guiding the migration of growing neurons during development.

This chapter focuses on the basic features of neurons and glia and on the electrical excitability of neurons. The molecular and cellular basis of synaptic transmission and signal transduction are covered in subsequent chapters.

THE NEURON

Neurons are highly asymmetric (polarized) cells that have three major components: a *cell body* (also known as a *soma* or perikaryon), a single long process called an *axon*, and a varying number of branching processes known as *dendrites* **2-2**. Aggregations of neuronal cell bodies form the gray matter of the brain (named for its appearance on freshly cut sections). Axons make up the white matter, whose appearance results from the myelin sheaths that insulate many axons and facilitate the conduction of action potentials. Although neurons share a common set of features, they have a variety of sizes and shapes **2-3** and serve very different functions within the networks in which they operate.

Overview of the Neuron

The cell body contains the nucleus and major cytoplasmic organelles such as the rough and smooth endoplasmic reticulum (ER) and Golgi apparatus **2-4**. It is primarily responsible for synthesizing and processing proteins, which are subsequently transported to their appropriate locations within the neuron. The nucleus contains genomic DNA that is transcribed into mRNA; mRNA is exported from the nucleus to the cytoplasm where it is translated into protein on ribosomes (Chapter 4). Although most mRNA remains in the cell body, some of it is transported to dendrites and axon terminals. Polyribosomes, which are multiple ribosomes arrayed on mRNA, and ER are found in dendrites, often right beneath synapses, where they presumably permit localized protein synthesis. Local control of protein synthesis may permit alterations to be made to specific synapses within a neuron, a mechanism which may underlie very precise changes in neural circuit function.

The cell body is the smallest part of the neuron; the bulk of cytoplasmic volume is distributed throughout the axon and the dendritic arbor. Yet, because it must produce components that sustain the rest of the neuron, the metabolic and synthetic demands upon the neuronal cell body are immense. Thus, the cell body contains large numbers of mitochondria, which are the sites of oxidative phosphorylation and provide the form of energy (adenosine triphosphatase [ATP]) used by all eukaryotic cells.

The axon is a fine tubular process that extends from the neuronal cell body; it conducts electrical impulses from the cell body to the axon terminals (presynaptic boutons) that form the presynaptic component of a synapse. *Projection neurons* are those that send axons to another region of the CNS or to the periphery, as opposed to *interneurons* whose axons remain within the CNS region of origin. Neurons generally have a single axon, the length of which varies from less than a millimeter for interneurons to more than a meter for motor neurons that innervate the extremities. The axons of long projection neurons typically are

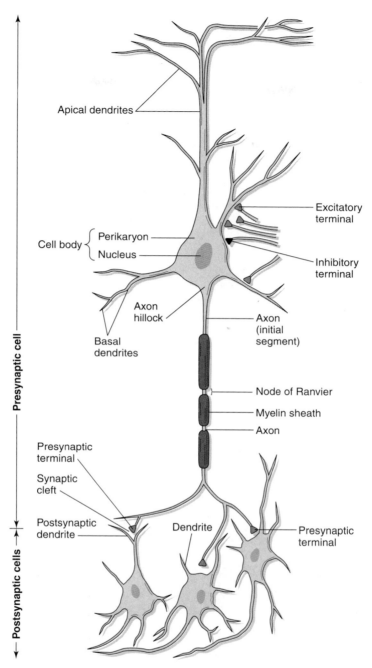

2–2 **Principal features of a typical vertebrate neuron.** Dendrites, which are the primary sites of synaptic contact, receive most of the incoming synaptic communication. The cell body contains the nucleus and is the site of gene transcription. The axon transmits information and often has multiple branches, the terminals of which form synapses with the dendrites of other neurons. (Reproduced, with permission, from Kandel ER, Schwartz JH, Jessell TM. *Principles of Neuroscience*, New York: McGraw-Hill; 2000:22.)

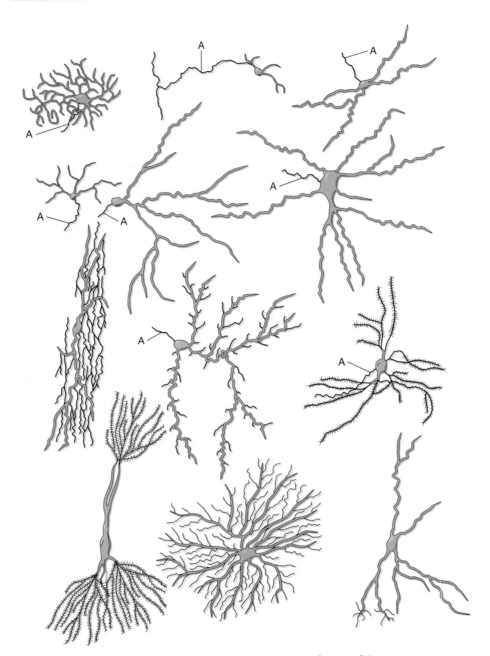

2-3 **Drawings of typical neurons in the CNS.** 'A' marks the axons of some of these neurons.

myelinated; those of local circuit neurons usually do not have myelin sheaths. The axon normally emerges from a region of the cell body called the axon hillock **2-2**, the region of the neuron from which an action potential is most often generated. As it approaches its terminal field of innervation, an axon may branch to varying degrees, depending upon the number of neurons with which it makes synaptic contact. Axons also may give rise to recurrent collaterals that often serve feedback regulatory functions.

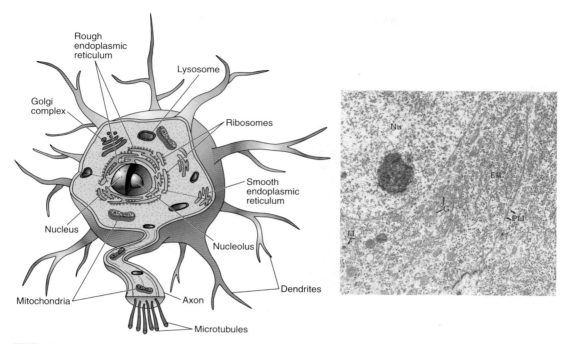

2-4 **Diagram and electron micrograph of intracellular organelles.** The nucleus (Nu) is the site of transcription of DNA to RNA. Proteins are synthesized in the endoplasmic reticulum (ER) and subsequently transported to the Golgi apparatus (G) where they undergo further modifications before they are transported to their final destination. Also shown are mitochondria (M), the energy storehouses for the cell, and the plasma membrane (PM). (Micrograph borrowed with permission from J Buchanan, Stanford University School of Medicine.)

Dendrites are multiple fine processes that extend from the neuronal cell body and, together with the cell body, serve as the primary structure for the reception of synaptic contacts from other neurons. The geometry of dendritic arbors can be very complex and indeed beautiful (see **2-3**). The precise location and extent of a dendritic arbor determine the role of a cell in a network. Many types of neurons have discrete spines protruding from their dendrites **2-5** . Such spines typically receive the major excitatory inputs directed to their respective cells. Moreover, the spines are thought to structurally and biochemically isolate synapses so that each synapse serves as a small, individual unit of information processing (Chapter 3). Dendritic spines are not fixed structures; neurons regulate the number and morphology of spines, in some cases over minutes and hours, in response to neural activity and environmental signals.

The main functions of the dendritic tree include the reception, processing, and integration of incoming synaptic communications. Dendrites are both electrically and biochemically quite complex. Dendrites, like

axons, contain voltage-dependent ion channels and thus can fire action potentials and actively propagate information to the soma. They also contain a wide variety of intracellular signaling molecules (Chapter 4) that are activated during synaptic communication and alter neuronal function.

The Cytoskeleton and the Transport of Proteins

The *cytoskeleton,* which represents the inner structure, or scaffold, of a neuron is formed by a system of interconnected molecular filaments termed *microtubules, intermediate filaments,* and *actin filaments.* Microtubules are made of polymers of tubulin, a globular protein that forms a heterodimer between α and β tubulin. Microtubules copurify with several microtubule-associated proteins (MAPs), which have significant roles in the assembly of microtubules, in cross-linking them to other filaments, and in transport functions. Intermediate filaments of neurons, called neurofilaments, are formed by three polypeptide subunits of low,

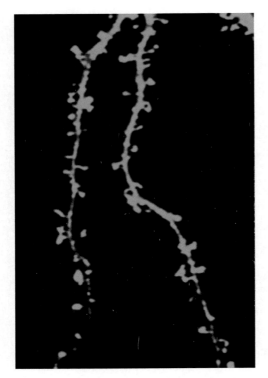

2–5 **Image of dendritic branches of a living hippocampal pyramidal neuron reveals a high density of dendritic spines.** This cell expresses green fluorescent protein (GFP) and was imaged using laser confocal fluorescence microscopy. (Image borrowed with permission from V Biou, Stanford University School of Medicine.)

middle, and high molecular masses. Actin filaments (also called microfilaments) are made of actin, a globular protein that self-assembles into a linear polymer. Microtubules and intermediate filaments are crosslinked to form a longitudinal scaffold for axons and dendrites. Actin microfilaments form a network underneath the entire surface membrane of the neuron; in dendrites and axons they are connected to microtubules and intermediate filaments. Actin microfilaments are heavily concentrated in dendritic spines and growth cones, both of which are dynamic structures that can respond to extracellular signals by changing shape.

The cytoskeleton not only has important structural functions, but also controls the transport of proteins between the cell body and its axonal and dendritic processes. Both fast anterograde and retrograde transport of proteins (100–400 mm/day) and slow anterograde transport (0.1–3.0 mm/day) occurs in axons.

Fast anterograde axonal transport involves the movement of transport vesicles, derived from the Golgi, along axonal microtubules. These vesicles contain many of the proteins necessary for the functioning of the presynaptic terminal.

The power to move vesicles along microtubules by fast axonal transport is derived from two force-generating proteins, *kinesin* and *dynein.* These proteins are ATPases that, by binding to microtubules, are stimulated to transport vesicles. Because microtubules have an intrinsic polarity, with plus ends pointing toward presynaptic terminals and minus ends pointing toward the cell body, they can serve as a compass to direct vesicle traffic. Kinesin and dynein also have an intrinsic polarity; kinesin moves vesicles only toward the plus end of microtubules and therefore is the motor protein for anterograde fast transport, and dynein moves them only toward the minus end and thus is the motor protein for retrograde fast transport. Retrograde axonal transport functions to return various membrane molecules to the soma for elimination and is also important for communicating information from nerve terminals to the soma.

The molecular mechanisms responsible for slow axonal transport and for the transport of proteins to dendrites are not well understood. Slow axonal transport appears to utilize the proteins that comprise the cytoskeleton itself—a dynamic rather than a static structure that is continually renewed. Proteins that are specifically directed toward dendrites rather than axons must be guided by molecular recognition signals that dictate the direction of transport. The dendritic cytoskeleton is different from that of axons. Unlike axons, in which the polarity of microtubules is fixed, dendrites have microtubules whose polarity varies because equal numbers of microtubules are oriented in each direction. The proteins associated with dendritic microtubules also differ from those of axonal microtubules; MAP2 is found only in dendrites and in the cell body, whereas the protein tau is found almost exclusively in axons. Perhaps these differences help guide the transport of specific proteins toward dendrites.

The Synapse

A synapse is a specialized structure involved in the transmission of information from one neuron to another. Synapses typically are composed of a single presynaptic element—the presynaptic terminal or bouton of an axon—and a postsynaptic element, which for excitatory synapses is often a dendritic spine. Although the *synaptic cleft* lies between these 2 elements, it is incorrect to think of the cleft as empty space that separates two independent structures. Instead, the presynaptic and postsynaptic elements of a synapse are tightly bound to one another and to the extracellular matrix by means of numerous proteins, such as cell adhesion molecules (CAMs), cadherins, and integrins, and by astrocytes. The synapse should therefore be considered an individual unit whose sole purpose is to transmit and process information.

Most synapses in the brain utilize chemical transmission. Neurotransmitters **2–1** are typically released from presynaptic terminals, diffuse across a synaptic cleft and bind to specialized receptor proteins on postsynaptic cells (Chapters 3 and 4). The presynaptic terminal contains specialized cellular structures that allow it to remain, to a certain extent, metabolically and functionally independent from the neuronal cell body. It contains large numbers of mitochondria to provide energy, enzymes to synthesize and degrade neurotransmitters, and synaptic vesicles to store substantial concentrations of neurotransmitters while waiting for a signal to be released. The postsynaptic dendritic membrane is markedly enriched with appropriate neurotransmitter receptors and elaborate intracellular signaling machinery.

Synapses that involve the innervation of a postsynaptic dendrite by a presynaptic nerve terminal represent just one anatomic arrangement of chemical synapses. Other arrangements, in particular, where substances are released by dendrites that act on nerve terminals, are described in **2–2**. Overall, chemical synapses are predominant in the CNS but do not represent the only form of synaptic transmission. In a small minority of cases, neurons are connected by means of a *gap junction* rather than separated by an intervening space. Gap junctions, which are formed by a large number of tightly packed proteins (connexons), produce so-called electrical synapses that permit electrical currents to flow directly between cells.

2–1   Identification of Neurotransmitters in the Brain

Our understanding of the molecular basis of neuropharmacology is significantly dependent on our ability to identify neurotransmitters in the mammalian brain. In theory, a substance that is released in response to stimulation of a neuron and that is capable of generating a measurable postsynaptic response, electrophysiologic or biochemical, might be classified as a neurotransmitter. However, to help elucidate the extraordinary complexity of neural signaling, more explicit criteria have been used to identify neurotransmitters.

Localization

A putative neurotransmitter must be localized to presynaptic terminals (or in some cases to dendrites or somas) in specific neural pathways **2–2**. Techniques for such localization include immunohistochemical staining and biochemical analysis of regional concentrations of the substance under study. The localization of enzymes required for the synthesis, degradation, or uptake of the substance helps to confirm the identification of a neurotransmitter.

Release

Classically, neurotransmitters are released in a Ca^{2+}-dependent manner, which can be established, eg, by depleting Ca^{2+} or blocking Ca^{2+} entry into neurons

(Chapter 3). In an intact brain, it can be determined whether stimulation of a pathway causes the release of a candidate neurotransmitter as measured in extracellular fluid by techniques such as *microdialysis* or, in the case of some substances, by electrochemical detection.

Synaptic Mimicry

The action of a suspected neurotransmitter should be mimicked by exogenous application of the substance. Such mimicry can be accomplished in vitro by application of the substance to reduced brain preparations, or in vivo by means of *microiontophoresis*. The actions of the substance can be evaluated by means of electrophysiologic, biochemical, or behavioral measurements.

Synaptic Pharmacology

Neurotransmitters act on receptors for which there may exist pharmacologic antagonists. Thus, if the action of a synaptically released substance is blocked by a selective receptor antagonist, the identity of the neurotransmitter is strongly suggested. Receptor agonists also may be used to demonstrate synaptic mimicry but may provide inaccurate results because several receptor subtypes can be coupled to the same postsynaptic effector mechanisms.

2-2   The Many Faces of Synaptic Transmission

A synapse was initially thought to involve a postsynaptic dendrite or cell body innervated by a presynaptic nerve terminal A. This classic definition described a synapse both structurally and functionally in terms of presynaptic and postsynaptic elements. Although such synapses, which can be termed *axodendritic* or *axosomatic,* are widespread in the CNS and may represent the predominant mode of synaptic transmission involving excitatory and inhibitory amino acids, we have learned that many additional types of synaptic transmission occur in the brain.

Axoaxonic synapses occur when neurotransmitters released from one nerve terminal acts on receptors located on other nearby nerve terminals B. Such nerve terminals may be functionally presynaptic in one synapse but functionally postsynaptic in another. Neurotransmitters also can act by means of autoreceptors located on the same terminals that release them C. Neurotransmitters can be released from cell bodies or dendrites (eg, nitric oxide, endogenous cannabinoids) and diffuse to act on neighboring nerve terminals D, resulting in a *dendroaxonic* synapse.

It is likely that several types of synaptic relationship coexist in most regions of the brain. Consider a hypothetical situation in which an excitatory amino acid nerve terminal innervates a dendritic spine by means of a classic axodendritic synapse E. In addition to acting on the dendritic spine, the released glutamate can affect further glutamate release by acting on autoreceptors at its own nerve terminals. Glutamate release is further modulated by nearby γ-aminobutyric acid (GABA)-ergic nerve terminals, which function as axoaxonic synapses with the glutamatergic terminals. Released monoamines or endogenous cannabinoids modify glutamate release from glutamatergic nerve terminals by means of actions on presynaptic receptors and modify postsynaptic responses to glutamate through actions on receptors near or on the dendritic spines.

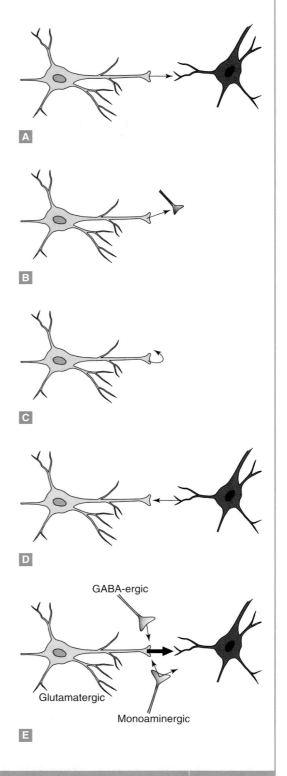

A

B

C

D

GABA-ergic

Glutamatergic

Monoaminergic

E

THE ELECTRICAL PROPERTIES OF NEURONS

Every heartbeat, every nerve impulse, every movement, and every thought is critically dependent on the tightly controlled and precisely timed flow of ions across cell membranes. A disruption of this flow, for example, by the puffer fish poison **tetrodotoxin,** can be fatal. Ion channel abnormalities are responsible for many human diseases (now called **channelopathies**). Mutations of ion channels can result in severe deficits in neuromuscular functioning, including **episodic ataxias** and **paralyses, myotonia, long QT syndrome** of the heart as well as **seizure disorders** **2-1**. Moreover, ion channels are also the targets of widely used and efficacious pharmacologic agents. For example, **phenytoin** and **carbamazepine,** which are used to treat **epilepsy,** act by altering Na^+ channel kinetics. **Lidocaine** and **procaine,** common local anesthetics, block voltage-gated Na^+ channels and prevent the conduction of nerve impulses that signal the occurrence of tissue damage and therefore pain. An awareness of ion channel structure and function is crucial for understanding neuropharmacology and neuronal disease processes.

Electrical Potential in Cells

An animal's nervous system receives information from the environment, integrates this information with past experience, and creates a behavioral response that promotes the survival of the organism. Sensory neurons receive information from both the external environment—for example, sounds and sights—and the internal environment, such as the sensation of hunger or the stretch of a muscle, and relay messages to other neurons. Neurons that receive these messages are responsible for directing appropriate signals to various locations that may include muscles, internal organs, glands, or other neurons. The swift communication of these signals typically benefits an organism. It can, for example, enable a prey's rapid response to the appearance of a predator, or produce a reflexive postural correction that is necessary to prevent a fall.

Neurons convey signals rapidly by alternately maintaining and varying their electrical potentials in relation to the extracellular environment. All neurons maintain a negative electrical potential (also known as a "membrane potential") relative to their extracellular environment. This negative potential provides a driving force for charged particles; in the absence of other forces, positive charges tend to be drawn into the cell, and negative charges tend to be repelled from the cell. When a neuron is activated by an external stimulus such as a chemical signal from another neuron, or by an event in the environment, it may *depolarize;* that is, its electrical potential may become less negative relative to the extracellular milieu. A neuron may, for example, depolarize from -70 mV to -50 mV. If a neuron undergoes significant depolarization, it may generate an action potential—a brief, all-or-none depolarization and repolarization of the membrane potential **2-6**. Such substantial, rapid depolarization will often stimulate a neuron to release neurotransmitters and thus convey information to other cells through chemical signals; for example, a signal conveyed to muscle cells may cause the contraction of a muscle, and a signal conveyed to an internal organ may stimulate or attenuate its activity.

How Neurons Maintain Electrical Potential

Two characteristics of nerve cells contribute to their ability to maintain an electrical potential. First, different types of ions are unequally distributed across the neuronal cell membrane. Generally, the neuron's interior contains a higher concentration of K^+ and lower concentrations of Na^+, Ca^{2+}, and Cl^- than does the extracellular space. These ionic gradients, which occur not only in neurons but in most cell types[1], are maintained through ion-specific pumps that require energy. Moreover, the neuron's interior contains many negatively charged, membrane-impermeable proteins that do not exist in the extracellular milieu.

Second, the neuronal cell membrane is differentially permeable to ions. In the resting state, most neurons are highly permeable to K^+, somewhat permeable to Cl^-, and very slightly permeable to Na^+ and Ca^{2+}. Because the cell membrane is a lipid bilayer, it would be completely impermeable to ions if it did not contain specialized proteins for ion transit. Ions strongly prefer interaction with the polar water molecules in intracellular and extracellular spaces to interaction with the hydrophobic lipid groups that comprise the bulk of the cell membrane. The selective permeability of the cell membrane depends on the numbers and states of its various ion channels. These neuronal properties—unequal permeability of ions across the cell membrane and unequal distribution of ions—are theoretically sufficient to maintain an electrical potential in a cell.

---

[1] Evolutionarily, the maintenance of ionic gradients may have developed from a drive to maintain an extracellular environment similar to that of seawater, where it is speculated that life began. Although higher in osmolarity than mammalian extracelluar fluid, seawater possesses a similar K^+ to Na^+ to Cl^- ratio.

■2-1■ Human Channelopathies

Family	Protein	Gene	G/L	Disease and Symptoms
Kir	Kir1.1 (ROMK)	*KCNJ1*	L	Bartter's syndrome (renal salt loss)
	Kir2.1 (IRK)	*KCNJ2*	L	Andersen's syndrome
	Kir6.2, K_{ATP} channel α-subunit	*KCNJ11*	L	Congenital hyperinsulinism
			G	Neonatal diabetes; DEND syndrome
	SUR1, β-cell K_{ATP} channel β-subunit	*SUR1*	L	Congenital hyperinsulinism
	SUR2, cardiac K_{ATP} channel β-subunit	*SUR2*	L	Dilated cardiomyopathy
K_v	K_v1.1, neuronal α-subunit	*KCNA1*	L	Episodic ataxia type 1, myokymia, neuromyotonia
	K_v7.1	*KCNQ1*	L	Long QT syndrome 1 and possible deafness; Atrial fibrillation; Jervell-Large-Nielsen syndrome
			G	Short QT syndrome
	K_v7.2	*KCNQ2*	L	Benign neonatal febrile convulsions
	K_v7.3	*KCNQ3*	L	Benign neonatal febrile convulsions
	K_v7.4	*KCNQ4*	L	Nonsyndromic deafness
	K_v11.1	*KCNH2*	L	Long QT syndrome 2
			G	Short QT syndrome
	MinK, I_{ks} cardiac β-subunit	*KCNE1*	L	Long QT syndrome 5 Jervell-Lange-Nielsen syndrome
	MIRP1, I_{kc} cardiac β-subunit	*KCNE2*	L	Long QT syndrome 6
TRP	TRPP2 (Polycystin 2, PKD2)	*TRPP2*		Autsosomal dominant polycystic kidney disease
	TRPC6	*TRPC6*	G	Focal segmental glomerulosclerosis, defective Mg^{2+} reabsorption
	TRPML1 (Mucolipin)	*Mcoln1*		Mucolipidosis IV
CNG	Retinal cGMP gated α1-subunit	*CNGA1*	L	Retinitis pigmentosa
	Retinal cGMP gated α3-subunit	*CNGA3*	L	Achromatopsia-2
	Retinal cGMP gated β3-subunit	*CNGB3*	L	Achromatopsia-3
K_{ca}	BK channel α-subunit	*KCMNA1*	G	Generalized epilepsy with paroxysmal dyskinesia
Na_v	Na_v1.1, neuronal α-subunit	*SCN1A*	G	Generalized epilepsy with febrile seizures type 2
			L	Severe myoclonic epilepsy of infancy
	Neuronal β-subunit	*SCN1B*	L	Generalized epilepsy with febrile seizures type 1
	Na_v1.2	*SCN2A*	G	Benign familial neonatal seizures
	Na_v1.4	*SCN4A*	G	Paramyotonia congenita; Hyperkalemic periodic paralysis; K^+-aggravated myotonia
			L	Hypokalemic periodic paralysis

(continued)

2-1 Human Channelopathies (*continued*)

Family	Protein	Gene	G/L	Disease and Symptoms
	Na$_v$1.5	SCN5A	G	Long QT syndrome 2, Brugada syndrome; Non-progressive congenital heart block; Progressive cardiac conduction defect
	Na$_v$1.9	SCN9A	G	Familial erythermalgia (pain)
Ca$_v$	Ca$_v$2.1	CACNA1A	L G E	Episodic ataxia type 2 Familial hemiplegic migraine Spinocerebellar ataxia type 6
	Ca$_v$1.4	CACNA1F		Congenital stationary night blindness
	Ca$_v$1.1	CACNA1S		Hypokalemic periodic paralysis; malignant hypothermia type 5
	Neuronal β4-subunit	CACNB4		Juvenile myoclonic epilepsy; Generalized epilepsy and praxis-induced seizures; Episodic ataxia type 3
	Ca$_v$1.2, α-subunit	CACNA1C		Timothy syndrome
	CFTR, epithelial Cl⁻ channel	CFTR	L	Cystic fibrosis
	Bestrophin, epithelial Cl⁻ channel β-subunit	BEST1	L	Vitelliform macular dystrophy (Best disease)
	ClC1, Cl⁻ channel skeletal muscle α-subunit	CLCN1	L L	Generalized myotonia (Becker's disease) Myotonia congenita (Thomson's disease)
	CLC2, Cl⁻ channel α-subunit	CLCN2	L	Several types of epilepsy
	ClC5, Cl⁻ transporter kidney	CLCN5	L	Dent's disease (X-linked) and other renal tubular disorders
	ClC7, Cl⁻ transporter	CLCN7	L	Osteopetrosis (dense bones), sometimes with blindness
	ClC-Ka, Cl⁻ channel kidney α-subunit	CLCNKA	L	Bartter's syndrome
	ClC-Kb, Cl⁻ channel kidney α-subunit	CLCNKB	L	Bartter's syndrome
	Barttin, Cl⁻ channel β-subunit		L	Bartter's syndrome with deafness

G, gain of function; L, loss of function; E, repeat expansion. The symptom of long and short QT syndrome is ventricular arrhythmia. The symptoms of Jervell-Lange-Nielsen syndrome include deafness and cardiac arrhythmias. Symptoms of autsosomal dominant polycystic kidney disease include cardiac septal defects. Achromatopsia is total color blindness. The symptoms of Timothy syndrome are multi-organ dysfunction including long QT syndrome and syndactyly. DEND syndrome is characterized by developmental delay, epilepsy, muscle weakness and neonatal diabetes. Anderson's syndrome is a multi-organ disorder that includes potassium-sensitive periodic paralysis and ventricular arrhythmia. Generalized myotonia (Becker's disease) and myotonia congenita (Thomson's disease) both result in skeletal muscle hyperexcitability. Bartter's syndrome results in renal salt loss. Congenital myasthenia results in muscle weakness. Hyperekplexia results in muscle contractures when startled. Mutations in ClC5 can cause kidney stones, hypophosphatemic rickets and low molecular weight proteinuria. For references see: www.ncbi.nlm.nih.gov/entrez/query.fcgi?ab=OMIM&omd=Limits (type in the gene name).

A Simple Cell Model

Consider a very simple model of a cell. The interior of the cell (*I*) contains 100 mM K⁺A⁻, where A⁻ is an impermeant anion such as a negatively charged protein. Exterior to the cell (*O*), the concentration of K⁺A⁻ is 5 mM **2-7** . To simplify this model, the effects of osmosis are ignored.

If the cell's lipid bilayer is impermeable to both K⁺ and A⁻, no movement of ions occurs across the bilayer, and the concentration of ions on each side of the bilayer remains constant. However, if the lipid bilayer of this cell became permeable to K⁺, and only to K⁺—for example, from the opening of K⁺-specific ion channels in the lipid bilayer—K⁺ ions but not A⁻ ions would be free to move across the lipid bilayer in both

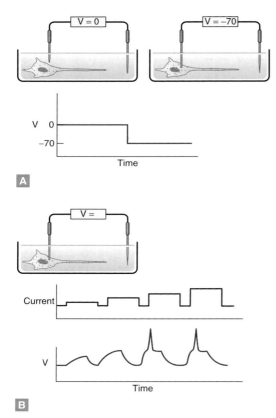

2-6 **Membrane potential.** **A.** As a sharp electrode penetrates a neuron, the difference in potential between the recording electrode and the bath drops from 0 to –70 mV. **B.** When small currents pass through the electrode, the potential of the cell changes in a passive manner. Larger currents elicit an all-or-none action potential.

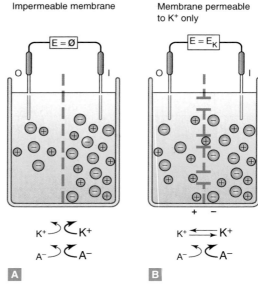

2-7 **A cell model.** **A.** If an impermeable membrane is placed between two compartments that contain different concentrations of the ionic solution K^+A^-, no movement of electrical charge can occur and the difference in potential between the two compartments (E) is zero. **B.** If the membrane becomes permeable to K^+, K^+ initially flows down its concentration gradient from *I* to *O*, creating an electrical potential that opposes the movement of K^+. The net movement of K^+ between *I* and *O* stops when the electrical force repelling K^+ equals the force of the concentration gradient; at this point K^+ has reached its equilibrium potential (E_k), which can be estimated with the Nernst equation.

directions. Because *I* contains 20 times more K^+ than *O*, many more K^+ ions would be likely to travel from *I* to *O* than from *O* to *I*. Consequently, a net efflux of K^+ from *I* to *O* would occur; because A^- would remain impermeable, it would not cross the membrane.

As soon as K^+ ions begin to move to *O*, however, a net positive charge develops in *O* because K^+ has left the cell without accompanying A^-. This net positive charge *repels* K^+ from *O*. Thus, two tendencies act in opposition to one another: (1) the tendency of K^+ to move out of *I* because more K^+ is present in *I* than in *O*, and (2) the tendency of K^+ to be drawn into *I* because of its relative negative potential.

Eventually, these two tendencies reach an equilibrium whereby the net efflux of K^+ from *I* (favored by

the concentration gradient) is equal to the net efflux of K^+ from *O* (promoted by the electrical potential). Only a minuscule fraction of K^+ must venture from *I* to *O* to create an electrical potential strong enough to balance the tendency of K^+ to leave *I* along its concentration gradient. As a consequence, a minuscule fraction of the A^- ions in *I* exist without accompanying K^+ ions, and this tiny separation of charge creates a negative potential of –75 mV in *I* relative to *O*. This negative charge within the cell exerts just enough force on the K^+ ions that the net flow of K^+ ions across the membrane is zero, despite the existing concentration gradient of K^+. The transmembrane electrical potential at which this equilibrium occurs (–75 mV) can be determined by the Nernst equation[2] and is termed the *equilibrium potential* (or the *Nernst potential*) for K^+.

A More Complicated Cell Model

A basic understanding of membrane potential drawn from the previous cell model can assist in understanding a model that more closely resembles a mammalian nerve cell. It involves: (1) a more complete complement of extracellular and intracellular ions, and (2) more realistic ionic permeabilities. **2-2** describes several features of this cell model. First, the net total charge on each side of the cell is zero, a condition that is necessary for electrical neutrality.[3] Second, the cell membrane is far more permeable to K^+ than to any other ion, which is the case for most neurons at rest. All other permeabilities are described relative to the permeability of K^+.

What is the electrical potential at which the net flux of charge across the cell membrane equals zero? If the cell were *only* permeable to K^+, the membrane potential would rest at the equilibrium potential of K^+, because all other ions would be trapped on one side of the cell and could not migrate to contribute to the generation of an electrical potential. However, the cell *is* permeable to other ions, although to a much lesser degree than it is to K^+. If the membrane were permeable *only* to Na^+, the resting potential would be at the equilibrium potential of Na^+. In this case, the cell interior would develop a *positive* potential relative to the exterior of the cell. The positive potential in the cell interior would repel Na^+ ions and balance the statistical tendency of these ions to flow down their concentration gradient and into the cell.

The true equilibrium potential for this cell model would be expected to lie somewhere between the equilibrium potentials for the various ions. The membrane permeability for each type of ion determines the relative contribution of each type of ion on the inside and outside of the membrane to the equilibrium potential. The equilibrium potential for this cell, -68 mV, lies

---

[2] The Nernst equation is $E_m = 58 \log (K_o/K_i)$ where E_m is the equilibrium membrane potential; K_o is the concentration of K^+ ions on the outside and K_i is the concentration of K^+ ions on the inside. The factor of 58 in this equation derives from several chemical values (eg, gas constant, temperature) as well as the valence of each ion and the conversion of natural logarithms to base 10 logarithms.

[3] Note that electrical neutrality cannot be achieved because a separation of charge persists across the cell membrane. It is also important to note that ionic concentrations in **2-2** are given in millimolar values, although a resting potential in a normal cell of -75 mV can be produced by a femtomolar net separation of charge. Moreover, both the cytoplasm of the cell and the extracellular milieu are electrically neutral, having an equal number of positive and negative charges; the difference in charge exists across the cell membrane, which acts as a capacitor.

2-2 **Idealized Free Ion Concentrations Inside and Outside a Nerve Cell**

Ion	Concentration Inside Cell (mM)	Concentration Outside Cell (mM)	Relative Permeability
K^+	100	5	1
Na^+	10	100	0.01
Cl^-	10	105	0.2
A^- (large anions)	100	0	0

between the equilibrium potentials estimated for K^+, Na^+, and Cl^-.[4] Because the membrane's permeability to K^+ is so much greater than its permeability to the other ions, the neuron's resulting membrane potential is much closer to the equilibrium potential of K^+ (-75 mV) than to that of Na^+ ($+58$ mV) or Cl^- (-59 mV).

Many electrophysiologic concepts and the roles of ion channels and ion channel-targeting drugs in physiologic processes can be understood intuitively by understanding the change in membrane potential caused by changing the permeability of the membrane to different types of ions via the opening and closing of ion channels. When only one type of ion channel opens, it drives the membrane potential of the cell toward the equilibrium potential of that ion. For example, if many of the Na^+ channels in this cell model were suddenly opened, causing Na^+ to be three times more permeable than K^+, the membrane potential would move toward the equilibrium potential for Na^+ (in this case $+19.6$ mV). If the Na^+ channels were to close suddenly, bringing the permeability ratio of Na^+ to K^+ back to its original value of 0.01, the membrane potential would return to -68 mV in response to the efflux of K^+ through the many open K^+ channels.

It also is important to emphasize that the equilibrium potential for a particular ion depends on the relative concentrations of that ion inside and outside the cell, which can vary considerably among different cell types and tissues. For example, the equilibrium potential for Cl^- can range from -60 to -90 mV.

Maintenance of Membrane Potential by ATP-Dependent Pumps

The equilibrium potential provides for an equal exchange of cations back and forth across the cell

---

[4] This can be calculated using the Goldman-Hodgkin-Katz equation. For details, see Hille 1992.

membrane: for every excess Na^+ ion that sneaks across the membrane, a K^+ ion moves out, holding the membrane stable at the predicted potential. This exchange occurs slowly enough that the ionic concentrations may be considered constant for short period of time. However, if a slow exchange of Na^+ for K^+ were allowed to continue for hours or days, the concentration gradients would eventually degenerate and the membrane potential would slowly begin to dissipate. *Na^+–K^+ pumps* maintain the ionic gradients across a cell membrane by extruding Na^+ from and pumping K^+ into the cell against their respective concentration gradients at the cost of energy 2-8. Each pump is a multimeric integral membrane protein consisting of transmembrane α subunits, which possess the catalytic and iontophoretic (ion pore-containing) domains of the pump, accessory transmembrane β subunits, which mediate the trafficking of the α subunit to the cell membrane, and tissue-specific regulatory subunits from the FXYD protein family.

The catalytic subunit of each pump has extracellular binding sites for K^+ and intracellular binding sites for Na^+ and ATP. ATP transfers its terminal phosphate to the catalytic subunit in a Na^+-dependent manner; because the pump is a protein that cleaves ATP by means of ion-dependent enzymatic activity, it often is referred to as an *Na^+/K^+-ATPase*. At the expense of the energy of hydrolysis of ATP, typically three Na^+ ions are transported out of the cell and two extracellular K^+ ions are transported in. Thus, the pump is *electrogenic*: it exports more positive charge than it imports. The phosphorylated catalytic subunit is subsequently hydrolyzed in the presence of K^+ ions, returning the catalytic subunit to its resting state. The resting potential of a cell with active Na^+–K^+ pumps is usually a few millivolts more negative than would be predicted on the basis of ion distribution and relative permeabilities alone.

The importance of Na^+–K^+ pumps in the maintenance of cellular membrane potential becomes quite evident when they are inhibited by pharmacologic

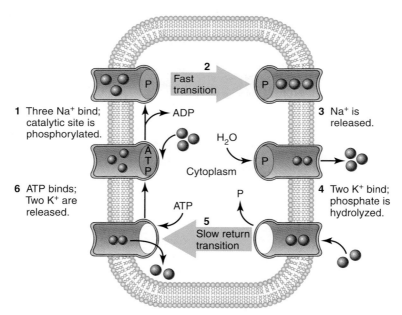

2-8 **The adenosine triphosphate (ATP)-dependent Na^+–K^+ pump.** The pump removes three Na^+ ions from the cell and introduces two K^+ ions. **1.** Three Na^+ ions bind to the interior face of the catalytic subunit, which subsequently is phosphorylated; **2.** through a conformational transition Na^+ ions become less tightly bound to the pump and obtain access to the extracellular space; **3.** Na^+ ions dissociate from the pump; **4.** when two K^+ ions bind to the pump it undergoes dephosphorylation; **5.** the pump changes conformation, providing the two bound K^+ ions with access to the cytoplasm; **6.** after ATP binds to the catalytic subunit, the two K^+ ions are released into the cytoplasm. ADP, adenosine diphosphate; P, phosphorylation.

agents. Cardiac glycosides such as **ouabain** and **digoxin,** which increase the contractile force of cardiac muscle and are used in the treatment of **congestive heart failure** and some cardiac **dysrhythmias,** are the best known inhibitors of the Na⁺–K⁺ pump. Normally, cardiac myocytes maintain low levels of intracellular Ca^{2+}, partly through a Na^+–Ca^{2+} pump that uses energy from the movement of Na^+ down its concentration gradient to transport Ca^{2+} out of the cell. Because cardiac glycosides inhibit Na^+–K^+ pumps and increase intracellular Na^+ concentrations, they make Na^+–Ca^{2+} pumps less effective. Consequently, intracellular Ca^{2+} concentrations increase, which increases the contractile force of cardiac muscle. These drugs also can slowly reduce the resting potential of neurons eventually to zero; in large neurons, this decline in potential occurs after several hours. This action of the drugs in the CNS accounts for common side effects of cardiac glycosides, including disturbed vision, confusion, and delirium.

Digoxin

BIOPHYSICAL PROPERTIES OF THE CELL MEMBRANE

In the cell model described previously, it was possible to create a potential across the membrane by making it selectively permeable to the ions distributed unequally across it. It also was possible to alter the potential of the membrane by changing the relative permeabilities of various ions, for example, by increasing the permeability of Na^+ relative to K^+. Likewise, the membrane's original potential could be restored by reinstating the original permeabilities. In addition to these features,

real neurons have two biophysical properties that affect the movement of charge and the development of potential across a neuronal membrane.

First, unlike the movement of charge in the cell model, charge is not transferred instantaneously from one neuronal compartment to another. Electrically, the membrane can be thought of as a *resistor and a capacitor* **2-9**. Resistance describes a membrane's ability to pass ions, and it is determined by the number and properties of the ion channels, and the thickness of the membrane. Thick membranes, such as myelinated axon membranes, are high resistors that are difficult to let ions through. Capacitance describes a membrane's ability to store charge; the larger the membrane's capacitance, the more charge required to raise a membrane's potential. Several properties such as size and, most significantly, thickness can affect a membrane's capacitance. A very large membrane area requires more stored charge to bring it to a given potential, or in other words it has a greater capacitance, than does a small membrane area. Very thick membranes are poor capacitors: because ions separated across a greater distance possess greater potential energy, fewer ions are required to reach a certain membrane potential. Because a myelin sheath increases a membrane's thickness, a myelinated axonal membrane is a high resistor and poor capacitor compared with a nonmyelinated membrane.

Sensory, Synaptic, and Action Potentials

Neurons exploit their ability to rapidly change their transmembrane potentials in order to receive information from the environment and to relay messages. Input from a variety of sources, including other neurons, can cause a neuron's membrane potential to fluctuate. If a neuron depolarizes enough or reaches threshold, it produces an *action potential*: a rapid, all-or-none depolarization that propagates down its axon. The firing of an axon generally leads to the release of neurotransmitter from the axon's terminals, which in turn conveys the neuron's signal to muscle cells, to effector organs such as glands, or to other neurons.

Receiving information Some neurons are equipped with specialized systems that enable them to receive information from the environment. Hair cells in the cochlea, for example, are sensitive to vibrational energy: vibrations cause the movement of tiny cilia on the surface of these cells. Such movement activates mechanosensitive ion channels that increase the membrane's permeability to Na^+ which in turn leads to depolarization of the hair cell. Photoreceptor cells in the

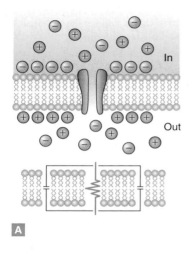

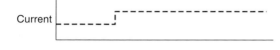

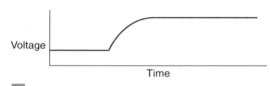

A

B

2-9 **The cell as a resistor-capacitor circuit. A.** The lipid bilayer of the cell's membrane separates charge and thus can be represented as a simple electrical circuit comprising resistance and capacitance. The number and state of the various ion channels in a cell membrane determine that membrane's *resistance,* or the ease with which ions can cross the membrane. Cell membranes with many open ion channels have low resistance; cell membranes with only a few open ion channels have high resistance. The *capacitance* of a membrane, or its ability to store charge, is determined by factors such as the area and thickness of the membrane. **B.** The opening of ion channels and the subsequent flow of current do not result in an instantaneous change in membrane potential. High-resistance and high-capacitance membranes require more time to develop a charge than low-resistance and low-capacitance membranes.

retina can respond to light because photons activate a series of chemical reactions that cause changes in the ionic permeability of the cell membrane, which in turn leads to changes in the membrane potential of the cell.

Neurons generally receive signals from other neurons through chemical neurotransmitters. Neurons typically release neurotransmitter at synapses where it binds to receptors on an adjacent neuron's cell membrane. The binding of neurotransmitter to a receptor routinely leads to changes in the receiving neuron's ion permeability. This change in permeability may occur directly; many neurotransmitter receptors are ligand-gated ion channels. However, changes in permeability also take place indirectly; many types of neurotransmitter receptors activate second messenger systems within a cell that in turn modify ion channels, causing changes in membrane potential (Chapters 3 and 4).

Integrating information The opening of ion channels in a localized area, such as a synapse, produces a transmembrane current that changes the membrane potential of a cell. However, this change in potential does not occur instantaneously or remain localized to the narrow region of membrane in which the current was generated. The integration of local changes in the transmembrane voltage of a neuron is affected by two basic types of summation: *spatial summation* and *temporal summation* **2-10** .

Neurons are "decision makers"—they must continually decide whether to respond to particular sets of stimuli by firing action potentials and in turn communicate with fellow neurons or with effector organs. A motor neuron in the spinal cord, for example, receives thousands of excitatory and inhibitory inputs from pathways that descend from the brain. These descending pathways deliver enormous amounts of information integrated from many areas of the brain, including motor planning, vestibular, and visual centers. The currents produced by excitatory and inhibitory inputs continually undergo summation to produce membrane potentials that fluctuate in time and space. A neuron reads fluctuating potentials at the base of its axon, the axon hillock, where it has a high concentration of voltage-dependent Na^+ channels. If the sum of these potentials produces a sufficient level of depolarization, an action potential is triggered.

Action potential and neurotransmitter release
An action potential is a rapidly propagating depolarization of the axonal membrane that can lead to the release of neurotransmitter from axon terminals. This phenomenon is best understood in terms of the responses of Na^+ channels to changes in voltage. In this section the Na^+ channel is discussed as an abstract

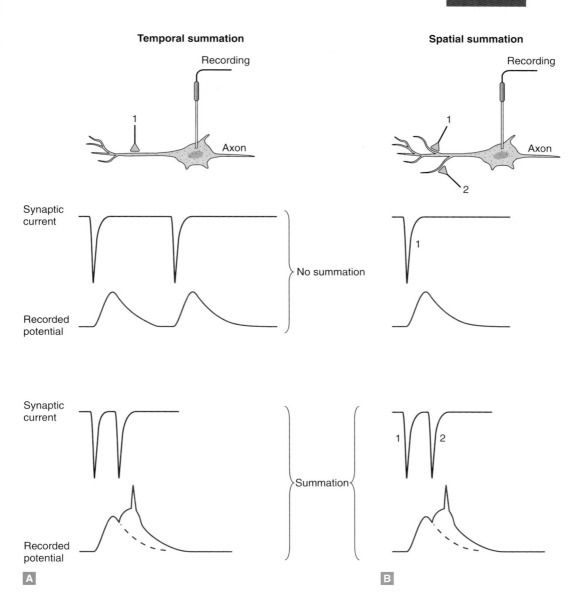

Temporal summation

Recording

1

Axon

Synaptic
current

Recorded
potential

No summation

Spatial summation

Recording

1

Axon

2

Synaptic
current

1

Recorded
potential

Synaptic
current

Summation

Recorded
potential

A

Synaptic
current

1   2

Recorded
potential

B

2–10 **Temporal and spatial summation of synaptic inputs. A.** Temporal summation occurs when repetitive synaptic input transpires so swiftly that synaptic potentials do not have time to decay. **B.** Spatial summation occurs when two independent inputs are activated within a finite window. Because of the passive electrical properties of the cell's membrane, they summate even though they were generated in different locations. (Adapted with permission from Kandel ER, Schwartz JH, Jessell TM. *Principles of Neural Science,* 4th ed. New York: McGraw-Hill; 2000:224.)

entity; its molecular structure is described in detail in the next section.

The opening of Na$^+$ channels (voltage gated or voltage dependent) upon membrane depolarization leads to an inward current that in turn causes further depolarization because the equilibrium potential of Na$^+$ is positive compared with the resting potential of the cell

membrane. Voltage-gated Na$^+$ channels continue to open and to permit further depolarization in a repetitive, self-perpetuating manner. In response to this positive feedback loop, the membrane of the cell's axon is quickly driven toward the equilibrium potential for Na$^+$.

However, two phenomena quickly return the membrane potential to its resting, hyperpolarized state **2–11**.

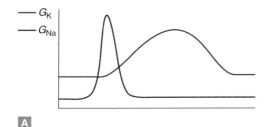

A

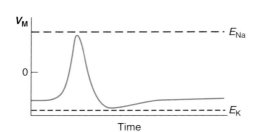

B

2-11 **Changes in membrane conductance during an action potential. A.** The first change is a rapid increase in Na⁺ conductance; this is followed by a slower, longer-lasting increase in K⁺ conductance. **B.** These changes result in a characteristic action potential: a sharp depolarization, from Na⁺ current moving inward, followed by a repolarization, from K⁺ current moving outward.

First, Na⁺ channels spontaneously close, or inactivate, after a brief period of time (1–2 ms), thus reducing the membrane's permeability to Na⁺ and minimizing the contribution of the Na⁺ gradient to the membrane's potential. Second, voltage-activated K⁺ channels open although their response to membrane depolarization is slower than that of Na⁺ channels. Subsequently, the transient influx of Na⁺ is rapidly overwhelmed by an outflow of K⁺ along its concentration gradient, and the membrane responds by resuming its resting potential near the K⁺ equilibrium potential. Although the automatic closing of the Na⁺ channels and the membrane's high resting conductance to K⁺ are sufficient to return the membrane to its resting potential, voltage-gated K⁺ channels accelerate the process. In fact, the amount and properties of the various K⁺ channels in a neuron play a critical role in determining the duration of a neuron's action potentials and the neuron's rate of firing.

Because there are Na⁺ channels along the length of the axon, the action potential propagates down the axon and invades the presynaptic nerve terminals, where it triggers

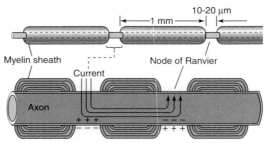

2-12 **Myelin and saltatory conduction along axons.** Current enters a myelinated axon at one node and exits at the next node, unlike the continuous exit of current that occurs in nonmyelinated axons. The myelin sheath greatly increases the resistance of the axonal membrane and decreases its capacitance.

the influx of Ca²⁺ by activating voltage-dependent Ca²⁺ channels and subsequently leads to the Ca²⁺-dependent release of neurotransmitter (Chapter 3). In nonmyelinated, small-diameter axons, action potential propagation is fairly slow because propagation is continuous and each segment of membrane must be depolarized to threshold. In myelinated axons, action potential propagation is *saltatory*: action potentials appear to jump from one node of Ranvier, a small gap in the myelin sheath, to the next at a much faster rate **2-12**. Because myelin increases the resistance and decreases the capacitance of the axonal membrane, current entering the axon at one node does not leak out of the internodal membrane but instead travels rapidly down the axon to depolarize the adjacent node until it reaches threshold. Disruption of myelination of axons under pathological conditions, such as **multiple sclerosis**, impairs the conductance of action potentials, and causes neurologic symptoms such as vision loss and muscle weakness.

Dendrites, the recipients of most incoming synaptic activity, are not electrically passive during this process; they contain a constellation of voltage-dependent Na⁺, Ca²⁺, and K⁺ channels and are capable of generating action potentials. Dendritic action potentials presumably amplify incoming synaptic signals so that they can be heard at the soma.

MOLECULAR PROPERTIES OF ION CHANNELS

Thus far, ion channels have been discussed only in the most abstract sense. However, modern advances in molecular biology, such as the isolation, cloning, and mutagenesis of ion channels, and in cell physiology, such as patch clamping techniques that allow the observation of single ion channels, have provided scientists with remarkably detailed knowledge of the operation of ion channels. The crystallization of bacterial ion pores and channels, including KcsA, a bacterial K^+ channel that is homologous to some human K^+ channels, also has yielded important functional and structural information. Consequently, we know the exact amino acid composition of hundreds of ion channels, have detailed models about how these channels assemble in cellular membranes, and understand which amino acids are responsible for features of ion channels such as selective permeability and the binding of pharmaceutical agents.

This section focuses on the voltage-gated–like (VGL) ion channel superfamily that includes but is not limited to voltage-gated Na^+, Ca^{2+}, and K^+ channels (Na_V, Ca_V, and K_V). The extended family members also include Ca^{2+}-activated K^+ channels (K_{Ca}), cyclic nucleotide–modulated ion channels (CNG and HCN), transient receptor potential channels (TRP), inward rectifier K^+ channels (K_{ir}), and 2-pore K^+ channels (K_{2P}). (Note that the term *rectifier* describes a channel that passes current much more efficiently in one direction; for example, an inward rectifier preferentially passes current into a cell.) Members of this gene family are principal players in regulating the electrical signals in neurons. We review these channels in considerable detail with the expectation that these proteins represent valuable targets for the development of future treatments for psychiatric and neurologic disorders. Another major family of ion channels, ligand-gated ion channels, that are responsible for translating chemical signals into electrical signals via generation of synaptic potentials, are discussed in subsequent chapters.

Structure of VGL Ion Channels

The fundamental features of an ion channel are its aqueous pore that controls ion permeation, the channel's gating mechanism, and its modulation. The relationship among the 143 protein members of this ion channel family is built on the amino acid sequences of the minimum pore region **2–13**. The founding members of this family are voltage-gated Na^+ channels. Their principal α subunit consists of four internally homologous domains that surround a central pore. Each of the domains contains six membrane-spanning α helices (S1-S6), and a membrane re-entrant loop between S5 and S6, also called SS1–SS2, that is believed to form a hairpin loop that dips down into the channel and forms the lining of the ion pore **2–14**.

Other voltage-gated channels display structures remarkably similar to those of the Na^+ channel. Most similar are the principal α subunits of Ca^{2+} channels, which also contain four internally homologous domains, each of which possesses six putative membrane-spanning regions **2–14**. Voltage-gated K^+ channels appear to be composed of subunits that correspond to only one of the four internally homologous domains of the Na^+ and Ca^{2+} channels. It is believed that four of these smaller subunits multimerize in the plasma membrane to form a channel that is similar in structure to the Na^+ and Ca^{2+} channels. Several other families of ion channels (K_{Ca}, CNG, HCN, and TRP) also have this tetrameric structure. However, although the inwardly rectifying K^+ channels are also tetramers, each of the subunits only has two transmembrane segments, named M1 and M2, which are analogous to the S5 and S6 segments of voltage-gated Na^+, Ca^{2+}, and K^+ channels. On the other hand, two of these pore motifs are linked together to generate the 2-pored K^+ channels. In mammalian cells, each of these channels is composed of several subunits in addition to their primary α subunits; the role of these accessory proteins is discussed in **2–3**.

Selectivity of Ion Channels

K^+ channels are 100 to 1000 times more permeable to K^+ than Na^+. Na^+ channels are 12 times more selective for Na^+ than for any other ion, and some Ca^{2+} channels are a thousand times more selective for Ca^{2+} than for other cations. A channel's ability to select one cation over another suggests remarkably sophisticated protein design, and how this is accomplished has been the focus of intense investigation.

Ions do not flow through ion channels like water through a pipe; such a model cannot explain how some channel pores are selective for Na^+ and others are selective for K^+. Instead, an ion binds transiently to one or more sites in a channel, with its permeability presumably determined by the amount of energy released during its binding to amino acid residues and by the energy required for its dissociation from some or all surrounding water molecules. The speed with which an ion can dissociate from a pore and escape from a channel is also likely to influence selectivity.

Crystallization of the bacterial KcsA K^+ channel has provided great insight into how ionic selectivity may be accomplished in K^+ channels. The selectivity filter is the narrowest part of the pore, formed by the SS1-SS2–like region of the KcsA channel, with a very conserved GYG sequence lying at the heart of the selectivity filter. Voltage-gated Na^+ and Ca^{2+} channels probably use a different strategy to achieve selectivity.

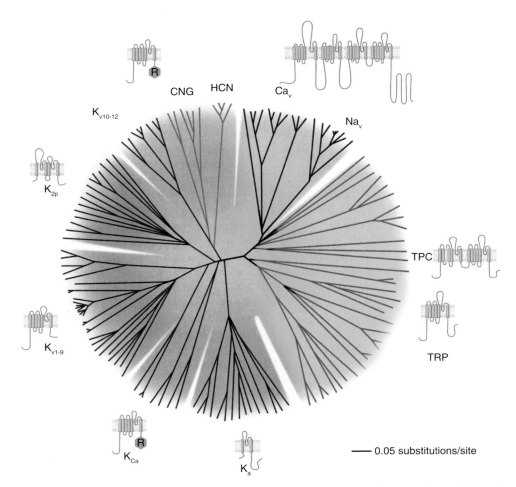

2-13 **Representation of the amino acid sequence relations of the minimal pore regions of the voltage-gated ion channel superfamily.** This global view of the 143 members of the structurally related ion channel genes highlights the seven major groups of ion channel families and their membrane topologies. Four-domain channels (Ca_V and Na_V) are shown as blue branches, K^+ selective channels are shown as red branches, cyclic nucleotide–gated channels are shown as magenta branches, and transient receptor potential (TRP) and related channels are shown as green branches. Background colors separate the ion channel proteins into related groups: light blue, Ca_V and Na_V; light green, TRP channels; light red, potassium channels, except K_V10–12, which have a cyclic nucleotide–binding domain and are more closely related to CNG and HCN channels; light orange, K_V10–12 channels and cyclic nucleotide–modulated CNG and HCN channels. Minimal pore regions bounded by the transmembrane segments M1 or S5 and M2 or S6 were aligned and refined manually for the 143 ion channel members; amino acid sequence positions with gaps in the alignment were omitted from the analyses. (Yu FH, Catterall WA. The VGL-chanome: A protein superfamily for electrical signaling and ionic homeostasis. *Sci STKE*. 2005;253:re15.)

Both types of channels use negatively charged residues, and perhaps some backbone carbonyls as well, to coordinate the cation.

Opening of Ion Channels

Na^+ channels responsible for propagating action potentials, K^+ channels responsible for terminating action potentials, and Ca^{2+} channels that admit Ca^{2+} to nerve terminals in response to action potentials are all voltage activated: they open when a membrane is depolarized. It is now known that voltage-activated ion channels display a gating charge, or a shift in the distribution of charge across the membrane, that occurs concomitantly with channel activation and is believed to result

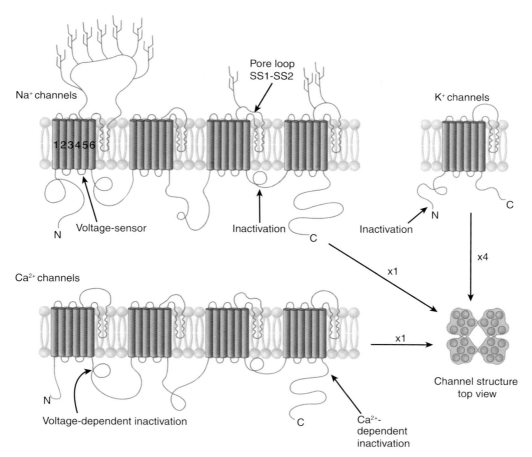

2-14 Structural similarities shared by voltage-dependent Na^+, Ca^{2+}, and K^+ channels. Each channel has subunits whose domains contain six membrane-spanning segments. The α subunit in both Ca^{2+} and Na^+ channels contains four domains. The subunit of the Shaker K^+ channel contains only one domain. The region that connects segments 5 and 6 in each domain (SS1–SS2) is believed to form the pore of each channel. The segment 4 in each domain is believed to be the voltage-sensor. The inactivation modules in Na^+, K^+, Ca^{2+} channels are located at different regions of the channels. (Adapted with permission from Barchi RL. Sodium channel gene defects in the periodic paralyses. *Curr Opin Neurobiol.* 1992;2:633; and Yu FH, Catterall WA. The VGL-chanome: A protein superfamily for electrical signaling and ionic homeostasis. *Sci STKE.* 2005;253 re15.)

from the movement of a putative voltage sensor within the ion channel itself. The S4 transmembrane domain, marked by a unique pattern of positively charged amino acids, may behave as a gating particle **2-14**. However, the exact conformational change that results from movement of the S4 domain and causes the opening of a channel remains controversial.

The addition of regulatory domains to the carboxyl terminus of K_{ir}, K_{Ca}, CNG, and HCN channels yields gating by binding of small intracellular ligands such as Ca^{2+}, ATP, and cyclic nucleotides or by interactions with protein ligands. Ligand binding to these domains is thought to rotate the S6 segment to open the pore. For K_{Ca} and HCN channels, ligand binding and membrane depolarization act in concert to open the pore.

Closing of Ion Channels

In some cases, the closing of a voltage-gated ion channel is simply the opposite of its opening: the channel undergoes conformational changes in response to a particular membrane voltage and subsequently returns to its resting conformation when the membrane voltage

---

The major pore-forming α subunits of Na^+, K^+, and Ca^{2+} channels are capable of conducting their own voltage-dependent, ion-selective current, and commonly contain the regulatory motifs modified by second messenger signaling as well as the binding sites for pharmacologic agents. However, many of these principal α subunits are physically associated with accessory subunits that modify their expression, functional properties, and subcellular localization. Unlike the structurally similar principal pore-forming subunits, the accessory subunits exhibit considerable diversity in amino acid sequence, size, post-translational modification, and postulated structure.

These accessory proteins are speculated to serve the following functions:

- They can facilitate channel trafficking to the plasma membrane or stabilize channels in the membrane.

- They can modulate activation and inactivation rates, normally toward faster gating kinetics.

- They can shift voltage dependence, normally toward more hyperpolarized potentials.

- Their phosphorylation can regulate channel properties **2-4**.

- They can influence ligand (toxins and pharmacologic agents) binding.

Importantly, mutations in some accessory subunits of ion channels are associated with familial diseases, such as **epilepsy** (eg, the neuronal Na^+ channel β subunit and the neuronal Ca^{2+} channel $β_4$ subunit) (Chapter 18), and **long QT syndrome** (the cardiac K^+ channel β subunits) **2-1**.

---

change subsides. This process is called *deactivation*. For example, the closure of voltage-gated ion channels such as the delayed rectifier K^+ channel, which restores an axon's resting potential after an action potential, does not appear to require additional regulatory mechanisms.

In response to depolarization, however, a voltage-gated Na^+ channel closes immediately after it is activated, even if the depolarization is maintained, such as during an action potential. This process of *inactivation* is distinctly different from that of *de*activation, the return of the Na^+ channel to its resting state. The "ball and chain" model of inactivation postulates the movement of a positively charged segment of a channel protein into an open ion channel, which prevents further conductance **2-14**. Site-directed mutagenesis indicates that the ball and chain portion of the Shaker K^+ channel (a prototype of K_V channels discussed below) is most likely its N terminus, and that of the Na^+ channel the cytoplasmic region between domains III and IV. In some Ca^{2+} channels, residues in the S6 segment of domain I, and the loop between domain I and II, appear to be functionally important in voltage-dependent inactivation. Some subtypes of Ca^{2+} channels also exhibit Ca^{2+}-dependent inactivation, which involves the C-terminal region **2-14**.

Several toxins and pharmaceutical agents act by modulating the process of inactivation. Some toxins selectively slow Na^+ channel inactivation, causing these channels to remain open for a longer period of time; a class of **scorpion toxins** that act in this manner can lead to spastic paralysis, seizures, and death. Other substances, including some drugs used in the treatment of **epilepsy** (eg, **phenytoin** and **carbamazepine**), selectively stabilize the inactivated state of the Na^+ channel, thereby decreasing neuronal excitability.

Types of Ion Channels

The voltage-dependent cation channels are similar enough in general architecture that it is possible to discuss their basic properties as a group. However, rapid advances in molecular biology, pharmacology, and electrophysiology have made it possible to distinguish hundreds of variations of ion channels. Distinct channels arise from different gene products, splice variants of the same gene transcript, posttranslational modifications, and combinations of individual channel subunits. The following sections of this chapter serve as an abbreviated catalogue of the various types and subtypes of voltage-gated cation channels and other types of cation channels from the VGL family **2-13**. The properties, molecular composition, and medical relevance of each are summarized in the most general terms; more information about each channel type can be found in the references listed at the end of the chapter.

Changes in the electrical properties of neurons, which are directly related to modifications of their ion channels, are crucial for the survival of an organism. In a threatening situation, for example, neurons that typically fire only a single action potential may respond by firing long trains of action potentials. The increased firing of such neurons can heighten awareness, provoke a stronger or more rapid behavioral response, or assist in forming a potent memory about a dangerous situation.

Among the most common means by which the excitability of neurons is altered is through the phosphorylation of ion channels, which involves the addition of free phosphate ($-PO_4^{3-}$) groups to particular amino acid residues of a channel protein (Chapter 4). This process changes the stable conformational state of a channel and in turn alters the magnitude and time course of the ionic currents it conducts. Phosphorylation thereby provides an excellent basis for ion channel flexibility; in seconds or less, the activation of second messenger systems in a neuron can lead to the phosphorylation of channel proteins and to equally swift changes in the electrical properties of the neuron. Depending on the channel, the phosphorylation site, the location of the phosphorylated amino acid residue, and the internal milieu of the cell, this process can alter the following biophysical properties:

- *Inactivation kinetics.* Protein kinase C phosphorylation of a single residue of an Na^+ channel's α subunit on the intracellular loop between transmembrane domains III and IV can slow the channel's inactivation. Similarly, phosphorylation of the rapidly inactivating K^+ channel known as $K_V3.4$ by protein kinase C causes the channel's inactivation to abate.

- *Current amplitude.* Activation of protein kinase A increases the amplitude of K^+ channel $K_V1.2$ currents; activation of protein kinase C decreases the amplitude of currents through Na^+ channels; and activation of protein kinase A

increases the amplitude of currents in KCNQ2 channels (a type of K_V channel). Mutations of this latter channel cause **benign familial neonatal convulsions** **2–1**.

- *Voltage dependence of channel responses.* Phosphorylation of L-type Ca^{2+} channels by protein kinase A not only slows channel inactivation but also shifts the channel's voltage dependence to more negative potentials.

- *Accumulation of channel protein in the plasma membrane.* Long-term protein kinase A treatment of oocytes expressing $K_V1.1$ K^+ channels increases the amplitude of currents expressed by these channels. This response is most likely caused by increased amounts of channel protein in the plasma membrane.

The effect of norepinephrine on hippocampal pyramidal cells illustrates how the phosphorylation of an ion channel protein can affect the behavior of a neuron, as shown in the figure. In the absence of norepinephrine, depolarization of a pyramidal cell results in a small number of action potentials. The activation of a Ca^{2+}-activated K^+ channel causes an after hyperpolarization (AHP), which limits the number of action potentials that occur in response to a depolarizing stimulus. In the presence of norepinephrine, depolarization of the pyramidal cell leads to a much more prolonged train of action potentials. Norepinephrine binds to the β-adrenergic receptor, which activates adenylyl cyclase, and leads to an accumulation of cAMP and activation of protein kinase A (Chapter 4). Protein kinase A in turn phosphorylates Ca^{2+}-activated K^+ channels and blocks their activity. Accordingly, norepinephrine increases the firing of a neuron by removing the hyperpolarizing currents, or AHP, that inhibit its activity. (Adapted with permission from Madison DV, Nicoll RA. Actions of noradrenaline recorded intracellularly in rat hippocampal CA1 pyramidal neurons in vitro. *J Physiol.* 1986; 372:221.)

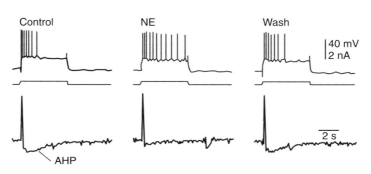

Sodium Channels

Na^+ channels are a relatively homogeneous group of ion channels. Variations do exist: in mammals, nine principal α subunit genes of Na^+ channels have been cloned, and they show different tissue distribution patterns, and different sensitivities to the typical Na^+ channel blocker **tetrodotoxin**. However, across species and tissue types, Na^+ channel properties are remarkably similar in terms of voltage dependence and activation-inactivation kinetics.

Tetrodotoxin

Pharmacology and toxicology of sodium channels
Toxins that bind to Na^+ channels are uncommon, but their effects can be dramatic. The isolation of the Na^+ channel was initially possible because it binds tightly and specifically to toxins such as **tetrodotoxin**, a heterocyclic compound found in many marine species, including the Japanese puffer fish, the globe fish, and the blue-ringed octopus. Approximately 200 humans experience tetrodotoxin poisoning each year, in most cases after consuming improperly prepared puffer fish. Symptoms of tetrodotoxin poisoning include facial numbness, headache, and increasing paralysis and respiratory distress. Although victims are completely paralyzed, they may be conscious and lucid until shortly before death, which generally occurs within 4 to 6 hours. Among those poisoned, the mortality rate is approximately 50%; survival is usually attributed to rapid treatment (gastric lavage) or the victim's ingestion of only a small amount of toxin. Because tetrodotoxin binds to the outside of the Na^+ channel at the S5–S6 loop of the α subunit, site-directed mutagenesis of amino acids in this region greatly reduces its ability to bind to the channel (see 2-14). Changes in amino acid sequence in this region in certain Na^+ channel subunits cause these channels to be resistant to tetrodotoxin to varying degrees.

Other Na^+ channel toxins act not by blocking the channel but by activating it, usually by slowing or eliminating its voltage-dependent inactivation, which

leads to the hyperexcitability of neurons and muscle tissue. Victims of these toxins, which have been isolated from **scorpion** and **sea anemone** species, may undergo convulsions and spastic paralysis.

Substances used to treat human disease generally have less dramatic effects on the Na^+ channel. **Phenytoin** and **carbamazepine,** which are used to treat **epilepsy,** act on Na^+ channels by slowing their recovery from an inactivated state. Because prolonged inactivation of these channels limits the firing rates of affected neurons, these drugs can prevent seizures. **Local anesthetics,** such as **cocaine,** and synthetic derivatives such as **lidocaine** and **procaine,** which are membrane permeable in their nonionized form, bind to the cytoplasmic side of the Na^+ channel and also cause Na^+ to bind to the inactivated state of the Na^+ channel, creating a use-dependent blockade of the channel.

Lidocaine

Procaine

The sodium channel in disease   Some inherited neurologic disorders, including certain **myotonias** and **periodic paralyses,** are linked to $Na_v1.4$ (also known as SkM1), the Na^+ channel in adult skeletal muscle. Although myotonia, which is characterized by muscle excitability, and periodic paralysis, which is characterized by muscle hypoexcitability, seem to be diametrically opposed, the underlying Na^+ channel defects are similar. Electrophysiologic studies indicate that both disorders involve slowed or impaired inactivation of the Na^+ channel. In individuals who experience periodic paralysis, the defect in Na^+ channel inactivation is severe enough that muscle remains at a depolarized potential and becomes refractory to further action potentials; in those who experience myotonia, the defect is less severe and results in repetitive firing. Mutations in neuronal and cardiac Na^+ channel subunits that slow or impair the inactivation of Na^+ channels are also linked to familial disorders such as

familial neonatal seizures, generalized epilepsy, and **long QT syndrome** ▆2-1▆.

Potassium Channels

K^+ channels generally act as a stabilizing force. Their diverse functions include setting a cell's resting potential, repolarizing the cell after an action potential, and controlling an action potential's rate of firing and shape. Proper K^+ channel functioning is critical not only to neuronal activity but also to the operation of many organ systems; mutations in K^+ channels lead to a variety of disorders, ranging from **ataxia** to **cardiac arrhythmias** ▆2-1▆. A malfunctioning K^+ channel generally causes some form of hyperexcitability in affected tissue; for example, the **long QT syndrome,** a delay in ventricular repolarization that can cause heart arrhythmias, results from a malfunction of the $K_V11.1$ (HERG) K^+ channel, which is responsible for repolarizing the ventricle after contraction. Indeed, binding to *HERG channels* is a common cause of cardiac side effects of many classes of medications and is now used as a routine screen during the drug discovery process. Mutations of the related $K_V7.2/7.3$ (KCNQ2/3) K^+ channel cause **benign familial neonatal convulsions,** which resolve as the affected child grows. Mutation of another K^+ channel $K_V1.1$, which is expressed at high levels in the cerebellum, is linked to a type of **episodic ataxia** believed to be caused by an abnormal increase in the firing of cerebellar cells. **Tetraethylammonium (TEA),** which selectively blocks most types of voltage-gated K^+ channels, has been a useful research tool.

Tetraethylammonium

Potassium channel classifications K^+ channels can be placed into two broad classes, six TM (transmembrane domain) and two TM channels ▆2-3▆. Six TM channels include voltage-gated K^+ channels (K_V1-12 families) and Ca^{2+}-activated K^+ channels ($K_{Ca}1$-5 families). Two TM channels are inwardly rectifying K^+ channels ($K_{ir}1$-7 families). The differences in these channels reflect the variety of ways that they can affect the firing properties of a neuron.

Voltage-gated K^+ channels subsequently have two different functional classes that are not categorized by subfamilies, *delayed rectifiers* and *A-type channels.* Delayed rectifiers undergo delayed activation after depolarization and inactivate slowly; they thereby facilitate repolarization by remaining open for a prolonged period of time. These channels also shape action potentials; blocking their activity increases the duration of action potentials which in turn depend solely on the inactivation of Na^+ channels for repolarization. *A-type channels,* also referred to as *Shaker-related channels* (after the first K^+ channel cloned from *Drosophila*), are transiently activated when a cell is depolarized after a period of hyperpolarization. They can function to decrease the frequency of action potential firing by prolonging the interspike interval.

Ca^{2+}-gated K^+ channels open in response to the binding of Ca^{2+}, which usually occurs after a depolarization-induced influx of Ca^{2+}. Generally, these channels can remain open for prolonged periods, such as a few seconds, and are responsible for several different types of long *after hyperpolarization* (AHP), which is a hyperpolarization of the membrane that occurs after an action potential or series of action potentials. A long AHP can profoundly affect the firing pattern of a neuron; for instance, when a steady stimulus produces a train of action potentials, an AHP often is generated in response and can gradually slow the rate of firing. This phenomenon, known as spike-frequency adaptation, occurs throughout the nervous system and has many functional consequences.

Sk channels (named for their small conductance) are a subtype of Ca^{2+}-gated K^+ channels that are important for AHPs; they have become attractive drug targets because of their roles in modulating neuronal firing. SK channels are blocked by **apamin,** a honeybee neurotoxin.

Inward rectifiers structurally resemble truncated Shaker-type channels that are missing S1–S4 segments; that is, they comprise only the putative pore-lining segments S5, S6, and SS1–SS2. As with the Shaker-type channels, four of these subunits are believed to multimerize to form a functional channel. Such rectifiers are described as anomalous because they open when the membrane is hyperpolarized and close as the membrane depolarizes. They most likely stabilize a membrane's potential when the potential is near rest, without inhibiting depolarization. By conducting outward current in the voltage range just slightly positive to E_K, they maintain a resting potential near E_K; however, if the cell is sufficiently depolarized they shut off, freeing the membrane to undergo further depolarization. This type of K^+ channel is found in the heart, in striated muscle, and in neurons.

Seven subfamilies of inward rectifiers—$K_{ir}1$-7—have been identified. Channels formed by members of the $K_{ir}3$ subfamily are especially noteworthy because of

2-3 **Blocking Agents for Potassium Channels**

Potassium Channel	Acting from Outside	Acting from Inside	Membrane-Permeant
6TM			
Delayed rectifier	TEA Cs^+, H^+, Ba^{2+} Capsaicin[a] Dendrotoxins[a] Noxioustoxin	TEA and QA Cs^+, Na^+, Li^+, Ba^{2+}	4-Aminopyridine Strychnine Quinidine
A	TEA Dendrotoxins	TEA	4-Aminopyridine Quinidine?
K(Ca)	TEA (BK) Cs^+ Apamin (SK)[a] Chlotrimazol (IK/SK)[a] Charybdotoxin (BK)[a]	TEA Na^+, Ba^{2+}	Quinidine
2TM			
Inward rectifier	TEA Cs^+, Rb^+, Na^+ Ba^{2+}, Sr^{2+}	H^+, Mg^{2+}[b] Spermine[b] Spermidine[b]	?
K_{ATP}	TEA Cs^+, Ba^{2+}	TEA Na^+, Mg^{2+}	Tolbutamide[c] Glibenclamide[c] Quinidine

Abbreviations: TEA, tetraethylammonium; QA, quaternary ammonium ions related to TEA.

[a]Acts on only some K channels in this class.

[b]Endogenous molecules that block outward current in K_{ir} channels.

[c]Unlike most other agents in this table, these sulfonylureas act allosterically by binding to accessory sulfonylurea receptor subunits (SUR) rather than by blocking the pore itself.

the role that G proteins play in their regulation (Chapter 4). G protein–coupled $K_{ir}3$ channels, termed GIRKs, are critical to many physiologic functions; for example, they mediate the slowing of heart rate by acetylcholine. The binding of acetylcholine to muscarinic acetylcholine receptors in the atrium activates a G protein and liberates its βγ complex, which in turn leads to the activation of a GIRK. The K^+ current produced by this activation slows the depolarization of sinoatrial cells to their firing threshold. This process explains the positive ionotropic and chronotropic effects of muscarinic cholinergic antagonists such as **atropine**. GIRKs are also expressed in the brain where, among other functions, they mediate a neuron's electrical responses to the activation of many types of G protein–coupled neurotransmitter receptors, especially those coupled with G proteins from the G_i family (Chapter 4).

K(ATP) channels ($K_{ir}6.2$), another atypical member of the K_{ir} family, play an important role in cellular and systemic metabolic regulation. Functionally, these channels are voltage insensitive; they close in the presence of high (100 μM–1 mM) intracellular ATP concentrations, and open when these concentrations are low, resulting in a more hyperpolarized membrane potential. They may serve as a protective function in neurons by reducing neural firing when neural energy reserves are depleted. Structurally, each of these ATP-sensitive K^+ channels is a multimeric complex comprising four $K_{ir}6.2$ subunits and one SUR (**sulfonylurea** receptor) protein. Sulfonylureas such as **tolbutamide** block K(ATP) channels and are used to treat adult-onset **diabetes**. The drugs act by increasing insulin secretion from pancreatic β cells. Mutations in $K_{ir}6.2$ channels cause congenital hyperinsulinemia **2-1**. **Iptakalim** is a structurally novel opener of K(ATP) channels, which shows promise as a neuroprotective agent in animal models. **Minoxidil**, used to restore hair growth, is also an activator of K(ATP) channels, although whether this action is related to its effects on hair growth remains unknown.

Tolbutamide

Calcium Channels

Ca^{2+} is an important signaling molecule that is present in low concentrations in extracellular fluid (1–5 mM)

and in minute concentrations in most cell interiors (approximately 0.1–0.2 μM). The opening of Ca^{2+} channels is the critical link between cell depolarization and Ca^{2+} entry, which can result in local intracellular Ca^{2+} concentrations as great as 100 μM. The subsequent binding of Ca^{2+} to intracellular molecules can lead to many significant responses, including muscle contraction; the triggering of neurotransmitter release from nerve terminals (Chapter 3); the activation of second messenger systems that cause many changes, including alterations in gene expression (Chapter 4); and, in extreme cases, neuronal self-destruction (Chapters 17 and 19). Some Ca^{2+} channels also impart electrical properties to the cells in which they are expressed; for example, such cells may show Ca^{2+} spikes—action potentials in which the depolarizing current is carried predominantly by Ca^{2+}.

Ca^{2+} channels are categorized in terms of their voltage dependence, kinetics (speed of activation and inactivation), and pharmacology. Ten Ca^{2+} channel genes have been isolated, many of which correspond to Ca^{2+} channel types that were originally classified according to their electrophysiologic properties **2-4**.

Verapamil

L channels L-type (*large* current or "*long* open time") Ca^{2+} channels are activated by large depolarizations (approximately –20 mV), can remain open for a long time before inactivating (500 ms or more), and are blocked by dihydropyridines. Four major L-channel subunits have been cloned: $Ca_V1.1–4$. The $Ca_V1.1$ (α1S) subunit resides exclusively in skeletal muscle, where it is abundant in transverse tubules; $Ca_V1.2$ (α1C) subunits are found in cardiac muscle, smooth muscle, the brain; and $Ca_V1.3$ (α1D) subunits predominate in cochlear hair cells, and endocrine and kidney cells, but also reside in the brain. $Ca_V1.4$ (α1F) subunits, the newest member of this gene family, are found only in the retina, and mutations in this gene are linked to **congenital stationary night blindness**.

Clinically, these channels are targets for **antianginal** and **antihypertensive** drugs. Organic L-type Ca^{2+} channel blockers, phenylalkylamines (eg,

2–4 Calcium Channels

Ca²⁺ Channel	Ca²⁺ current Type	Primary Localizations	Previous Name of α Subunits	Specific Blocker	Functions
$Ca_V1.1$	L	Skeletal muscle	α_{1S}	DHPs	Excitation-contraction coupling Calcium homeostasis Gene regulation
$Ca_V1.2$	L	Cardiac muscle Endocrine cells Neurons	α_{1C}	DHPs	Excitation-contraction coupling Hormone secretion Gene regulation
$Ca_V1.3$	L	Endocrine cells Neurons	α_{1D}	DHPs[a]	Hormone secretion Gene regulation
$Ca_V1.4$	L	Retina	α_{1F}	DHPs[a]	Tonic neurotransmitter release
$Ca_V2.1$	P/Q	Nerve terminals Dendrites	α_{1A}	ω-Agatoxin	Neurotransmitter release Dendritic Ca²⁺ transients
$Ca_V2.2$	N	Nerve terminals Dendrites	α_{1B}	ω-CTX-GVIA	Neurotransmitter release Dendritic Ca²⁺ transients
$Ca_V2.3$	R	Cell bodies Dendrites Nerve Terminals	α_{1E}	SNX-482	Ca²⁺-dependent action potentials Neurotransmitter release
$Ca_V3.1$	T	Cardiac muscle Skeletal muscle Neurons	α_{1G}	Mibefradil	Repetitive firing
$Ca_V3.2$	T	Cardiac muscle Neurons	α_{1H}	Mibefradil	Repetitive firing
$Ca_V3.3$	T	Neurons	α_{1I}	Mibefradil	Repetitive firing

[a]$Ca_V1.3$ and $Ca_V1.4$ are less sensitive to DHPs (dihydropyridines) compared to $Ca_V1.1$ and $Ca_V1.2$.

verapamil), dihydropyridines (**eg, nifedipine**), and benzo- thiazepines (**eg, diltiazem**), decrease myocardial contractile force and thereby reduce myocardial oxygen requirements, or reduce smooth muscle contractility and thereby decrease arterial and intraventricular pressure. L-type Ca²⁺ channels are located primarily on the cell bodies and proximal dendrites of neurons. They admit Ca²⁺ to the cell body during periods of strong depolarization, and this influx causes second messenger activation and changes in gene transcription. Yet substances that block these channels rarely have noticeable neurologic side effects, despite the fact that some—for example, **nimodipine**—can cross the blood-brain barrier. One possibility is that one of the neuronal L-type Ca²⁺ channels, $Ca_V1.3$ channels, are less sensitive to these typical L channel blockers.

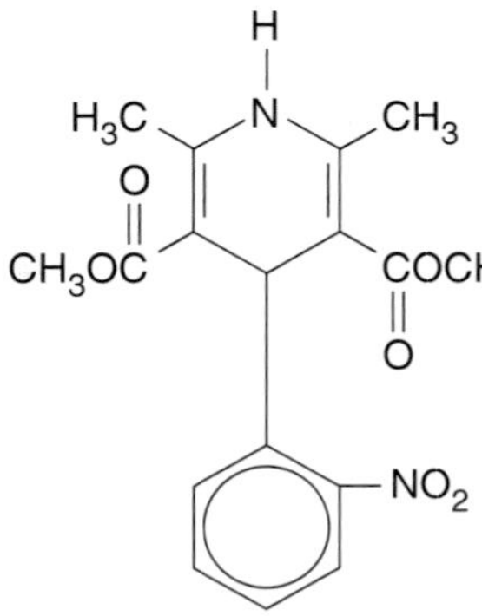

Nifedipine

T channels T-type (*t*iny current or *t*ransient) Ca²⁺ channels are activated by depolarizations near resting potential; half-maximal activation of these channels occurs at approximately −40 mV. They exhibit voltage-dependent inactivation such that depolarization produced by their activation ultimately triggers their inactivation. Because of this self-limiting property, these channels are excellent oscillators; in fact, they are believed to provide a pacemaker current in thalamic neurons that generate the rhythmic cortical discharge associated with **absence seizures** (**petit mal**). **Ethosuximide**, which blocks T-type current, is an effective therapy for these seizures (Chapter 18). The recent cloning of T-type channel subunits $Ca_V3.1$-3 ($\alpha1G$, H, I) should facilitate the development of drugs that interact more specifically with this important Ca^{2+} channel subtype.

P/Q, N, and R channels The α subunits of these channels belong to one subfamily $Ca_V2.1,3$ ($\alpha1A$, B and E). The Ca_V2 channels are high-voltage activated, not sensitive to L channel blockers, yet can be blocked with high affinity by peptide toxins derived from **spiders** and **sea snails** **2–4**. This subfamily of Ca^{2+} channels is best known for their regulation of neurotransmitter and hormone release: Ca^{2+} flows into nerve terminals through these channels in a voltage-dependent manner that triggers this release (Chapter 3). P/Q ($Ca_V2.1$) and N ($Ca_V2.2$) channels contribute most of the Ca^{2+} influx that triggers neurotransmitter and hormone release. P/Q type channels also control neurotransmitter release at neuromuscular junctions, whereas N type channels control neurotransmitter release in sympathetic neurons. A synthetic peptide blocker of N type Ca^{2+} channels (**ziconotide**) is under

development for treating patients unresponsive to intrathecal opiates for relief of **chronic pain**. $Ca_V2.3$ channels underlie a subpopulation of R (resistant)-type Ca^{2+} channels. The functions of $Ca_V2.3$ channels are less well defined, but may include neurotransmitter and hormone release and the generation of dendritic calcium transients.

Mutations of the human $Ca_V2.1$ ($\alpha1A$) gene have been linked to **familial hemiplegic migraine**, **spinalcerebellar ataxia**, and **episodic ataxia**. Although this gene is richly expressed in Purkinje cells, how the mutant P/Q channels cause the abnormalities seen in these disorders is still under study.

Cyclic Nucleotide–Regulated Channels

The family of cyclic nucleotide-regulated channels includes the cyclic nucleotide–gated (CNG) channels and the hyperpolarization-activated cyclic nucleotide–gated (HCN) channels. These channels are six TM segment channels, structually similar to voltage-gated K^+ channels. They are nonselective cation channels, in that monovalent ions (K^+, Na^+) can pass through with no discrimination, and divalent ions (Ca^{2+}) can pass as well.

The activation of CNG channels is mediated by the direct binding of cGMP or cAMP to the C-terminal region of the channel protein. These channels are expressed in the cilia of olfactory neurons and in outer segments of rod and cone photoreceptors, where they transduce odorant signals and photons into electrical signals **2–5**. Photoreceptor channels

---

2–5   **Signal Transduction in CNG Channels**

The role that cGMP-gated channels play in converting light energy, in the form of photons, to an electrical signal that the nervous system can interpret is well understood. Photons activate the light-sensing pigment rhodopsin (which is highly homologous in structure to a G protein-coupled receptor) in the outer segments of rods in the retina. Photoactivated rhodopsin in turn activates a phosphodiesterase that causes the breakdown of cGMP (Chapter 4). This transient fall in the cytosolic concentration of cGMP results in the closure of tonically activated cGMP-gated channels, which causes hyperpolarization of the photoreceptor cell. Rods respond to this hyperpolarization by releasing less transmitter,

thereby informing other cells in the retina that a light signal has been received.

A similar process transduces odorant signals. Activation of odorant receptors, which are G protein coupled, stimulates adenylyl cyclase and the production of cAMP (Chapter 4). The increase in cAMP activates cAMP-gated channels, which causes depolarization of the olfactory neurons. Resulting action potentials in these neurons signal efferent neurons that an olfactory stimulus has been received. In contrast to the channels involved in photoreception, which are activated preferentially by cGMP, olfactory channels can be opened by either cAMP or cGMP.

strongly discriminate between cGMP and cAMP, whereas the olfactory channels are almost equally sensitive to both ligands.

CNG channels are heterotetramers composed of homologous A subunits (CNGA1-4) and B subunits (CNGB1-3). Each subunit binds a single molecule of cAMP or cGMP. Although the binding of only one subunit can cause a channel to open, maximum activation of the channel requires the binding of all four subunits to cyclic nucleotide. Mutations in CNG genes are linked to **retinitis pigmentosa** and **achromatopsia** **2-1**.

In mammals, the HCN family comprises four members (HCN1–4). They are expressed in neurons, cardiac pacemaking cells, and photoreceptors. In contrast to most other VGL channels, HCN channels open upon hyperpolarization and close at positive potentials. The currents carried by these channels are also known as I_h, I_f, or I_q currents. cAMP and cGMP can bind to the C-terminal region of HCN channels and enhance the channel activity by shifting the activation curve to more positive voltages. Because their activation causes the cell to depolarize, often beyond spike threshold, these channels help drive a repetitive cycle of rhythmic firing and, hence, are called "pacemaker channels." Mutations in HCN4 are associated with **sick sinus node disease** **2-1**.

Given the key role of HCN channels in cardiac pacemaking, these channels are promising pharmacological targets for the development of drugs used in the treatment of cardiac arrhythmias and ischemic heart disease. For example, **ivabradine**, a heart rate-lowering agent, is a use-dependent blocker of HCN channels. Similar compounds include **zetabradine** and **cilobradine**. The effect of cAMP on these channels is exploited by several common drugs used to modify heart rate; for example, **propranolol,** a β-adrenergic antagonist, reduces cellular cAMP levels, which decreases heart rate in part by inhibiting I_h channels. Because the rhythmic activity of neurons is integral to functions such as arousal, maintenance of the sleep-wake cycle, and respiratory rate, these pacemaker channels are important targets for future drug development. Indeed, antagonists of these channels are currently undergoing evaluation for use in the treatment of cardiovascular and neuropsychiatric disorders.

TRP Channels

TRP channels are named after their role in *Drosophila* phototransduction. Mutations in the channel caused the response to light to be transient, and resulted in a decrease in the level of light-induced Ca^{2+} influx. To date, some 28 genes have been identified in mammals encoding TRP channels. They are divided into six subfamilies (TRPC, TRPV, TRPM, TRPP, TRPA, TRPML), all of which are six TM domain channels that lack the complete set of positively charged residues in S4 which act as voltage sensors. TRP channels are permeable to Ca^{2+} and Na^+, and, in some cases, Mg^{2+}. No single activation mechanism is shared by all TRP channels. In general, TRP channels can be described as Ca^{2+} permeable cation channels with polymodal activation mechanisms, including *receptor activation* (ie, certain G protein–coupled receptors and receptor tyrosine kinases activate phospholipases that can subsequently modulate TRP channel activity), *ligand activation* (ie, exogenous small organic molecules, endogenous lipids or products of lipid metabolism, purine nucleotides, inorganic ions), and *direct activation* (ie, change of temperature, mechanical stimuli, conformational coupling to IP$_3$ [inositol triphosphate] receptors, channel phosphorylation). Because most TRP channels are responsive to multiple stimuli, they can integrate these stimuli, and couple them to downstream signal amplification cascades through elevation of intracellular Ca^{2+} and membrane depolarization.

TRP channels are of particular importance in sensory perception, including vision, taste, smell, hearing, mechanosensation, and thermosensation. As just one example, TRPV1 is activated by **capsaicin**, the active ingredient in hot pepper. TRP channels, particularly their involvement in pain, are discussed in greater detail in Chapter 11 (see **11-1**). TRP channels also allow individual cells to sense changes in the local environment, such as alterations in fluid flow and mechanical stress. As cellular sensors, TRP channels are proposed to participate in various physiologic processes, such as regulating vessel tone, fertilization, Mg^{2+} absorption, and neurite outgrowth. Mutations in TRP channels are associated with diseases such as **hypomagnesemia**, **polycystic kidney disease**, and a neurodegenerative disease, **mucolipidosis** **2-1**.

Chloride Channels

While this chapter has focused on cation channels, neurons and most other cells are also permeable to Cl^-. Cl^- channels are critical for many physiologic processes, and mutations of these channels have been implicated in a variety of diseases (see **2-1**).

Cl^- channels serve two primary functions. First, they dampen electrical excitability. In most cells, including neurons and myocytes, the intracellular concentration of Cl^- is close to, but below, its electrochemical equilibrium. In a manner similar to that of K^+ channels, Cl^- channels provide a force—the concentration gradient of Cl^-—that pulls the cell toward the equilibrium potential of Cl^-, which is generally a hyperpolarized value. As a result, the inactivation of Cl^- channels can lead to hyperexcitability; for example, mutations in the Cl^- channel protein CLC-1 in skeletal muscle lead to muscle hyperexcitability, which results in **myotonia**. Similarly, the binding of **strychnine** to Cl^--conducting glycine receptors on, among other cells, motor neurons of the spinal cord can lead to violent convulsions and death (Chapter 5).

Cl^- channels also control the osmotic flow of water across the cell membrane. Some Cl^- channels that regulate osmotic balance are in fact activated by the swelling of a cell; activation of these channels allows Cl^- to exit the swollen cell, accompanied by cations and water. These channels play an important role in secretory cells, such as those of the mucosal epithelium, and in the kidney. Indeed, the so-called **loop diuretics,** such as **furosemide,** block Cl^- channels in the ascending loop of Henle and are widely used in the treatment of **congestive heart failure**.

As might be expected, the channels that permit Cl^- to cross plasma membranes differ in molecular composition from the voltage-gated cation channels. Cl^- channels comprise three molecular varieties 2–15. *Ligand-gated Cl^- channels* are among the most important in the brain; they act as signaling proteins for the inhibitory neurotransmitters γ-aminobutyric acid (GABA) and glycine and are discussed further in Chapter 5. *CLC channels,* which are believed to function as multimers of CLC proteins, are a family of homologous proteins characterized by 12 presumptive transmembrane domains (see 2–15). Nine CLCs have been cloned (CLC-1-7, CLC-Ka and CLC-Kb), among them CLC-1, 2, Ka, and Kb reside on plasma membranes to control Cl^- flux and membrane potential, and CLC3-5, possibly 6 and 7 as well, are located on the membrane of intracellular vesicles and are thought to be important in maintaining the pH of these vesicles. Human mutations

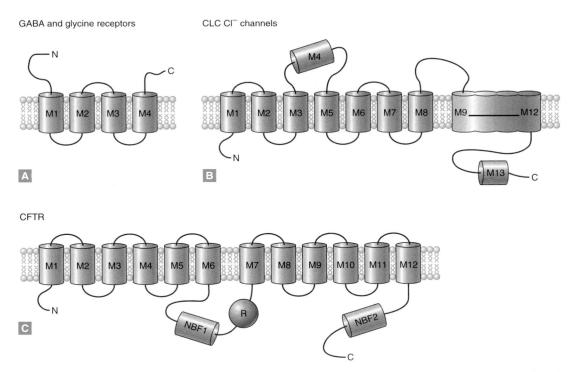

GABA and glycine receptors   CLC Cl^- channels

CFTR

2–15 Structural models of three Cl^- channel families. **A.** Topological model of γ-aminobutyric acid (GABA) and glycine receptor channels (see Chapter 5). **B.** CLC channel. **C.** CFTR channel. TM, transmembrane domains; NBF, nucleotide-binding fold; R, regulatory (phosphorylation) domain. (Adapted with permission from Jentsch TJ. Chloride channels: A molecular perspective. *Curr Opin Neurobiol.* 1996;6:304.)

in CLC channels are linked to several diseases, including several **renal disorders**, **neurodegeneration**, and possibly **epilepsy** 2-1 .

Cystic fibrosis *transmembrane conductance regulator (CFTR) channels* are activated by the binding of ATP to two nucleotide-binding domains and by the phosphorylation of key serine residues on the regulatory domain (see 2-15 ; also see 2-4 for a discussion of ion channel phosphorylation). Like CLC channels, CFTRs are believed to possess 12 transmembrane domains; however, CFTR channels are distinguished from CLC channels by features such as their nucleotide binding domains. The CFTR is among the most intensively studied ion channels because mutations of this channel cause **cystic fibrosis,** a relatively common hereditary disease that affects one in 3000 Caucasian newborns. In individuals with cystic fibrosis, the loss of CFTR Cl⁻ channels in several types of epithelial cells limits the egress of Cl⁻ ions into the lumen. Through mechanisms that are not completely understood, the disease also affects epithelial Na⁺ channels, whose malfunctioning causes the production of a thick, desiccated mucus. This abnormal secretion leads to obstruction of the biliary and pancreatic tracts and to a greatly increased incidence of pulmonary disease.

GLIA

Astroctyes

Astrocytes constitute between 25% and 50% of the cellular volume of most brain regions. Although a subset of these cells is morphologically reminiscent of stars as their name implies, their form varies widely. In gray matter, the predominant form is the protoplasmic astrocyte, whereas in white matter the predominant form is the fibrous astrocyte. In addition to their shape, astrocytes can be identified by the unique intermediate filaments composed of glial fibrillary acidic protein (GFAP) that fill their processes. Accordingly, antibodies to GFAP robustly stain astrocytes but not neurons.

Partly because of their high concentration of filaments, astrocytes give structure to the brain. Their processes extend to the pia mater, one of the membranes that cover the brain, to the ependyma, which lines the brain's ventricular system, and to the serosal surface of capillaries that penetrate the brain parenchyma. Moreover, astrocytes extend processes to the cell bodies of neurons and form sheaths around breaks in myelin (nodes of Ranvier) and around many synapses as well 2-16 . Astrocytes also help to keep the brain isolated

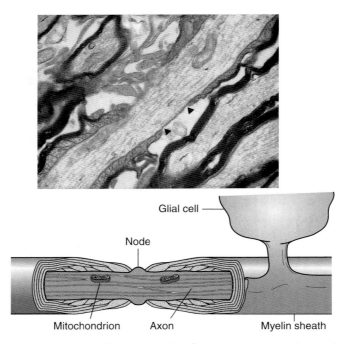

2-16 Electron micrograph and diagram of a single node of Ranvier. A break in the myelin sheath at the node (*between arrowheads in photomicrograph*) exposes the axonal plasma membrane to the extracellular space. (Image borrowed with permission from J. Kocsis, Yale University.)

from the general circulation. They play a central role in building and maintaining the blood-brain barrier by inducing endothelial cells that line capillaries in the brain to form tight junctions between cells.

Astrocytes serve many functions in the brain. *Radial glia*, which are the embryonic precursors of astrocytes, provide a scaffolding, or path, for the migration of neurons—a critical event in the development of the mature architecture of the brain. Astrocytes also synthesize adhesion molecules and extracellular matrix proteins, including CAMs, fibronectin, and laminin. These proteins are involved in neuronal migration and may regulate axonal pathfinding. As previously mentioned, astrocytes also elaborate neurotrophic factors and cytokines throughout life—molecules that are involved in the development and maintenance of both neurons and glia (Chapter 8).

Because astrocytes take up excess neurotransmitters and ions, including K^+, that are a product of neurotransmitter release and receptor activation, they help maintain the extracellular milieu that surrounds neurons during synaptic transmission. Among transporters that promote the reuptake of excitatory amino acid neurotransmitters, the highest density are found on astrocytes. Astrocytes also may play a heretofore unappreciated role in neuronal communication because they can be coupled to each other by means of gap junctions and can generate intracellular Ca^{2+} waves in response to activity in neurons. Moreover, some astrocytes express proteins normally considered neuronal, such as ion channels and neurotransmitter receptors. Although the physiologic significance of these properties remains unclear, they suggest that astrocytes can alter their function in response to neuronal activity in their vicinity. In fact, evidence is accumulating that astrocytes can influence synaptic function via the uptake of neurotransmitters such as glutamate and the activity-dependent release of a number of different factors.

Astrocytes also may be involved in disease. After **brain injury, inflammation**, and some types of **infection**, and in response to neurodegenerative processes such as **Alzheimer disease,** astrocytes hypertrophy and may proliferate. Such *reactive gliosis* is accompanied by alterations in gene expression in the reactive glia and the elaboration of cytokines and other soluble factors. Some of these factors recruit additional glia to respond to injury, which under extreme circumstances can result in damage to large numbers of nearby neurons.

Oligodendrocytes and Schwann Cells

Oligodendrocytes in the CNS and Schwann cells in the peripheral nervous system produce and ensheathe axons with myelin. By forming a relatively thick layer of insulation, myelin enables rapid electrical conduction down axons by markedly diminishing the capacitance of the neuronal membrane and increasing its resistance. Whereas Schwann cells can produce only one myelin sheath, oligodendrocytes can produce several of them. This is accomplished by the oligodendrocyte membrane wrapping itself in multiple layers around the axon (see 2-16). As mentioned previously, the axons express a high level of voltage-gated Na^+ channels at their nodes of Ranvier, small gaps in myelin between each myelinated segment, which permit the regeneration of an action potential.

Although the major chemical components of myelin in the CNS differ from those of myelin in the peripheral nervous system, both types contain hydrophobic proteolipids that function as insulators. Thus, the destruction of myelin sheaths can lead to marked deficits in nerve conduction velocity and a variety of sensory and motor deficits. Such deficits are characteristic of **multiple sclerosis,** a disease that involves the destruction of oligodendrocytes and the subsequent loss of myelin, presumably in response to an autoimmune mechanism (Chapter 8).

Microglia

Microglia are an important component of the defense mechanisms against infectious diseases of the CNS. Although the source of microglial cells remains controversial, it is believed that they are derived primarily from monocytic progenitor cells of bone marrow that enter the brain and undergo differentiation; thus, many microglia appear to be related to peripheral macrophages. Evidence suggests that some microglia also may be derived from glial lineages, although this pathway remains incompletely characterized. Like astrocytes, microglia respond to insult and injury with alterations in their morphology and number and thereby are important for tissue defense and repair. However, as with immune cells in other tissues, excessive activation of microglia can be deleterious and may contribute to inflammatory, and perhaps neurodegenerative, disorders of the CNS. Microglia are, for example, major mediators of the CNS effects of **human immunodeficiency virus (HIV) infection.**

CEREBRAL BLOOD FLOW

Compared with other organs in the human body, the brain consumes a disproportionate share of energy and oxygen and consequently is richly vascularized. Its vascular bed is supplied by perforating arteries that branch into the subarachnoid space and subsequently enter the brain parenchyma. These arterioles in the brain's gray matter, which is more densely vascularized than the white matter, give rise to a large number of capillary beds. These in turn drain into a venous network that terminates in large venous sinuses before returning blood to the general circulation.

The strict local control of cerebral circulation correlates well with neural activity. This correlation is the basis of current **brain imaging** techniques that utilize cerebral blood flow, such as **positron emission tomography** (**PET**) with ^{15}O water, or that rely on blood oxygenation, such as **magnetic resonance imaging** (**MRI**) with endogenous blood oxygen level–dependent contrast (BOLD), as a surrogate to gauge neural activity. The chemical signals that couple neural activity to regulation of the vasculature remain an important matter of investigation.

Because presynaptic nerve terminals exhibit tremendous metabolic activity and contain a large fraction of the mitochondria in the brain, imaging signals related to blood flow or to the use of oxygen or glucose may reflect the functioning of nerve terminals rather than the activity of cell bodies or dendrites. This tendency greatly complicates the interpretation of brain imaging studies; for example, strong imaging signals that result from increased activity of inhibitory nerve terminals may reflect a decrease in the activity of postsynaptic cell bodies. This type of problem challenges scientists to better understand the biologic processes that underlie images of the living human brain and to develop markers that more closely approximate the firing of neurons.

Blood-Brain Barrier

Signaling in the nervous system depends on precise concentrations of extracellular ions and on the carefully controlled release, reuptake, and metabolism of neurotransmitters. If the brain were not isolated from the general circulation, changes in ion concentration related to diet or hydration status would routinely disrupt neural function in profound ways. Ingestion of common nutrients, such as amino acids, that also serve as neurotransmitters or their precursors, or the release of peripheral hormones, would wreak havoc on brain function.

These catastrophic occurrences are prevented by the existence of a blood-brain barrier that creates an isolated homeostatic milieu for the brain and spinal cord. This barrier is formed by tight junctions between endothelial cells of capillaries in cerebral vascular beds, which restrict the passage of soluble molecules **2–17**. The endothelial cells line the lumen of

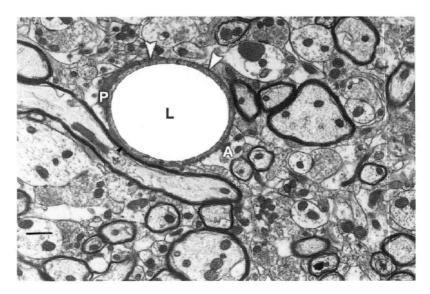

2–17 Electron micrograph of a capillary that forms part of the blood-brain barrier. In contrast to peripheral tissues, where small gaps (fenestrations) between endothelial cells of capillary walls allow small substances to pass freely, endothelial cells in the CNS form tight junctions without fenestrations, which occlude passive diffusion. These tight junctions, together with pericytes (P), the associated basement membrane, and astrocyte foot processes (A), form the blood-brain barrier. The exterior wall of the capillary is marked by arrowheads. L, lumen. (Reproduced with permission from Zigmond MJ, Bloom FE, Landis SC, et al., eds. *Fundamental Neuroscience*. New York: Academic Press; 1999.)

the vessels and are surrounded by a continuous basal lamina. Potential space around the capillaries is taken up by pericytes that surround the capillary walls (see 2-17); these cells are involved in secretion of proteins that contribute to the basement membrane. Because the end feet (terminal processes) of perivascular astrocytes intercalate between the pericytes and contact the basal lamina, they are believed to be involved in the formation and maintenance of the tight junctions between the cerebral endothelial cells 2-18. In contrast, small spaces between endothelial cells in the general circulation permit blood solutes to enter the surrounding tissues.

Only highly lipophilic molecules can diffuse passively through the membranes of vascular cells to enter the brain; thus, any peripherally administered drug that targets the CNS must be relatively lipophilic. In contrast, hydrophilic molecules are generally excluded from the brain; only water-soluble

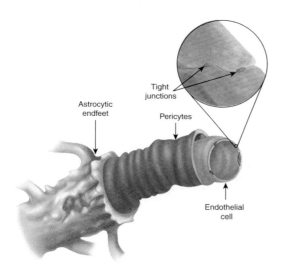

2-18 Schematic representation of surrounding pericytes (covering about 20%–30% of the capillary surface) and astrocytic endfeet projecting on the endothelial cells of the cerebral capillaries that induce and maintain the blood-brain barrier. In contrast, endothelial cells of peripheral capillaries do not form a tight barrier because they lack the specific input of these brain cells. See text for details. (Reprinted with permission from Miller G. *Science*. 2002;297:1116–1118. Illustration by C. Slayden. © 2002 AAAS.)

molecules that are recognized by ATP-dependent transport processes, such as glucose, amino acids, and nucleosides, can enter the CNS. Some other substances gain access to the brain by means of receptor-mediated processes (eg, iron-transferrin, insulin, and lipoproteins; 2-6, 2-19). Many additional substances (eg, leptin) appear to penetrate the brain, although the underlying mechanisms remain poorly understood.

Some areas of the brain that surround the cerebral ventricles, including the area postrema of the medulla, the circumventricular organs, and regions of hypothalamus, lack a blood-brain barrier. These regions have fenestrated capillaries that allow peptides, hydrophilic molecules, and other solutes to enter the brain. In these periventricular regions, the brain is able to sample the general circulation, detect circulating hormones and cytokines, and subsequently direct adaptive responses to these signals. The area postrema, for example, contains chemoreceptors that trigger **vomiting** in response to circulating toxins.

In addition to the physical impediment provided by the blood-brain barrier, transmembrane pumps are found in the CNS that can rapidly transport drugs out of the CNS, even if the drugs have penetrated the blood-brain barrier. One such family of pumps, the **P-glycoproteins**, was first investigated as a cause of resistance to cancer chemotherapy agents; P-glycoproteins are expressed in cells at the blood-brain barrier.

Because the blood-brain barrier excludes all but small, highly lipophilic substances from the CNS, many potential pharmacotherapeutic agents cannot be used successfully. Accordingly, neuropharmacologic research continues to focus on developing strategies for penetrating the blood-brain barrier to improve drug delivery (see 2-6). Increasingly drugs can be screened to see whether they are substrates for P-glycoprotein pumps and thus unlikely to achieve therapeutic concentrations in neurons. There are also attempts to generate **inhibitors of P-glycoproteins** as a means of enhancing the actions of certain drugs in the CNS. Certain L-type Ca^{2+} channel blockers, for instance, inhibit P-glycoproteins. Use of such drugs could be beneficial if planned as a strategy to increase brain concentrations of a drug, but can cause toxicity if a patient inadvertently takes a penetrant CNS drug at regular doses which is normally removed from the CNS by P-glycoproteins.

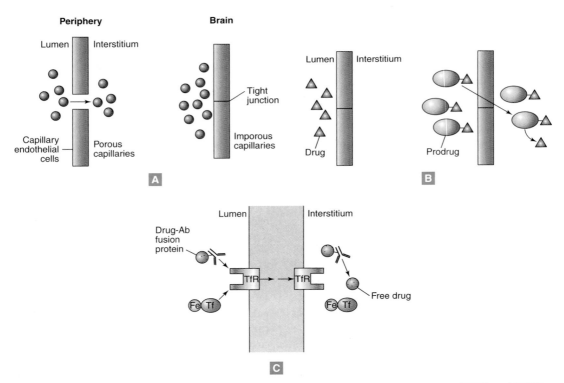

2-19 Schematic illustrations of the blood-brain barrier. **A.** The blood-brain barrier shown in **2-17** and **2-18** is depicted. **B.** *Left,* A hydrophilic drug that cannot penetrate the blood-brain barrier. *Right,* The drug is converted into a hypothetical prodrug after it is coupled to a large lipophilic entity. The resulting prodrug is able to cross the blood-brain barrier; after it enters the brain, it is cleaved into free drug. **C.** Hypothetical use of the transferrin receptor (TfR) to transport a drug into the CNS. Fe-transferrin (Fe-Tf) complexes bind to the TfR. An anti-TfR antibody (Ab), to which a peptide drug is fused, also binds to the receptor. The entire Fe-Tf-TfR-Ab-drug complex is internalized by the endothelial cell, transported across the cell, and incorporated into the opposing cell membrane, where Fe-Tf and Ab-drug are released into the interstitial fluid. Free drug is subsequently cleaved from the Ab-drug complex.

2-6 Overcoming the Blood-Brain Barrier

Although the blood-brain barrier provides essential protection for the brain, it also impedes the delivery of drugs for the treatment of neuropsychiatric disorders. Many small molecules with potentially useful biologic activities are hydrophilic and thus unable to penetrate the brain. Moreover, many of the brain's intercellular messengers are neuropeptides or relatively large proteins such as neurotrophic factors. These substances, as well as their structural analogs, are almost completely excluded from the CNS by the blood-brain barrier. Consequently, an important research area is focused on devising novel ways to penetrate the blood-brain barrier to deliver agents to the brain.

Invasive methods are perhaps the most straightforward. The introduction of a shunt into the cerebrospinal fluid (CSF), through intracerebroventricular or intrathecal cannulae, enables most substances to be administered to the CNS. Such shunts can be introduced by means of a relatively benign surgical procedure and are most commonly used in the treatment of **hydrocephalus** (excessive CSF pressure) to allow the flow of CSF into the abdominal cavity. In recent years, early

(Continued)

2-6 ▪ **Overcoming the Blood-Brain Barrier (*Continued*)**

clinical trials have gotten underway to deliver genes encoding a protein of interest directly into a brain area by use of viral vectors. Such viral-mediated gene transfer (a form of **gene therapy**) remains highly experimental but could prove one day to be a fundamentally novel method for correcting disease-related abnormalities in the brain.

Another general approach to penetrating the blood-brain barrier is to administer a substance that disrupts the barrier temporarily; **mannitol's** osmotic properties, for example, are able to force apart the tight junctions on endothelial cells. Such disruption is followed by peripheral administration of a drug, which would be able to penetrate the compromised barrier. However, substances such as mannitol have a transient effect; the tight junctions that help form the barrier typically are restored within a couple of hours. Recently it has been possible to temporarily open the blood-brain barrier with selective agents that open tight junctions, including **cereport,** which activates bradykinin B$_2$ receptors. (Bradykinin is a peptide that serves transmitter functions in the brain and periphery; see Chapter 7.)

A drug also can be delivered into the brain when it is coupled with a large lipophilic moiety; such coupling enables the drug to passively cross the blood-brain barrier. After it enters the brain, the lipophilic moiety is cleaved, resulting in the release of free drug. This prodrug concept (see **2-19**) is appealing and conceptually quite simple, but to date has not yielded much success.

Still another strategy for penetrating the blood-brain barrier exploits several receptor-mediated processes that normally transport needed substances into or out of the CNS. The best understood process of this sort involves the transferrin receptor, which is located on the luminal surface of capillary endothelial cells and binds to Fe-transferrin complexes (see **2-19**). The Fe-transferrin-transferrin receptor complex is subsequently internalized into the endothelial cells and transported to the opposite or basal aspect of the cell where it is incorporated into the cell membrane. When it faces the interstitial side of the capillary wall, Fe-transferrin is free to diffuse into the brain's extracellular fluid. Investigators are currently attempting to construct antibodies that bind to the transferrin receptor in a way that does not disrupt the receptor's ability to bind Fe-transferrin. Neuropeptides and larger proteins, such as neurotrophic factors, could then be linked to these antibodies. Evidence suggests that the entire complex (Fe-transferrin-transferrin receptor-antibody-neuropeptide) may be effectively transported across the capillary wall.

SELECTED READING

Neurons and Glia

Auld DS, Robitaille R. Glial cells and neurotransmission: an inclusive view of synaptic function. *Neuron.* 2003;40:389–400.

Cowan WM, Sudhof TC, Stevens CF. *Synapses.* Baltimore: Johns Hopkins University Press; 2000.

Fields RD, Stevens-Graham B. New insights into neuron-glia communication. *Science.* 2002;298:556–562.

Volterra A, Meldolesi J. Astrocytes, from brain glue to communication elements: the revolution continues. *Nature Rev Neurosci.* 2005;6:626–640.

Electrical Properties and Ion Channels

Ashcroft FM. From molecule to malady. *Nature.* 2006;440:440–447.

Beaumont V, Zucker RS. Enhancement of synaptic transmission by cyclic AMP modulation of presynaptic I$_h$ channels. *Nature Neurosci.* 2000; 3:133–141.

Catterall WA. Structure and regulation of voltage-gated Ca^{2+} channels. *Annu Rev Cell Dev Biol.* 2000;16: 521–555.

Catterall WA. From ionic currents to molecular mechanisms: the structure and function of voltage-gated sodium channels. *Neuron.* 2000;26:13–25.

Choe S, Kreusch A, Pfaffinger PJ. Toward the three-dimensional structure of voltage-gated potassium channels. *Trends Biochem Sci.* 1999;24: 345–349.

Doyle DA, Cabral JM, Pfuetzner RA, et al. The structure of the potassium channel: molecular basis of K$^+$ conduction and selectivity. *Science.* 1998;180:69–77.

Ertel EA, Campbell KP, Harpold MM, et al. Nomenclature of voltage-gated calcium channels. *Neuron.* 2000;25: 533–535.

Gouaux E, MacKinnon R. Principles of selective ion transport in channels and pumps. *Science.* 2005;310:1461–1465.

Hausser M. Spruston N, Stuart GJ. Diversity and dynamics of dendritic signaling. *Science.* 2000;290:739–744.

Hille B. *Ionic Channels of Excitable Membranes.* 3rd ed. Sunderland, MA: Sinauer Press; 2001.

Jan LY, Jan YN. Voltage-sensitive ion channels. *Cell.* 1989;56:13–25.

Jentsch TJ. Neuronal KCNQ potassium channels: physiology and role in disease. *Nature Rev Neurosci.* 2000;1:21–30.

Jentsch TJ, Neagoe I, Scheel O. CLC chloride channels and transporters. Curr Opin Neurobiol. 2005;15:319–325.

Jentsch TJ, Poet M, Fuhrmann JC, et al. Physiological functions of CLC Cl⁻ channels gleaned from human genetic disease and mouse models. *Annu Rev Physiol.* 2005;67:779–807.

Johnston D, Wu SM-S. *Foundations of Cellular Neurophysiology.* Cambridge, MA: MIT Press; 1995.

IUPHAR Compendium of Voltage-Gated Ion Channels. *Pharmacol Rev.* 2005.

Lai HC, Jan LY. The distribution and targeting of neuronal voltage-dependent ion channels. *Nature Rev Neurosci.* 2006;7:548–562.

MacKinnon R. Nobel Lecture: Potassium channels and the atomic basis of selective ion conduction. *Biosci Rep.* 2004;24:75–100.

Miller C. ClC chloride channels viewed through a transporter lens. *Nature* 2006;440:484–489.

Montell C. The TRP superfamily of cation channels. *Sci STKE.* 2005;272: re3.

Ramsey IS, Delling M, Clapham DE. An introduction to TRP channels. *Annu Rev Physiol.* 2006;68:619–647.

Yu FH, Catterall WA. The VGL-chanome: a protein superfamily specialized for electrical signaling and ionic homeostasis. *Sci STKE.* 2004;253: re15.

Blood-Brain Barrier

Abbott NJ, Ronnback L, Hansson E. Astrocyte-endothelial interactions at the blood-brain barrier. *Nature Rev Neurosci.* 2006;7:41–52.

De Boer AG, Gaillard PJ. Drug targeting to the brain. *Annu Rev Pharmacol Toxicol.* 2007;47:323–355.

Fromm MF. Importance of P-glycoprotein at blood–tissue barriers. *Trends Pharmacol Sci.* 2004;25:423–429.

Pan W, Kastin AJ. Polypeptide delivery across the blood-brain barrier. *Curr Drug Targets—CNS Neurol Dis.* 2004;3:131–136.

Uhr M, Grauer MT, Holsboer F. Differential enhancement of antidepresssant penetration into the brain of mice with abdb1ab (mdr1ab) P-glycoprotein gene disruption. *Biol Psychiatry.* 2003;54:840–846.

Synaptic Transmission

- Synaptic transmission is a signal transduction process that begins with the action potential-dependent release of a neurotransmitter from a presynaptic terminal. The neurotransmitter then binds to and activates postsynaptic receptors that modify the electrical and biochemical properties of the postsynaptic cell.

- The major classes of neurotransmitters are amino acid transmitters, such as glutamate and GABA; monoamines, including dopamine, norepinephrine, and serotonin; peptides; diffusible gases, such as nitric oxide; lipid-derived molecules, such as endocannabinoids; and nucleosides, such as adenosine.

- Neurotransmitters are stored in small organelles called synaptic vesicles that fuse with the presynaptic terminal membrane and release their contents when an action potential invades the terminal and causes a rise in calcium due to activation of voltage-dependent calcium channels.

- A single neurotransmitter typically activates several different subtypes of receptors.

- Neurotransmitter receptors are classified as ligand-gated ion channels or G protein–coupled receptors.

- After being released, most neurotransmitters are transported back into the presynaptic terminal or into glia by specialized proteins called plasma membrane transporters. A different family of transporters is responsible for pumping neurotransmitter into synaptic vesicles.

- Neurotransmitter transporters are important targets of many antidepressant medications and psychostimulant drugs such as cocaine.

- The proteins that are responsible for the fusion of synaptic vesicles with the presynaptic plasma membrane, a process known as exocytosis, have been identified and extensively characterized. Some of these proteins are the targets of bacterial toxins, such as tetanus and botulinum toxin.

- After exocytosis, synaptic vesicles are recycled and used again by repackaging them with neurotransmitter.

When we think, feel, or move, information passes rapidly between neurons across specialized gaps called synapses. When we learn and remember, synapses undergo significant activity-dependent alterations. Given the centrality of synaptic transmission to the function of the nervous system, it is not surprising that the large majority of drugs used to treat neuropsychiatric illnesses act on different protein components of specific synapses. This chapter explores the biochemical basis of synaptic transmission and explains how this process is regulated.

THE SYNAPSE

Neurons are morphologically specialized to receive, process, and send information **3-1**. As discussed in Chapter 2, the key structure across which information is transferred, by use of chemical neurotransmitters, is the synapse. Synaptic transmission is a result of three types of processes that convert electrical information into a chemical signal and then back again: (1) electrical information in the axon of a presynaptic neuron is converted to a chemical signal in its nerve terminal, (2) this chemical signal is transmitted to another cell across a synapse, and (3) the chemical message received by the postsynaptic cell is converted into an electrical signal. It should be noted that a small percentage of synapses are gap junctions, morphological connections between two neurons that permit the direct flow of electrical current from cell to cell (Chapter 2). These electrical junctions are morphologically distinct from chemical synapses. Because virtually all pharmacologic agents act at chemical synapses rather than at gap junctions, chemical synapses are the sole focus of this chapter.

Most types of communication between neurons must be precise and rapid. Fast and accurate information exchange is partly ensured by restricting the process within a synapse. The synapse was originally defined by three distinct elements: a presynaptic nerve terminal or bouton, its postsynaptic target, and the space between them known as the synaptic cleft. Over the past several decades, extensive investigation has revealed additional details, including presynaptic structures specialized to release chemical neurotransmitters from the nerve terminal, and postsynaptic structures involved in processing these signals **3-1** and **3-2**. On the presynaptic side of the synapse, in the active zone of the nerve terminal, neurotransmitter is released from vesicles that cluster near the plasma membrane. On the other side of the synapse are postsynaptic specializations, the composition of which

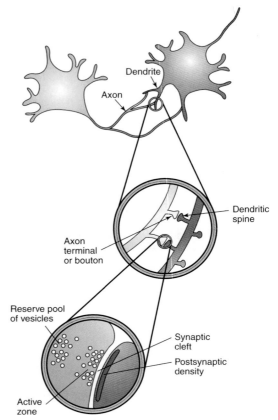

3-1 **At the interface between an axon and a postsynaptic cell, known as the synaptic cleft, an axon terminal, or synaptic bouton, innervates a dendritic spine.** In the active zone of the presynaptic terminal, synaptic vesicles cluster against the plasma membrane. A reserve pool of synaptic vesicles lies nearby, and the postsynaptic density lies opposite the active zone within the dendritic spine.

varies with the type of neurotransmitter released from the presynaptic terminal. The postsynaptic density, which is detected at excitatory synapses, is the best-characterized postsynaptic specialization. It is easily identified in electron micrographs **3-2** as a proteinaceous matrix of fine filaments just under the plasma membrane of postsynaptic dendritic spines. The proteins that comprise this structure, such as postsynaptic density protein 95 (PSD95), act as a scaffold to cluster and organize molecules involved in postsynaptic signaling. The synaptic cleft itself is bound by extracellular matrix proteins and cell adhesion molecules that may function to strengthen or weaken synaptic contacts.

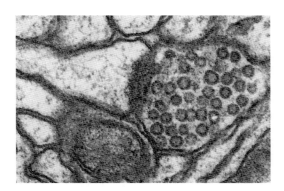

3-2 **Electron micrograph of an excitatory synapse.** Two primary components are evident: a presynaptic terminal (*right*) and the postsynaptic target, with a dendritic spine to the left. A depolarization-dependent influx of Ca^{2+} into the terminal causes synaptic vesicles, visible as uniform spherical organelles, to fuse with the plasma membrane, thereby releasing neurotransmitter into the synaptic cleft. Released transmitter subsequently binds to postsynaptic receptors. The postsynaptic density, the site at which receptors are located, is visible as the dark, electron-dense region adjacent to the plasma membrane at the end of the dendritic spine. (Image kindly provided by K. Harris from Synapse Web: synapses.clm.utexas.edu)

Neurotransmitters

Neurotransmitters are often classified by their chemical makeup, although there is only a rough correlation between these classes and neurotransmitter function **3-1**. The major chemical groupings are amino acid transmitters, such as glutamate and γ-aminobutyric acid (GABA); monoamines, including dopamine, norepinephrine, and serotonin; peptides; diffusible gases, such as nitric oxide; nucleosides, such as adenosine; and lipid-derived signaling molecules, such as endogenous cannabinoids (endocannabinoids). Historically, it was believed that only one type of transmitter could be synthesized and released from a cell, but we now know that a single neuron may utilize multiple neurotransmitters. Examples include corelease of monoamines such as norepinephrine with peptides such as neuropeptide Y, but some neurons also release more than one small molecule neurotransmitter, and some neurons release multiple neuropeptides (Chapter 7). The biosynthesis, metabolism, and functions of the different types of neurotransmitters, as well as the receptors that mediate their signaling, are discussed extensively in subsequent chapters. This chapter focuses predominantly on the mechanisms underlying neurotransmitter release.

Storage and Release of Neurotransmitters

With the exception of the diffusible gases and lipid-derived signaling molecules, most chemical transmitters are stored in secretory vesicles. Like other cellular organelles, these vesicles have a limiting membrane composed of a phospholipid bilayer and an aqueous lumen **3-1**. The lumen is filled with thousands of transmitter molecules that sometimes reach near-molar concentrations. During synaptic transmission, secretory vesicles fuse with the plasma membrane, allowing communication between the aqueous interior of the vesicle and the extracellular space. The most abundant form of secretory vesicle in the central nervous system (CNS) is the so-called small synaptic vesicle. These vesicles cluster in the active zone of the nerve terminal and are released rapidly when the nerve terminal depolarizes.

The amount of transmitter in each vesicle is called a quantum. Because transmitter release proceeds through the fusion of individual vesicles with the presynaptic terminal plasma membrane, the release process is known as quantal release.

Postsynaptic Signaling

After a neurotransmitter diffuses across the synaptic cleft to the postsynaptic neuron, receptors embedded in the postsynaptic membrane bind to the neurotransmitter and cause an electrical or biochemical alteration in the postsynaptic cell. *Excitatory* signals cause the membrane to *depolarize* so that positive charge flows into the cell, and *inhibitory* signals cause the membrane to *hyperpolarize*, whereby positive charge flows out of the cell or negative charge flows into the cell. These electrical signals are integrated in the dendrites and cell body and, if depolarization is sufficient, an all-or-none action potential fires and transmits an electrical impulse along the axon (Chapter 2). Whether synaptic transmission is fast, occurring within several milliseconds, or slow—taking place in seconds or minutes—depends on the type of receptor targeted by the neurotransmitter **3-3**.

Fast Synaptic Transmission

Fast synaptic transmission is mediated by transmitter- or ligand-gated ion channels, also called ionotropic receptors. The most extensively studied of these is the

3-1 Chemical Neurotransmitters

Transmitter Type	Representative Example	Structure
Biogenic amines	Monoamines: Dopamine	(3,4-dihydroxyphenyl ring)—CH_2—CH_2—NH_2
	Acetylcholine	CH_3—$\overset{\overset{O}{\|\|}}{C}$—O—$CH_2$—$CH_2$—$\overset{+}{N}(CH_3)_3$
Amino acids	γ-aminobutyric acid (GABA)	CH_2—CH_2—CH_2—COOH, with NH_2 on first CH_2
	Glutamate	COOH—$\overset{\overset{NH_2}{\|}}{CH}$—$CH_2$—$CH_2$—COOH
Peptides	Leu-enkephalin	Tyr–Gly–Gly–Phe–Leu
Nucleosides	Adenosine	(adenine + ribose structure)
Gases	Nitric oxide	·N=O
Lipid-derived	Anandamide	(arachidonoyl chain)—$CONHCH_2CH_2OH$

nicotinic acetylcholine receptor, which is composed of five subunits that enclose a central aqueous pore. When acetylcholine binds to this receptor, the pore opens transiently (1 to 10 ms) and allows the passage of approximately 20,000 positively charged Na^+ ions. The vast majority of excitatory and inhibitory synapses in the brain utilize ionotropic receptors for the amino acids glutamate and GABA (Chapter 5). Molecular cloning has revealed that the basic design of most, if not all, ligand-gated channels is similar to that of voltage-gated channels (Chapters 2 and 5).

Slow Synaptic Transmission

Many of the neurotransmitters involved in fast synaptic transmission also induce slower synaptic responses when they activate receptors coupled to heterotrimeric guanine nucleotide–binding proteins (G proteins). These receptors are often termed metabotropic receptors. Most other types of neurotransmitters, including the monoamines and neuropeptides, also activate G protein–coupled receptors. When a neurotransmitter binds to a G protein–coupled receptor, the receptor

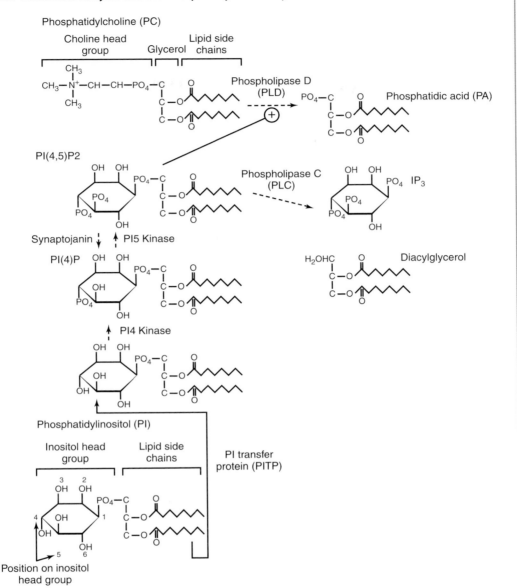

Position on inositol
head group

Membrane bilayers serve to compartmentalize cells; however, they are fluid and flexible. As a result, membrane-defined vesicles can fuse with a plasma membrane and can form by budding from parent organelles. Furthermore, the membrane bilayers surrounding different organelles vary in terms of their phospholipid composition, and the head groups of the component lipids can be altered enzymatically. The 1, 4, and 5 positions of the inositol head groups may be linked to phosphate groups by reactions that are catalyzed by different lipid kinases (see figure). In addition, lipid phosphatases can remove phosphate from the inositol ring. A growing number of observations link phosphatidylinositol (PI) phosphorylation to membrane fusion events.

Because phospholipases can cleave chemical bonds in phospholipids, they play an important role in cell signaling and membrane trafficking. Two products of phospholipase C and D (PLC and PLD) are shown in the figure. The products of PLC, inositol triphosphate (IP_3) and diacylglycerol (DAG), are important second messengers and play a role in cell signaling as discussed in Chapter 4. In contrast, the product of PLD, phosphatidic acid (PA), appears to be involved in membrane trafficking. Studies have revealed that IP_3 can activate PLD, thus indicating the complex functional interaction between these pathways.

Ligand-gated ion channel

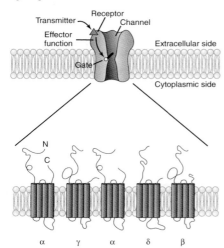

G protein-coupled receptor

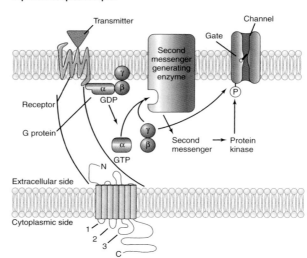

3-3 **Ligand-gated channels and G protein-coupled receptors.** Ligand-gated ion channels, which mediate fast synaptic transmission, are composed of one or more subunits (eg, $\alpha\ \beta\ \gamma\ \delta$) embedded in the plasma membrane that form a central, gated pore. In response to the binding of transmitter, this type of receptor undergoes a conformational change, opening the gate and allowing ions to diffuse passively along concentration gradients through a hydrophilic opening in an otherwise hydrophobic bilayer. G protein–coupled receptors, which mediate slow synaptic transmission, transduce neurotransmitter signals through a different mechanism. These proteins do not form gated pores in the membrane; rather, the binding of transmitter induces a conformational change that allows the receptor to activate a heterotrimeric G protein (Chapter 4). The activated G protein dissociates into a free α subunit bound to GTP and a free $\beta\gamma$ subunit dimer. Both can activate enzymes that synthesize second messengers; in addition, $\beta\gamma$ dimers directly regulate certain ion channels. Second messengers also regulate ion channels, most often by activating protein kinases, which subsequently phosphorylate such channels (P). 1 2 3, cytoplasmic domains of G protein–coupled receptor. (Adapted with permission from Kandel ER, Schwartz JH, Jessell TM. *Principles of Neural Science*, 4th ed. New York: McGraw-Hill; 2000:184.)

activates an associated G protein. The α subunit of the G protein subsequently dissociates from its $\beta\gamma$ subunits, with both α and $\beta\gamma$ subunits then activating downstream molecules, including specific types of ion channels (Chapter 4). These biochemical steps mediate slow synaptic transmission because they generally require more time to develop compared with the opening of a ligand-gated channel. Stimulation of G protein–coupled receptors does not always produce excitatory or inhibitory transmission; in some cases it modulates the actions of other neurotransmitters, such as glutamate.

In addition to regulating ion channels, G protein α and $\beta\gamma$ subunits activate several enzymes that regulate the formation of second messengers such as cAMP, cGMP, and diacylglycerol (DAG). G proteins also regulate the flow of the second messenger Ca^{2+} into neurons. Once formed, second messengers stimulate or inhibit protein kinases or protein phosphatases, whose subsequent phosphorylation or dephosphorylation of ion channels results in the generation of postsynaptic electrical signals. Some second messengers, such as cAMP and cGMP, and G protein subunits (α and $\beta\gamma$) can directly bind to and modify the activity of specific ion channels. Moreover, these second messenger cascades regulate gene transcription and protein synthesis, which may alter the types and amounts of ion channels expressed by a neuron. Such activities can have long-lasting effects on neuronal function (Chapter 4). Thus, the involvement of G protein–coupled receptors greatly increases the complexity and flexibility of the types of electrical signals that can be generated by neurotransmitters.

Receptor Subtypes

Ligand-gated ion channels and G protein–coupled receptors each comprise multiple subtypes. A single neurotransmitter can activate a variety of these receptor subtypes, and several members of the same receptor family can colocalize at a single synapse; consequently, the signal received by a postsynaptic neuron can vary considerably and may be quite complex. Ultimately, the actions of any individual neurotransmitter are dictated by the receptor subtype to which it binds and by the subsynaptic localization of that receptor.

Before the advent of molecular cloning techniques, receptor subtypes were grouped according to their pharmacologic profiles, including their responses to particular agonists and antagonists. More recently, cloned receptors have been grouped more precisely on the basis of structural and functional similarities and according to their cellular localization. Some receptor subtypes tend to be located in particular cell types or subcellular regions. Presynaptic localization does not exclude postsynaptic localization, and the presence of some receptor subtypes—for example, the serotonin $5HT_{1a}$ receptor—in both presynaptic terminals and postsynaptic cells further increases the complexity of synaptic communication. The activation of receptors located in the presynaptic bouton typically modifies the release of neurotransmitter. Presynaptic receptors that respond to the transmitter released by that terminal are called *autoreceptors;* presynaptic receptors that respond to other transmitters are sometimes called *heteroreceptors.* Variations in signaling pathways activated by different receptor subtypes underscore the central role of receptors in dictating the actions of the transmitters that bind to them.

NEUROTRANSMITTER STORAGE, REUPTAKE, AND RELEASE

The Role of Calcium Ions

Our current understanding of synaptic transmission is based on work performed in the 1950s, which uncovered the role of Ca^{2+} in neurotransmitter release at the neuromuscular junction (NMJ). The NMJ comprises a presynaptic motor nerve terminal and a postsynaptic specialization on the muscle cell known as an end plate. Although the NMJ differs significantly from a synapse in the CNS, it is similar enough to serve as a model. When the motor nerve of the NMJ is electrically stimulated, it releases a chemical message that produces an electrical signal in the muscle cell, called the excitatory postsynaptic current, which in turn causes contraction of the muscle. When this contractile process is paralyzed, the relationship between

chemical transmission and the electrical response can be studied in isolation. The chemical transmitter at the vertebrate NMJ is acetylcholine, identified in 1921 as the first known chemical neurotransmitter.

Early studies of the NMJ found that the action potential per se was not required for acetylcholine release. Rather, the action potential caused the nerve terminal to depolarize, which in turn caused the release of transmitter. This was demonstrated by eliminating the action potential with **tetrodotoxin**, which blocks voltage-gated Na^+ channels (Chapter 2), and changing the voltage in the nerve terminal with an electrode, which makes it possible to depolarize the terminal and induce transmitter release directly. It was subsequently discovered that eliminating extracellular Ca^{2+} prevented the release of neurotransmitter; it was therefore concluded that the entry of Ca^{2+} into the nerve terminal triggered transmitter release. We now know that the opening of voltage-gated Ca^{2+} channels in response to depolarization (Chapter 2) causes a rapid increase in the intracellular concentration of Ca^{2+}, which in turn causes the release of neurotransmitter.

Quantal Release

Related studies of the NMJ revealed that, in the absence of presynaptic stimulation, the postsynaptic cell exhibited small, spontaneous electrical responses. Equally important was the discovery that these miniature end plate potentials (MEPPs or *minis*) were all approximately the same size. Indeed, when the nerve was stimulated to evoke larger postsynaptic currents, the resulting end plate potentials were always integral sums of the MEPPs 3-4 . These findings led to the hypothesis that a single MEPP represents the postsynaptic response to the smallest amount of transmitter released by a presynaptic cell, thus giving birth to the idea of quantal release.

The precise physical equivalent of a quantum remained to be determined, but two pieces of evidence suggested that this elemental unit represented the transmitter contained in a single synaptic vesicle. First, electron micrographs revealed clusters of regular round vesicles lined up at the presynaptic membrane (see 3-2). Second, these vesicles sometimes appeared to be fused with the plasma membrane and, in the process of opening their lumen to the extracellular space, such vesicles look like the Greek letter Ω and are called omega profiles. Thus, small vesicles at the site of transmitter release appeared capable of releasing their contents into the synaptic cleft by fusing with the plasma membrane. Whether these synaptic vesicles contained neurotransmitter was unclear; however, biochemical studies demonstrated that synaptic

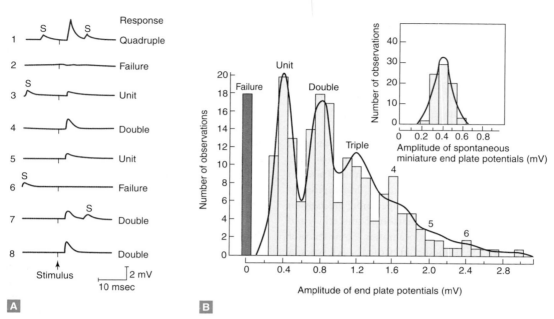

3–4 **Synaptic responses recorded during electrophysiologic experiments in the 1950s and 1960s.** These experiments demonstrated that neurotransmitter is released from presynaptic terminals in discrete packages or quanta. Moreover, they determined that the postsynaptic response does not have a fixed amplitude but occurs in discrete steps, each of which represents the response to transmitter released from a single vesicle. **A.** Spontaneous miniature end plate potentials (S), which are electrical recordings of postsynaptic electrical activity in the absence of an external stimulus, and synaptic responses (end plate potentials) evoked by a weak stimulus. The recorded end plate potentials are generated by the release of one to four quanta of neurotransmitter; occasionally a weak stimulus fails to trigger such a release. **B.** A histogram that indicates the amplitude of the end plate potentials reveals peaks that are multiple integrals of the miniature end plate potentials (*inset*). (Reproduced with permission from Kandel ER, Schwartz JH, Jessell TM. *Principles of Neural Science*, 4th ed. New York: McGraw-Hill; 2000:260.)

vesicles at the NMJ contained acetylcholine. These findings validated the theory that a synaptic vesicle represents the anatomic equivalent of electrophysiologically defined quanta. Fittingly, the process of transmitter release was subsequently referred to as *exocytosis*.

Although morphologic studies indicate that there are tens to hundreds of synaptic vesicles in each nerve terminal, neurotransmitter is not released every time an action potential invades this structure. Instead, neurotransmitter release is a stochastic or probabilistic process: In response to an action potential it sometimes occurs and sometimes fails to occur. The probability of transmitter release can vary widely from synapse to synapse and can be modified by the activation of presynaptic neurotransmitter receptors, by drugs, and by recent synaptic activity.

The quantal hypothesis has stood the test of time. With few exceptions, studies have confirmed that neurotransmitter is released from the nerve terminal in synaptic vesicles. Whether these packets of neurotransmitter are always the same size has been technically difficult to determine; however, variations among quanta most likely exist. Indeed, some of the first synaptic vesicles isolated from the NMJ revealed cholinergic vesicles that contained varying amounts of transmitter. In the CNS, quantal size may vary even more than it does at the NMJ. Variations in the postsynaptic response to each quantum and evidence indicating that different populations of synaptic vesicles may differ in the amount of neurotransmitter they store strongly support this theory. Although investigators have yet to determine the mechanisms underlying variations in synaptic vesicle content, they most likely involve the proteins that synthesize neurotransmitters and transport them into synaptic vesicles.

Packaging and Transport of Neurotransmitters

Small-molecule neurotransmitters such as the monoamines and amino acid transmitters are synthesized in the cytoplasm of the neuron; the enzymes that convert precursors into mature neurotransmitters are discussed in subsequent chapters on individual neurotransmitters. Because they are synthesized in the cytoplasm, these neurotransmitters must be transported across the synaptic vesicle membrane into its lumen. The process of vesicular transport serves to package neurotransmitters for regulated exocytotic release.

Purified secretory vesicles express distinct proteins called vesicular transporters that mediate the pumping or transport of monoamines, such as dopamine, norepinephrine, and serotonin; acetylcholine; GABA and glycine; and glutamate into the vesicles **3-5** and **3-2**. Vesicular transport of all monoamines is mediated by

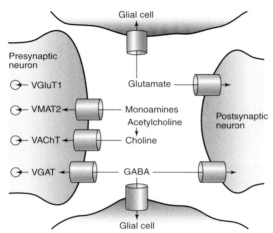

3-5 **Transmitter fates.** Mechanisms for terminating the action of transmitters include transport into the presynaptic terminal, uptake by glia or postsynaptic cells, enzymatic degradation, and passive diffusion away from the synapse. For monoamines, neurotransmission is terminated by transport across the plasma membrane. In contrast, acetylcholine is degraded in the synaptic cleft by acetylcholinesterase and transported into the presynaptic terminal as choline. The actions of the amino acid transmitters glutamate and γ-aminobutyric acid (GABA) are terminated by active transport into postsynaptic neurons or glia; GABA also can be transported into presynaptic terminals. After reaching a presynaptic terminal, a neurotransmitter may be degraded (not shown) or recycled into synaptic vesicles. Vesicular transporters include proteins specific for GABA (VGAT), acetylcholine (VAChT), monoamines (VMAT2), and glutamate (VGluT1). Acetylcholine must be resynthesized from choline and acetylCoA before it is transported by VAChT.

a single protein, termed *vesicular monoamine transporter 2* (VMAT2). The active transport of monoamines and acetylcholine is driven by the pH gradient (ΔpH) across the vesicle membrane, which propels the exchange of two luminal protons for one cytoplasmic transmitter molecule. In contrast, glutamate transport depends primarily on an electrochemical gradient ($\Delta\Psi$), and GABA transport depends on both ΔpH and $\Delta\Psi$. The transporter for purine transmitters such as adenosine has not yet been identified.

Drugs that inhibit vesicular transport have significant behavioral effects. **Reserpine** inhibits the vesicular transport of monoamines and causes their depletion at the synapse (Chapter 6). As a result, reserpine can decrease blood pressure, but its side effects, including **depression** in some patients, limited its clinical use. **Amphetamines**, which act on both vesicular and plasma membrane transporters (see below) release vesicular monoamine stores, first into the cytoplasm and then into the synapse (Chapter 6), resulting in potent psychostimulant effects. Because of their central role in synaptic transmission, vesicular transporters are potential targets for the development of novel psychoactive drugs.

Termination of Neurotransmitter Action

After exocytosis, neurotransmitter is inactivated, either by enzymatic degradation or by active transport out of the synaptic cleft. The latter process may include transport across the plasma membrane of the presynaptic terminal, postsynaptic neurons, or neighboring glia **3-5**. Like vesicular transport, plasma membrane transport requires specific transport proteins. However, unlike vesicular transport, it depends on energy provided by the Na^+ gradient across the plasma membrane. These transport activities have been important targets of therapeutic drugs since the early 1960s, when it was discovered that **cocaine** and many **antidepressants** act initially by inhibiting the plasma membrane transport of monoamines such as dopamine, norepinephrine, or serotonin (Chapters 6, 14, and 15).

Most of the proteins responsible for plasma membrane transport of neurotransmitter have been identified through molecular cloning and belong to one of two families. One family includes transporters for GABA and for monoamine transmitters. Transporters of dopamine, norepinephrine, or serotonin are expressed only in their specific monoaminergic cell populations. Plasma membrane transporters of both monoamines and GABA use the cotransport of Na^+ and Cl^- ions to

3-2 **Molecularly Cloned Neurotransmitter Transporters[1]**

Amine/GABA Family

Transporter	Transmitter	Localization
GAT-1	GABA	Neurons (presynaptic and postsynaptic); glia
GAT-2	GABA	Glia
GAT-3	GABA	Glia
GAT-4	GABA	Glia
DAT	Dopamine	Dopaminergic neurons
SERT	Serotonin	Serotonergic neurons
NET	Norepinephrine	Noradrenergic and adrenergic neurons

Glutamate Family

Animal Homologs of Human Transporters	Transmitter[2]	Localization
EAAT1 (GLAST1, rat)	Glutamate	Neurons
EAAT2 (GLT-1, rat)	Glutamate	Astrocytes
EAAT3 (EAAC1, rabbit)	Glutamate	Astrocytes; Bergmann glia
EAAT4	Glutamate	Purkinje cells
EAAT5	Glutamate	Retina

Vesicular Transporters

Transporters	Transmitter	Localization
VGAT	GABA; glycine	Synaptic vesicles
VMAT1	Monoamines	Non-neuronal vesicles
VMAT2	Monoamines	Synaptic vesicles; dense core vesicles
VAChT	Acetylcholine	Synaptic vesicles
VGluT1	Glutamate	Synaptic vesicles

[1]The plasma membrane choline transporter (CHT) is distinct from other neurotransmitter transporters in that it is a member of the sugar/glucose transporter family (GluT, or SLC2 for solute carrier family 2). Within the central and peripheral nervous systems, the CHT is expressed within cholinergic neurons only.
[2]All known glutamate transporters also transport aspartate. However, aspartate's role as a neurotransmitter is not well established (Chapter 5).

drive transmitter into the cytosol. A second family of plasma membrane transporters includes at least 4 structurally related glutamate transporters. In contrast to monoamine and GABA transporters, glutamate transporters drive transmitter uptake through cotransport of Na^+ and H^+ into the cell and the countertransport of K^+ out of the cell. In addition, glutamate transporters may function as Cl^- channels, an activity that appears to be uncoupled from transmitter transport.

Differences in the subcellular localization of plasma membrane transporters have important functional ramifications (see **3-5**). The monoamine transporters are concentrated in the plasma membranes of presynaptic terminals; thus, in addition to terminating synaptic transmission, plasma membrane transport of monoamines also serves to recycle them for another round of exocytosis. Four isoforms of the GABA transporter have been identified, and at least 1 (GAT-1) is found in the presynaptic terminals of GABAergic neurons. However, other GAT isoforms are located on glia and possibly postsynaptic neurons, which suggests that a portion of exocytosed GABA is not recycled. Likewise, glutamate transporters are located primarily on glia and to a lesser extent on postsynaptic neurons thus, the bulk of exocytosed glutamate also does not appear to be recycled; rather, each round of glutamatergic transmission uses transmitter synthesized de novo.

Degradative enzymes play an important role in the termination of synaptic transmission as well. Enzymes that inactivate monoamines in this manner are located in the extracellular space of the synaptic cleft, as well as intracellularly. At the NMJ and in the CNS, acetylcholine is rapidly inactivated by acetylcholinesterases in the synaptic cleft; the metabolite choline is subsequently transported into the presynaptic terminal by a plasma membrane choline transporter, for recycling. Acetylcholine itself is not transported across the plasma membrane (see 3-5).

The fate of exocytosed transmitter also may include diffusion out of the synaptic cleft. Electrophysiologic studies suggest that glutamate may diffuse out of the synaptic cleft and bind to receptors at adjacent synapses in a process that may serve to alter the spatial specificity of synaptic transmission. In contrast, monoamine plasma membrane transporters can be concentrated at the boundaries of the active zone of a presynaptic nerve terminal and may act to restrict diffusion of transmitter to adjacent synapses.

Synaptic Vesicles and Large Dense Core Vesicles

Many neurons express a distinct class of secretory vesicles called large dense core vesicles (LDCVs), which release neurotransmitter but differ from small synaptic vesicles. Synaptic vesicles are smaller (approximately 40 nm in diameter) and more abundant and cluster at active zones in the nerve terminal. In contrast, LDCVs are slightly larger (80–120 nm) and contain neuropeptides (Chapter 7). In the adrenal medulla and certain cultured cells, LDCVs also contain monoamine transmitters in their lumen, although in the CNS most synaptically released monoamine is derived from small synaptic vesicles. LDCVs also contain aggregates of soluble proteins that appear as a dense core in electron micrographs—hence, their name. Unlike synaptic vesicles, LDCVs are not closely linked to the active zone and are released from other sites in the cell. Although both types of vesicles use similar machinery for exocytosis, the release of neurotransmitter from LDCVs occurs in response to different concentrations of intracellular Ca^{2+} and to different patterns of presynaptic activity compared with release from small synaptic vesicles.

BIOCHEMISTRY OF NEUROTRANSMITTER RELEASE: THE EXOCYTOTIC CYCLE

The cornerstone of presynaptic function is the quantal release of transmitter through exocytosis. The quantal release of transmitter must be localized and rapid, repeatable at high frequencies, and amenable to up-regulation or down-regulation over time. Rapid release is necessary to allow communication between neurons within milliseconds, and temporal precision is necessary to preserve the timing of the electrical information encoded in an action potential. Thus, exocytosis must be precisely coordinated with the influx of Ca^{2+} induced by depolarization of the nerve terminal. Terminals must be capable of sustained firing and neurotransmitter release because communication between neurons often involves repeated trains of stimuli. Finally, exocytosis must be a highly regulated process to accommodate the neural plasticity that underlies learning and memory. These requirements are satisfied by the following five steps in the cycle of exocytotic release 3-6 :

1. *Docking.* Synaptic vesicles release neurotransmitter only at the active zone of a nerve terminal, exactly opposite the signal transduction machinery of the postsynaptic cell. This arrangement minimizes the time required for transmitter to reach the postsynaptic cell and also enhances the precision of communication between the two cells. Because the active zone occupies a relatively restricted area along the plasma membrane of the nerve terminal, vesicles must be specifically targeted to this region through a process referred to as docking.

2. *Priming.* Morphologic analyses indicate that approximately 10 to 30 vesicles are docked at the active zone of CNS synapses. However, most of these vesicles are not capable of Ca^{2+}-induced release and must undergo an active maturation process known as priming, which requires adenosine triphosphate (ATP) hydrolysis. Primed vesicles release neurotransmitter within a millisecond of Ca^{2+} influx into the cell. The speed of this release suggests that priming may initiate a partial fusion of the synaptic vesicle with the plasma membrane. Moreover, the energy obtained from ATP hydrolysis may be used to alter the conformation of proteins involved in exocytosis.

3. *Fusion/Exocytosis.* Fusion of the synaptic vesicle with the presynaptic plasma membrane requires deformation of the two apposing membranes. Because this event is tightly linked to the influx of Ca^{2+}, the underlying protein machinery is believed to involve a Ca^{2+} sensor. Fusion of the membranes allows exocytosis: extrusion of vesicle contents into the synaptic cleft.

4. *Endocytosis.* After the synaptic vesicle fuses with the plasma membrane and releases its contents, the vesicle membrane is recycled by a process of internalization known as endocytosis. As with other endocytotic processes, the internalization of synaptic vesicles is facilitated by a protein lattice that coats the internal face of the plasma membrane.

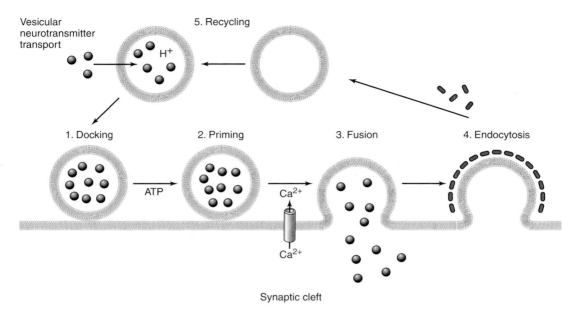

Vesicular neurotransmitter transport

5. Recycling

H⁺

1. Docking   2. Priming   3. Fusion   4. Endocytosis

ATP

Ca²⁺

Ca²⁺

Synaptic cleft

3–6 **The exocytotic cycle.** The exocytotic cycle consists of several distinct steps: (**1**) docking of synaptic vesicles at the plasma membrane of the active zone; (**2**) priming, an ATP-dependent step that prepares each vesicle for release; (**3**) fusion/exocytosis, the release of neurotransmitter triggered by the influx of Ca²⁺ through voltage-gated channels in the plasma membrane; (**4**) endocytosis, retrieval of vesicle membrane facilitated by a protein coat (*dashed line*) that subsequently dissociates from each vesicle; and (**5**) recycling, whereby vesicles move through an endosome intermediate (not shown) or invaginations from the plasma membrane.

5. *Recycling.* This mechanism conserves synaptic vesicle membrane and helps to maintain a pool of release-competent vesicles. Two major models of synaptic vesicle recycling have been proposed. In the first, vesicles fuse with larger endosomes after endocytosis; subsequently, synaptic vesicles bud from these endosomes to engage in another round of exocytosis. According to the second model, synaptic vesicles bud directly from deep invaginations of the plasma membrane that are distinct from endosomes. Although synaptic vesicles recycle according to the first model in some neuroendocrine cells in culture, the latter process is believed to predominate in the CNS. A third process, which may occur intermittently at individual presynaptic terminals, is "kiss and run" exocytosis during which vesicles never completely fuse with the plasma membrane; in this model transmitter leaks out through a pore that opens between the lumen of the vesicle and the extracellular space.

The entire exocytotic cycle lasts approximately 30 to 60 seconds. Exocytosis occurs within 1 ms and endocytosis occurs within 5 seconds; the other steps of the cycle occupy the remaining time. The speed of exocytosis, which is truly breathtaking, is required for the overall efficiency of information processing in the nervous system.

Proteins Involved in the Exocytotic Cycle

Until the 1990s, the mechanisms underlying vesicle release and recycling remained obscure, partly because the proteins involved in these processes were not known. During the past 15 years many of these proteins have been identified. Thus, the component of synaptic transmission that was for decades represented by a black box, namely the triggering of exocytosis by Ca²⁺ entry, is gradually being replaced by a series of precisely defined molecular events.

The Function of SNARES: Vesicle Docking or Fusion?

The morphologic differences between vesicles docked at the active zone of a nerve terminal and those that are undocked suggest that neurons contain mechanisms for segregating these pools and for targeting vesicles to the active zone. Initial experiments suggested that a group of proteins known as SNAREs might be involved in this process. SNAREs include three synaptic proteins that were first isolated biochemically and have since become integral to our understanding of vesicle fusion and transmitter release: synaptobrevin, also known as vesicle-associated membrane protein (VAMP); syntaxin; and synaptosomal-associated protein of 25 kDa (SNAP-25), each of which have several isoforms. Synaptobrevins are 18 kDa and span the vesicle membrane, with one transmembrane domain near the C terminus. Syntaxins are 35 kDa and are also integral membrane proteins. In contrast, SNAP-25 is anchored to the membrane by lipid groups (long-chain fatty acids) attached to central cysteine residues. At the active zone, syntaxin and SNAP-25 localize in the plasma membrane and are known as t-SNAREs (*t* for target membranes). In contrast, synaptobrevin is localized primarily in the vesicular membrane and thus has been labeled a v-SNARE, or vesicle SNARE.

Three important findings led to the hypothesis that these proteins are involved in exocytosis at the presynaptic terminal. First, several **bacterial toxins** known to cause neurologic symptoms were proven to inhibit exocytosis and to cleave specific SNARE proteins `3-2`. Likewise, the **black widow spider toxin** (α-latrotoxin) affects transmitter release by acting on proteins in the presynaptic nerve terminal. Second, mutation of yeast homologs of the SNAREs causes defects in membrane trafficking. These two lines of investigation implicated the SNAREs in synaptic transmission, but did not address the mechanism through which they might promote exocytosis. The third finding, which emerged from in vitro biochemical studies, was that syntaxin, synaptobrevin, and SNAP-25 spontaneously form a thermodynamically stable 1:1:1 complex. Because syntaxin and SNAP-25 are located primarily in the plasma membrane, and synaptobrevin is located primarily in the vesicle membrane, it was proposed that the association of these proteins might serve to target synaptic vesicles to the plasma membrane during the docking step of the exocytotic cycle. This postulate, known as the SNARE hypothesis, has been influential in the study of membrane trafficking in general as well as the molecular mechanisms underlying synaptic transmission.

Subsequent evidence has indicated that SNAREs play a direct role in membrane fusion, with other molecules facilitating docking. Genetic deletion of syntaxin in *Drosophila* decreases exocytosis, but does not decrease the number of docked vesicles in nerve terminals. Similarly, the injection of **tetanus toxin** (see `3-2`) or

fragments of SNARE proteins into the presynaptic terminal of the giant axon of the squid lead to an increased number of docked vesicles. A decrease in the number of docked vesicles would be expected if the SNAREs were required for docking. These findings therefore suggest that the SNAREs may function predominantly at a later step in the exocytotic cycle, namely, fusion.

This hypothesis is supported by several lines of evidence. SNAREs that have been reconstituted into lipid vesicles have been assayed for vesicle fusion with the use of fluorescent dyes. Vesicles containing equimolar amounts of syntaxin and SNAP-25 fused with vesicles containing synaptobrevin, indicating that v-SNAREs and t-SNAREs alone can generate fusion between lipid bilayers. The mechanism for fusion has been suggested by in vitro experiments in which SNAREs bind to each other in parallel with the C terminus of each SNARE similarly oriented. Thus, like viral hairpin proteins, which mediate the entry of viruses into cells, the SNAREs (or SNAREpins) may change their conformation or binding properties to allow fusion between opposing bilayers `3-7` and `3-8`. The favorable thermodynamics of SNARE complex formation may drive the fusion of two such bilayers over the energy barrier that normally prevents the intermingling of bilayers.

Disassembly of the SNAREs by NSF

Because association of the SNAREs appears to drive fusion of the vesicle membrane with the plasma membrane, dissociation of the SNAREs must occur before the vesicle can be reclaimed from the plasma membrane to embark on a new exocytotic cycle. *N*-ethylmaleimide sensitive factor (NSF) and the soluble NSF attachment proteins (SNAPs) may perform this function (see `3-7`). [1] NSF is a soluble tetramer composed of 76-kDa subunits and requires SNAPs to bind to vesicle membranes and participate in exocytosis. A key finding in the search for the molecular composition of the exocytotic apparatus was the discovery that both NSF and the SNAPs also bind with high affinity to the SNAREs, including syntaxin, synaptobrevin, and SNAP-25. Remarkably, the aggregate composed of these proteins can be dissociated into its component proteins by the addition of ATP. This occurs because NSF is an ATPase; by hydrolyzing ATP, NSF generates the energy to dissociate the thermodynamically stable complex of NSF, SNAPs, and SNARES.

---

[1]Note that SNAPs (soluble NSF attachment proteins) are not related to SNAP-25 (synaptosomal-associated protein of 25 kDa). The name SNARE comes from "SNAP receptors" because SNAREs were found to bind SNAPs.

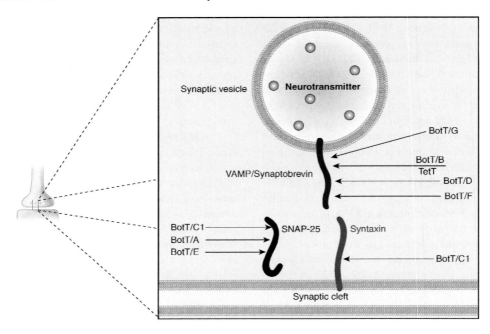

Botulism and tetanus are neurologic disorders caused by toxins from pathogenic bacteria. **Botulism,** which occurs after the ingestion of contaminated food, is caused by *Clostridium botulinum.* This strain secretes an armamentarium of seven potent neurotoxins (A, B, C1, D, E, F, and G), each of which affects exocytosis by cleaving several specific synaptic vesicle proteins, including synaptobrevin, syntaxin, and SNAP-25 (see figure and table). The toxins thereby induce an asymmetric descending paralysis due to inactivation of cranial and peripheral nerves. Because of its ability to cause paralysis in muscle, localized injections of **botulinum toxin,** colloquially known as "**Botox,**" are used therapeutically to treat **blepharospasm,** spasms of the muscle surrounding the tear duct, and **dystonia,** abnormal skeletal muscle tone, as well as for cosmetic purposes.

Tetanus is caused when *Clostridium tetanus* contaminates a wound. Tetanus toxin is also a protease that targets synaptic vesicle proteins (eg, synaptobrevin) and inhibits exocytosis. The result is a poisoning of both motor neurons and inhibitory neurons, which causes increased muscle tone and spasms; it often strikes the masseter muscles first, resulting in **lockjaw.**

Black widow spider venom contains α-**latrotoxin,** a 130-kD protein that induces a profound paralysis by causing a massive release and subsequent depletion of acetylcholine at the neuromuscular junction. The targets of α-latrotoxin are shown in the table.

Each of these toxins functions as a protease that breaks apart its specific protein target and thereby prevents its normal functioning. The discovery of targets for these toxins was a major breakthrough in our understanding of the molecular basis of exocytosis because it led to the identification of several proteins that play key roles in this process.

Toxin	Neural Target[1]
Botulinum neurotoxin	
A	SNAP-25
B	Synaptobrevin
C1	Syntaxin, SNAP-25
D	Synaptobrevin
E	SNAP-25
F	Synaptobrevin
G	Synaptobrevin
Tetanus toxin	Synaptobrevin
α-Latrotoxin	Neurexin1; CIRL/latrophilin

[1]Some clostridial toxins also cleave a non-neuronal form of synaptobrevin known as cellubrevin.

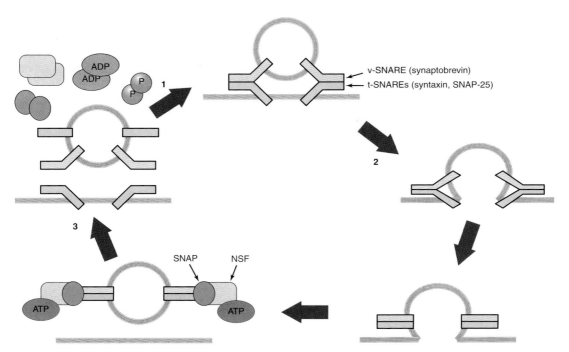

3-7 **Model of the cycle whereby SNAREs induce membrane fusion and NSF dissociates the SNARE complex to initiate another round of fusion.** This cycle includes the following steps: **1.** SNAREs form a stable complex. v- and t-SNAREs engage partners on opposite membranes in a parallel fashion with respect to their membrane anchors. **2.** SNAREs induce fusion. This fusion of the vesicle with the plasma membrane may be homologous to membrane fusion by viral hairpin proteins that assist the entry of viruses into cells. **3.** NSF dissociates the SNARE complex. After binding to the SNAREs with the aid of a SNAP, NSF dissociates the complex with energy derived from adenosine triphosphate (ATP) hydrolysis into adenosine diphosphate (ADP) and free phosphate (P).

Disassembly is likely to occur when SNAREs occupy the same membrane. Indeed, t-SNAREs and v-SNAREs have been found to coexist on synaptic vesicle membranes. These observations suggest the following model: SNAREs induce fusion between a vesicle membrane and a plasma membrane by fastening together in parallel; to allow another round of exocytosis, NSF uses energy obtained from ATP hydrolysis to unzip the stable SNAREs **3-7** and **3-8**.

Synaptotagmin: The Ca^{2+} Sensor for Transmitter Release

Unlike most membrane trafficking events, which appear to proceed constitutively, neurotransmitter release is triggered by Ca^{2+}. Thus, an important goal in the study of synaptic transmission has been to identify the mechanism by which exocytotic machinery senses Ca^{2+} influx. Several lines of evidence suggest that the 65-kDa protein synaptotagmin is a primary mediator of this process. Investigators first proposed this

possibility after the elucidation of synaptotagmin's primary structure revealed so-called C2 domains similar to those found in protein kinase C, a Ca^{2+} and phospholipid-dependent kinase (Chapter 4). Synaptotagmin contains two C2 domains, C2A and C2B **3-9**, each of which binds two Ca^{2+} atoms. Extensive NMR and crystallographic analyses reveal that these domains form a novel Ca^{2+}-binding motif composed primarily of β sheets. Such binding does not induce a conformational change but is believed to induce a significant shift in electrostatic potential, or charge, in the Ca^{2+} binding domain, which may function to regulate the interaction of synaptotagmin with other molecules involved in vesicle fusion.

Because there are many different forms of synaptotagmin, a variety of methods have been used to determine whether the predominant form, synaptotagmin I, is a Ca^{2+} sensor in vivo. Most convincingly, studies of synaptotagmin mutations in *Drosophila, C. elegans,* and mice have confirmed that synaptotagmin I plays an important role in exocytosis. Knockout and

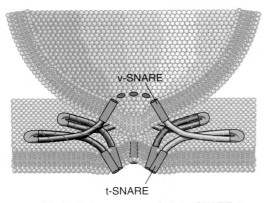

3-8 **Proposed topology of SNAREpins, including the v-SNARE synaptobrevin and the t-SNAREs syntaxin and SNAP-25.** Viral hairpin proteins are proposed to form similar structures to induce the fusion of apposing lipid membranes. (Reproduced with permission from Weber T, Zemelman BV, McNew JA, et al. SNAREpins: Minimal machinery for membrane fusion. *Cell* 1998;92:759.)

common variants being RIM1α and RIM2α) and *Munc-13s* as well as the extraordinarily large proteins *bassoon* and *piccolo*. While the exact functions of each of these proteins is not yet known, genetic deletion studies indicate that the activity-dependent regulation of transmitter release is impaired in their absence. Furthermore, individual presynaptic terminals express different complements of these active zone proteins and this likely contributes to significant differences in their functions.

Rab proteins are a large family of small GTP-binding proteins that are crucial in regulating many types of intracellular membrane transport (Chapter 4). Rab3a plays a particularly important role in regulating synaptic vesicle trafficking and exocytosis. It undergoes a cycle of association with and dissociation from synaptic vesicles in parallel with their exocytosis and endocytosis. It appears to function at a late stage in synaptic vesicle exocytosis after docking. Importantly, it directly interacts with RIM1α, and both Rab3a and RIM1α are required for the long-lasting, activity-dependent enhancement of transmitter release (termed presynaptic long-term potentiation, or LTP) that occurs at some

knockin mice have provided particularly useful information. In synaptotagmin I knockouts, fast Ca^{2+}-dependent transmitter release is strongly suppressed, while a second, slower phase of transmitter release, which is also Ca^{2+}-dependent, is not affected. This second phase of release may be mediated by other synaptotagmin isoforms. Furthermore, genetically modifying the affinity of synaptotagmin I for Ca^{2+} has an exactly parallel effect on the Ca^{2+} sensitivity of transmitter release. Other parameters of transmitter release remain unchanged in these mice, thus verifying that synaptotagmin I regulates only one step of the exocytotic cycle: fast Ca^{2+}-triggered fusion.

Additional Proteins Involved in Neurotransmitter Release

Thus far we have only mentioned a small number of the 100 or so proteins that are involved in neurotransmitter release and its regulation. The active zone, the site at which vesicles dock and fuse with the presynaptic plasma membrane, is a highly organized macromolecular complex containing so-called "scaffolding" proteins, which, via their multiple protein–protein interaction domains, are critical for the appropriate positioning of the proteins that are key components of the vesicle cycling and fusion machinery. These include families of proteins termed *RIMs* (the most

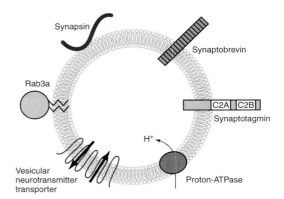

3-9 **Synaptic vesicle proteins.** Proteins involved in transmitter packaging and exocytosis include the proton-ATPase, which generates a proton gradient across the vesicle membrane, and vesicular transporters, which use the proton gradient to actively transport neurotransmitter into the lumen of vesicles. Synaptobrevin is involved in vesicle fusion and possibly targeting, and synaptotagmin functions as a Ca^{2+} sensor, binding Ca^{2+} ions with C2 domains encoded in the primary structure of the protein. The small G protein Rab3a, which is bound to vesicles by a lipid anchor, functions to regulate the exocytotic cycle. Synapsins associate peripherally with vesicles and may segregate them into storage pools.

presynaptic terminals following their repetitive activation. In addition to Rab3a, presynaptic terminals contain one or more of three other Rab3 isoforms termed Rab3b, c, and d, the exact functions of which are unknown.

Although we have emphasized the central function of the SNAREs, synaptobrevin, syntaxin, and SNAP-25, in mediating vesicle exocytosis, this process is highly regulated due to the participation of several additional proteins. Among the most important of these are *complexins*, which bind to SNARE complexes and prevent membrane fusion until they are displaced by synaptotagmin 1 in a Ca^{2+}-dependent manner to allow synaptic vesicle fusion. Another important protein is *Munc-18*, which binds to syntaxin and thereby regulates the SNARE-dependent fusion of synaptic vesicles.

The number of docked synaptic vesicles at individual presynaptic terminals is small, on the order of 3 to 10. Thus, during prolonged bursts of activity there are mechanisms in place to replenish these vesicles from another pool of vesicles called the "reserve" pool. *Synapsins* are a family of proteins that bind to synaptic vesicles and tether them to the presynaptic actin cytoskeleton. They are believed to be important for regulating the trafficking of vesicles between the "reserve" pool and the "readily releasable" pool of vesicles which are docked at the presynaptic plasma membrane. When phosphorylated by protein kinases such as protein kinase A, synapsins dissociate from synaptic vesicles, a biochemical change that contributes to short-term, activity-dependent change in neurotransmitter release.

Endocytosis and Recycling

Clathrin-mediated endocytosis After fusion and exocytosis, synaptic vesicle proteins are reclaimed from the plasma membrane through clathrin-mediated endocytosis **3–10**. Clathrin is composed of two highly conserved subunits that self-assemble into structures called triskelions, each of which consists of three light-chain and three heavy-chain subunits. It forms a proteinaceous coat that helps shape the membrane into a bud that is subsequently pulled away from the inner surface of the plasma membrane. Clathrin is linked to membranes through heteromeric adapter proteins (APs), each of which comprises a large central domain and two projecting ears. The two sides of the central domain and both ears are composed of α and β subunits; two smaller σ and μ subunits also bind to the central domain. At least four types of adapters are known to exist, and each localizes in a different subcellular organelle; the adapter at the plasma membrane is called AP-2. Each type of adapter protein may

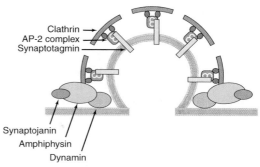

3–10 **The endocytotic machinery.** Clathrin-mediated endocytosis allows synaptic vesicles to be retrieved from the nerve terminal. Because the protein machinery required for this process is complex, only a few of the major components are shown in this figure. Clathrin and the heteromeric AP-2 adaptor complex form the coat around the budding vesicle, which may be linked to the vesicle membrane by synaptotagmin. Dynamin is a pinchase that pinches or severs the neck of the budding vesicle. Amphiphysin, which plays a central role in the coordination of endocytosis, binds to several proteins, including dynamin, AP-2, clathrin, and the phospholipid phosphatase synaptojanin. The locations of both synaptojanin and amphiphysin may differ from those in this figure, which primarily serves to show protein–protein interactions.

contain cell type–specific subunits. A neuron-specific subunit known as β3b, or β-NAP, was originally isolated as the antigen responsible for a so-called **paraneoplastic syndrome**, or **tumor-induced autoimmunity syndrome,** which results in cerebellar degeneration.

To ensure that other types of proteins are not mistakenly recruited into synaptic vesicles, adapters bind to highly specific proteins at the plasma membrane. The only synaptic vesicle protein known to bind AP-2 is synaptotagmin. Thus, this protein may play a dual role: it may serve as a Ca^{2+} sensor during exocytosis and as a tag during endocytosis. However, different isoforms of synaptotagmin may be involved in these processes.

After endocytosis, the clathrin coat is removed from the membrane to allow further trafficking and recycling to the existing pool of synaptic vesicles. The molecular chaperone heat shock protein 70c (*hsp70c*) likely is involved in disassembling clathrin, with the assistance of additional tissue-specific cofactors.

Endocytic machinery An important component of the biochemical machinery underlying endocytosis is the protein *dynamin*. This protein cycles between phosphorylated and dephosphorylated states during the exocytotic cycle. Biochemical assays have revealed that dynamin encodes a GTPase activity that was linked to endocytosis after the discovery of a mutation in the *Drosophila dynamin* gene known as *shibere*. Flies containing this mutation were isolated more than 25 years ago and display defects in cell signaling. Electron micrographs of the nerve terminals of mutant flies revealed hundreds of vesicles attached to each plasma membrane by short ring-coated necks. Discovery of the shibere phenotype suggested that these rings, which are oligomers of shibere protein, may function to pinch off the neck of a vesicle as it buds from the plasma membrane. Recent findings strongly suggest that dynamin is intimately involved in the endocytosis of synaptic vesicles and that GTP hydrolysis helps to drive this process. Thus, as originally suggested by the *shibere* mutant, dynamin, with the assistance of proteins that are located in the necks of budding vesicles, appears to function as a "pinchase" to sever or pinch off the necks of coated vesicles as they bud from the plasma membrane. Dynamin-mediated endocytosis has also been implicated in the down-regulation of G protein–coupled receptors in response to sustained receptor activation (Chapters 4 and 6).

Vesicle recycling   After endocytosis, synaptic vesicles are recycled. As mentioned previously, the biogenesis and recycling of synaptic vesicles may involve budding from both plasma membrane invaginations and endosomal compartments discrete from the plasma membrane. Although the contribution of each pathway to vesicle formation in neurons remains unclear, some of the molecular components of the endosomal pathway have been determined with the use of model neuroendocrine cells. Like endocytosis at the plasma membrane, the budding of synaptic vesicles from endosomes involves protein coats formed from heteromeric APs. However, endosomal budding employs a different AP protein (AP-3) and does not require clathrin. Interestingly, mutations in one of the large subunits of AP-3 (δ3) may disrupt vesicle trafficking in both mice and humans. The phenotypes of *mocha*, a δ3 mutation in mice, include an increase in baseline electrical activity in the brain and a unique hypersynchronized 6- to 7-Hz EEG pattern. In humans, a similar mutation results in a form of **Hermansky–Pudlak syndrome (HPS)**, which is notable for defects in storage granules. Moreover, tumor-related antibodies to a neuronally expressed β subunit of AP-3 (known as β3b or β-NAP) induce **cerebellar degeneration**. Such findings suggest that defects in secretory vesicle biogenesis

and its regulation may underlie other neuropsychiatric syndromes.

Complexity and Specialization

During the past two decades, many of the molecules responsible for the quantal release of neurotransmitter have been identified, and some of the protein–protein interactions underlying this complex process and its intricate regulation have been teased apart. Yet, this chapter presents a simplified view. Neurons express multiple isoforms of many of the proteins described here; for example, more than 10 isoforms of synaptotagmin have been isolated, and each may regulate a different aspect of synaptic transmission. Isoforms of other synaptic proteins exhibit striking cell type–specific distributions in the brain. Furthermore, almost all of the molecular understanding of the process of synaptic vesicle exocyotsis and endocytosis derives from the study of excitatory synapses that utilize the neurotransmitter glutamate. Whether the presynaptic release of the major inhibitory neurotransmitter GABA or modulatory transmitters such as monoamines involve identical molecular machinery remains to be determined.

Given that most if not all neuropsychiatric disorders can be conceptualized as being due to dysfunctions in synaptic transmission, elucidating the detailed molecular mechanisms underlying this fundamental signal transduction process is likely to reveal a great deal about the pathophysiology, and perhaps even the pathogenesis, of such brain disorders. Furthermore, it is anticipated that several proteins involved in neurotransmitter release or the termination of transmitter action will be important targets of therapeutic agents. Indeed, the many isoforms of these proteins should facilitate the design of drugs that act on specific neuronal cell types or synaptic processes.

SELECTED READING

Bazalakova MH, Blakely RD. The high-affinity choline transporter: a critical protein for sustaining cholinergic signaling as revealed in studies of genetically altered mice. *Handbook Exp Pharmacol*. 2006;175: 525–544.

Bellocchio EE, Reimer RJ, Fremeau RT, Edwards RH. Uptake of glutamate into synaptic vesicles by an inorganic phosphate transporter. *Science*. 2000;289:957–960.

Chaudhry FA, Boulland JL, Jenstad M, Bredahl MK, Edwards RH. Pharmacology of neurotransmitter transport into secretory vesicles. *Handbook Exp Pharmacol*. 2008;184:77–106.

Cowan WM, Sudhof TC, Stevens CF. *Synapses.* Baltimore: Johns Hopkins University Press; 2000.

Fernandez-Chacon R, Konigstorfer A, Gerber SH, et al. Synaptotagmin I functions as a calcium regulator of release probability. *Nature.* 2001;410:41–49.

Geppert M, Sudhof TC. RAB3 and synaptotagmin: The yin and yang of synaptic membrane fusion. *Annu Rev Neurosci.* 1998;21:75–95.

Greengard P. The neurobiology of slow synaptic transmission. *Science.* 2001;294:1024–1030.

Hilfiker S, Pieribone VA, Czernik AJ, et al. Synapsins as regulators of neurotransmitter release. *Phil Trans Royal Soc London Biol Sci.* 1999;354:269–279.

Jahn R, Scheller RH. SNARES—engines for membrane fusion. *Nature Rev Mol Cell Biol.* 2006;7:631–643.

Katz B. The *Release of Neural Transmitter Substances.* Liverpool: Liverpool University Press; 1969.

Kennedy MB. Signal processing machines at the postsynaptic density. *Science.* 2000;290:750–754.

Kuromi H, Kidokoro Y. Two distinct pools of synaptic vesicles in single presynaptic boutons in a temperature sensitive *Drosophila* mutant, shibere. *Neuron.* 1998;20:917–925.

Liu Y, Edwards RH. The role of vesicular transport proteins in synaptic transmission and neural degeneration. *Annu Rev Neurosci.* 1997;20:125–156.

Murthy VN, De Camilli P. Cell biology of the presynaptic terminal. *Annu Rev Neurosci.* 2003;26:701–728.

Neher E. Vesicle pools and Ca^{2+} microdomains: New tools for understanding their roles in neurotransmitter release. *Neuron.* 1998;20:389–399.

Rizo J, Sudhof TC. Snares and Munc18 in synaptic vesicle fusion. *Nature Rev Neurosci.* 2002;3: 641–653.

Scales SJ, Scheller RH. Lipid membranes shape up. *Nature.* 1999;401:123–124.

Seal RP, Amara SG. Excitatory amino acid transporters: A family in flux. *Annu Rev Pharmacol Toxicol.* 1999;39:431–456.

Slepnev VI, De Camilli P. Accessory factors in clathrin-dependent synaptic vesicle endocytosis. *Nature Rev Neurosci.* 2000;1:161–172.

Sollner T, Whiteheart SW, Brunner M, et al. SNAP receptors implicated in vesicle targeting and fusion. *Nature.* 1993;362:318–324.

Sudhof TC. The synaptic vesicle cycle. *Annu Rev Neurosci.* 2004;27:509–547.

Takamori S, Holt M, Stenius K, et al. Molecular anatomy of a trafficking organelle. *Cell.* 2006;127: 831–846.

Takamori S, Rhee JS, Rosenmund C, Jahn R. Identification of a vesicular glutamate transporter that defines a glutamatergic phenotype in neurons. *Nature.* 2000;407:189–194.

Tang J, Maximov A, Shin OH, Dai H, Rizo J, Sudhof TC. A complexin/synaptotagmin 1 switch controls fast synaptic vesicle exocytosis. *Cell.* 2006;126:1175–1187.

Weber T, Zemelman BV, McNew JA, et al. SNAREpins: Minimal machinery for membrane fusion. *Cell.* 1998;92:759–772.

CHAPTER 4

Signal Transduction in the Brain

KEY CONCEPTS

- Signal transduction refers to the processes by which signals between cells carried by neurotransmitters, hormones, trophic factors, and cytokines are converted into biochemical signals within cells.

- Neurotransmitter receptors can be divided into two classes by their signal transduction mechanism—one class involving activation of an ion channel that is intrinsic to the receptor and the other involving activation of G proteins.

- Signal transduction can alter neuronal function on vastly different time scales ranging from very rapid (millisecond) changes in membrane potential produced by ligand-gated channels to changes over seconds produced by intracellular second messengers and protein kinases.

- Many critical drugs that act on the nervous system are agonists or antagonists at G protein-coupled receptors.

- Although second messengers such as cyclic nucleotides and Ca^{2+} may directly gate ion channels, their major role in intracellular signaling systems is to regulate protein kinases that phosphorylate other proteins.

- The brain contains four major serine-threonine protein phosphatases, which reverse the actions of second messenger-dependent protein kinases.

- Neurotrophins, such as nerve growth factor and brain-derived neurotrophic factor, interact with a family of receptors-receptor tyrosine kinases (Trks).

- Certain cytokines, act on receptors that activate tyrosine kinases called Janus kinases, which in turn activate a family of transcription factors called signal transducers and activators of transcription (STATs).

- Many intracellular signaling pathways ultimately regulate gene expression.

- Transcription is stimulated when an activator protein displaces nucleosomes, the major component of chromatin, permitting a complex of proteins, called general transcription factors, to bind DNA at a core promoter and recruit RNA polymerase.

- DNA binding sites for regulatory proteins are called regulatory elements, and the proteins that bind them are called transcription factors.

- Each gene has a unique pattern of cellular expression and response to physiologic signals based on the combinatorial interaction of regulatory elements found within its regulatory region.

- Eukaryotic cells increase the diversity of proteins that can be produced from a single gene by alternatively splicing the exons within the primary transcript.

- Mature (spliced) messenger RNAs are transported from the nucleus into the cytoplasm, where they are translated to proteins on organelles called ribosomes.

- During and after translation, proteins are processed by cleavage into smaller proteins and by a variety of covalent modifications such as glycosylation.

Signal transduction refers to the processes by which intercellular signals such as neurotransmitters, neurotrophic factors, circulating hormones, and cytokines produce intracellular biochemical alterations that in turn modify neuronal functioning including the regulation of gene expression. Intercellular signals and their receptors, generally located in the neuronal plasma membrane, represent only a small amount of all information processing in the brain. An understanding of the complex biochemical mechanisms that operate inside neurons and ultimately mediate the actions of all intercellular signals is required to appreciate not only the ways in which the brain responds to drugs and other stimuli but also the ways in which it continuously adapts to a host of environmental changes.

OVERVIEW OF SIGNAL TRANSDUCTION PATHWAYS

Four general patterns of signal transduction occur in the brain **4-1** . One pattern **4-1A** , discussed briefly in Chapter 3, involves the binding of neurotransmitter to a multimeric plasma membrane receptor complex that contains a ligand-gated ion channel. Protein–protein interactions tether such ion channels, or receptor ionophores, at proper subcellular locations and often to other signaling proteins. This mechanism of signal transduction is used primarily by the amino acid neurotransmitters at their ionotropic receptors (Chapter 5) as well as by acetylcholine at nicotinic receptors (Chapter 6), serotonin at $5HT_3$ receptors (Chapter 6), adenosine triphosphate (ATP) at certain purinergic receptors (Chapter 8), and heat at certain vanilloid receptors (Chapter 11). The structural features of ligand-gated ion channels are discussed in detail in the chapters devoted to these transmitters.

A second pattern, also briefly described in Chapter 3, is characterized by the binding of neurotransmitters to plasma membrane receptors that couple with guanine nucleotide–binding proteins or G proteins **4-1B** . Most neurotransmitters bind to this superfamily of G protein–coupled receptors, as do several cytokines. All such receptors have a seven-transmembrane domain structure, whose N terminus faces the extracellular space and whose C terminus faces the cytoplasm; other structural features of these receptors are discussed in detail in Chapter 6, wherein the β-adrenergic receptor is presented as a prototype. The binding of ligands to these receptors initiates a range of biologic effects on target neurons, which include direct G protein regulation of certain ion channels (see **4-1B** , *left*) and the triggering of complex cascades of

intracellular messengers. Activation of intracellular messenger pathways leads to the generation of second messengers and the regulation of protein phosphorylation, and ultimately to diverse physiologic responses to extracellular stimuli **4-2** , including regulation of ion channels (see **4-1B** , *right*). As will be become evident, protein phosphorylation is the major molecular currency of intracellular signal transduction pathways. Protein phosphorylation describes a process by which protein kinases add phosphate groups to specific target proteins, and protein phosphatases remove these phosphate groups. Phosphate groups, because of their large size and negative charge, alter the conformation and overall charge of a protein and hence its function.

A third pattern of signal transduction involves the direct activation of a class of protein kinases, called protein tyrosine kinases, which phosphorylate proteins on tyrosine residues **4-1C** . This type of signaling is used by most types of neurotrophic factors and cytokines. In some cases the neurotrophic factor receptor and the protein tyrosine kinase reside in a single protein; in other cases the receptor must recruit cytoplasmic protein tyrosine kinases to effect their signaling. Activation of the protein tyrosine kinase triggers cascades of further protein phosphorylation that ultimately lead to the many effects of neurotrophic factors on brain function, including the regulation of ion channels.

A fourth pattern characterizes transduction by all known steroid hormones and certain other lipophilic extracellular signals that cross the plasma membrane and activate receptors in the neuronal cytoplasm **4-1D** . Upon binding their ligand, these cytoplasmic receptors translocate to the nucleus, where they bind DNA and function as transcription factors. Thus these receptors can be considered ligand-activated transcription factors.

G PROTEINS AND SECOND MESSENGERS

G Proteins

G proteins perform a central function in the process of transmembrane signaling in the nervous system. These proteins were named because of their ability to bind the guanine nucleotides, guanosine triphosphate (GTP) and guanosine diphosphate (GDP). G proteins couple receptors to specific intracellular effector systems (see **4-1**). Three major types of G protein are involved in the transduction of signals produced by neurotransmitter binding: Gs, $G_{i/o}$, and G_q **4-1** . Other subtypes serve more specialized funcions in

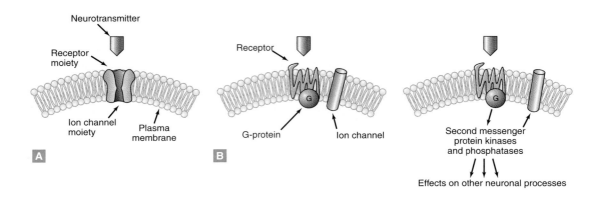

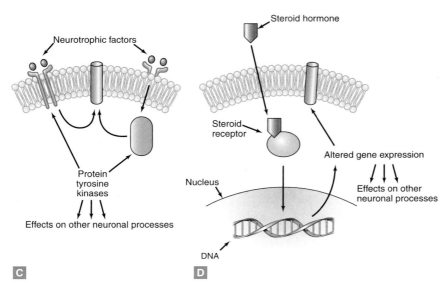

4-1 **General patterns of signal transduction in the brain. A.** Neurotransmitter activation of a receptor that contains an ion channel. **B.** Neurotransmitter activation of a G protein–coupled receptor. After it is activated, the G protein can directly regulate an ion channel (*left*), or trigger the regulation of second messenger–dependent protein kinases and protein phosphatases, which can in turn regulate other ion channels and many neuronal processes (*right*). **C.** Neurotrophic factor activation of a receptor that contains protein tyrosine kinase activity or that activates such a kinase indirectly. **D.** Steroid hormone activation of a cytoplasmic receptor. After the receptor is bound by hormone, it translocates to the nucleus and regulates gene expression.

discrete cell types. Each type of G protein is a heterotrimer composed of single α, β, and γ subunits. Individual α_s, α_i, α_q, etc. subunits are primarily responsible for the unique functions of the G proteins that contain them **4-1**. Additionally, several types of β and γ subunits complex with one another and differentially associate with subtypes of α subunits to confer still greater degrees of specificity on intracellular signaling proteins. The functional cycle of G proteins is

shown schematically in **4-3**. All eukaryotic cells also contain a distinct class of monomeric guanine nucleotide–binding proteins that subserve several critical roles in the regulation of cell function; these are termed *small-molecular-weight G proteins* and are described in **4-1**.

Several bacterial toxins produce their pathogenic effects by regulating the activity of specific G proteins through a process termed *ADP-ribosylation* (see **4-1**).

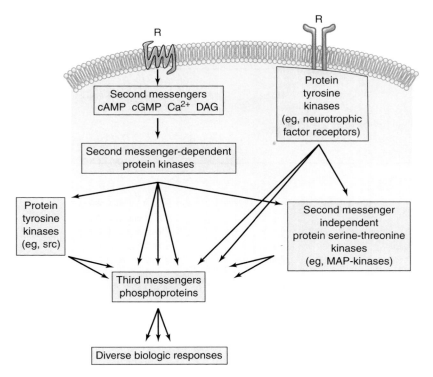

4-2 **Signal transduction pathways in neurons**. Extracellular signals, or first messengers, produce biologic responses in target neurons through a series of intracellular signals. Many activate second messenger pathways resulting in the phosphorylation of diverse types of proteins that can be considered third messengers, which mediate the biologic responses of the first messengers. First messengers also produce biologic responses through the activation of protein tyrosine kinases, some of which are physically linked to plasma membrane receptors (R), whereas others are cytoplasmic.

This process involves the addition of an ADP-ribose group from nicotinamide adenine dinucleotide (NAD) to an amino acid residue in the G protein. **Cholera toxin** ADP-ribosylates and irreversibly activates $G_{\alpha s}$ by inhibiting its GTPase activity, whereas **pertussis toxin** ADP-ribosylates and inactivates $G_{\alpha i}$ and $G_{\alpha o}$ by stabilizing their association with $\beta\gamma$ subunits. **Diphtheria toxin** ADP-ribosylates and inactivates a small G protein, known as eukaryotic elongation factor 2, which regulates ribosomal function (see **4-1**). G proteins also are the targets of certain insect venoms. The best characterized is **mastoparan,** a 10 amino acid–long peptide contained in wasp venom. The peptide stimulates the GTPase activity of $G_{\alpha i}$ subunits, thereby shortening the duration of the GTP-bound activated subunits.

G protein function can be regulated by several modulatory proteins. A neurotransmitter receptor may be seen as one type of modulatory protein, specifically a guanine nucleotide exchange factor, because it triggers the release of GDP from the α subunit. *Regulators of G protein signaling* (RGS proteins) activate the GTPase activity intrinsic to the α subunits of G proteins; thus, these proteins inhibit G protein function by shortening the duration of the signals from both the activated GTP-α subunit and the free $\beta\gamma$ subunits. All G protein α subunits, except for $G_{\alpha s}$, are known to be regulated in this manner. More than 20 subtypes of RGS proteins, each with a characteristic expression pattern in the brain, have been identified. Phosducin is another modulatory protein that binds to $\beta\gamma$ subunits and thereby competes with these subunits for binding to α subunits and possibly to effector proteins.

G Protein Regulation of Ion Channels

Many types of neurotransmitter receptors regulate ion channels by means of G proteins. The process by which this regulation occurs is best established for

4–1 Heterotrimeric G Protein α Subunits in Brain

Class	Molecular Mass (kDa)	Toxin-Mediated ADP-Ribosylation	Effector Protein(s)
G_s family			
$G_{\alpha s1}$	52	Cholera	Adenylyl cyclase (activation)
$G_{\alpha s2}$	52		
$G_{\alpha s3}$	45		
$G_{\alpha s4}$	45		
$G_{\alpha olf}$	45		
G_i family			
$G_{\alpha i1}$	41	Pertussis	Adenylyl cyclase (inhibition)
$G_{\alpha i2}$	40		?K$^+$ channel (activation)
$G_{\alpha i3}$	41		?Ca^{2+} channel (inhibition)
			?Phospholipase C (activation)
			?Phospholipase A$_2$
$G_{\alpha o1}$	39	Pertussis	?K$^+$ channel (activation)
$G_{\alpha o2}$	39		?Ca^{2+} channel (inhibition)
$G_{\alpha t1}$	39	Cholera and	Phosphodiesterase in rods and cones (activation)
$G_{\alpha t2}$	40	pertussis	
$G_{\alpha gust}$	41	Unknown	Phosphodiesterase in taste epithelium (activation)
$G_{\alpha z}$	41	None	?Adenylyl cyclase (inhibition)
G_q family	41–43		
$G_{\alpha q}$		None	Phospholipase C (activation)
$G_{\alpha 11}$			Unknown
$G_{\alpha 14}$			
$G_{\alpha 15}$			
$G_{\alpha 16}$			
G_{12} family	44	None	Unknown
$G_{\alpha 12}$			
$G_{\alpha 13}$			

neurotransmitter receptors that couple to $G_{\alpha i}$ or $G_{\alpha o}$. Via G protein coupling, these receptors activate inwardly rectifying K$^+$ channels (GIRKs) or inhibit voltage-gated Ca^{2+} channels, depending on the cell type involved. This regulation occurs primarily through the βγ subunits of G proteins, which directly open, or gate, GIRKs and limit the opening of Ca^{2+} channels in response to membrane depolarization.

Second Messengers

G proteins also transduce the activation of neurotransmitter receptors by neurotransmitter binding to altered intracellular levels of second messengers in target neurons. Prominent second messengers in the brain include cyclic adenosine monophosphate (cAMP), cyclic guanosine monophosphate (cGMP), Ca^{2+}, nitric oxide (NO), and the major metabolites of both phosphatidylinositol—inositol triphosphate (IP$_3$) and diacylglycerol (DAG)—and arachidonic acid, such as prostaglandins. Altered levels of second messengers mediate the effects of receptor activation on many types of ion channels and on numerous physiologic responses.

Cyclic nucleotides   cAMP and cGMP are classified as cyclic nucleotides because they are synthesized from ATP and GTP, respectively, through the formation of a cyclic phosphodiester ring **4–4**. Neurotransmitter receptors coupled via G_s stimulate cAMP levels via activation of *adenylyl cyclase*, the enzyme responsible for the synthesis of cAMP **4–5**. In contrast, receptors coupled via G_i inhibit adenylyl cyclase. Nine forms of adenylyl cyclase (types I–IX) have been identified, each of which exhibits a distinctive pattern of expression in brain and peripheral tissues **4–6**. All but type IX are activated by the natural plant molecule, **forskolin**.

Neurotransmitters regulate cGMP levels by means of two mechanisms. A very small number of plasma

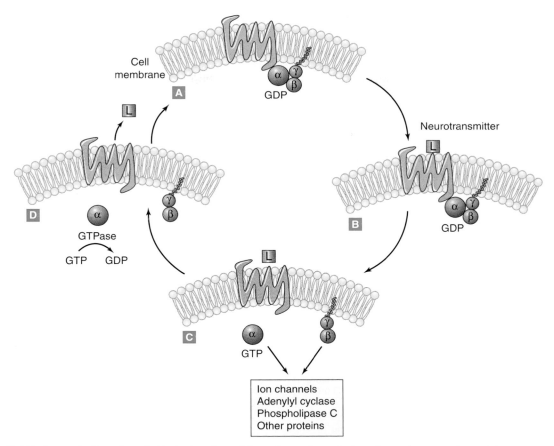

4–3 **G protein function.** **A.** Under basal conditions, G proteins exist in cell membranes as heterotrimers composed of single α, β, and γ subunits. The α subunits are bound to GDP, and the G protein heterotrimer is anchored to the plasma membrane by an isoprenyl (acyl) group attached to C-terminal cysteine residues of the γ subunit. **B.** After the receptor (R) is activated by its ligand (eg, neurotransmitter), it physically associates with the α subunit, causing the latter to release GDP. Subsequently, GTP (present in the cell at higher concentrations than GDP) binds to the α subunit. **C.** GTP binding causes the dissociation of the α subunit from its βγ subunits and from the receptor. Free α subunits, bound to GTP, are functionally active and directly regulate a number of effector proteins, such as ion channels, adenylyl cyclase, and phospholipase C. Free βγ subunits are also biologically active and directly regulate some of the same effector proteins. **D.** GTPase activity intrinsic to the α subunit degrades GTP to form GDP, and in turn causes the reassociation of the α and βγ subunits. This reassociation, in conjunction with the dissociation of the ligand from the receptor, restores the basal state.

membrane receptors, such as atrial natriuretic peptide receptors, contain *guanylyl cyclase* that is activated when a ligand binds to the receptor. In most cases, however, guanylyl cyclase is a cytosolic enzyme that is activated by NO (see **4–5**). NO, in turn, is generated via nitric oxide synthase (NOS), which is activated by Ca^{2+} in conjunction with the Ca^{2+}-binding protein calmodulin. Accordingly, neurotransmitters that increase intracellular Ca^{2+} levels typically increase cGMP levels by generating nitric oxide. **Organic nitrates** that are used as vasodilators in the treatment of ischemic heart disease

work by generating free NO in vascular smooth muscle, which increases cellular cGMP levels and in turn leads to muscle relaxation. Because NO is a soluble gas, it can diffuse out of the neuron in which it is synthesized and stimulate guanylyl cyclase in neighboring cells, thereby increasing cGMP levels. Thus, NO functions as both an intercellular and intracellular messenger in the brain. The potential utility of **NOS inhibitors** in the treatment of stroke is described in Chapter 19.

cAMP and cGMP are enzymatically degraded by *phosphodiesterases* (PDEs), which are expressed in

A large superfamily of small G proteins, so named because of their low molecular mass (20–35 kDa), serve critical functions in the cell. Like the α subunits of heterotrimeric G proteins, small G proteins bind guanine nucleotides, possess intrinsic GTPase activity, and cycle through GDP-bound and GTP-bound forms **4-3**. All classes of G protein undergo a change in their affinity for target molecules as they shift from GDP- to GTP-bound forms, most likely because such a shift causes them to undergo a large conformational change. This enables small G proteins to function as molecular switches that control several cellular processes (see table).

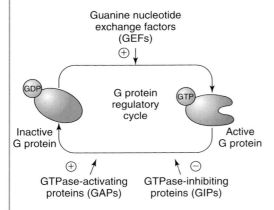

Among the best characterized small G proteins are those that comprise the Ras family, a series of related proteins of approximately 21 kDa. Their activity is highly regulated by a variety of associated proteins (see figure). Guanine nucleotide exchange factors (GEFs) increase the activity of Ras proteins by stimulating the release of GDP from their inactive forms and facilitating their binding to GTP. In contrast, GTPase-activating proteins (GAPs) bind to Ras proteins, thereby stimulating their intrinsic GTPase activity and reducing their functional activity. A mutation in one type of GAP results in **neurofibromatosis**, a disease characterized by the uncontrolled growth of glial cells that express myelin. Conversely, GTPase inhibitory proteins (GIPs) bind to Ras proteins and inhibit their GTPase activity.

Ras proteins and heterotrimeric G proteins interact with their related proteins in strikingly analogous ways. For example, G protein–coupled receptors provide essentially the same function for heterotrimeric G proteins that GEFs perform for Ras proteins. Likewise, GTPase-activating and GTPase-inhibiting proteins modify Ras proteins in much the same way that RGS proteins and βγ subunits regulate heterotrimeric G proteins. However, there are important differences as well. Because Ras proteins are characterized by far less intrinsic GTPase activity than heterotrimeric G protein α subunits, GAPs exert a more profound effect on the functioning of the Ras system and are essentially responsible for turning it on and off.

Numerous types of cell signals, including most neurotrophic factors, converge on Ras and related proteins to regulate MAP-kinase pathways, which in turn produce diverse effects on cell function. The mechanisms involved in these cascades are presented in greater detail in the text.

Rab proteins, which are involved in membrane vesicle trafficking, represent another small G protein family. Rab subtypes, particularly Rab3, have been implicated in the regulation of exocytosis and neurotransmitter release at nerve terminals (Chapter 3). ARF is a small G protein involved in functioning of the Golgi apparatus. It appears to control the binding of a protein coat to budding vesicles, including synaptic vesicles that mediate neurotransmitter release at the synapse.

Examples of Small G Proteins

Class	Proposed Cellular Function
Ras	Signal transduction (control of growth factor and MAP-kinase pathways)
Rac, Cdc42	Signal transduction (control of cellular stress responses and MAP-kinase pathways)
Rab	Vesicle trafficking and exocytosis in synaptic vesicles
Rho	Assembly of cytoskeletal structures (e.g., actin microfilaments)
ARF	Assembly and function of Golgi complex ADP-ribosylation of $G_{\alpha s}$
EF-2	Regulation of protein synthesis at ribosomes
Ran	Nuclear-cytoplasmic trafficking of RNA and protein

CdC42, cell division cycle 42; ARF, ADP-ribosylation factor; EF-2, eukaryotic elongation factor 2.

4-4 **Cyclic AMP (cAMP) synthesis and degradation.** The metabolism of cGMP is analogous to that shown for cAMP: guanylyl cyclase catalyzes the synthesis of cGMP from GTP, and phosphodiesterase hydrolyzes cGMP into 5'-GMP.

numerous forms in brain and other tissues. As outlined in **4-2**, these enzymes differ in their relative selectivity for cAMP and cGMP and in their regulation by other cellular signals, such as by the cyclic nucleotides themselves or by Ca^{2+}/calmodulin. At high concentrations, **caffeine** and related methylxanthines inhibit phosphodiesterase activity, which may contribute to some of the pharmacologic effects of these drugs, particularly at higher doses.

Nonselective PDE inhibitors, which affect many forms of the enzyme, are associated with pervasive side effects, but progress has been made in the development of selective PDE inhibitors. **Sildenafil** (Viagra) and related drugs, specific inhibitors of PDE type V,

are prescribed for the treatment of **erectile dysfunction.** PDE type V is concentrated in vascular smooth muscle and especially, but not exclusively, in the vasculature of the penis. Considerable effort also has been made toward developing PDE inhibitors that are selective for isoforms of the enzyme expressed predominantly in the brain. **Rolipram,** for instance, inhibits all isoforms of PDE type IV; this drug initially showed promise as an **antidepressant,** but its clinical utility was limited by side effects such as nausea. However, because the type IV enzyme comprises many subtypes (see **4-2**), an inhibitor of one subtype may lead to the development of an effective antidepressant without rolipram's side effects.

Calcium The regulation of intracellular Ca^{2+} levels by neurotransmitter receptors occurs via two major mechanisms **4-7**. Neurotransmitter receptor activation can alter the flux of extracellular Ca^{2+} into neurons in several ways: (1) Ca^{2+} passes directly through certain subtypes of ligand-gated channels, such as activated nicotinic cholinergic and N-methyl-D-aspartate (NMDA) glutamate receptors (Chapters 5 and 6); (2) specific voltage-gated Ca^{2+} channels are inhibited by G_i, as previously outlined; (3) the depolarization of a neuron, which causes the activation of voltage-gated Ca^{2+} channels, leads to large increases in intracellular Ca^{2+} levels (Chapter 2); or (4) the activation of other second messenger systems may alter Ca^{2+} channel properties; for example, cAMP and neurotransmitters that act through cAMP can modulate voltage-gated Ca^{2+} channels by regulating their phosphorylation.

The second major mechanism by which neurotransmitters can increase intracellular levels of free Ca^{2+} is through regulation of the phosphatidylinositol system and subsequent actions on intracellular Ca^{2+} stores (see **4-7**). Such regulation is possible because many types of neurotransmitter receptors are coupled through G proteins to an enzyme termed *phospholipase C* (PLC). Receptor activation of is mediated most often by subtypes of G_q, whose $\beta\gamma$ subunits are primarily responsible for this regulation.

Phospholipase C and the phosphatidylinositol pathway Phospholipase C catalyzes the breakdown of phosphatidylinositol, which results in the generation of two lipid molecules that function as second messengers in the brain: IP_3 and DAG (**4-8** and **4-9**). The most important forms of PLC in the brain are designated β and γ **4-10**. The β form is predominantly responsible for mediating the effects of neurotransmitters that are coupled to G_q, and the γ form is

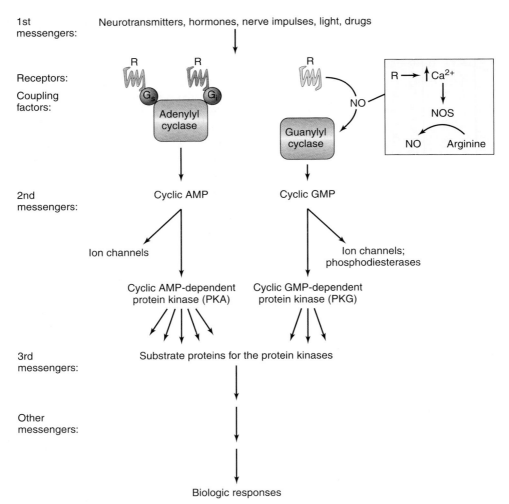

4-5 **Cyclic AMP (cAMP) and cyclic GMP (cGMP) second messenger systems.** Most extracellular messengers influence these systems through interactions with neurotransmitter receptors (R); others, including many drugs such as phosphodiesterase inhibitors that inhibit the breakdown of cAMP and cGMP, influence these second messenger systems directly. G proteins (G_s or $G_{i/o}$) are coupling factors that mediate the ability of neurotransmitter receptors to activate or inhibit adenylyl cyclase, the enzyme that catalyzes the synthesis of cAMP. Neurotransmitters typically increase cGMP levels by elevating cellular Ca^{2+} levels (see **4-7**). Increased Ca^{2+} levels trigger the activation of nitric oxide synthase (NOS), which converts arginine to nitric oxide (NO). NO subsequently activates guanylyl cyclase, which catalyzes the synthesis of cGMP. After they are synthesized, the second messengers activate cAMP-dependent protein kinase and cGMP-dependent protein kinase, respectively. PKA and PKG phosphorylate an array of substrate proteins (or third messengers), whose altered physiologic activity provokes biologic responses to extracellular messengers, either directly or indirectly (eg, through intervening fourth, fifth, or sixth messengers). Alternatively, cAMP and cGMP directly gate certain types of ion channels, and cGMP can directly activate phosphodiesterases, for example, in the retina.

predominantly responsible for mediating the effects of neurotrophic factors on this enzyme.

PLC action on phosphatidylinositol results in the generation of free inositol-1-phosphate which, through

a series of lipid phosphorylation events, is converted into active IP_3 or inositol-1,4,5-triphosphate **4-9**. IP_3 is subsequently recycled by means of successive dephosphorylation into inositol, which cells use to replenish

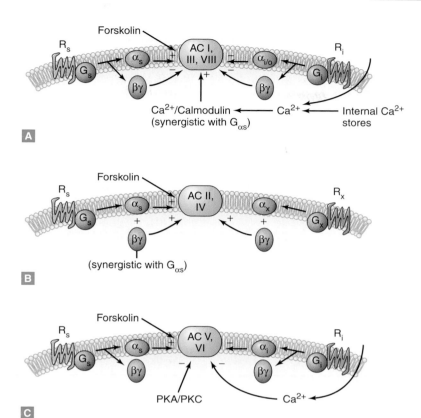

4-6 **Regulation of adenylyl cyclase (AC) activity.** Although most forms of the enzyme are activated by $G_{\alpha s}$ and forskolin, they vary in their regulation by Ca^{2+} and G protein $\beta\gamma$ subunits. **A.** Because adenylyl cyclase types I, III, and VIII are stimulated by Ca^{2+}/calmodulin, these enzymes typically are activated by an increase in cellular Ca^{2+} levels. $G_{\alpha s}$ interacts synergistically with Ca^{2+}/calmodulin and, in the presence of activated $G_{\alpha s}$, type I adenylyl cyclase is inhibited by $\beta\gamma$ subunits. $G_{\alpha i}$ has been proven to mediate neurotransmitter inhibition of these adenylyl cyclases. **B.** Adenylyl cyclase types II and IV are not sensitive to Ca^{2+}/calmodulin and, in the presence of activated $G_{\alpha s}$, are stimulated synergistically by $\beta\gamma$ complexes. The source of the $\beta\gamma$ complexes could be $G_{\alpha s}$ itself or any of several other types of G proteins (eg, G_i, G_o, G_q), depicted as G_x in the figure. **C.** Types V and VI are inhibited in response to phosphorylation by cAMP-dependent protein kinase (PKA) or protein kinase C (PKC). They are also inhibited by free Ca^{2+} and by $G_{\alpha i}$, but are not influenced by $\beta\gamma$ subunits.

phosphatidylinositol in their membranes. **Lithium,** which remains an important drug in the treatment of **mania** and other mood disorders, inhibits several of these inositol phosphatases although it is not known whether this action is related to the drug's clinical effects. IP_3 acts on an IP_3 receptor, which functions to release Ca^{2+} from intracellular organelles such as the endoplasmic reticulum. **Thapsigargan** inhibits this effect. Some organelles also contain a related **ryanodine** receptor, which triggers the release of Ca^{2+} from intracellular stores in response to a rise in Ca^{2+} itself. This process is inhibited by **rapamycin**. DAG, the other

metabolite of phosphatidylinositol, functions as a second messenger in cells by activating protein kinase C, as will be discussed below.

Arachidonic acid metabolites   The prostaglandin and leukotriene families of intracellular messengers play important roles in the regulation of signal transduction in the brain and elsewhere. Prostaglandins and leukotrienes are generated by a complex biochemical cascade, depicted in **4-11**, initiated by phospholipase A_2, which cleaves membrane phospholipids to yield free arachidonic acid. Next, arachidonic acid is

4-2   **Classification and Selected Properties of Cyclic Nucleotide Phosphodiesterases**

Family	Regulatory and Kinetic Characteristics	Genes Described	Selective Inhibitors[1]
I	Ca^{2+}/calmodulin-stimulated; regulated by Ca^{2+}/calmodulin and phosphorylation; have a low affinity for cAMP and cGMP except for PDE1C gene product, which has high affinity for cAMP	PDE1A (59-61 kDa) PDE1B (63 kDa) PDE1C (67 kDa, 75 kDa in brain)	Trifluoperazine Vinpocetine 8-methoxymethyl-3-isobutyl-1-methylxanthine
II	cGMP-stimulated; regulated by cGMP; have low affinity for cAMP and cGMP	PDE2 (105 kDa, soluble and particulate)	EHNA
III	cGMP-inhibited; regulated by phosphorylation and cGMP; high affinity, cGMP > cAMP	PDE3A PDE3B (110-135 kDa)	Milrinone Enoximone Amrinone[2]
IV	cAMP-specific; regulated by phosphorylation and cAMP; high affinity, cAMP >>> cGMP	PDE4A PDE4B PDE4C PDE4D (short and long forms of each)	Rolipram Ro20-1724
V	cGMP-binding; cGMP-specific	PDE5 (smooth muscle)	Sildenafil Vardenafil Tadalafil
VI	Retina cGMP specific; regulated by transducin; high affinity, cGMP >>> cAMP	PDE6A (α subtype) PDE6B (rod β subtype) PDE6C (cone β subtype)	—
VII	cAMP-specific; rolipram insensitive	PDE7A	—

[1]A number of compounds, particularly the methylxanthines (eg, theophylline, isobutylmethylxanthine, caffeine) also inhibit most major forms of PDE.
[2]These compounds represent a small portion of the known specific inhibitors of PDE III.
PDE, phosphodiesterase; EHNA, erythro-9-(2-hydroxy-3-nonyl) adenine

cleaved by *cyclooxygenase* to yield, after numerous enzymatic steps, several types of prostaglandins and other cyclic endoperoxides, such as prostacyclins and thromboxanes, or it is cleaved by *lipoxygenase* to yield the leukotrienes **4-11**.

The varied biologic activities of these endoperoxides and leukotrienes serve to regulate adenylyl cyclase, guanylyl cyclase, ion channels, protein kinases, and other cellular proteins, either directly or by serving as the endogenous ligands for G protein–coupled receptors.

Receptors for the leukotrienes are termed *BLT* or *LT receptors*, and those for prostaglandins and thromboxanes are termed *prostanoid receptors*. Several prostanoid receptors are known, and each is named for the arachidonic acid metabolite with the highest affinity for that receptor. EP receptors, for example, are activated preferentially by prostaglandin E_2 (PGE$_2$). All

LT receptors are coupled by G_q and presumably act by stimulating the PLC pathway. In contrast, the numerous subtypes of prostanoid receptors are coupled by either G_q, G_s, or G_i.

Aspirin, acetaminophen, and all nonsteroidal anti-inflammatory drugs (**NSAIDs**) such as **ibuprofen** exert their antipyretic, analgesic, and anti-inflammatory effects by inhibiting cyclooxygenase, which has both constitutive (COX$_1$) and inducible (COX$_2$) forms. COX$_1$ is expressed in many locations, including the upper gastrointestinal tract, where nonselective COX inhibitors block the protective functions of prostaglandins. Such interference increases the risk of peptic ulceration, a common side effect of these drugs. Selective COX$_2$ inhibitors, such as **rofecoxib,** that are analgesic and anti-inflammatory but with less disturbance of the gastrointestinal tract were in wide use until recent reports of cardiovascular toxicity (Chapter 11).

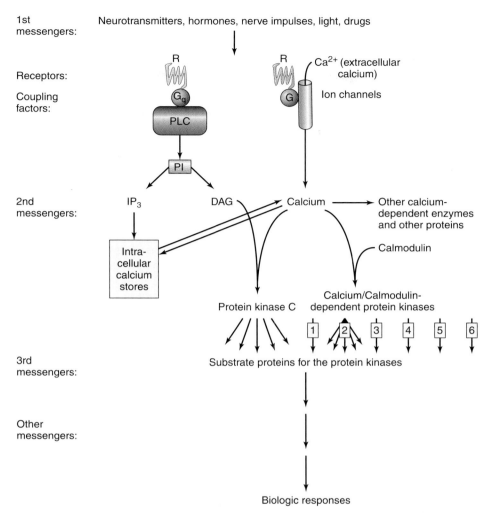

4-7 **Ca^{2+} and phosphatidylinositol second messenger systems**. Most extracellular messengers act on these systems, as they do on the cAMP and cGMP systems, through interactions with neurotransmitter receptors (R). However, some drugs, such as Ca^{2+} channel blockers and lithium, can influence these systems directly. G proteins (typically G$_q$) are coupling factors that mediate the ability of neurotransmitter receptors to regulate phospholipase C (PLC), which metabolizes phosphatidylinositol (PI) to form inositol triphosphate (IP$_3$) and diacylglycerol (DAG). IP$_3$ acts to increase intracellular levels of free Ca^{2+}, also a second messenger in the brain, by releasing Ca^{2+} from internal stores. Increased levels of intracellular Ca^{2+} also result from the flux of Ca^{2+} across the plasma membrane stimulated by nerve impulses and certain neurotransmitters. The brain contains two major classes of Ca^{2+}-dependent protein kinases. One is activated by Ca^{2+} in conjunction with the Ca^{2+}-binding protein calmodulin (CaM-kinase), and the other, protein kinase C, is activated by Ca^{2+} in conjunction with diacylglycerol and various phospholipids. Many of these kinases have broad substrate specificities (as indicated by the multiple arrows in the figure). Phosphorylation of substrate proteins, or third messengers, by these various Ca^{2+}-dependent protein kinases, alters their physiologic activity and either directly or indirectly triggers biologic responses to extracellular messengers.

4-8 The chemical structure of phosphatidylinositol and its generation of diacyglycerol and inositol 1,4,5-triphosphate (IP$_3$), a reaction catalyzed by phospholipase C.

PROTEIN PHOSPHORYLATION: A FINAL COMMON PATHWAY IN THE REGULATION OF NEURONAL FUNCTION

Most of the effects of intracellular second messengers are produced through their regulation of protein phosphorylation. Protein phosphorylation may inactivate a neurotransmitter receptor, cause an ion channel to open more or less readily, or enable the synthesis of a neurotransmitter much more rapidly. In addition, second messengers have a much smaller number of effects via their direct binding to specific effectors; for example, cAMP and cGMP bind to and directly gate ion channels in some neurons, Ca^{2+} binds to and directly regulates the activity of several enzymes, and cGMP binds to and directly activates phosphodiesterase in the retina.

Second Messenger–Dependent Protein Phosphorylation Cascades

Among the best characterized protein kinases in the brain are those activated by the second messengers cAMP, cGMP, Ca^{2+}, and diacylglycerol. All of these protein kinases, named for the second messengers that activate them, phosphorylate substrate proteins on serine or threonine residues, and thus are referred to as protein serine–threonine kinases.

The brain contains one major type of cAMP-dependent protein kinase (termed *protein kinase A* or *PKA*) and of cGMP-dependent protein kinase (termed *protein kinase G* or *PKG*). The structure and function of these enzymes are shown in **4-12**. Virtually all cellular actions of cAMP in eukaryotic cells, except for those related to cyclic nucleotide–gated channels (Chapter 2), are mediated by the activation of PKA (see **4-5**). PKA's integral role in these cellular processes stems from its ubiquitous expression and its ability to phosphorylate a wide array of substrate proteins, including many types of ion channels, receptors, cytoskeletal proteins, and nuclear transcription factors. It is believed that many of the cellular actions of cGMP are mediated by the activation of PKG (see **4-5**), however; less is known about the function of PKG, in part because it is not as widely expressed as PKA.

There are two major classes of Ca^{2+}-dependent protein kinases (see **4-7**). One class is activated by Ca^{2+} in conjunction with calmodulin and is referred to as Ca^{2+}/calmodulin-dependent protein kinase or *CaM-kinase*. The other is activated by Ca^{2+} in conjunction with diacylglycerol and other lipids and is referred to as *protein kinase C* (PKC). The **phorbol esters,** which activate all known PKC isoforms, have been a valuable tool in PKC research. The brain contains several forms of each of these enzymes, which exhibit very different regulatory properties and are expressed in distinct neuronal cell types throughout the nervous system. Examples of this diversity are shown in **4-3** and **4-4**, while some of the unique structural properties of PKC enzymes are depicted in **4-12**.

Certain CaM-kinases engage in complex modes of regulation. CaM-kinase II, for example, can autophosphorylate itself and in turn create a form

4-3 Ca^{2+}/Calmodulin-Dependent Protein Kinases

CaM-kinase I	Synapsin, others
CaM-kinase II	Many
CaM-kinase III	Eucaryotic elongation factor-2
CaM-kinase IV	CREB, others
Myosin light chain kinase	Myosin light chain
Phosphorylase kinase	Phosphorylase

4–4 **Protein Kinase C Family**

Subtype	Localization
Regulated by Ca^{2+} and DAG	
α	Ubiquitous
βI/βII	Occurs in many tissues; moderately concentrated in brain
γ	Highly concentrated in brain tissue
Ca^{2+}-independent; but regulated by DAG	
δ	Occurs in many tissues; may occur in brain
ε	May be highly concentrated in brain tissue
η	Unknown
θ	Unknown
Ca^{2+}- and DAG-independent, but enzymes are homologous to PKC	
ι	Unknown
ζ	Occurs in some tissues; moderately concentrated in brain
PRKs	Unknown

Note: Cloning studies have revealed an increasing number of PKC-homologous enzymes, with very different regulatory properties. Three classic forms of PKCs require Ca^{2+} and DAG for their activation. Several other forms are Ca^{2+}-independent, yet are activated by DAG; these forms are missing a portion of the C2 domain (see **4–12**). Some forms are not regulated by Ca^{2+} or DAG; these are missing portions of their C1 and C2 domains. PRKs, PKC-related kinases.

of the enzyme that remains active even after Ca^{2+} levels have returned to normal. Such a sustained period of kinase activation may represent a molecular mechanism that contributes to learning and memory (Chapter 13). In addition, CaM-kinases I and IV can be activated by a newly identified kinase known as CaM-kinase kinase, which in turn is activated by Ca^{2+}/calmodulin and inhibited by PKA phosphorylation.

Protein kinase-anchoring proteins An interesting regulatory feature of protein kinases has been uncovered in recent years: their localization in distinct subcellular regions in neurons is controlled by specific anchoring proteins. Such proteins are believed to sequester each type of kinase to the region of a neuron, such as the postsynaptic specialization or cell nucleus, that requires its function, and to bring the kinases in close approximation to some of their protein substrates. Examples include the A kinase–anchoring proteins (AKAPs) for PKA and receptors for activated C kinase (RACKs) for PKC.

Protein kinase inhibitors There has been intense interest in the development of protein kinase inhibitors for use as research tools and as potential therapeutic agents. The most specific of these are peptide inhibitors, which are directed at the active site of a particular enzyme. The prototype, a naturally occurring 17-kDa protein known as protein kinase inhibitor (PKI), is a highly specific inhibitor of PKA that is expressed in many tissues. Small molecule protein kinase inhibitors have been explored in the treatment of numerous diseases. Their development is furthest along for several cancers, and remains more hypothetical for neurodegenerative disorders, such as Alzheimer disease (Chapter 17). Examples of protein kinase inhibitors used experimentally in neuroscience research are listed in **4–5**.

4–5 **Examples of Protein Kinase Inhibitors**

Inhibitor	Target(s)[1]
Rp-cAMPS[2]	PKA
H7[3]	PKC, PKA, PKG, and others
H89[3]	PKA, PKG
Bisindolymaleimide I	PKC
Calphostin	PKC
R59949[4]	PKC
Chelerythrine	PKC
KN-62	CaM-Ks
Roscovitine	Cdk-5
Staurosporine	PKC, PTKs
Genistein	PTKs
Tyrphostins	PTKs
PP1	Src family PTKs

[1]Most of these inhibitors show relative specificity at the stated target but are not perfectly selective.

[2]Although this compound is an inhibitor of the type-I regulatory subunit, it is a partial agonist at the type-II subunit. The stereoisomer of the compound, Sp-cAMPS, is an activator of PKA.

[3]Examples of a large series of isoquinoline inhibitors that show varying specificity at different protein kinases.

[4]One of a series of DAG site inhibitors.

PKA, protein kinase A; PKG, protein kinase G; PKC, protein kinase C; CaM-K, Ca^{2+}/calmodulin-dependent protein kinase; Cdk-5, cyclin-dependent kinase type 5; PTK, protein tyrosine kinase; PP1, 4-amino-5-(4-methylphenyl)-7-(*t*-butyl) pyrazole[3,4-D]pyrimidine.

Protein phosphatases   The brain contains four major types of protein phosphatases that undo the actions of the second messenger–dependent protein kinases. These protein phosphatases, termed *protein serine–threonine phosphatases*, differ in their regional distribution in the brain and in their regulatory properties. These enzymes, which are summarized in ■ 4–6 ■, are termed *protein phosphatases 1, 2A, 2B, and 2C*. This terminology is based on the biochemical properties of these enzymes as they were first identified.

Neurotransmitters can regulate protein phosphatases, and in turn influence protein phosphorylation, by means of two known mechanisms. Phosphatase 2B, also referred to as calcineurin, is activated directly when it is bound to Ca^{2+}/calmodulin. Thus, neurotransmitters that alter cellular Ca^{2+} levels can influence the phosphorylation of cellular proteins by influencing calcineurin activity. Calcineurin activity is also regulated by immunophilins. This class of proteins, including cyclophilin and FKBP (FK506 binding protein), was originally discovered in lymphocytes and is the target of several important immunosuppressive agents, such as **cyclosporin** and **FK506.** Immunophilins are also expressed in the brain, although little is known about their physiologic

regulation of neuronal function. However, when they are bound to FK506 and related drugs, the immunophilins inhibit calcineurin activity.

The other mechanism of protein phosphatase regulation is indirect and involves a class of proteins referred to as *protein phosphatase inhibitors*, examples of which are listed in ■ 4–6 ■. Among these, the best known are *phosphatase inhibitors 1* and *2* and *dopamine- and cAMP-regulated phosphoprotein of 32 kDa* (DARPP-32). DARPP-32 is especially concentrated in neurons of the striatum, which receive dense dopaminergic innervation. These proteins are highly potent inhibitors of protein phosphatase 1, the predominant protein serine–threonine phosphatase in mammalian cells. Phosphorylation of most of these inhibitor proteins by PKA or by other protein kinases greatly enhances their inhibitory activity. In neurons that contain these inhibitors, neurotransmitters that alter cellular cAMP levels can influence the phosphorylation of cellular proteins by altering protein phosphatase 1 activity as well as by activating PKA. This process is illustrated in ■ 4–13 ■.

Studies of the physiologic functions of phosphatases have been facilitated by the identification of natural small molecules that are relatively specific phosphatase inhibitors. Among these, the best known is **okadaic acid,** which inhibits protein phosphatases 1 and 2A.

The anchoring of protein phosphatases to specific cellular domains by a series of regulatory subunits, which can be tissue-specific, represents another level of regulation. For example, a recently described protein, termed *spinophilin*, may function as a protein phosphatase 1–anchoring protein that selectively tethers the enzyme to dendritic spines. In contrast, the protein phosphatase 1 nuclear targeting subunit (PNUTS) may target the same phosphatase to the cell nucleus.

■ 4–6 ■   Protein Serine-Threonine Phosphatases

Class	Inhibitor Proteins
PP1	
$\alpha;\ \beta;\ \gamma1;\ \gamma2$	Inhibitor 1; inhibitor 2; DARPP-32; and NIPP-1
PP2A	Inhibitor 1^{2A}; inhibitor 2^{2A}
PP2B (calcineurin)	Immunophilins: cyclosporin A-cyclophilin FK506-FK506 binding protein
PP2C	
PP4	
PP5	
Dual-function phosphatases (VH1 family) MKP (MAP-kinase phosphatases) Cdc25	

PP1, protein phosphatase; DARPP-32, dopamine and cAMP-regulated phosphoprotein of 32 kDa; NIPP-1, nuclear inhibitor of PP1; VH, vaccinia virus; Cdc25, cell division cycle protein 25.

NEUROTROPHIC FACTOR-REGULATED PROTEIN PHOSPHORYLATION CASCADES

Significant progress has been made in the delineation of intracellular signal transduction pathways for neurotrophic factors, which are discussed in detail in Chapter 8. As mentioned previously, most of these pathways involve the activation of protein tyrosine kinases, which occurs by different mechanisms, depending on the neurotrophic factor involved. These pathways illustrate the extraordinary complexity of intracellular regulation, and keeping

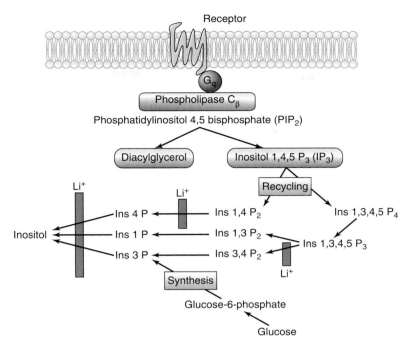

4-9 **The phosphatidylinositol cycle: actions of lithium.** Many neurotransmitter receptors are linked by G_q (or another G protein) to phospholipase Cβ, which hydrolyzes phosphatidylinositol-4, 5–bisphosphate (PIP_2) to generate two second messengers: diacylglycerol and inositol 1,4,5–triphosphate (IP_3). IP_3 acts to release Ca^{2+} from intracellular stores and subsequently is metabolized to forms that may not participate in neural signal transduction, including inositol 1,3,4,5-tetraphosphate (Ins 1,3,4,5 P_4). These forms are eventually metabolized to produce three inositol monophosphates, which differ only in terms of the carbon atom to which the phosphate group is linked. Synthesis of inositol from glucose-6-phosphate also must pass through an inositol monophosphate intermediate. All inositol monophosphates are metabolized by inositol monophosphate phosphatase, an enzyme that is inhibited by therapeutic concentrations of lithium (Li^+). Thus, in the presence of lithium, these monophosphates cannot be dephosphorylated to yield free inositol, which is required to regenerate phosphatidylinositol-4,5 bisphosphate. Lithium also inhibits inositol polyphosphate-1-phosphatase, an enzyme required for other metabolic steps in the recycling pathway.

track of them can be daunting, even for scientists who study them. Although neurotrophic factors and their signaling pathways typically have been studied because of their central role in neural development and differentiation, research has confirmed that they are critical for mediating responses to a wide array of external stimuli throughout the adult life of an organism.

Neurotrophin Signaling Pathways

Neurotrophic factor signal transduction cascades are best established for the neurotrophins, as summarized in **4-14** (Chapter 8). Neurotrophins bind to a plasma membrane receptor, termed *Trk*, and in turn trigger the dimerization, phosphorylation, and intrinsic protein tyrosine kinase activity of Trk. Once activated, Trk

signals via three main intracellular pathways—the Ras-Raf-ERK, IRS-PI3-kinase-Akt, and PLCγ pathways **4-14**— which are distinguished by several features. First, the Ras-Raf-ERK and IRS-PI3-kinase-Akt pathways involve cascades of multiple serine–threonine protein kinases which phosphorylate and activate successive kinases. An example of these cascades is shown in **4-15**. This leads to an extraordinary level of amplification in the cell. Second, all three pathways culminate in the phosphorylation of numerous cell proteins, which mediate the diverse effects of neurotrophins on neuronal function. Third, each of these pathways utilizes highly specific modes of protein–protein interactions, termed *src homology (SH2) domains*. Elaboration of SH2 domains in neurotrophin signaling led to a series of major discoveries of diverse types of

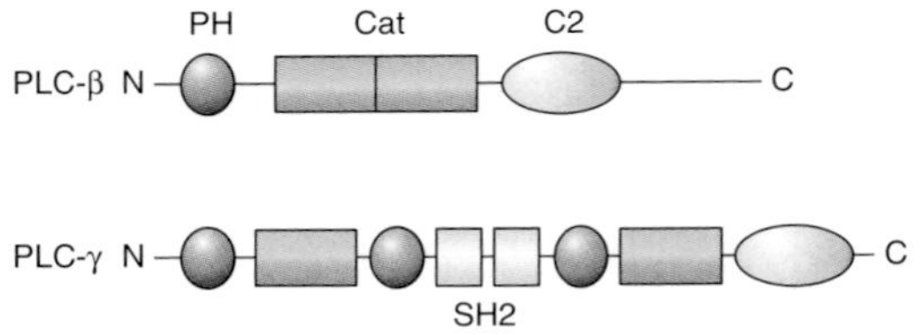

4-10 Structure of phospholipase C (PLC). The two major forms of PLC in the brain are PLCβ and PLCγ. PLCβ mediates the ability of G protein–coupled receptors (linked by G_q) to stimulate the phosphatidylinositol pathway (see 4-7). PLCγ mediates the ability of neurotrophic factors to stimulate the pathway (see 4-14). Both forms contain a pleckstrin homology domain (PH) on the N terminus that anchors the enyzme to the plasma membrane, a catalytic domain (Cat) composed of two homologous units, and a C2 domain that binds to and is activated by Ca^{2+}. PLCβ contains a larger C-terminal domain, which enables it to couple to G proteins, whereas PLCγ contains two additional PH domains and two SH2 domains, which enable it to couple to neurotrophin receptors.

protein–protein interaction domains (eg, PDZ, leucine zipper domains) that are integral to cell signaling 4-2.

A pathway that is functionally parallel to the Ras-Raf-ERK pathway in neurotrophin signaling is activated by certain cytokines and noxious stimuli 4-15. Tumor necrosis factor-α or UV light, for example, leads to the activation of the small G protein Rac. In response, Rac activates a cascade of protein kinases which culminates in the phosphorylation and activation of Jun N-terminal kinase (JNK). JNK phosphorylates the transcription factors Jun and activating transcription factor-2 (ATF2) and thereby enables them to regulate gene expression. Because this pathway is involved in responses to cellular stress, JNK is often referred to as a stress-activated protein kinase, or SAP-kinase. Another SAP-kinase is a 38-kDa protein known as p38.

JAK–STAT Pathway

Another prominent family of cytokines and hormones employs a very different mechanism of signal transduction. This family includes ciliary neurotrophic factor (CNTF) and leptin, among many others (Chapter 8). Each interacts with a specific plasma membrane α receptor named for the ligand (eg, CNTF α receptor). The α subunits of these receptors subsequently form heterotrimeric complexes with other proteins (Chapter 8). After these complexes are formed, the tripartite receptor associates with a protein tyrosine kinase called Janus kinase (JAK), which normally exists in the cytoplasm in its inactive form. The association of JAK with the receptor complex leads to JAK's activation and to the phosphorylation and activation of a family of transcription factors called *signal transducers and activators of transcription* (STATs). The activation of STATs in turn leads to many of the long-term effects of the cytokine on cell function.

GDNF Signaling Pathway

A similar pattern characterizes signaling by glial cell line-derived neurotrophic factor (GDNF) and the related neurotrophic factors known as neurturin and persephin. These factors are distant relatives of the transforming growth factor-β family and are of particular interest because of their potent neurotrophic effects on dopaminergic neurons. GDNF, neurturin, and persephin each bind to a unique receptor that dimerizes and interacts with the protein tyrosine kinase Ret (Chapter 8), which then mediates the diverse actions of these neurotrophic factors on cell function.

Cytoplasmic Protein Tyrosine Kinases

The first protein tyrosine kinase discovered was Src, which we now know is a prototype of a large family of such kinases that exist in the cell cytoplasm and in general are not physically part of a plasma membrane receptor complex. Src family members that are expressed at high levels in neurons include Fyn, Yes, Lck, and Lyn, in addition to Src itself. By phosphorylating many types of substrates, such as ion channels, glutamate receptor subunits, synaptic vesicle proteins, and transcription factors, Src family kinases have been implicated in the regulation of numerous neuronal processes, including synaptic transmission, neurotransmitter release, cell survival, and gene expression.

Protein Tyrosine Phosphatases

Interestingly, many more types of protein tyrosine phosphatases occur in the brain than do types of protein serine–threonine phosphatases. Some protein tyrosine phosphatases are selective for ERK and related MAP-kinases. Other enzymes are membrane associated and contain extracellular domains that may represent recognition sites for as yet unknown intercellular signals. Still other forms of protein tyrosine phosphatases are soluble and are present throughout the neuronal cytoplasm. Certain membrane- and cytosol-associated forms that exhibit highly restricted distributions in the nervous system may subserve specialized functions. For example, the striatal-enriched phosphatases (STEPs) are

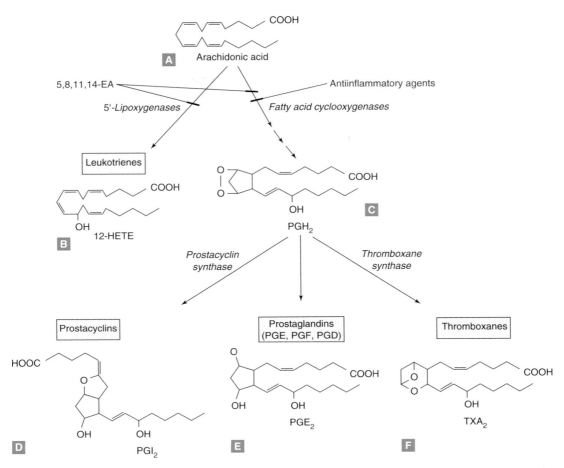

4-11 **Arachidonic acid signaling pathways.** **A.** Arachidonic acid gives rise to many important signaling molecules, which are products of two main pathways. **B.** One involves 5'-lipoxygenase and gives rise to the leukotrienes. **C.** The other involves the action of cyclooxygenase and gives rise to three families of signals: prostacyclins **D**, prostaglandins **E**, and thromboxanes **F**. Cyclooxygenases are inhibited by nonsteroidal anti-inflammatory agents. 5,8,11,14-Eicosatetraenoic acid (EA) is a lipoxygenase inhibitor that also inhibits cyclooxygenases.

expressed at high levels in striatal medium spiny neurons and contribute to the unique features of these cells. Although inhibitors of protein tyrosine phosphatases might be expected to promote the survival of neurons, this remains an unproven hypothesis. **Vanadate**, which inhibits most if not all protein tyrosine phosphatases, has been used as an experimental tool to study these enzymes in neural phenomena.

Other Protein Phosphorylation Cascades

Second messenger-dependent protein kinases and the protein kinases that function in neurotrophic factor signaling cascades represent a relatively small fraction

of the ~100 forms of protein kinases that have been identified in mammalian cells **4-7**. Research is now revealing how most of these other kinases affect neural functioning. G protein receptor kinases (GRKs), for example, phosphorylate G protein–coupled receptors and mediate receptor desensitization **4-3**. Many protein kinases were first characterized according to their role in basic cellular functions, such as cell division or intermediary metabolism (eg, glycogen synthase kinases, casein kinases, and cyclin-dependent kinases); however, recent evidence indicates that several of these enzymes operate in particular signal transduction cascades in the brain. Cyclin-dependent kinase-5 (Cdk-5), for example, is believed to be one of the protein kinases responsible for the hyperphosphorylation

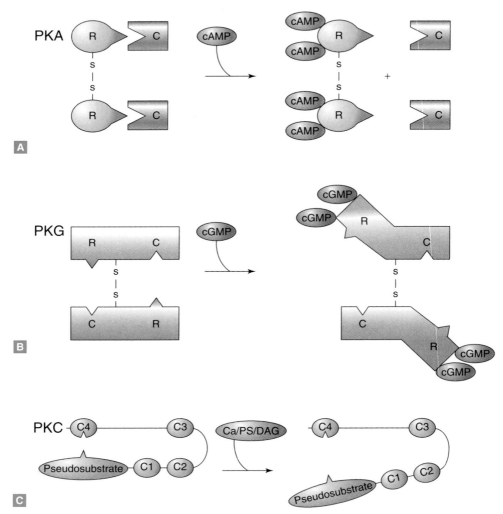

4-12 **Activation of protein kinases. A.** The PKA holoenzyme, which is inactive, is a dimer composed of two reg-ulatory subunits (R) joined by disulfide bonds, each of which is associated with a catalytic subunit (C). Two mole-cules of cAMP bind to each regulatory subunit, causing it to dissociate from the catalytic subunit, which in turn becomes active. **B.** PKG is activated in a similar manner, although its regulatory and catalytic domains exist within a single polypeptide chain. Regulatory subunits of PKA and regulatory domains of PKG may be autophosphory-lated in response to activation by cAMP or cGMP, respectively; such autophosphorylation promotes further disso-ciation and activation of the enzymes. **C.** PKC is a single polypeptide chain that comprises several identifiable domains. C1 binds diacylglycerol (DAG) and phorbol esters, C2 binds Ca^{2+} and phosphatidylserine (PS), C3 binds ATP, and C4 contains the active, or catalytic, site. The pseudosubstrate site is functionally analogous to the regula-tory domain of PKA and PKG in that it inhibits catalytic activity of the enzyme. In response to the binding of Ca^{2+}, PS, and DAG, this inhibition is relieved, and PKC is activated.

of a microtubule-associated protein in the brain known as tau; such hyperphosphorylation con-tributes to several types of dementia, including **Alzheimer disease** and **Pick disease** (Chapter 17).

Another substrate for Cdk-5 in the brain is DARPP-32. As previously discussed, phosphorylation of DARPP-32 by PKA converts it into an inhibitor of pro-tein phosphatase 1. Recent research has shown that phosphorylation of DARPP-32 by Cdk-5 on a different amino acid residue converts DARPP-32 into an inhibitor of PKA. Thus DARPP-32 can serve as a switch, alternately inhibiting the phosphorylation or dephosphorylation

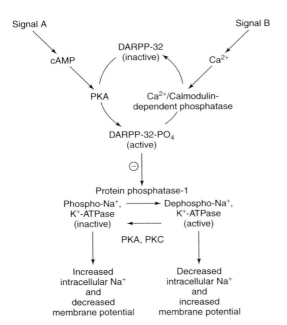

4-13 **Proposed physiologic role of DARPP-32.** The figure illustrates how DARPP-32 might integrate cellular cAMP and Ca^{2+} signals. DARPP-32 is converted by cAMP into an active phosphatase inhibitor by activation of PKA, which phosphorylates DARPP-32, whereas Ca^{2+} has the opposite effect by activating a phosphatase that dephosphorylates DARPP-32. Phosphorylated (active) DARPP-32, by inhibiting protein phosphatase 1, may increase the phosphorylation state of numerous phosphoproteins, for example, the Na^+,K^+-ATPase shown here, to regulate numerous physiologic processes. (Borrowed from P Greengard, The Rockefeller University, with permission.)

of various phosphoproteins, depending on the level of activity of PKA versus Cdk-5 in the neuron.

Another serine–threonine kinase of increasing interest to neuropharmacologists is glycogen synthase kinase 3β (GSK3β). As will be described in greater detail in Chapter 14, GSK3β is part of the wnt signaling pathway that is implicated in the regulation of neuronal survival. The kinase is potently inhibited by **lithium;** however, it remains uncertain whether this is related to lithium's mood stabilizing properties.

Centrality of Protein Phosphorylation

The final step of most signal transduction pathways is the regulation of phosphoproteins, which include an array of substrate proteins for each protein kinase and protein phosphatase involved in phosphorylation. It is now well established that protein phosphorylation underlies the regulation of diverse aspects of neuronal function **4-8**. The phosphorylation of neuronal proteins influences the regulation of ion channel activity; neurotransmitter receptor sensitivity; neurotransmitter synthesis, release, and reuptake; axoplasmic transport; the elaboration of dendritic and axonal processes; and the differentiation of neurons. Many forms of neural plasticity, including learning and memory, are similarly governed by the phosphorylation of neuronal proteins.

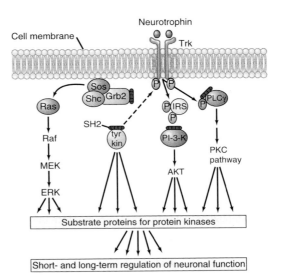

4-14 Intracellular pathways of neurotrophins in the brain. The activation of a neurotrophin receptor (Trk) stimulates protein tyrosine kinase activity and results in the autophosphorylation of the receptor. The phosphorylated receptor subsequently associates with other proteins, such as Grb2, Shc, and Sos, to activate the small G protein Ras, which in turn leads to the activation of Raf, a protein serine–threonine kinase. Raf phosphorylates and activates a MAP-kinase kinase (MEK), which subsequently activates a MAP-kinase (ERK) by phosphorylating it on threonine and tyrosine residues. In alternative pathways, Trks (1) attract by means of SH2 domains, phosphorylate, and activate phospholipase C (PLCγ); (2) activate phosphatidylinositol-3-kinase (PI-3-K) by means of insulin receptor substrate (IRS) proteins, which contain SH2 domains and act as linker proteins; or (3) activate other cytoplasmic protein tyrosine kinases that lack a receptor domain. P represents phosphorylation of the indicated proteins on tyrosine residues.

Mammalian signaling			
ERK pathway	SAP-kinase pathway	General scheme	Yeast signaling
RAS ↓	Rac, Cdc-42 ↓	Small G protein ↓	Cdc-42
? ↓	PAK ↓	MAP-kinase kinase kinase kinases ↓	Ste20
Raf ↓	MEKK ↓	MAP-kinase kinase kinases ↓	Ste11
MEK ↓	SEK ↓	MAP-kinase kinases ↓	Ste7
ERK ↓	SAP-kinase (JNK) ↓	MAP-kinases ↓	Fus3, Kss1
RSK	MAPKAP kinase	MAP-kinase activated kinases	

4-15 **MAP-kinase pathways.** Pathways originally delineated in yeast (*right*) are compared with homologous pathways more recently identified in mammalian cells (*left*). MEK, MAP-kinase and ERK kinase; ERK, extracellular signal–regulated kinase; RSK, ribosomal S6 kinase; SEK, SAP-kinase kinase; SAP-kinase, stress-activated protein kinase; JNK, Jun kinase; MAPKAP-kinase, MAP-kinase activated protein kinase.

Although proteins are covalently modified in many ways—for example, by ADP-ribosylation, acylation, carboxymethylation, tyrosine sulfation, and glycosylation—none of these mechanisms is as widespread or as readily subject to regulation by synaptic and hormonal stimuli as phosphorylation.

HETEROGENEITY IN BRAIN SIGNAL TRANSDUCTION PATHWAYS

Molecular biologic research has revealed a degree of heterogeneity in intracellular messenger pathways not suspected by classic biochemical, pharmacologic, or physiologic studies. Moreover, individual subtypes of intracellular signaling proteins possess unique regulatory properties and exhibit varying levels of expression in different neuronal cell types. Such heterogeneity has raised the specter of developing new medications that target intracellular messenger proteins. This point can be illustrated by consideration of RGS proteins. With more than 20 RGS subtypes known, many of which show highly restricted patterns of expression within the brain, it is conceivable that drugs aimed at antagonizing one particular subtype could exert a potent and clinically

useful effect on the signaling of G protein–coupled receptors within brain regions of interest.

SIGNALING TO THE CELL NUCLEUS: THE DYNAMIC REGULATION OF GENE EXPRESSION

All living cells depend on the regulation of gene expression by extracellular signals for their development, homeostasis, and adaptation to the environment. Indeed, many signal transduction pathways function primarily to modify transcription factors that alter the expression of specific genes. Thus, neurotransmitters, growth factors, and drugs change patterns of gene expression in cells and in turn affect many aspects of nervous system functioning, including the formation of long-term memories. Many drugs that require prolonged administration, such as antidepressants and antipsychotics, trigger changes in gene expression that are thought to be therapeutic adaptations to the initial action of the drug.

The mechanisms underlying the control of gene expression are becoming increasingly well understood. These are subject to various forms of dynamic regulation in the cell, including structural changes in chromatin, transcription of DNA into RNA **4-16**, splicing of RNA into mRNA, editing and other covalent modifications of mRNA, translation of mRNA into protein, and posttranslational modification of a protein into its mature, functional form. Although we have learned the molecular details of some these regulatory processes, such information has not yet been exploited for the medical treatment of CNS disorders. This section provides a detailed overview of the regulation of gene expression in cells, underscoring its profound impact on neural and behavioral plasticity. Central to this section is the belief that the therapeutic effects of drugs that influence the CNS often depend on alterations in gene expression, as well as the expectation that novel therapeutic agents for neuropsychiatric disorders will one day target some of the mechanisms that govern the transcription and translation of genes into mature proteins.

Regulation of Gene Expression by Chromatin

In eukaryotic cells, DNA is contained within a discrete organelle called the nucleus, which is the site of DNA replication and transcription. Transcriptionally quiescent regions of DNA are tightly packed into a coil, whereas regions characterized by active transcription may be more than a 1000-fold more extended.

4–2   **Protein-Protein Interactions as Novel Drug Targets**

Noncatalytic protein-protein interactions are important for the regulation of enzyme activity, in the transport and subcellular localization of proteins, and in the formation of specialized multiprotein complexes. These protein interactions regulate diverse neuronal functions, including signal transduction, gene expression, cytoskeletal organization, synaptic connectivity, and neurotransmission. During the past decade, researchers have identified protein subregions, or domains, that are responsible for binding to other proteins with high affinity and specificity (see table). Many of these sites of protein-protein interaction are modular and contain distinct three-dimensional structures that retain their binding capacity even when they are separated from the rest of the protein. Domains with similar amino acid sequences, structures, and binding activities have been found in proteins that are otherwise unrelated, and these domain families have been given special names.

Because of their functional importance, their specificity, and their variety, protein-protein domains are extremely attractive targets for experimental and therapeutic drugs. Cell-permeable peptides and synthetic nonpeptide agents that block protein-protein interactions are currently being developed, as are agents that facilitate these interactions. This exciting and rapidly expanding field should become an increasingly integral part of basic and clinical neuropharmacology.

Selected Protein-Protein Interaction Domains

Domain	Interaction	Domain-Containing Proteins	Binding-Target Proteins	Functions
Leucine zipper	Hydrophobically binds other leucine zipper domains	Fos Jun CREB	Jun Fos CREB	Homodimers or heterodimers of transcription factors
Pleckstrin homology	Binds to inositol lipids, $G_{\beta\gamma}$ subunits, and PKC	Pleckstrin IRSs PLCs GRKs AKT/PKB Sos Dynamin	$G_{\beta\gamma}$ PKC	Targets proteins to membrane; permits regulation of enzyme activity by inositol lipids, and perhaps by $G_{\beta\gamma}$, PKC.
PDZ	Binds to C-terminal in consensus S/TXV, or to other PDZ domains	PSD95 GRIP Homer nNos	Shaker K^+ channels, NMDARs, AMPARs, mGluRs	Allows ion channel clustering; forms signal transduction complexes
Phosphotyrosine binding/interacting	Binds phosphotyrosines in NPXpY consensus	IRSs Shc	RTKs, JAKs	Forms signal transduction complexes
Regulator of G protein signaling	Binds to specific G protein α subunits	RGS family	$G_{\alpha i}/G_{\alpha o}$ $G_{\alpha q}$ $G_{\alpha t}$ (transducin)	Down-regulates signaling through G proteins by increasing their GTPase activity

Selected Protein-Protein Interaction Domains (*Continued*)

Domain	Interaction	Domain-Containing Proteins	Binding-Target Proteins	Functions
Src homology 2	Binds phosphotyrosines in YXXphi consensus, both intermolecular and intra-molecular interactions occur	Src family PTKs PLCγ PI-3-K RasGAP PTP1C Shc Grb2 STATs	IRSs RTKs	Forms signal transduction complexes; allows regulation of enzyme activity by tyrosine kinases
Src homology 3	Binds polyproline sequences, with PXXP consensus	Src family PTKs PLCg PI-3-K RasGAP Grb2 Amphiphysin	Sos Shc Dynamin	Forms signal transduction complexes
WW	Binds polyproline sequences, with XPPXY consensus	FE65 YAP	WBPs	Unknown

RGS, regulator of G protein signaling; SH, src homology; PTB, phosphotyrosine binding; YAP, Yes-associated protein (Yes is a PTK); Grb2, growth factor receptor binding protein 2; PLC, phospholipase C; PI-3-K, phosphoinositol-3-kinase; STAT, signal transducer and activator of transcription; JAK, janus kinase; RTK, receptor tyrosine kinase; PTK, protein tyrosine kinase; Shc, src homology containing protein; NMDAR, NMDA glutamate receptor; AMPAR, AMPA glutamate receptor; mGluR, metabotropic gluta-mate receptor; PSD, postsynaptic density; nNOS, neuronal nitric oxide synthase; IRS, insulin receptor substrate; WBP, WW domain binding protein; GRK, G protein-coupled receptor kinase; GAP, GTPase activating protein; PTP, protein tyrosine phosphatase.

Chromosomes are extremely long molecules of DNA, which are wrapped around histone proteins to form nucleosomes, the major subunits of chromatin. Chromatin plays a critical role in transcriptional regula-tion, because it can repress gene expression by inhibit-ing the ability of transcription factors to access DNA. In fact, chromatin ensures that genes are inactive unless their expression is required 4-17. To activate gene expression, cells must attenuate nucleosome-mediated repression of an appropriate subset of genes by means of activator proteins that modify chromatin structure. This activation process, which involves transcription factors, histones, and many other regulatory proteins, remodels chromatin and opens up regions of DNA to permit their transcription into RNA.

Activation or repression of chromatin is mediated in part via the covalent modification of histone proteins, including their acetylation, phosphorylation, and methylation, among other chemical changes (eg, ubiqui-tylation, glycosylation) 4-18 and 4-19. Histone acety-lation is associated with an opening of chromatin and activation of gene expression. Histone methylation is associated with either gene activation or repression depending on the amino acid residue underoing methy-lation. DNA itself can undergo methylation, which mediates more profound repression of gene expression. The molecular mechanisms mediating most of these changes in chromatin structure remain poorly understood, although considerable detail is now avail-able for histone acetylation, which is catalyzed by histone acetyltransferases (HATs) and reversed by histone deacetylases (HDACs). Regulation of histone acetylation has been implicated in recent years in a wide range of neuroscientific phenomena, including learning and memory and the actions of several classes of psychotropic drug. Indeed, there is a great deal of interest in the poten-tial therapeutic utility of HDAC inhibitors, which have been shown to promote learning and memory and exert antidepressant-like effects in animal models. Most avail-able **HDAC inhibitors,** for example, **sodium butyrate**, **tri-chostatin A**, **SAHA (Vorinostat)**, and **MS-275** are highly nonspecific, but work is underway to synthesize small molecule inhibitors specific for certain HDAC subtypes. HAT's represent another putative drug target, although

■■4–7■■ Major Classes of Protein Serine–Threonine Kinases[1]

Second messenger-dependent protein kinases
  cAMP kinase
  cGMP kinase
  Ca^{2+}/calmodulin kinases
  Protein kinase C

MAP kinases
  ERKs
  JNKs or SAP-kinases

MAP kinase-regulating kinases
  MEKs
  SEKs
  Raf
  MEKK

Cyclin-dependent protein kinases (Cdks)
  Cdk-2
  Cdk-5

Cdk regulating kinases
  Cdk-activating kinase (CAK)
  CAK-kinase

G protein receptor kinases (GRKs)

Others
  Ribosomal S6 kinases (RSKs)
  Casein kinases

[1]This list is not intended to be comprehensive. These protein kinases, are present in many cell types and are included here because their multiple functions in the nervous system include the regulation of neuron-specific phenomena. Not included are other protein kinases present in diverse tissues (including brain) that play a role in generalized cellular processes, such as intermediary metabolism, but that may not play a role in neuron-specific phenomena. ERK, extracellular signal-regulated kinase; JNK, Jun kinase; SAP-kinase, stress-activated kinase; MEK, MAP-kinase or ERK kinase; SEK, SAP-kinase or ERK kinase; MEKK, MEK kinase; Cdc-2, cell division cycle-protein 2; Cdk-5, cyclin-dependent kinase type 5; CAK, Cdk-activating kinase.

less explored to date than HDAC's. **Curcumin**, a major ingredient in the curry spice, turmeric, is an inhibitor of HAT activity, among many other actions, and is purported to have beneficial **anti-cancer** and **anti-inflammatory** effects in open trials.

Research has demonstrated that genetic defects in the remodeling of chromatin cause several neurologic and psychiatric syndromes ■■4–9■■. An example is **Rett syndrome,** an **autism**-like disorder, caused by mutation in a gene that controls DNA methylation ■■4–4■■.

Regulated Steps of Transcription

Genes contain a coding region that specifies the sequence of the encoded mRNA and its protein along with much longer regulatory regions that determine when, where, and to what extent that gene is expressed. These regulatory regions have been termed *promoter* or *enhancer* regions. The best characterized regulatory regions of genes are located immediately upstream from (or 5′ to) their coding regions. However, DNA sequences located 3′ of the coding region, and even within the coding region, have been shown to contain regulatory information. Only a small percentage of chromosomal DNA in the human genome (approximately 4%) is responsible for encoding the roughly 30 000 genes that encode RNA strands. Among RNA strands, only a minority—for example, rRNA, tRNA, and snRNA—have cellular functions themselves; most RNA is mRNA that serves as an intermediate between DNA and protein. The spacing of genes on chromosomes is far from uniform: some chromosomal regions, and indeed whole chromosomes, are gene rich or gene poor. Intergenic regions alternately consist of unique sequences and long stretches of tandemly repeated sequences referred to as *satellite DNA*. Whether this extragenic DNA performs a structural or regulatory role or simply represents parasitic DNA that is replicated in conjunction with functional regions of DNA is currently a matter of debate.

Transcription occurs in regions of open chromatin, where a complex of proteins, called general transcription factors, binds DNA at a core promoter and recruits RNA polymerase (see ■■4–17■■). The construction of this protein complex at the transcription start site and the first steps of RNA synthesis are referred to as *transcription*

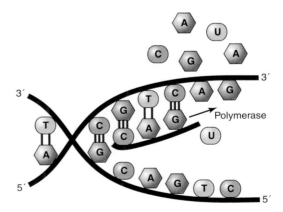

■■4–16■■ Complementary base pairing of DNA. A DNA double helix unwinds, allowing the transcription of a new, complementary strand of RNA catalyzed by an RNA polymerase in the 5′ to 3′ direction.

One of the dramatic features of G protein–coupled receptors is their rapid desensitization in response to agonist stimulation. An important mechanism underlying this desensitization is phosphorylation of the receptor by a second messenger–activated kinase such as PKA and by a β-adrenergic receptor kinase (β-ARK) that has been renamed G protein receptor kinase (GRK; see figure).

The details of GRK action are best established for the β-adrenergic receptor. Agonist binding to the receptor stimulates G_s, which leads to the activation of adenylyl cyclase, increased levels of cAMP, and the activation of PKA. The activation of PKA subsequently triggers many of the physiologic effects of β-adrenergic receptor stimulation through the phosphorylation of numerous substrate proteins. However, among the proteins phosphorylated by the kinase is the receptor itself, which is phosphorylated on several serine residues in its cytoplasmic domains. This process reduces the subsequent ability of agonists to activate the receptor. For example, phosphorylation of the receptor may trigger its endocytosis or internalization from the plasma membrane, sequestering it from further agonist binding. An internalized receptor may be returned to the plasma membrane after its dephosphorylation or may undergo proteolysis during periods of prolonged agonist exposure (see **6–15**).

Phosphorylation of the β-adrenergic receptor by PKA can be viewed as an example of negative feedback: activation of the receptor stimulates intracellular cascades that reduce further receptor activation. Phosphorylation of the receptor by PKA also can mediate *heterologous desensitization* of the receptor; any neurotransmitter–receptor system that works through cAMP may stimulate β-adrenergic

receptor phosphorylation by means of PKA and lead to receptor desensitization. Thus this process enables one neurotransmitter–receptor system to affect another.

The β-adrenergic receptor is also phosphorylated on several distinct serine residues by GRKs, protein serine–threonine kinases that are constitutively active and not regulated by second messengers (see part B of figure). This kinase can phosphorylate the receptor only when the receptor is bound to agonist because such binding alters the receptor's conformation in such a way that it becomes a good substrate for the kinase. After it undergoes phosphorylation by GRK, the receptor is able to bind a protein known as β-arrestin, which effectively sequesters the receptor and prevents its further interaction with the ligand or G protein. Recent studies indicate that the βγ subunits of G proteins are required to bring GRK, a predominantly cytosolic enzyme, into close association with the plasma membrane–associated receptors occupied by ligand. This process represents an elegant mechanism by which GRK is specifically recruited to receptors that have been recently activated, as evidenced by nearby free βγ complexes.

Phosphorylation of the β-adrenergic receptor by GRK, like its phosphorylation by the cAMP-dependent enzyme, can be viewed as negative feedback. However, unlike phosphorylation by PKA, phosphorylation by GRK represents an example of *homologous desensitization*: only the β-adrenergic receptor molecules occupied by the agonist are affected in this process.

This model of receptor desensitization has been shown to operate for many types of G protein–coupled receptors.

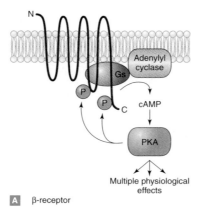

A β-receptor

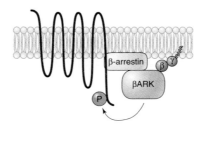

B β-receptor

4-8 Neuronal Proteins Regulated by Phosphorylation

Regulated Protein	Protein Kinase	Effect
Enzymes involved in neurotransmitter biosynthesis and degradation		
Tyrosine hydroxylase	PKA, PKC, CaM-KII	Increase in enzyme activity
Tryptophan hydroxylase	CaM-KII	Increase in enzyme activity
G protein-coupled receptors		
β-adrenergic receptor	PKA, GRKII	Receptor desensitization
Opioid receptors	GRKII	Receptor desensitization
Neurotransmitter-gated ion channels		
GluR1 (AMPA subunit)	PKA	Increase in response
NMDAR1 (NMDA subunit)	PKC, tyrosine kinase	Increase in response
Ion channels		
Voltage-gated Na^+ channel	PKA, PKC	Decrease in channel conductance
Voltage-gated Ca^{2+} channel	PKA	Increase in channel conductance
Enzymes and other proteins involved in the regulation of second messengers		
Phospholipase Cγ	Tyrosine kinase	Increase in enzyme activity
IP_3 receptor	PKA	Increase in Ca^{2+} release
Protein kinases		
PKA	PKA	Increase in dissociation and activity
CaM-K1 and IV	CaM-KK	Increase in enzyme activity
Trk	Trk	Increase in signaling
Protein phosphatase inhibitors		
DARPP-32	PKA, PKG	Increase in inhibitory activity
Inhibitor 1	PKA	Increase in inhibitory activity
Inhibitor 2	GSK3	Decrease in inhibitory activity
Cytoskeletal proteins		
MAP-2	PKA	Promotion of microtubule assembly
Tau	Cdk-5 and others	Increase in aggregation
Myosin light chain	MLC-K	Increase in binding to actin
Synaptic vesicle proteins		
Synapsin	PKA, CaM-KII	Increase in neurotransmitter release
Transcription factors		
CREB	PKA, CaM-KIV, RSK	Increase in transactivation
STAT proteins	JAK	Increase in transactivation

This list is not intended to be comprehensive but instead indicates the diverse types of neuronal proteins that are regulated by phosphorylation.
PKA, protein kinase A; PKC, protein kinase C; CaM-K, Ca^{2+}/calmodulin-dependent protein kinases; GRK, G protein-coupled receptor kinase; CaM-KK, CaM-K kinase; Trk, Trk receptor; PKG, protein kinase G; GSK3, glycogen synthase kinase 3; MAP-2, microtubule-associated protein-2; MLC-K, myosin light chain kinase; RSK, ribosomal S6 kinase; STAT, signal transducers and activators of transcription; JAK, Janus kinase.

initiation. For many genes, transcription initiation occurs at a so-called TATA box (a sequence rich in T and A nucleotides). In the elongation step, RNA polymerase transcribes RNA across the length of a gene. The final step in the transcription of RNA is termination.

Posttranscriptional Regulation

The resulting nuclear RNA engages in a posttranscriptional process called *splicing*, which removes internal sequences that will not be translated into protein in that particular cell **4-20**. Alternative splicing provides

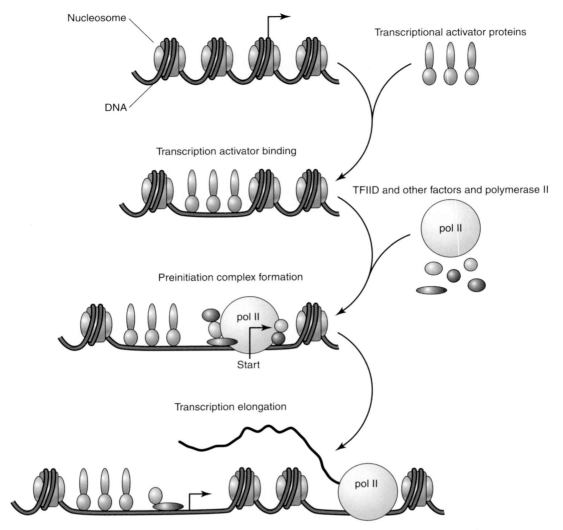

4-17 **Inhibition of gene expression by the nucleosomal structure of chromatin.** To activate the transcription of DNA into RNA, activator proteins (see **4-18**) must displace nucleosomes. This permits general transcription factors (collectively called TFIID) and RNA polymerase (pol) II to bind to the transcription initiation site in a gene (start arrow). Still more nucleosomes must be displaced to permit transcription elongation.

a mechanism by which a single gene can give rise to several mRNAs and proteins. This is because different exons (sequences of genes that are retained in mRNAs) can be used to construct the mature mRNA depending on the cell type and stage of development involved. In fact, some genes are heavily spliced, with numerous mRNAs formed through alternative splicing. One of the most extraordinary examples is *neurexin*: three neurexin genes are thought to give rise to hundreds of neurexin proteins through alternative splicing, which help control the formation of specific

contacts in the developing nervous system. Thus, the true molecular diversity of mammalian cells is significantly underrepresented by the approximately 30 000 genes contained in the genome.

Subsequently the mature mRNA is exported from the nucleus into the cytoplasm. All mRNA molecules contain untranslated regions (UTRs) at their 5′ and 3′ ends that affect mRNA stability and translatability. For example, a poly(A) tail is coupled to mRNA by means of an endonucleolytic cleavage step that produces the 3′ end of a mature mRNA molecule. While the stability

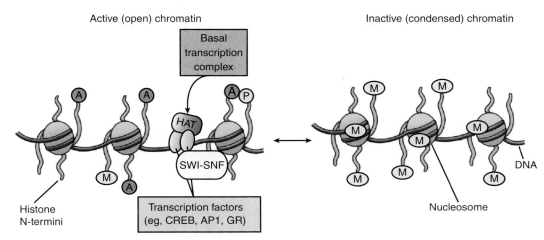

4-18 **Transition between activated and inhibited chromatin.** The first step in gene activation is the binding of a transcription factor, which recruits other proteins, including HATs and SWI-SNF complexes, to the gene. HATs acetylate nearby histones on their N-termini (A), leading to the loosening of the chromatin. SWI-SNF are ATPase–containing complexes that provide the molecular motors to move nucleosomes across DNA as transcription is initiated and continues. In contrast, inhibited chromatin is typically enriched in methylation of particular residues in histones at their N-termini (M). (Methylation of other sites is associated with gene activation.) H3 can also be phosphorylated (P), a modification associated with gene activation. GR, glucocorticoid receptor.

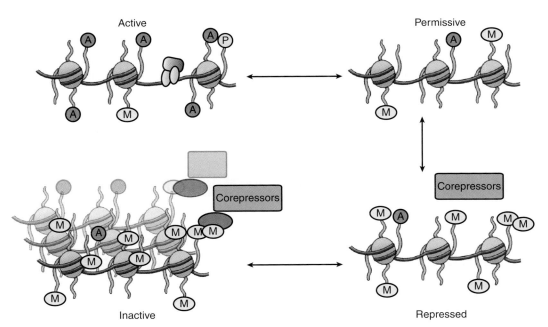

4-19 **Chromatin exists as a continuum from activated to inactivated states.** The most tightly (and perhaps irreversibly) inhibited chromatin involves methylation of the DNA itself and the recruitment of many repressor proteins (eg, MeCP2). Less inhibited chromatin is in more permissive states, sufficiently loosely bound to allow transcription factors to initiate gene activation as shown in **4-18**

4-9   **Examples of Diseases of Chromatin Remodeling**

Disease	Chromatin Defect	Clinical Features
Rubinstein-Taybi syndrome	Heterozygous mutations in *CBP* (CREB binding protein)	Autosomal dominant inheritance Mental retardation Abnormal facial features, blunted growth
Fragile X syndrome	Hypermethylation of DNA at the *FMR1* and *FMR2* (Fragile X mental retardation-1,2) promoters, caused by trinucleotide repeat expansion	X-linked inheritance Most common inherited form of mental retardation, signs of autistic behavior Macrocephaly, long and narrow face with large ears, macroorchidism, hypotonia
Coffin-Lowry syndrome	Mutation in *RSK2* (ribosomal S6 kinase-2), which can interact with CREB and CBP and can phosphorylate H3 in vitro	X-linked inheritance Psychomotor retardation Craniofacial and skeletal abnormalities
Rett syndrome	Mutations in *MeCP2*	X-linked, affecting predominantly girls Pervasive developmental disorder associated with cognitive decline and autistic-like behavior
α-Thalassemia/mental retardation syndrome, X-linked (ATR-X)	Mutations in *ATRX* gene, encoding the X-linked helicase-2 (XH2) — a member of SWI/SNF family of proteins Defective chromatin remodeling thought to down-regulate the α-globin locus	X-linked inheritance Mental retardation Hemolytic anemia, splenomegaly, facial, skeletal, and genital anomalies
Immunodeficiency—centromeric instability—facial anomalies syndrome (ICF)	Mutations in *Dnmt3B* (DNA methyltransferase 3B) Hypomethylation at centromeric regions of chromosomes 1, 9, and 16	Autosomal recessive Mild mental retardation Marked immunodeficiency, facial anomalies
Myotonic dystrophy	Abnormal CTG repeat expansion at the 3'UTR of the *DM1-Protein Kinase* gene favors chromatin condensation, affecting expression of many neighboring genes	Autosomal dominant Mild mental retardation, myotonia, abnormal cardiac conduction, insulin-dependent diabetes, testicular atrophy, premature balding
Prader-Willi syndrome	Rare forms caused by abnormal imprinting (DNA methylation) of paternal chromosomal region 15q11-13	Mild mental retardation, endocrine abnormalities
Angelman syndrome	Rare forms caused by abnormal imprinting (DNA methylation) of maternal chromosomal region 15q11-13	Cortical atrophy, cerebellar dysmyelination, cognitive abnormalities

and translatability of an mRNA molecule are regulated by its polyadenylation, the underlying mechanisms remain poorly understood. Eukaryotic mRNAs are also modified at their 5′ ends with the addition of a modified guanosine cap. This cap increases the stability of the mRNA and promotes efficient protein synthesis by binding protein factors that are required to initiate the assembly of a translation-competent ribosome.

The translation of mRNA into protein is governed by the genetic code. The sequence of nucleotides in a molecule of mRNA is read on ribosomes in serial order and in groups of three. Each triplet of nucleotides, called a *codon*, specifies a single amino acid. The translation of mRNA into protein is mediated by tRNAs, which recognize the three bases in a codon and carry the corresponding amino acid. Translation initiation always occurs at the codon AUG (specifying methionine), and translation is terminated when the ribosome reaches a stop codon in the mRNA.

Finally, the newly synthesized protein may undergo a variety of chemical modifications and cleavages. Such

4-4 Rett Syndrome

Rett syndrome is a pervasive developmental disorder that occurs predominantly in females and shares certain clinical features with **autism-spectrum disorders.** Infants appear normal at birth and show normal developmental milestones until approximately 6 months of age, when severe developmental arrest occurs. Thereafter, patients are afflicted by gross deterioration in mental, social, and motor functioning.

The vast majority of cases of Rett syndrome are caused by loss-of-function mutations in the gene that encodes methyl-CpG-binding protein 2 (MECP2), which is located on the X chromosome. MECP2, through interactions with Sin3A (a transcriptional repressor) and certain histone deacetylases, binds to methylated CpG dinucleotides in the genome and represses gene transcription. Thus,

MECP2 is part of the normal mechanisms by which methylation of DNA causes repression of gene expression. Such mechanisms are implicated in the phenomenon of *genetic imprinting*, which explains why certain traits are preferentially inherited from the mother or father independent of the dominance or recessiveness of the trait. For example, if a paternal gene is highly methylated, it remains inactive in the offspring, regardless of whether it is dominant or recessive.

A major goal of future research is to determine how loss of MECP2 leads to the pervasive developmental arrest that is characteristic of patients with Rett syndrome. Research also is needed to determine which genes are overexpressed in the absence of MECP2, and why developmental arrest occurs during mid-infancy.

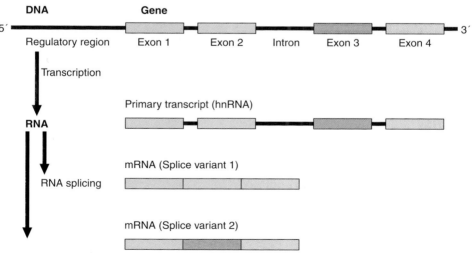

4-20 **Transcription and RNA splicing.** Horizontal red lines represent DNA regulatory regions and introns. Colored rectangles represent exons. The region to the left of the first exon is the 5′ regulatory region of the gene, but regulatory elements are also found in introns and sometimes even downstream of the last exon. The primary transcript, also known as heterogeneous RNA (hnRNA), contains both exons and introns and (in the example shown) gives rise to two alternatively spliced mRNAs: one containing exons 1, 2, and 4, and one containing exons 1, 3, and 4. If these splice variants were exported from the nucleus and translated in the cytoplasm, they would give rise to distinct proteins.

cleavages can yield multiple protein or polypeptide products from a single mRNA. One of the best-characterized examples is the pro-opiomelanocortin gene, whose single mRNA gives rise to several hormones, including β-endorphin, α-melanocyte-stimulating hormone (α-MSH), and adrenocorticotropin (ACTH), among other biologically active products (Chapter 7). A protein must also be targeted to the appropriate cellular compartment, which is determined by the protein's amino acid sequence, by its covalent modification (eg, glycosylation, phosphorylation, etc.), and by the presence of other proteins in the cell that serve scaffolding or anchoring functions. Details regarding posttranslational alterations and the associated sorting of proteins to different cellular locations are addressed in subsequent chapters in this book.

The stability of a protein, like that of an mRNA molecule, is highly regulated. Some proteins, such as those in the Fos family of transcription factors (see below), are highly unstable because they contain specific amino acid sequences, termed degrons, that serve as substrates for proteolytic enzymes, or proteases. As well, the stability of certain proteins depends on their association with other proteins. Many cellular proteins undergo proteolysis by means of the *ubiquitin–proteasome* pathway, whereby specific enzymes add ubiquitin groups to the targeted protein. This addition tags the protein for proteolysis by proteasomes, which are large multiprotein complexes. Abnormal functioning of proteasomes is implicated in neurodegenerative disorders, such as **Parkinson disease** (Chapter 17). Specific inhibitors of proteasomes, such as **leu-leu-leu** and **lactacystin**, are used experimentally to study the role of proteasomes in cell regulation.

Micro RNAs

Recent research has demonstrated that small RNAs, termed microRNAs or miRNAs, are encoded by the genome and transported to the cytoplasm where they serve a regulatory function by binding to specific mRNAs and inhibiting their translation. The molecular details by which this occurs are now well known 4–21. Several hundred miRNAs have been identified in mammalian cells to date and, interestingly, many show dynamic regulation in neurons in response to a host of stimuli. Accordingly, miRNAs represent a newly discovered mechanism of gene regulation, the role of which in neurologic and psychiatric disorders has not yet been explored. Down-regulation of mRNA translation via miRNA is termed *RNA interference* (or *RNAi*), and such regulation is now being exploited experimentally, where miRNAs are used to knock down a target mRNA of

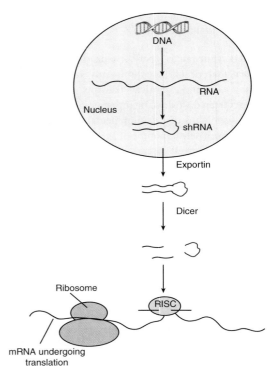

4–21 **Mechanism of RNA interference.** MicroRNA's are transcribed from DNA, typically by RNA polymerase III. Due to complementary sequences at their two ends, they form hairpin loops, which gives rise to shRNAs (small hairpin RNAs). shRNAs are transported to the cytoplasm by exportin, where they are cleaved by dicer, to generate free RNAis (RNA interference), which bind to complementary sequences in mRNAs and, with a protein complex called RISC, inhibits protein translation.

interest in neurons or even in the brain in vivo in order to understand the biological activity of the encoded protein. There is even interest in the possible utility of miRNAs, perhaps delivered via viral vectors, in the treatment of a wide range of human disorders.

REGULATION OF GENE EXPRESSION BY EXTRACELLULAR SIGNALS

All of the steps of gene expression, from RNA transcription to protein translation to posttranslational modifications of proteins, offer critical control points for dynamic regulation. However, by far the best understood is regulation of gene transcription, which is the focus of the remainder of this chapter. The precise control of transcription by extracellular signals such as neurotransmitters, growth factors, and cytokines permits the regulation of processes such as cell proliferation and differentiation and assists cells in adapting to their environments. Each cell in an organism contains a complete copy of that organism's genome. However, selective expression of this common genome is required for the formation of distinct cell types during development, including the formation of thousands of types of neurons in the brain. In the fully differentiated adult brain, a subset of an organism's genes remains accessible for expression and the rate of their expression is under constant control in response to the external environment. Indeed, such regulation of gene transcription is now thought to be a key mechanism for neural and behavioral plasticity.

Transcription Factors: Key Regulators of Gene Expression

The rate of transcription of a given gene is determined first by the state of its nearby chromatin. Many genes are inaccessible for transcription in neurons due to their presence in silenced chromatin. Conversely, many neural genes are not expressed in nonneural cells due to the action of the transcriptional repressor, REST (also

called NRSF). Other genes available for transcription exist in varying states of activation (see **4–19**), some being actively transcribed, others not transcribed but in a permissive state, that is, able to be turned on in response to the right stimulus. The activation of such permissive genes involves several steps which are only briefly summarized here. The key step is the binding of a class of protein, named transcription factors, to short DNA sequences, called *response elements*, present along the regulatory regions of genes. The regions of genes where transcription factors bind are often termed *promoters* or *enhancers*. Transcription factor binding provides part of the thermodynamic energy to spread nucleosomes apart. The factors also recruit to the gene enzymes that modify histones, such as HATs, which further loosens the nucleosome complex. More than 100 proteins may bind to the vicinity of an activated gene. This basal transcription apparatus contains RNA polymerase (more specifically, RNA polymerase II for virtually all genes that encode mRNAs) and a host of proteins that move nucleosomes along a strand of DNA, allowing for its transcription into RNA.

Transcription factors typically contain physically distinct functional domains **4–22**. These domains contribute to the categorization of transcription factors into various families. Many transcription factors are active only when they form dimers or higher-order complexes. Multimerization domains are diverse and include so-called leucine zippers (see **4–2**). Whether

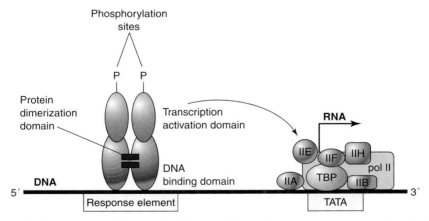

4–22 **A generalized polymerase II promoter.** Two regulatory elements, including a hypothetical activator, or response element, and the TATA box are located on a stretch of DNA (*red line*). The TATA element binds the TATA binding protein (TBP), which associates with multiple general transcription factors (TFIIA, B, E, F, and H). This basal transcription apparatus recruits RNA polymerase (pol) II and also forms the substrate for interactions with various activator proteins, which typically contain DNA-binding domains, dimerization domains, and transcription activation domains. Several of these proteins may be modified by phosphorylation.

transcription factor dimers are homodimers or heterodimers, both partners commonly contribute to the DNA binding domain and to the activation domain.

Interestingly, dimerization sometimes can be a mechanism for the negative control of transcription, as illustrated by the CREB (cAMP response element binding protein) family of transcription factors. CREB normally binds to its cAMP response elements (CREs) as homodimers. However, another gene, CREM (cAMP response element modulator), encodes a truncated protein ICER (inducible cAMP repressor), which can dimerize with CREB. However, because ICER lacks an activation domain, the resulting CREB-ICER dimers cannot activate transcription. ICER is thus an endogenous inhibitor of CREB-mediated transcription.

Although transcription factors may directly contact several proteins in the basal transcription complex, they sometimes interact with this apparatus through the mediation of coactivator or adapter proteins (see **4-22**). In either scenario, transcription factors that bind at a distance from the core promoter can interact with the basal transcription apparatus because the DNA forms loops that bring distant regions in contact with each other.

Many activator proteins become involved in the assembly of the mature transcription apparatus only after modification, such as phosphorylation, has occurred in response to extracellular signals. This, too, is illustrated by CREB. CREB can activate transcription only when it is phosphorylated on a particular serine residue (ser133) because phosphorylation of this residue permits CREB to interact with an adapter protein known as CREB-binding protein (CBP), which in turn contacts and activates the basal transcription apparatus in part via its HAT activity. Interestingly, mutations in CBP cause **Rubinstein-Taybi** syndrome, an autosomal dominant disorder characterized by mental retardation, bone and palatal abnormalities, and cardiac dysfunction **4-9**.

Transcription Factors: Targets of Signaling Pathways

Two major mechanisms of transcriptional regulation by extracellular signals are illustrated in **4-23**. One of these mechanisms involves transcription factors that are present at significant levels under basal conditions and are rapidly stimulated by signaling cascades to activate or repress the transcription of responsive target genes. By means of the other major mechanism, transcription factors that are expressed at very low levels under basal conditions are induced by a physiologic signal that enables them to regulate the expression of a series of genes.

A critical step in the extracellular regulation of gene expression is the transduction of signals from the cell membrane to the nucleus, which can be accomplished by several mechanisms. Some transcription factors translocate to the nucleus in response to their activation. These include steroid hormone receptors, whose translocation is triggered by the binding of their ligand, and NF-κB, a transcription factor retained in the cytoplasm by a binding protein (IκB) that masks its nuclear localization signal. Signal-regulated phosphorylation of IκB by IκK (I kappa kinase) leads to the dissociation of NF-κB, which in turn is permitted to enter the nucleus to bind DNA; IκB subsequently undergoes proteolysis in the cytoplasm **4-24**. Other transcription factors must be phosphorylated or dephosphorylated directly before they can bind to DNA; for example, the phosphorylation of STATs by protein tyrosine kinases in the cytoplasm permits their multimerization, which in turn permits nuclear translocation and the construction of an effective DNA binding site in the multimer.

Some transcription factors are already bound to their cognate regulatory elements in the nucleus under basal conditions and are converted into transcriptional activators by phosphorylation. CREB, for example, is bound to CREs before cell stimulation **4-25**. The critical nuclear translocation step for CREB involves the activation of protein kinases such as protein kinase A, which, after entering the nucleus, phosphorylates CREB. Alternatively, CREB activation can involve the nuclear translocation of second messengers, such as Ca^{2+} bound to calmodulin. After entering the nucleus, these second messengers activate Ca^{2+}/calmodulin-dependent protein kinase type IV which in turn phosphorylates CREB **4-25**. As previously mentioned, phosphorylation converts CREB into a transcriptional activator by permitting it to recruit CBP into the transcription complex.

The remainder of this chapter focuses on several transcription factor families that have received a great deal of attention as mediators of neural and behavioral plasticity in the adult.

CREB Family of Transcription Factors

CREB regulates transcription by binding to CREs present in a subset of genes. As their name suggests, CREs enable cAMP to activate genes and have more recently been shown to confer responsiveness of genes to Ca^{2+} and to the MAP-kinase pathway as well. CREs have been identified in many genes expressed in the nervous system, including those that encode neuropeptides, neurotransmitter synthetic enzymes, signaling proteins, and other transcription factors.

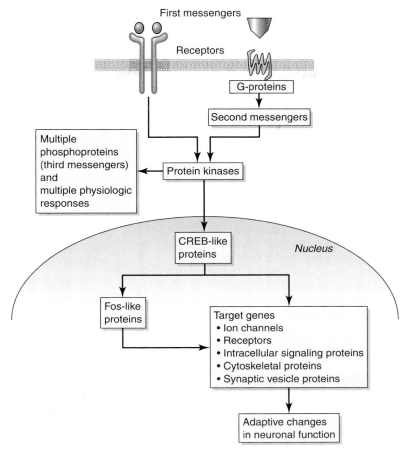

4-23 **Intracellular pathways underlying the regulation of gene expression.** The stimulation of neurotransmitter, hormone, or neurotrophic factor receptors activates specific second messenger and protein phosphorylation pathways, which produce effects on neuronal function through the phosphorylation of numerous proteins. Changes in gene expression occur by means of two basic mechanisms. When constitutively expressed transcription factors, such as CREB, are phosphorylated by protein kinases, their transcriptional activity is altered and this causes changes in the expression of specific target genes. Among the target genes are those that encode other transcription factors, such as Fos family proteins. Once induced, these transcription factors alter the expression of still other target genes.

The consensus CRE sequence, TGACGTCA, illustrates the palindromic nature of many transcription factor binding sites: the DNA sequence of the site's two complementary DNA strands, which run in opposite directions, are identical **4-26**. Many regulatory elements are perfect or approximate palindromes because many transcription factors bind to DNA as dimers, whereby each member is responsible for recognizing half of the binding site. While the idealized CRE site is a palindrome, several (nonpalindromic) variations in the sequence exist in CREB-regulated genes.

Regulation of CREB by cAMP, Ca²⁺, and growth factors cAMP, Ca²⁺, and growth factors activate CREB by causing its phosphorylation at ser133. cAMP activates protein kinase A, whereas Ca²⁺ activates Ca²⁺/calmodulin-dependent protein kinase IV, both of which phosphorylate ser133 **4-25**. CREB is also phosphorylated on ser133 by a growth factor–activated kinase, known as ribosomal S6 kinase (specifically RSK-90), which is phosphorylated and activated by MAP-kinases. The activation of CREB thereby illustrates a striking convergence of

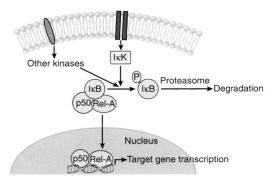

4-24 **Regulation of NFκB.** An active NFκB transcription factor complex (composed of p50 and Rel-A) is retained in the cytoplasm, where it is inactive, by IκB. Cellular signals activate NFκB via phosphorylation of IκB, which leads to its rapid degradation. p50-Rel-A is then free to enter the nucleus where it binds to its specific response elements and regulates the transcription of specific target genes. Phosphorylation of IκB is catalyzed in most cases by IκK (I kappa kinase), which in turn is activated via receptors for inflammatory cytokines, such as tumor necrosis factor. Other cellular kinases can also lead to NFκB activation via indirect actions that lead to IκK activation.

several signaling pathways on the phosphorylation of a single amino acid residue in the protein. As mentioned earlier, such phosphorylation of CREB activates it by enabling its interaction with CBP. CREB contains sites other than ser133 that can be phosphorylated, which may assist in fine-tuning the regulation of CREB-mediated transcription.

CREB mediation of neural plasticity   The activation of a single transcription factor by convergent signaling pathways is particularly important in the nervous system because it may represent a mechanism for long-term neural adaptations. A case in point is learning and memory, which depend on the temporally coordinated arrival of two different signals that subsequently must be integrated in target neurons and their circuits. CREB has been shown to be important for learning and memory in several species. Genetic knockout of CREB in *Aplysia*, *Drosophila*, and rodents impairs the formation of new memory, while overexpression of wildtype or constitutively active forms of CREB causes the opposite effects. Likewise, CREB is required for cellular models of learning and memory, such as long-term potentiation. The role of CREB in these processes is discussed in greater detail in Chapter 13.

CREB-like proteins   CREB, like many transcription factors, is a member of a large family of related proteins. Other members of this family may compensate for CREB when it is inactivated, and also provide independent forms of positive and negative gene regulation. Among the proteins that are closely related to CREB are *activating transcription factors* (ATFs) and *CRE modulators* (CREMs), which are generated by distinct genes. Several alternative splice forms of CREB, ATFs, and CREMs have been identified. All of these proteins bind CREs as dimers, and many can heterodimerize with CREB itself. The similarities between ATF1 and

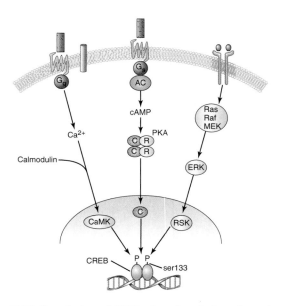

4-25 **Regulation of CREB phosphorylation.** Several signaling pathways converge on the phosphorylation of CREB at a single serine residue (ser133). Neurotransmitters that stimulate adenylyl cyclase (AC) increase CREB phosphorylation by activating protein kinase A (PKA). Activated PKA catalytic subunits translocate to the nucleus, where they phosphorylate (P) ser133. Neurotransmitters that inhibit adenylyl cyclase cause the opposite cascade and inhibit CREB phosphorylation. Increased Ca^{2+} permeates the nucleus, where it activates Ca^{2+}/calmodulin-dependent protein kinases (CaMK), particularly CaMK IV, which phosphorylate ser133. Growth factor regulated pathways also lead to CREB phosphorylation by means of the Ras–Raf–MEK pathway that leads to the activation of extracellular signal–regulated kinases (ERKs). ERKs translocate to the nucleus and phosphorylate and activate ribosomal S6 kinase (RSK), which in turn phosphorylates ser133.

Cyclic AMP response element

$\longrightarrow$

5´ TGACGTCA 3´
3´ ACTGCAGT 5´

$\longleftarrow$

AP-1 element

5´ TGACTCA 3´
3´ ACTGAGT 5´

4-26 **The palindromic structure of consensus CREs and AP-1 elements.** Palindromes or near palindromes are common features of regulatory elements that bind transcription factors as dimers. In general, perfect palindromes are the strongest binding sites for these factors. An intact CGTCA sequence (*arrows*) may be an absolute requirement for CREs.

CREB are especially striking because both are activated by cAMP and Ca^{2+} signaling pathways. Many ATF proteins and CREM isoforms also appear to activate transcription; however, some CREMs, such as ICER, act to repress it, as stated earlier.

The dimerization domain used by CREB proteins, and several other families of transcription factors, is called a leucine zipper, mentioned above. This domain is composed of an α helix in which every seventh residue is a leucine; the leucines line up along one face of the α helix 2 turns apart. The aligned leucines of the two dimerization partners interact hydrophobically to stabilize the dimer. The many proteins, in addition to CREB, that utilize these mechanisms of dimerization belong to a superfamily known as basic-leucine zipper, or bZIP, proteins.

AP-1 Family of Transcription Factors

AP-1 (activator protein-1) transcription factors are indispensable in the regulation of neural gene expression by extracellular signals. AP-1 proteins bind DNA, as heterodimers or homodimers, to the DNA sequence TGACTCA, which is called the AP-1 sequence. This consensus sequence is a heptamer that forms a palindrome flanking a central C or G base (see **4-26**). Although it differs from the CRE sequence by only a single base, AP-1 sites strongly prefer AP-1 proteins as opposed to CREB, which requires an intact CGTCA sequence. As a result, this single base difference between CRE and AP-1 sites significantly influences which transcription factors, and hence which intracellular signaling pathways, can regulate a particular gene. Many genes expressed in the nervous system contain AP-1 sites in their regulatory regions. Among these are genes that encode neuropeptides,

neurotransmitter receptors, neurotransmitter synthetic enzymes, and cytoskeletal proteins.

AP-1 transcription factors bind to DNA as dimers that comprise two families of proteins, Fos and Jun, both of which are bZIP proteins. The known members of the Fos family are c-Fos, FRA1, FRA2, and FosB and its alternative spliced variant ΔFosB. The known members of the Jun family are c-Jun, JunB, and JunD. Most AP-1 complexes are formed by one Fos family member and one Jun family member. Unlike Fos proteins, certain Jun proteins also can form homodimers that bind to AP-1 sites, albeit with far lower affinity than Fos-Jun heterodimers. Transcriptional regulation is further complicated by the fact that some AP-1 proteins can heterodimerize, by means of the leucine zipper, with members of the CREB–ATF family. AP-1 proteins also can form higher order complexes with apparently unrelated families of transcription factors. They can, for example, complex with and inhibit the transcriptional activity of steroid hormone receptors.

Among Fos and Jun proteins, only JunD is expressed constitutively at high levels in many cell types. The other AP-1 proteins tend to be expressed at low or even undetectable levels under basal conditions, but with stimulation may be induced to high levels of expression. Thus, unlike regulation by constitutively expressed transcription factors such as CREB, regulation by most Fos/Jun heterodimers requires new transcription and translation of the transcription factors themselves. Most AP-1 proteins have short half-lives, which means that they exert highly transient effects of some stimulus on gene expression. An exception is ΔFosB which, unlike all other Fos family proteins, is highly stable and thereby can mediate relatively persistent changes in gene expression **4-27**. Accordingly, ΔFosB has been implicated in long-lasting neural and behavioral plasticity, in particular, drug addiction (Chapter 15).

Activation of cellular genes by AP-1 The genes that encode most AP-1 transcription factors are termed immediate early genes (IEGs). IEGs, a prototype of which is the c-Fos gene, are activated rapidly (within minutes) and transiently and do not require new protein synthesis. Late response genes, in contrast, are induced or repressed more slowly (over hours) and depend on the synthesis of new proteins. The term IEG initially applied to viral genes in eukaryotic cells that are activated immediately after infection by commandeering host cell transcription factors. Viral IEGs generally encode transcription factors that activate the late expression of viral genes.

The application of IEG terminology to nonviral genes has created some confusion. Many cellular genes

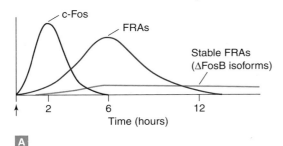

A

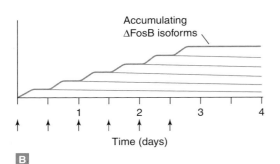

B

4-27 **Changes in the composition of AP-1 complexes over time. A.** Several waves of Fos family proteins are induced by acute stimuli in neurons. c-Fos, which is induced most rapidly, degrades within several hours; several others, such as FosB, ΔFosB, FRA1, and FRA2, are induced somewhat later and persist somewhat longer than c-Fos. A portion of the acutely induced ΔFosB is stabilized by phosphorylation, which allows the protein to persist in the brain. **B.** With repeated stimulation, each stimulus induces a low level of stabilized ΔFosB isoforms, as indicated by the horizontal lines. The result is a gradual increase in total ΔFosB levels, as indicated by the stepped line; such an increase gradually induces significant levels of a long-lasting AP-1 complex, which may underlie long-lasting forms of neural plasticity in the brain.

are induced independently of protein synthesis but with a time course whose duration is between that of classic IEGs and late response genes. Moreover, many cellular genes that are regulated as IEGs encode proteins that are not transcription factors; for example, any gene induced by CREB could potentially show temporal features of induction of an IEG. Despite these complications, the concept of IEG-encoded transcription factors has assisted our understanding of gene regulation in the nervous system. In addition, several IEGs (in particular, c-Fos itself) have been used as cellular markers of neural activation because of their rapid induction from low basal levels in response

to neuronal depolarization and various second messenger and growth factor pathways **4-28**.

Activation by multiple signaling pathways   The best characterized cellular IEG is c-Fos. Because this gene contains binding sites for CREB **4-29**, it is not surprising that it can be activated rapidly by neurotransmitters or drugs that stimulate the cAMP or Ca^{2+} pathways. The c-Fos gene also can be induced by the Ras/MAP-kinase pathway, discussed earlier in this chapter. This activation may occur in part via phosphorylation and activation of CREB by RSK. However, growth factor induction of c-Fos also occurs via a CREB-independent mechanism: subtypes of ERK translocate into the nucleus where they phosphorylate the transcription factor Elk-1 (also called the ternary complex factor, or TCF). Elk-1 subsequently complexes with the serum response factor (SRF) to bind to and activate the serum response element (SRE) in the c-Fos gene (see **4-29**). SREs are also present in many other growth factor-inducible genes.

Still another mechanism of c-Fos induction involves cytokine-activated signaling pathways that trigger the activation of STATs. As previously mentioned, STATs are activated in response to their phosphorylation by protein tyrosine kinases, JAKs, which in turn are activated by a variety of cytokines and other signals, as stated earlier. After they are activated, they form multimeric complexes, translocate to the nucleus, and bind to their specific DNA response elements, called STAT sites. The c-Fos gene (see **4-29**) contains a STAT site (also called SIE [SIF-inducible element]), which mediates the induction of the gene by cytokines. STAT sites are found in many genes expressed in the nervous system.

Regulation by phosphorylation   Several AP-1 proteins are regulated at the posttranslational level by phosphorylation. The best studied example is c-Jun, which is phosphorylated in response to the activation of a MAP-kinase signaling pathway, called SAP-kinases or Jun N-terminal kinases (JNKs), by some form of cellular stress (see **4-15**). JNKs phosphorylate c-Jun in its transcriptional activation domain, and thereby increase its ability to activate transcription. This process has been implicated in the modulation of synaptic transmission and may, under unique circumstances, trigger the activation of apoptosis (programmed cell death) pathways (Chapter 17).

Steroid Hormone Receptor Superfamily

Steroid hormones (eg, **glucocorticoids, estrogen, testosterone,** and **mineralocorticoids**) and related

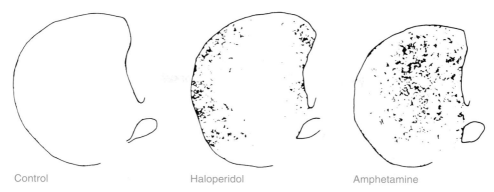

Control   Haloperidol   Amphetamine

4–28 **Example of using c-Fos induction to map patterns of neuronal activation in the brain.** Acute administration of cocaine (a drug of abuse; see Chapter 15) or haloperidol (an antipsychotic drug; see Chapter 16) induces c-Fos in striatum, but with different patterns. Cocaine induces c-Fos more medially, while haloperidol induces c-Fos more laterally. These findings have provided insight into the subtypes of striatal neurons affected by these 2 drug treatments.

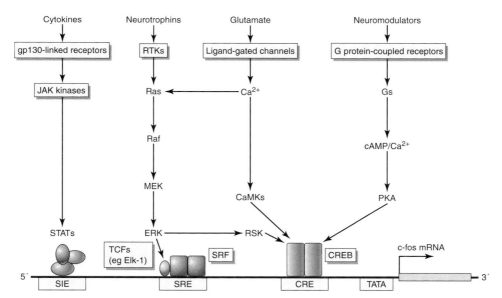

4–29 **Regulatory region of the c-Fos gene.** A CRE site binds CREB, a serum response element (SRE) binds serum response factor (SRF) and ternary complex factor (TCF or Elk-1), and a SIF-inducible element (SIE) binds STAT proteins; these three elements represent a small number of all known transcription factor–binding sites. Proteins that bind at these sites are constitutively present in cells and are activated by phosphorylation. CREB can be activated by protein kinase A, Ca^{2+}/calmodulin-dependent protein kinases (CaMKs), or ribosomal S6 kinases (RSKs); Elk-1 can be activated by the MAP-kinases ERK1 and ERK2; and the STAT proteins can be activated by the JAK protein tyrosine kinases. Because the activation of c-Fos by any of multiple signaling pathways requires only signal-induced phosphorylation rather than new protein synthesis, it can be triggered rapidly by a wide array of stimuli. RTKs, receptor tyrosine kinases; STATs, signal transducers and activators of transcription; JAK, Janus kinase.

signals (**retinoids, thyroid hormones,** and **vitamin D₃**) are small, lipid-soluble ligands that diffuse readily across cell membranes. Unlike the receptors for peptide hormones, which are located in the cell membrane, the receptors for these ligands are localized in the cytoplasm. In response to ligand binding, steroid hormone receptors translocate to the nucleus, where they regulate the expression of certain genes by binding to specific hormone response elements (HREs) in their regulatory regions. Thus, these receptors are sometimes referred to as the nuclear receptor superfamily. Steroid, thyroid, and retinoid hormones and their nuclear receptors are critical for nervous system function, and are extremely important in CNS pharmacology (Chapters 10 and 14).

The mechanisms by which the glucocorticoid receptor (GR) operates are representative of those utilized by most receptors in this superfamily. Under basal conditions, the GR is retained in the cytoplasm by a large multiprotein complex of chaperone proteins,

including the heat shock protein Hsp90 and the immunophilin Hsp56. After it is bound by glucocorticoid, the GR dissociates from its chaperones, translocates to the nucleus, and subsequently binds to glucocorticoid response elements (GREs). GREs typically are 15 bases in length and consist of 2 palindromic half sites. GRs and related nuclear receptors have a modular structure similar to that of other transcription factors **4–30**. The DNA-binding domain of the GR is characterized by multiple cysteines organized around a central zinc ion, an arrangement often referred to as a zinc finger. Many other transcription factors possess this DNA-binding domain.

GREs can confer either positive or negative regulation on the genes to which they are linked (see **4–30**). A well-characterized negative GRE is located in the proopiomelanocortin gene mentioned above (Chapters 7 and 10); the GRE permits glucocorticoids to repress the gene, which encodes (ACTH), and thus

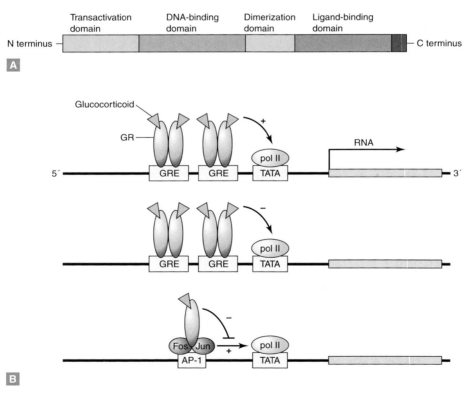

4–30 **The glucocorticoid receptor (GR). A.** GR domains. **B.** Transcriptional regulation by glucocorticoids and the GR. The idealized promoters represented here contain two glucocorticoid response elements (GREs) or one AP-1 site. GRs act on GREs to activate (*top*) or inhibit (*center*) transcription, and also inhibit AP-1-mediated transcription by binding directly to a Fos-Jun dimer (*bottom*). The TATA box binds the general transcription factors required for activation.

acts as an important feedback mechanism by inhibiting further glucocorticoid synthesis.

GRs are responsible for many important physiologic actions that do not appear to be mediated by DNA binding. Rather, they can interfere with transcriptional activity mediated by other transcription factors—particularly those mediated by AP-1 and NF-κB proteins (see 4–30). Glucocorticoids can also interfere with NF-κB activity by inducing expression of IκB, the protein that holds NF-κB in the cytoplasm.

Additional members of the nuclear hormone receptor superfamily have been identified in recent years. Some respond to cholesterol and are important in the regulation of intermediary metabolism. The endogenous ligands for many others are not yet known. Yet there is indirect evidence for their involvement in neural functioning. Nerve growth factor inducible factor B (NGFI-B) and Nurr1, for example, are regulated in the brain by exposure to certain psychotropic drugs, including **cocaine** and **antipsychotic** agents.

Other Transcription Factors

The CREB, AP-1, NF-κB, STAT, and steroid hormone receptor families represent just a small portion of the transcription factors that are expressed in neurons and glia. However, other transcription factors are undoubtedly involved in neural signaling. C/EBP (CAATT enhancing binding protein) and its family members are known to mediate some of the effects of the cAMP pathway on gene expression. Egr family members (eg, Egr-1/Zif268/NGFI-A) are zinc finger transcription factors that, like c-Fos, are induced rapidly and transiently in the brain by stimuli whose temporal features resemble those of IEGs. The induction of Egr family proteins has been correlated with induction of hippocampal long-term potentiation (Chapter 13); however, the target genes of these proteins remain poorly characterized. Circadian genes, the prototype of which is Clock, are transcription factors that control diurnal variations in cell function through the regulation of gene expression (Chapter 12).

The functional mechanisms addressed in this chapter are far more intricate than their descriptions suggest. Regulatory regions of genes are often far longer than the coding regions of genes, and regulatory information is contained not only in the 5′ promoter regions of genes but also in transcribed sequences and in 3′ untranscribed regions. Moreover, within the 5′ regions, this chapter focuses on a relatively small number of response elements. Any given gene likely contains many regulatory sites, and these sites do not

---

4–5 **Trancription Factors as Drug Targets**

Most medications used in neurology and psychiatry act directly on neurotransmitter receptors or on proteins that influence levels of neurotransmitters, such as transporters and synthetic enzymes. Collectively, these proteins represent a minute fraction of all proteins expressed in neurons. This diversity currently is being exploited for the development of pharmaceutical agents.

Transcription factors and other proteins involved in the regulation of gene expression may represent viable targets for drugs, particularly if they are expressed in a limited number of cell types or if they exhibit unique temporal patterns (see ΔFosB in 4–27). Conversely, transcription factors such as CREB or c-Fos would not be useful for this purpose because they are ubiquitous. However, efforts to exploit any of these proteins should not be hampered by their location in the nucleus; most drugs that penetrate the blood–brain barrier also cross cell and nuclear membranes.

Although it remains unclear whether protein–DNA binding sites represent suitable targets for drugs, we know that protein–protein interaction domains can be targeted by small molecules. Because most transcription factors bind DNA as dimers or multimeric complexes, these interaction domains may possess the diversity and specificity characteristic of successful pharmaceutical targets. An example is provided by the **thiazolidinedione** drugs, which are used to treat adult-onset (insulin-resistant) **diabetes.** These drugs bind to and activate peroxisome proliferator-activated receptor-γ (PPARγ), a member of the steroid hormone superfamily of nuclear receptors. The PPARγ–thiazolidinedione complex dimerizes with retinoid X receptor (RXR)—another member of the nuclear receptor family—and the dimer binds to target response elements in DNA. Among the genes that contain such response elements are those that encode for proteins that enhance sensitivity to insulin.

function in isolation but influence one another. Consequently the temporal and spatial synthesis of multiple signaling pathways affects the expression of most genes. Unraveling this complexity is a daunting task, particularly in vivo, but is likely to yield important clues for understanding neural and behavioral plasticity. One goal of future research, outlined in **4-5**, is to take advantage of the enormous complexity and specificity of these mechanisms to generate agents that act more rapidly and more effectively in the treatment of neuropsychiatric disorders.

SELECTED READING

Alarcon JM, Malleret G, Touzani K, et al. Chromatin acetylation, memory, and LTP are impaired in CBP+/− mice: a model for the cognitive deficit in Rubinstein-Taybi syndrome and its amelioration. *Neuron.* 2004;42:947–959.

Alonso A, Sasin J, Bottini N, et al. Protein tyrosine phosphatases in the human genome. *Cell.* 2004;117: 699–711.

Carlezon WA Jr, Duman RS, Nestler EJ. The many faces of CREB. *Trends Neurosci.* 2005;28:436–445.

Chasse SA, Dohlman HG. RGS proteins: G protein-coupled receptors meet their match. *Assay Drug Dev Technol.* 2003;1:357–364.

Cooper DM, Crossthwaite AJ. Higher-order organization and regulation of adenylyl cyclases. *Trends Pharmacol Sci.* 2006;27:426–431.

Felsenfeld G, Groudine M. Controlling the double helix. *Nature.* 2003;421:448–453.

Impey S, McCorkle SR, Cha-Molstad H, et al. Defining the CREB regulon: a genome-wide analysis of transcription factor regulator regions. *Cell.* 2004;119: 1041–1054.

Kaplan DR, Miller FD. Neurotrophin signal transduction in the nervous system. *Curr Opin Neurobiol.* 2000;10:381–391.

Karin M, Yamamoto Y, Wang QM. The IKK NF-kappa B system: a treasure trove for drug development. *Nature Rev Drug Disc.* 2004;3:17–26.

Lachner M, O'Sullivan RJ, Jenuwein T. An epigenetic road map for histone lysine methylation. *J Cell Sci.* 2003;116:2117–2124.

Levenson JM, Sweatt JD. Epigenetic mechanisms in memory formation. *Nature Rev Neurosci.* 2005;6: 108–118.

Mayr B, Montminy M. Transcriptional regulation by the phosphorylation-dependent factor CREB. *Nature Rev Mol Cell Biol.* 2001;2:599–609.

Mehats C, Andersen CB, Filopanti M, Jin SL, Conti M. Cyclic nucleotide phosphodiesterases and their role in endocrine cell signaling. *Trends Endocrinol Metab.* 2002;13:29–35.

Moretti P, Zoghbi HY. MeCP2 dysfunction in Rett syndrome and related disorders. *Curr Opin Gen Dev.* 2006;16:276–281.

Persengiev SP, Green MR. The role of ATF/CREB family members in cell growth, survival and apoptosis. *Apoptosis.* 2003;8:225–228.

Pierce KL, Lefkowitz RJ. Classical and new roles of beta-arrestins in the regulation of G-protein-coupled receptors. *Nature Rev Neurosci.* 2001;2:727–733.

Preininger AM, Hamm HE. G protein signaling: insights from new structures. *Sci STKE.* 2004;218:re3.

Siegel GJ, Albers RW, Brady ST, Price DL. *Basic Neurochemistry*, 7th ed. New York: Academic Press; 2006:335–346.

Smith FD, Langeberg LK, Scott JD. The where's and when's of kinase anchoring. *Trends Biochem Sci.* 2006;31:316–323.

Soderling SH, Beavo JA. Regulation of cAMP and cGMP signaling: new phosphodiesterases and new functions. *Curr Opin Cell Biol.* 2000;12:174–179.

Soderling TR, Stull JT. Structure and regulation of calcium/calmodulin-dependent protein kinases. *Chem Rev.* 2001;101:2341–2352.

Sunahara RK, Dessauer CW, Gilman AG. Complexity and diversity of mammalian adenylyl cyclases. *Annu Rev Pharmacol Toxicol.* 1996;36:461–480.

Susio J, Levin DB, de Amorim GV, Bakker S, Macleod PM. Syndromes of disordered chromatin remodeling. *Clin Genet.* 2003;64:83–95.

Svenningsson P, Nishi A, Fisone G, Girault JA, Nairn AC, Greengard P. DARPP-32: an integrator of neurotransmission. *Annu Rev Pharmacol Toxicol.* 2004;44: 269–296.

Thomas GM, Huganir RL. MAPK cascade signalling and synaptic plasticity. *Nature Rev Neurosci.* 2004;5:173-183.

Tsankova N, Renthal W, Kumar A, Nestler EJ. 2007. Epigenetic mechanisms and psychiatry disorders. *Nature Rev Neurosci.* 2007;8:355–367.

Van Aelst L, Cline HT. Rho GTPases and activity-dependent dendrite development. *Curr Opin Neurobiol.* 2004;14:297–304.

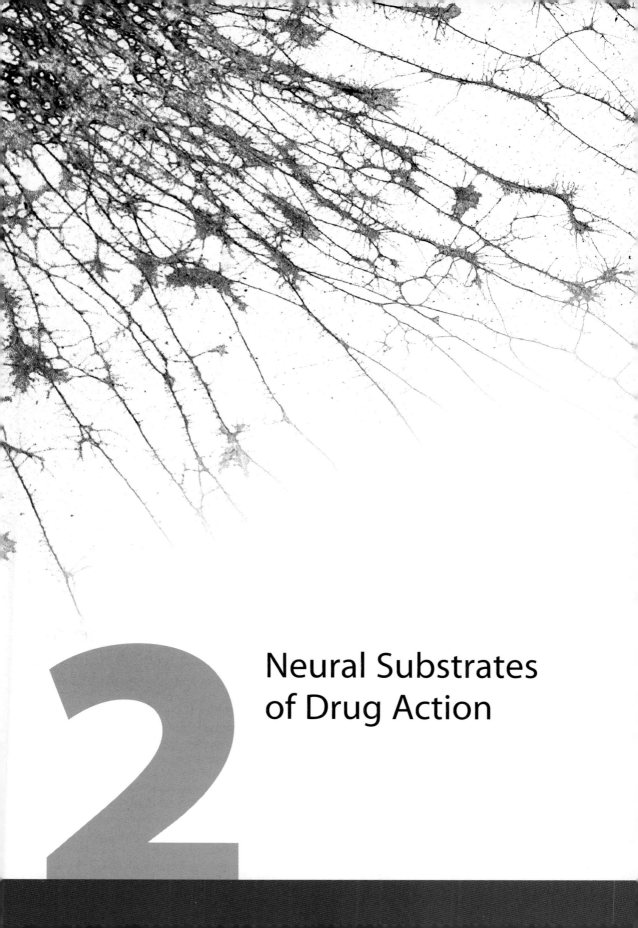

2

Neural Substrates
of Drug Action

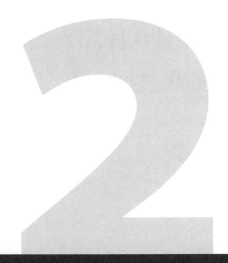

CHAPTER 5

Excitatory and Inhibitory Amino Acids

KEY CONCEPTS

- The major excitatory neurotransmitter in the brain is glutamate; the major inhibitory neurotransmitter is GABA.

- Glutamate receptors comprise two large families, ligand-gated ion channels called ionotropic receptors and G protein-coupled receptors called metabotropic receptors.

- Ionotropic glutamate receptors are divided into three classes—AMPA receptors, kainate receptors, and NMDA receptors—which are named after synthetic ligands that activate them. Individual excitatory synapses typically express several different subtypes of ionotropic glutamate receptors as well as metabotropic receptors.

- In contrast to AMPA receptors and kainate receptors, the NMDA receptor has two important biophysical properties. Because it is highly permeable to calcium and is voltage dependent, it allows calcium entry only if the cell is depolarized.

- AMPA receptors mediate the vast majority of excitatory synaptic transmission in the brain, whereas NMDA receptors play an important role in triggering synaptic plasticity and, when overactivated, in triggering excitotoxicity.

- The eight different subtypes of metabotropic glutamate receptors, when localized to the presynaptic terminal, inhibit neurotransmitter release, and when localized to the postsynaptic membrane, exert complex modulatory effects through specific signal transduction cascades.

- The most extensively studied form of synaptic plasticity is long-term potentiation (LTP) in the hippocampus, which is triggered by strong activation of NMDA receptors and the consequent large rise in postsynaptic calcium concentration.

- Long-term depression (LTD), a long-lasting decrease in synaptic strength, also occurs at most excitatory and some inhibitory synapses in the brain.

- The $GABA_A$ receptor, a ligand-gated chloride channel, and the $GABA_B$ receptor, a G protein–coupled receptor, are the two major classes of GABA receptors.

- $GABA_A$ receptors, which are highly heterogeneous, mediate the bulk of inhibitory synaptic transmission in the brain. A number of drugs, most notably benzodiazepines and barbiturates, bind to $GABA_A$ receptors and enhance their function.

- $GABA_B$ receptors are localized both presynaptically, where they inhibit neurotransmitter release, and postsynaptically, where they mediate a slow, inhibitory synaptic response.

- Glycine, like GABA, is an inhibitory neurotransmitter that activates receptors that are ligand-gated chloride channels. It is critical in inhibitory neurotransmission in the spinal cord and brainstem.

Amino acids are the building blocks of proteins involved in normal intermediary metabolism, but they can also function as neurotransmitters. The amino acids glutamate and, to a much lesser extent, aspartate mediate most of the fast excitatory synaptic transmission in the brain; likewise, the amino acids γ-aminobutyric acid (GABA) and, to a lesser extent, glycine mediate most fast inhibitory synaptic transmission. Excitatory amino acids are utilized by nearly every information-bearing circuit in the brain and have been implicated in such diverse pathologic processes as **epilepsy, ischemic brain damage, anxiety,** and **addiction**. In addition, they are necessary for the development of normal synaptic connections. Consequently, amino acid neurotransmitters have been the subject of intensive research during the past two decades.

GLUTAMATE

The Major Excitatory Neurotransmitter

Long before glutamate's role in neurotransmission was established, investigators observed that glutamate excites most neurons in the CNS. In fact, it is responsible for most neurotransmitter action at excitatory amino acid receptors. Glutamate is present in high concentrations in the adult CNS and is released in a Ca^{2+}-dependent manner by electrical stimulation. Enzymes responsible for glutamate synthesis and degradation are located in both neurons and glial cells, as are high-affinity glutamate receptors and excitatory amino acid reuptake transporters (EAATs), which terminate the synaptic actions of glutamate. Many of these reuptake and receptor proteins also respond to aspartate, which is believed to mediate transmission at a small number of central excitatory synapses.

Synthetic and Degradative Pathways

Glutamate and aspartate are charged amino acids and therefore do not cross the blood–brain barrier. As a result, they must be synthesized in the brain from glucose and a variety of other precursors. Glutamate, which is the reduced form of glutamic acid, is in a metabolic pool with α-oxoglutaric acid and glutamine. Glutamate that is destined to be used for neurotransmission is packaged into synaptic vesicles and released from nerve terminals in response to nerve impulses **5-1**. After it is released, glutamate is primarily taken up by glial cells, where it is converted into glutamine by glutamine synthetase. The resulting glutamine is transported out of glia by system N-1 (SN1), a Na^+- and H^+-dependent pump that is homologous to the vesicular GABA transporter (VGAT). Glutamine is subsequently taken up by neurons, by means of a transport process that remains poorly described, and is converted back into glutamate by glutaminase. As discussed later in this chapter, glutamine also replenishes the transmitter pool of GABA.

Release and Reuptake

Synaptic vesicles actively accumulate glutamate through a Mg^{2+}- and adenosine triphosphate (ATP)-dependent uptake process that is driven by an electrical gradient across their membranes. During uptake, concentrations of glutamate in these vesicles likely exceed 20 mM. Substances that destroy the electrochemical gradient across vesicular membranes prevent the transporters from concentrating this amino acid. The three isoforms of the vesicular glutamate transporter, VGluT1-3, are highly selective with a high affinity for glutamate and a low affinity for aspartate. When an action potential arrives in the presynaptic terminal of a neuron, it initiates a complex cascade that results in the fusion of synaptic vesicles with the presynaptic membrane and the release of glutamate into the synaptic cleft (Chapter 3). Glutamate then freely diffuses across this narrow cleft to interact with its corresponding receptors on the postsynaptic face of an adjacent cell.

The reuptake of glutamate and aspartate serves to control the extracellular concentrations of these amino acids in the CNS. Na^+-dependent glutamate plasma membrane transporters are coupled to electrochemical gradients for Na^+, K^+, and H^+ **5-1**. Because such coupling permits the transport of glutamate and aspartate against their concentration gradients, glutamate transporters are capable of decreasing extracellular glutamate concentrations to submicromolar levels. These transporters take up glutamate and aspartate with similar affinity and maximum velocity (V_{max}). Glutamate transport is electrogenic resulting in the net inward movement of positive charge during each transport cycle.

Four principal members of the high-affinity Na^+-dependent family of glutamate plasma membrane transporters have been cloned from rat and salamander: GLAST (glutamate-aspartate transporter), GLT-1 (glutamate transporter-1), EAAC1 (excitatory amino acid carrier-1), and sEAAT5 (salamander excitatory amino acid transporter-5). The human homologs of these transporters are EAAT1, EAAT2, EAAT3, and EAAT5, respectively; in addition, EAAT4 has been cloned from human motor cortex. Each of these

Presynaptic neuron

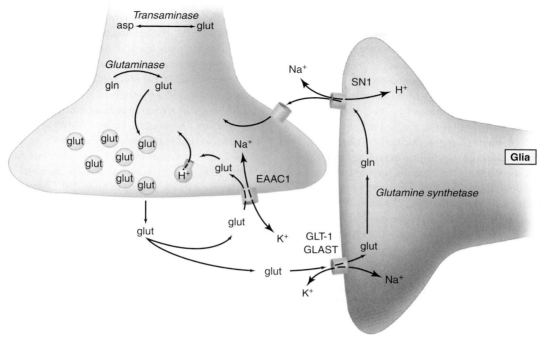

5–1 **Synthesis and degradation of the neurotransmitter pool of glutamate.** In the mitochondrial compartment of glutamatergic nerve terminals, glutamine (gln) is converted to glutamate (glut) by the enzyme glutaminase. Alternatively, glutamate is synthesized by the transamination of aspartate (asp) by transaminase. Newly synthesized glutamate is packaged into synaptic vesicles by means of a Mg^{2+}- and ATP-dependent proton gradient–coupled uptake process. After it is released from nerve terminals, most of it is taken up into glial cells, where it is converted into glutamine by glutamine synthetase. Glutamine is then pumped out of the glia by SN1 and taken up by nerve terminals, where it is converted back to glutamate to replenish the transmitter pool. Uptake of glutamate into glial (and, to a lesser extent, neural) compartments is achieved by the Na^+-dependent glutamate transporters GLT-1, GLAST, and EAAC1.

transporters belongs to a large superfamily whose members transport a wide range of neurotransmitters and related substances. The transporters GLAST and GLT-1, which are expressed by glial cells, appear to be responsible for the majority of glutamate reuptake in the CNS (see **5–1**).

Several pathologic conditions, such as **ischemia,** can lead to the accumulation of glutamate or aspartate in extracellular spaces, which results in the excessive activation of glutamate receptors (Chapters 17 and 19). Such activation can in turn cause a variety of pathologic changes and can, in its extreme form, result in cell death. Glutamate transporters limit the concentrations of free glutamate and aspartate in extracellular spaces, and thereby prevent the excessive stimulation

of glutamate receptors. Consequently, agents capable of facilitating transporter function might limit the damage caused by ischemia and other neurologic insults that cause extracellular glutamate to increase. Currently, however, only inhibitors of glutamate transporters are available. Two such inhibitors are D,L-threo-3-hydroxyaspartate (**THA**), a broad-spectrum antagonist of glutamate and aspartate transport, and dihydrokainate (**DHK**), an inhibitor selective for the glial GLT-1 transporter. Although these drugs are useful experimental tools, they have no apparent clinical use.

Glutamate Receptors

Glutamate receptors comprise two large families: the ionotropic and the metabotropic receptors. Ionotropic glutamate receptors contain associated ion channels that are gated by agonist binding. Three classes of ionotropic glutamate receptors, N-methyl-D-aspartate (**NMDA**), α-amino-3-hydroxy-5-methyl-4-isoxazole propionic acid (**AMPA**), and **kainate** receptors, were originally named based on the ability of these drugs to serve as selective agonists **5–1**.

Metabotropic glutamate receptors belong to the large superfamily of G protein-coupled receptors. These receptors, which are characterized by seven transmembrane domains, couple to G proteins and in turn mediate the biologic effects of receptor activation (Chapter 4). The term *metabotropic* was used to indicate that these receptors affect cellular biochemical ("metabolic") processes, and do not form ion channels. However, metabotropic glutamate receptors, like other G protein-coupled receptors, can exert profound effects on neuronal function through the regulation of other ion channels, second messenger cascades, and protein phosphorylation.

5–1 Glutamate Receptors

Ionotropic

Functional Classes	Gene Families	Agonists	Antagonists
AMPA	GluR1	Glutamate	CNQX
	GluR2	AMPA	NBQX
	GluR3	Kainate	GYK153655
	GluR4	(S)-5-fluorowillardine	
Kainate	GluR5	Glutamate	CNQX
	GluR6	Kainate	LY294486
	GluR7	ATPA	
	KA1		
	KA2		
NMDA	NR1	Glutamate	D-AP5, D-APV
	NR2A	Aspartate	2R-CPPene
	NR2B	NMDA	MK-801
	NR2C		Ketamine
	NR2D		Phencyclidine

Metabotropic

Group I	mGluR1	1S, 3R-ACPD	AIDA
	mGluR5	DHPG	CBPG
Group II	mGluR2	1S, 3R-ACPD	EGLU
	mGluR3	DCG-IV	PCCG-4
		APDC	
Group III	mGluR4	L-AP4	MAP4
	mGluR6	1S, 3R-ACPD	MPPG
	mGluR7		
	mGluR8		

Mediation of fast excitatory transmission

Synaptically released glutamate interacts with postsynaptic receptors located on immediately adjacent cells or on the presynaptic nerve terminals from which glutamate is released. The binding of glutamate to AMPA and NMDA receptors opens postsynaptic cation channels and initiates a two-component excitatory postsynaptic current (EPSC) at most central synapses **5–2**. Considerable evidence suggests that AMPA and NMDA receptors colocalize at most functional excitatory synapses. However, the ratio of AMPA to NMDA receptors at individual synapses can vary greatly; indeed, some synapses may contain only NMDA or AMPA receptors. In contrast, smaller numbers of kainate receptors are present in most CNS regions.

The activation of an AMPA receptor mediates a synaptic current that has a rapid onset and decay, whereas the current mediated by an NMDA receptor has a slower onset and a decay that lasts as long as several hundred milliseconds (see **5–2**). The decay time of the NMDA receptor-mediated current is approximately 100 times longer than the mean open time of its channel. Such prolonged activation is believed to be caused by glutamate's high affinity ($K_d = 3$–$8\ \mu M$) for and consequent slow dissociation from these receptors. In contrast, glutamate has a much lower affinity for AMPA receptors ($K_d = 200\ \mu M$), from which it rapidly dissociates.

AMPA receptors will respond to single vesicles of glutamate. NDMA receptors, however, because of their special voltage dependence (described later in this chapter), require coordinated input from many synapses for substantial activation. This allows NMDA receptors to act as coincidence detectors that can sense the activity of many independent synaptic inputs converging on the same cell **5–3**.

AMPA Receptors

Current is carried through AMPA receptors primarily by the movement of Na^+ from the extracellular space into the intracellular compartment. However, because the reversal potential of current (the membrane potential at which net current flow is zero; see Chapter 2) through AMPA channels is close to 0 mV, an outward current carried by K^+ must counterbalance the inward flow of Na^+ ions. The resulting current-voltage relationship for these AMPA receptors is roughly linear (see **5–2**).

Some AMPA receptors, on both neurons and astrocytes, are also permeable to Ca^{2+}. The translocation of Ca^{2+} from the extracellular space to the intracellular compartment plays a key role in the regulation of several second messenger systems. Thus the permeability

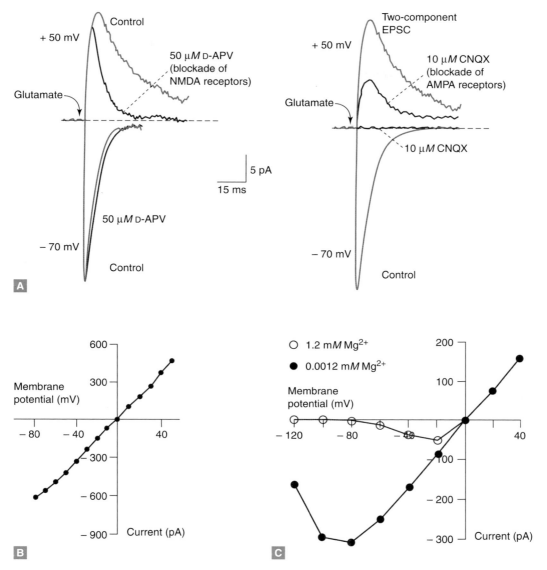

5-2 Synaptically released glutamate interacts with postsynaptic AMPA and NMDA receptors. **A.** Excitatory post-synaptic currents (EPSCs) caused by glutamate in a hippocampal neuron. When glutamate binds to NMDA and AMPA receptors, postsynaptic cation channels open, initiating a two-component EPSC. These components can be pharmacologically separated. Blockade of NMDA receptors by the antagonist D-APV (*left*) reveals a rapid AMPA receptor–mediated component of the EPSC. Conversely, blockade of AMPA receptors by CNQX (*right*) reveals a slowly rising and decaying NMDA receptor–mediated component of the EPSC at positive voltages. In contrast, application of D-APV at negative voltages (lower left) reveals little NMDA receptor contribution to the EPSC due to the profound block of these channels by Mg^{2+} ions. **B.** The current–voltage relationship for AMPA receptors. This relationship is roughly linear and reverses at approximately 0 mV, indicating that the channels do not discriminate well between Na^+ and K^+ ions. **C.** The current–voltage relationship for NMDA receptors. The concentration of Mg^{2+} in the extracellular fluid of the brain (approximately 1 mM) is sufficient to virtually abolish ion flux through NMDA receptor channels at membrane potentials close to resting potential (approximately −70 mV). As the membrane potential becomes less negative or even positive, the affinity of Mg^{2+} for its binding site decreases, permitting the passage of ionic current. Removal of extracellular Mg^{2+} linearizes the current–voltage relationship and permits significant current flow at negative voltages.

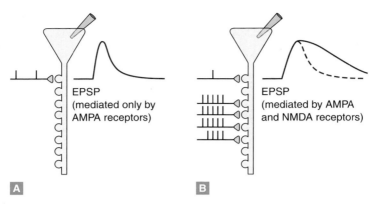

5-3 **The NMDA glutamate receptor as a coincidence detector.** **A.** A single synaptic input results in the generation of a short-lasting excitatory postsynaptic potential (EPSP) that is mediated entirely by AMPA receptors. **B.** When multiple inputs occur simultaneously, the same single synaptic input generates a longer-lasting EPSP that is mediated by both AMPA and NMDA receptors. Thus the NMDA receptor can "sense" the activity in adjacent inputs.

of some AMPA receptors to Ca^{2+} may have great functional importance, particularly in cells that do not contain NMDA receptors (which can always flux Ca^{2+}). AMPA receptor channels that are permeable to Ca^{2+} exhibit an inwardly rectifying type of current–voltage relationship; they pass current readily in the inward direction but not in the outward direction. This occurs because intracellular **polyamines** such as **spermine** and **spermidine**, which associate with the channel, prohibit outward current from passing through.

All AMPA receptors can be blocked selectively by certain quinoxaline diones, the most notable of which is 6-nitro-7-sulphamobenzo-quinoxaline 2,3-dione (**NBQX;** see **5-1**). NBQX is a potent competitive antagonist of AMPA receptors; which is reasonably selective for AMPA receptors over kainate receptors. Drugs in the 2,3-benzodiazepine class, such as **GYKI 53655,** are noncompetitive, selective antagonists of AMPA receptors and show promise as neuroprotective drugs for the treatment of **stroke.** Because it has minimal effects on kainate or NMDA receptors, this class of drug permits unequivocal separation of the AMPA receptors from other categories of glutamate receptors.

AMPA and kainite receptors desensitize within milliseconds of exposure to agonist and can be reliably distinguished from one another by their response to two drugs, **cyclothiazide** and the lectin **concanavalin A.** Cyclothiazide relieves AMPA receptor desensitization but does not affect kainate receptors. In contrast, concanavalin A relieves the desensitization of kainate receptors, most likely by interacting with surface sugar chains, but does not have significant effects on AMPA receptors.

The possibility that enhancement of AMPA receptor function may be beneficial therapeutically has received increased attention with the development of a family of compounds termed **AMPAkines** or **AMPA potentiators.** They enhance AMPA receptor–mediated excitatory synaptic transmission by slowing deactivation or desensitization of the receptors, with the former mechanism appearing to be more functionally important. Clinical trials are currently being conducted in a wide range of neuropsychiatric disorders (eg, **Alzheimer disease**, **attention deficit hyperactivity disorder** or **ADHD**) to determine whether this class of compound may be clinically useful.

Molecular composition of AMPA receptors
Three families of ionotropic glutamate receptor subunits, encoded by at least 16 genes, assemble to form functional AMPA, NMDA, or kainate receptors (see **5-1**). Within each family there is greater than 80% identity at the amino acid level over membrane spanning domains. Between families, a lower degree of identity exists (~50%). Ionotropic glutamate receptors are believed to exist as tetramers. Different subunit combinations produce functionally different glutamate receptors. Moreover, there are striking regional differences in the expression of genes that encode these subunits.

Four subunits, termed GluR1 through GluR4 (also known as GluRA through GluRD), coassemble to form AMPA receptors. Each of these subunits is encoded by a distinct gene, and each exists in two forms, termed *flip* and *flop*. The flip and flop forms, which are generated by alternative splicing, exhibit region-specific patterns of expression in the brain, and give rise to receptors that differ in desensitization rates. The best characterized AMPA receptor subunit is GluR1, which is predicted to be 889 amino acids long; other ionotropic receptor subunits, such as those of nicotinic, $GABA_A$, or glycine receptors, are approximately 420 amino acids long. The extra length of GluRs results from unusually large N-terminal extracellular domains.

AMPA and kainate glutamate receptor families have a topology that differs from that of certain other ligand-gated ion channels, such as $GABA_A$ and glycine receptors 5-4. Glutamate receptor subunits possess

only three transmembrane spanning domains. What appears to be an abridged transmembrane domain (TM), located between TM2 and TM3 in glutamate subunits, is a reentrant loop whose ends both face the cytoplasm. Homology mapping of glutamate receptors suggests that agonist binding requires portions of both the large N terminus and the short region between TM1 and TM2 (see 5-4).

AMPA receptors lacking the GluR2 subunit are highly permeable to Ca^{2+} ions and are commonly found on GABAergic inhibitory interneurons throughout the brain. This Ca^{2+} permeability has been traced to a single amino acid in the reentrant loop of GluR2, which is known as the Q/R site (see 5-4). In GluR1, GluR3, and GluR4, a glutamine (Q) resides at this position, but in GluR2 an arginine (R) is present. When heteromeric receptors contain GluR2 they are relatively impermeable to Ca^{2+}, most likely because the positive charge of the arginine residue repels Ca^{2+} from the channel pore. The replacement of glutamine with arginine in GluR2 occurs because of a process called *RNA editing*: the gene for GluR2 encodes a glutamine, and the unedited form of GluR2 is expressed in various regions of the brain during development. However, virtually all of the GluR2 mRNA present in adult mammalian brain is edited to a codon that encodes arginine at this site. This editing changes a single base within GluR2 transcripts. Inhibition of such RNA editing in mice by molecular genetic means can be lethal, presumably because many AMPA receptors that normally are Ca^{2+} impermeable become Ca^{2+} permeable, making cells vulnerable to the neurotoxic effects of excessive intracellular Ca^{2+}.

In addition to Ca^{2+} permeability, the Q/R site of GluR2 influences the single channel conductance properties of associated AMPA receptors and the sensitivity of the receptor complex to blockage by **polyamine spider toxins** and endogenous **polyamines**. AMPA receptors that do not contain edited GluR2 show greater overall conductance. In addition, there is voltage-dependent inhibition of outward current flow by endogenous intracellular polyamines at positive membrane potentials giving rise to the inward rectification that is characteristic of GluR2-lacking AMPA receptors.

The flip and flop splice variants of receptor subunits GluR1 through GluR4, together with the products of Q/R editing, yield a wide range of AMPA receptor subunit proteins. This diversity provides neurons with an extraordinary degree of flexibility in the construction of AMPA receptors. The degree of AMPA receptor heterogeneity employed by neurons in vivo remains unknown. Ca^{2+}-permeable AMPA receptors

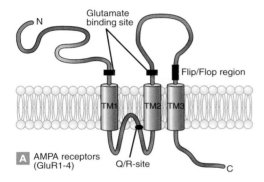

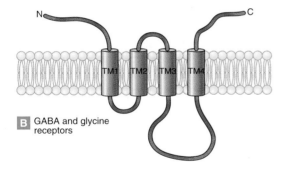

5-4 Membrane topology of AMPA glutamate, $GABA_A$, and glycine receptors. A. AMPA glutamate receptor subunits (GluR1-4) possess only three transmembrane spanning domains. The channel lining domain between TM1 and TM2 is a reentrant loop with both ends facing the cytoplasm. The Q/R site, which controls the Ca^{2+} permeability of AMPA receptor subunits, is located in this loop. The flip-flop site, located extracellularly between TM2 and TM3, yields two splice variants of each subunit. The glutamate binding site of AMPA receptors is formed by several amino acids in the N-terminal and extracellular loop. **B.** In contrast to AMPA receptors, $GABA_A$ and glycine receptors possess four putative membrane-spanning domains.

lacking the GluR2 subunit are consistently found at excitatory synapses on GABAergic inhibitory interneurons, whereas most principal cells (ie, projection neurons) express Ca^{2+}-impermeable AMPA receptors that contain the edited form of GluR2. The physiologic significance of these differences has not been completely characterized, but there is growing evidence that the number of GluR2-lacking AMPA receptors at particular synapses is subject to dynamic regulation and may be an important mechanism of neural and behavioral plasticity.

Kainate Receptors

Kainate receptors, like AMPA receptors, are cation-selective ligand-gated ion channels that strongly depolarize neurons when activated. They are found on presynaptic terminals, of both excitatory and inhibitory synapses, where their activation can modify neurotransmitter release, both because of their depolarizing actions and because, depending on their molecular composition, they are permeable to Ca^{2+}. Depending on the synapse and the degree of activation, presynaptic kainate receptors can either facilitate or depress transmitter release. Kainate receptors are also found postsynaptically on certain neurons, where they normally generate slow, small, but functionally important, postsynaptic potentials. In the hippocampus and cortex, they may be particularly important in the early development of neural circuits. Recent data suggest that kainate receptors can also be metabotropic, initiating a G protein signaling cascade independent of its ionotropic signaling.

Kainate receptors are comprised of a distinct array of subunits. The subunits GluR5 through GluR7 coassemble with KA1 or KA2 subunits to form functional kainate receptors. Homomeric GluR5, GluR6, and GluR7 receptors expressed in mammalian cell lines bind kainate with an affinity of approximately 80 to 100 nM. These homomeric receptors may correspond to low-affinity kainate binding sites previously identified in membrane fractions of the brain. In contrast, homomeric KA1 receptors bind kainate with an affinity of 4 nM and may correspond to high-affinity kainate binding sites in the brain. However, when they are expressed alone, KA1 and KA2 are virtually inactive because they lack functional channels. Consequently, it is believed that they serve as modulatory subunits that confer high-affinity kainate binding on channels formed by GluR5 through GluR7. GluR5 and GluR6 exist in several splice variants, and also undergo Q/R editing, meaning that kainate channels can vary in their Ca^{2+} permeability.

Selective kainate receptor antagonists are under development; those currently available, such as **LY382884**

5-1, are primarily selective for the GluR5 subunit. **LU97175** generally antagonizes kainate receptors, although it is most potent for GluR7 containing receptors. **SYM 2081** is potent agonist for GluR5 and GluR6 containing kainate receptors, and rapidly desensitizes the receptors; it can therefore be used as an antagonist. However, **GYKI 53655** remains the most valuable agent for determining whether a given synaptic current is mediated by AMPA or kainate receptors, as stated earlier.

Kainate receptors are believed to contribute to the development of **temporal lobe epilepsy**, and genetic studies have linked alleles of GluR6 to **Huntington disease** (in which it might be a disease modifier), **autism**, and **schizophrenia**. However, the role of kainate receptors in normal neuronal function, let alone in the development of complex neuropathologies, remains uncertain.

NMDA Receptors

NMDA receptors have several properties that set them apart from other ligand-gated receptors. At membrane potentials more negative than approximately −50 mV, the Mg^{2+} in the extracellular fluid of the brain virtually abolishes ion flux through NMDA receptor channels, even in the presence of glutamate. Thus, at the resting membrane potentials which are typical of most neurons, approximately −60 to −70 mV, the activation of these receptors results in little current flow. This is because the entry of Mg^{2+} into the channel pore blocks the movement of monovalent ions across the channel.

In the presence of Mg^{2+} ions, the receptor's current–voltage relationship has a region of slope-negativity that produces a characteristic J shape when plotted (see **5-2**). As the receptor's membrane potential becomes less negative (more depolarized), the affinity of Mg^{2+} for its binding site decreases, and the blocking action of Mg^{2+} becomes ineffective; consequently, ionic current can pass through the channel as the cell membrane depolarizes.

As previously mentioned, NMDA receptors can be thought of as coincidence detectors capable of sensing simultaneous activity at a number of adjacent synapses (see **5-3**). They possess this capability because they function (ie, pass current) only when they are stimulated by presynaptically released glutamate at a time when the postsynaptic cell is depolarized by activity in adjacent synapses. Repetitive stimulation is required because the depolarization produced by single inputs is not sufficient to relieve the blockage of the NMDA receptor channel by Mg^{2+}.

The activation of NMDA receptors, like that of AMPA receptors, produces a nonspecific increase in permeability to the monovalent cations Na^+ and K^+. However, unlike most AMPA and kainate receptors in the adult CNS, NMDA receptors are highly permeable to Ca^{2+}. Although their activation results in appreciable current and tends to depolarize the cell membrane toward the threshold for action potential firing, such activity is unlikely to represent the primary function of these receptors. Instead, NMDA receptors likely provide one of the most significant mechanisms by which synaptic activity can increase the level of intracellular Ca^{2+} at individual synapses. The major endogenous agonist for NMDA receptors is glutamate itself although there is some evidence that aspartate can also activate this receptor. Numerous competitive antagonists of the agonist recognition site are available, notably D-2-amino-5-phosphonopentanoic acid (**AP-5** or **APV**) and 3-(2-carboxypiperazin-4-yl)1-propenyl-1-phosphonic acid (**CPP**). These compounds are not useful clinically because they are polar and penetrate the blood–brain barrier poorly.

The NMDA receptor is unique among all neurotransmitter receptors in that its activation requires the simultaneous binding of two different agonists. In addition to the binding of glutamate at the conventional agonist-binding site, the binding of glycine appears to be required for receptor activation **5-5** . Because neither of these agonists alone can open this ion channel, glutamate and glycine are referred to as coagonists of the NMDA receptor. The physiologic significance of the glycine binding site is unclear because the normal extracellular concentration of glycine is believed to be saturating. However, recent evidence suggests that D-*serine* may be the endogenous agonist for this site. D-Serine, made through the conversion of L-serine by serine racemase, is subject to regulated release and specific reuptake primarily from glial cells. Thus, the glial

environment of neurons may have a critical influence on NMDA receptor synaptic function.

The glycine site on the NMDA receptor may prove to be an important drug target. **Cycloserine,** originally developed as an antitubercular drug, is a weak partial agonist at this site and thus can modulate NMDA receptor function in vitro and in vivo. Cycloserine is reported to enhance the effects of **antipsychotic** drugs in patients with **schizophrenia**. More specific agonists, such as **HA966,** have been used in laboratory animals but are not yet available for clinical investigation. Derivatives of **kynurenic acid,** such as 5,7-dichlorokynurenic acid (**5,7-DCK**) and **quinolinecarboxylic acid,** are also competitive antagonists at the glycine site. It is important to note that the glycine site on NMDA receptors is distinct from the **strychnine**-sensitive glycine receptor, which mediates the independent neurotransmitter functions of glycine.

Another important site on the NMDA glutamate receptor binds **phencyclidine** (**PCP**) and related drugs such as **MK801** and **ketamine** **5-5** . These drugs, which bind at or near the Mg^{2+}-binding site, occlude the NMDA receptor channel. Thus they act as noncompetitive receptor antagonists, and their actions, like those of Mg^{2+}, are somewhat voltage dependent. These drugs exert potent effects on the brain. At lower concentrations they are **psychotomimetic** and produce effects, such as cognitive impairment, hallucinations, and delusions that are similar to some of the symptoms of **schizophrenia** (Chapter 16). At higher doses, these drugs are **dissociative anesthetics**. Many are used predominantly in veterinary practice. However, **ketamine** has been used successfully as a pediatric anesthetic because children are less likely than adults to exhibit psychotic-like side effects. Interestingly, doses of **ethanol** associated with the upper range of intoxication in humans exert effects on NMDA receptors that are similar to those produced by PCP and related drugs.

In addition, NMDA receptors have one or more modulatory sites that bind **polyamines**. The occupancy of one of these sites relieves tonic proton block and thereby potentiates NMDA receptor activation. At higher concentrations, however, polyamines act on an extracellular site to produce a voltage-dependent block of the ion channel and consequently inhibit receptor activation.

Because they mediate a large number of important physiologic functions, and also contribute to cell damage and death when they are overactivated (Chapters 17 and 19), NMDA receptors have been a prominent target for therapeutic drugs. Many drugs that target these receptors have been developed and tested in clinical trials

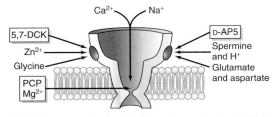

5-5 **Pharmacologic binding sites of the NMDA receptor.** Sites for drugs that promote receptor function (Na^+ and Ca^{2+} influx) appear in normal type, and sites for drugs that inhibit receptor function appear in boxes. 5,7-DCK; 5,7-dichlorokynurenic acid.

for conditions such as **stroke** or **head trauma** in which excitotoxicity may play a significant role. However, compounds with clear efficacy and tolerable side effects have yet to be identified. The large number of modulatory sites on the NMDA receptor increases the likelihood that clinically useful compounds will be discovered.

Molecular composition of NMDA receptors Two families of NMDA receptor subunits have been identified. One family is represented by a single gene (NR1) that encodes proteins composed of approximately 900 amino acids; the other is represented by four genes (NR2A–NR2D; see **5-1**) that encode proteins composed of approximately 1450 amino acids. Although homomeric NR1 receptors appear to possess all of the pharmacologic features characteristic of bona fide NMDA receptors, recent evidence suggests that the physiologically relevant glutamate-binding site is located on the NR2 subunit. Moreover, the very small currents supported by homomeric NR1 receptors increase by more than 100-fold when such receptors are coexpressed with NR2 subunits. It is therefore believed that NMDA receptors in the brain exist as NR1–NR2 heteromeric complexes. Some neurons also express the NR3A or NR3B subunit, which modulates NMDA receptor function, decreasing both the conductance and the Ca^{2+} permeability of the channel. The physiological significance of the NR3 subunit is not understood.

More than nine splice variants of NR1 have been cloned. These variants differ with regard to their regional patterns of expression in the CNS, their regulation (eg, by phosphorylation, polyamines, and Zn^{2+}), the electrophysiologic properties of channels they form, and their affinity for elements of the neuronal cytoskeleton. Such distinguishing features suggest that these variants may be involved in different components of the synapse.

The subtype of NR2 subunit that combines with NR1 subunits can influence the biophysical and pharmacologic properties of endogenous NMDA receptors. During early postnatal development, many synaptic NMDA receptors are composed of NR1 and NR2B. This subunit combination yields a receptor that produces very long-lasting synaptic responses and one that is strongly inhibited by the NMDA receptor antagonist **ifenprodil**. Gradually during the first few weeks of brain development, it is thought that the NR2B subunit is replaced by NR2A (and perhaps NR2C), yielding a receptor that produces shorter synaptic currents and that is no longer sensitive to ifenprodil. There is also evidence that different synapses in the adult brain preferentially express NR1–NR2A vs. NR1–NR2B NMDA receptors, which makes the development of selective agonists and antagonists a high priority.

In addition to the many regulatory mechanisms that have been described for NMDA receptors (see **5-5**), an interesting form of Ca^{2+}-dependent inactivation of these receptors is brought about by the Ca^{2+}-binding protein calmodulin. In response to Ca^{2+} entry, calmodulin interacts with the C-terminal domain of the NR1 subunit, reducing the frequency with which the receptor channel opens and also the length of time that it remains open. In addition, calcineurin, a Ca^{2+}/calmodulin-dependent protein phosphatase (Chapter 4), inactivates NMDA receptors by dephosphorylating them. Thus, one form of NMDA receptor modulation may occur through a 2-step process, whereby the receptor undergoes dephosphorylation and subsequent binding to Ca^{2+}-calmodulin.

Finally, there are reports that the dopamine D_1 receptor can interact directly with the NMDA receptor and inhibit its function. This effect is mediated by a direct protein–protein interaction and is independent of G protein and second messenger cascades. Further work is needed to understand whether this mechanism of NMDA receptor regulation is widespread and functionally significant.

Metabotropic Glutamate Receptors

Eight metabotropic glutamate receptors, termed mGluR1 through mGluR8, have been cloned (see **5-1**). mGluRs are considerably larger than other G protein–coupled receptors, and a comparison of their amino acid sequences with those of other receptors reveals little homology or common features. mGluRs are therefore considered to constitute a separate family of receptors. Like other G protein-coupled receptors, mGluRs contain seven membrane-spanning domains; however, like the ionotropic receptors, they also possess an unusually large N-terminal extracellular domain that precedes the membrane-spanning segments **5-6**.

There are three functional groups of mGluRs based on amino acid sequence homology, agonist pharmacology, and the signal transduction pathways to which they are coupled. Group I includes mGluR1 and mGluR5, which are generally found on postsynaptic neurons adjacent to excitatory synapses. Group II is composed of mGluR2 and mGluR3, while group III comprises mGluR4, mGluR6, MGluR7, and mGluR8. Group II and III mGluRs are often found on presynaptic terminals where they modulate transmitter release. Members of each group share approximately 70% sequence homology, with approximately 45% homology exhibited between groups. Alternatively spliced variants also have been described for mGluR1, mGluR4, mGluR5, and mGluR7.

The classification of mGluRs into three groups is supported by their signal transduction mechanisms.

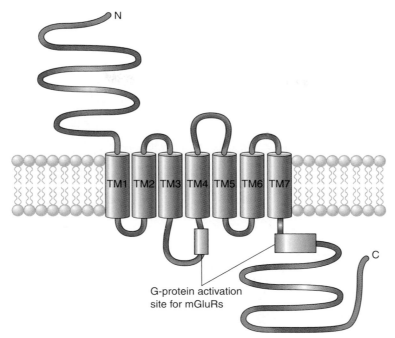

5-6 **Proposed membrane topology of mGluRs and GABA$_B$ receptors.** mGluRs and GABA$_B$ receptors contain seven transmembrane domains and are members of the G protein-coupled receptor superfamily. These receptors can be distinguished from most other G protein-coupled receptors by their unusually large extracellular N-terminal domains. In mGluRs, the second intracellular loop and the intracellular C-terminal domain determine the specificity of G protein coupling.

Group I mGluRs stimulate phospholipase C activity by means of the G protein G$_q$, and thereby release Ca^{2+} from cytoplasmic stores through IP$_3$ (Chapter 4). Yet group I mGluRs vary in their ability to increase intracellular Ca^{2+} levels, most likely because each receptor has a different affinity for G$_q$. Activation of phospholipase C leads to the formation of not only IP$_3$ but also diacylglycerol, which, in conjunction with increases in intracellular Ca^{2+}, activates protein kinase C. In contrast to group I mGluRs, groups II and III mGluRs inhibit adenylyl cyclase and regulate specific K$^+$ and Ca^{2+} ion channels, actions believed to be mediated via coupling to G$_{i/o}$.

Glutamate activates all of the mGluRs, with potencies that range from 2 nM for mGluR8 to 1 μM for mGluR7. Highly selective agonists for each of the three groups also have been identified **5-1**. 3,5-Dihydroxyphenylglycine (**DHPG**) appears to be a selective group I agonist; **LY354740** is a highly selective agonist for group II mGluRs; and L-amino-4-phosphonobutyrate (**L-AP4**) is a selective agonist of the group III mGluRs. mGluR antagonists have been developed for the various subtypes, but few antagonize a whole group. **LY341495** at low concentrations will inhibit group II mGluRs, but at high concentrations will inhibit all mGluRs. 2-methyl-6-(phenylethynyl)-pyridine (**MPEP**) is a group I antagonist with some selectivity for mGluRs.

Modulation of ion channel activity mGluRs located on the postsynaptic membrane modulate a variety of ligand- and voltage-gated ion channels expressed on central neurons **5-7**. The activation of each of the three groups of mGluRs has been found to inhibit L-type voltage-gated Ca^{2+} channels, and groups I and II are capable of inhibiting N-type Ca^{2+} channels. Additionally, mGluR activation can close voltage-gated K$^+$ channels, resulting in a slow depolarization and neuronal excitation. The exact mechanism by which mGluRs inhibit K$^+$ currents is not yet clear. In cerebellar granule cells, mGluRs increase the activity of Ca^{2+}-dependent K$^+$ channels, termed *BK channels*, and thereby reduce cell excitability. In some cells, mGluRs also activate G protein-coupled, inwardly rectifying K$^+$ (GIRK) channels. Thus, postsynaptic mGluRs can have a wide range of effects, depending on the cell type involved and the mGluR subtype that is activated.

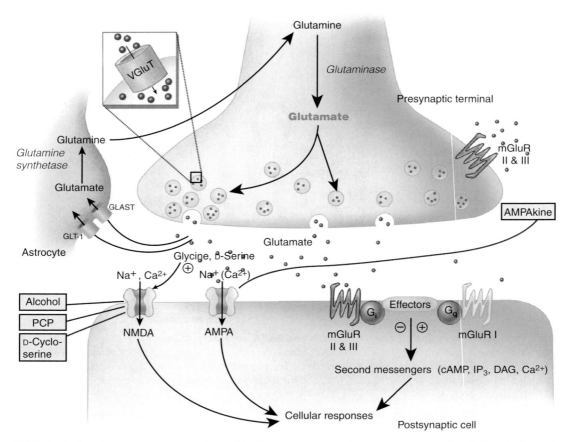

5-7 **Typical excitatory synapse.** AMPA and NMDA receptors which are ionotropic, and mGluRs, which are G protein-coupled, are all localized in the postsynaptic spine but have different subcellular locations (not depicted in figure). mGluRs are also located on the presynaptic terminal, where they act as inhibitory autoreceptors, in part by reducing Ca^{2+} influx. Not shown are kainate receptors, which can have either postsynaptic or presynaptic locations, depending on the synapse.

mGluR-mediated presynaptic inhibition at excitatory synapses Several types of mGluRs are located on the presynaptic terminals of central neurons and the activation of presynaptic mGluRs blocks both excitatory glutamatergic and inhibitory GABAergic synaptic transmission in many CNS regions **5-7**. In the hippocampus, mossy fiber-evoked EPSPs on CA3 pyramidal neurons are blocked by **DCG-IV**, which acts on presynaptic group II mGluRs located on granule cell terminals. Similar effects have been observed throughout the cerebral neocortex. In contrast, synaptic transmission between Schaeffer collaterals and CA1 pyramidal cells is resistant to DCG-IV but is reduced by **L-AP4**, a group III mGluRs agonist. One mechanism by

which activation of mGluRs decreases neurotransmitter release may involve the inhibition of voltage-gated Ca^{2+} channels on the presynaptic nerve terminal membrane. Such activity has been observed directly at certain glutamatergic synapses, where mGluR agonists suppress voltage-gated P/Q-type Ca^{2+} channels and thereby inhibit transmitter release. Accordingly, mGluRs most likely function as inhibitory autoreceptors at many glutamatergic nerve terminals.

The numerous effects that mGluRs can have on both postsynaptic cells and presynaptic terminals is confusing, especially because the conditions under which these receptors are physiologically activated are not always clear. Yet the diversity that characterizes mGluRs and their actions promises to further the development of subtype-specific drugs for the treatment of neuropsychiatric disorders. Several drugs that target specific presynaptic mGluRs are under evaluation for the treatment of **anxiety disorders** and **schizophrenia.** A recent study, for example, reported significant antipsychotic effects of a group II mGluR agonist, a promising finding which now requires replication (Chapter 16). mGluR ligands also may be useful in the treatment of **epilepsy.**

Synaptic Clustering of Glutamate Receptors

Effective synaptic communication requires the precise localization of high concentrations of appropriate presynaptic and postsynaptic proteins at the synapse. On the postsynaptic side of the synapse, neurons must be able to target glutamate receptors to excitatory but not inhibitory synapses and must ensure that the receptors are appropriately clustered opposite presynaptic

---

5–1 **PDZ Proteins and Synaptic Clustering of Glutamate Receptors**

Immunocytochemical and ultrastructural studies have revealed that individual excitatory synapses can contain profoundly different densities of AMPA, NMDA, kainite, and metabotropic glutamate receptors. Furthermore, their localization in dendritic spines usually differs. The ionotropic receptors (AMPA and NMDA) are located in the central part of the postsynaptic density opposite presynaptic release sites. In contrast, mGluRs are located at the periphery of synapses. This subsynaptic segregation of ionotropic and metabotropic receptors may permit the differential activation of these receptors based on patterns of presynaptic activity. A series of proteins have been identified in recent years that assist in clustering glutamate receptors at synapses. Most of these contain several PDZ domains, structures known to mediate many intracellular protein–protein interactions.

The first of these proteins to be isolated was *postsynaptic density protein of 95 kDa* (PSD-95); as its name implies, this protein occurs in high concentrations in the postsynaptic density, the most prominent structural specialization of the postsynaptic membrane of excitatory synapses. PSD-95 is a member of a family of related scaffolding proteins, including PSD-93, SAP-97, and SAP-102. These proteins all contains three PDZ domains, two of which can interact with the C-terminus of NMDA receptors. PSD-95 and related family members are believed to be critical components of the molecular mechanism responsible for the clustering of NMDA and AMPA receptors at synapses (see figure).

In contrast to NMDA receptors, AMPA receptors and mGluRs do not bind directly to PSD-95 but instead bind to their cognate PDZ-containing proteins. AMPA receptors bind to a protein known alternately as *stargazin or transmembrane AMPA receptor regulatory protein* (TARP). This protein links AMPA receptors to PSD-95, and regulates the trafficking of AMPA receptors to the cell surface and the synapse. This trafficking has been shown to be critical for certain forms of synaptic plasticity, such as long-term potentiation or LTP **5–8**. *Homer*, a protein that binds to the C-terminus of group I mGluRs, contains a single PDZ-like domain. Interestingly, expression of some splice variants of Homer can be regulated by neuronal activity; thus nerve impulses may influence the efficacy of mGluR synaptic transmission by regulating receptor clustering at physiologic sites.

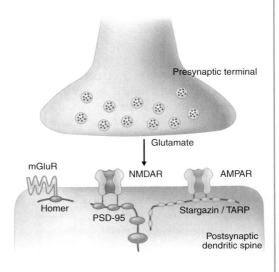

terminals that release glutamate. Several members of the protein family involved in this clustering contain single or multiple copies of an amino acid sequence termed the *PDZ domain*, which is important for mediating many important protein-protein interactions 5–1. Evidence supports the evolving hypothesis that each subtype of glutamate receptor interacts with distinct proteins at the synapse. Accordingly, the subcellular localization of each type of receptor may be independently regulated under physiologic conditions. Although these mechanisms remain poorly understood, they appear to be important for certain forms of neural plasticity.

Role of Glutamate in Neural Plasticity

The high permeability of NMDA receptor channels to divalent cations, especially to Ca^{2+}, has many implications for cell function. The concentration of Ca^{2+} in the cell interior typically is heavily buffered to approximately 100 nM and is tightly regulated by several mechanisms, including storage in intracellular organelles. Ca^{2+} entry through NMDA receptor channels can lead to a transient increase in intracellular Ca^{2+} concentrations to the micromolar range. Such an increase can in turn result in the activation of many Ca^{2+}-dependent enzymes, including Ca^{2+}/calmodulin-dependent protein kinases (CaM-kinases), calcineurin (protein phosphatase 2B), protein kinase C, phospholipase A_2, phospholipase C, nitric oxide synthase, and several proteases (Chapter 4).

One of the most important consequences of NMDA receptor activation is the generation of often long-lasting changes in synaptic function termed *synaptic plasticity*. Many forms of synaptic plasticity have been discovered in the mammalian CNS, but long-term potentiation (*LTP*) and long-term depression (*LTD*) of excitatory synaptic responses in CA1 pyramidal cells in the hippocampus have been the most extensively characterized. LTP and LTD are activity-dependent alterations in synaptic efficacy that can last weeks or months in vivo. Changes in receptor number (eg, via altered receptor trafficking 5–1 or transcription) or changes in receptor function (eg, due to phosphorylation 5–2), contribute to these changes in synaptic strength. The bidirectional control of synaptic strength by LTP and LTD is believed to underlie some forms of learning and memory in the mammalian brain.

The best understood form of long-lasting synaptic plasticity is NMDA receptor–dependent LTP, which is found in many regions of the mammalian brain but has been most extensively studied in the hippocampus because of its key role in learning and memory

(Chapter 13). The triggering of this form of LTP requires activation of NMDA receptors by synaptically released glutamate when the postsynaptic membrane is already strongly depolarized. This depolarization relieves the voltage-dependent block of the NMDA receptor channel by Mg^{2+}, and allows Ca^{2+} to enter the postsynaptic dendritic spine when the receptor is activated by glutamate. The rise in postsynaptic Ca^{2+} concentration, the critical trigger for LTP, activates complex intracellular signaling cascades that include several protein kinases, most notably CaM-kinase II 5–8A. The primary mechanism underlying the increase in synaptic strength during LTP is a change in AMPA receptor trafficking that results in an increased number of AMPA receptors in the postsynaptic plasma membrane. Within a few hours, the maintenance of LTP requires protein synthesis and there is growing evidence that LTP is accompanied by observable enlargements of dendritic spines. Such structural changes may be essential to cement the information storage process initiated at synapses upon LTP induction.

At many excitatory synapses throughout the brain, weaker activation of NMDA receptors can elicit the opposite phenomenon, NMDA receptor–dependent LTD, which is thought to result from a smaller rise in postsynaptic Ca^{2+} than is required for LTP 5–8B. This more modest change in postsynaptic Ca^{2+} activates serine/threonine phosphatases, which dephosphorylate critical synaptic substrates including AMPA receptors themselves. The depression of synaptic strength during NMDA receptor–dependent LTD is due to the removal of synaptic AMPA receptors via dynamin- and clathrin–dependent endocytosis. An intriguing feature of NMDA receptor–dependent LTD is that NMDA receptor–mediated synaptic responses are also depressed via mechanisms distinct from those responsible for the LTD of AMPA receptor–mediated responses.

Surprisingly, activation of postsynaptic mGluRs can also lead to a form of LTD that was first described in the cerebellum but also occurs in the hippocampus and neocortex. At the cerebellar parallel fiber synapse, LTD requires both postsynaptic Ca^{2+} influx through voltage-gated Ca^{2+} channels and postsynaptic group I mGluR activation, while at other synapses activation of postsynaptic mGluRs alone appears to be sufficient. In most cases, however, this form of LTD is mediated by clathrin-dependent endocytosis of synaptic AMPA receptors 5–8C. At certain developmental stages, rapid protein synthesis is required for both mGluR-triggered AMPA receptor endocytosis and LTD. There is evidence from mouse models that this form of LTD may be relevant to **Fragile X mental retardation syndrome**. FMRP (Fragile X mental retardation protein),

5–2 Modulation of Glutamate and GABA Receptors by Phosphorylation

Among synapses in the brain, the most ubiquitous are excitatory synapses that utilize glutamate and inhibitory synapses that utilize GABA. Consequently, the modulation of glutamate and GABA receptors by intracellular second messenger cascades is believed to be of paramount importance for a host of normal brain functions.

The functioning of all subtypes of ionotropic glutamate receptors, including that of AMPA, NMDA, and kainate receptors, can be dramatically altered by phosphorylation. The AMPA receptor subunit GluR1 is phosphorylated by three major protein serine–threonine kinases: protein kinase A, protein kinase C, and Ca^{2+}/calmodulin-dependent protein kinase II (CaM-kinase II). All three kinases increase the current elicited by agonist activation of GluR1-containing AMPA receptors by phosphorylating distinct residues in their intracellular C-terminus. Similarly, when the kainate receptor subunit GluR6 is phosphorylated by protein kinase A, these receptors become more responsive.

Phosphorylation/dephosphorylation of these receptors or closely associated proteins (see 5–1) also can dramatically influence their trafficking to synapses or their removal from synapses. Such modulation may underlie activity-dependent forms of synaptic plasticity believed to be involved in learning and memory 5–8 .

The modulation of NMDA receptor function appears to involve both serine–threonine kinases and protein tyrosine kinases. Activation of the tyrosine kinase Src, for example, causes an increase in NMDA-induced currents. The biochemical mechanism responsible for this process is unclear but may involve phosphorylation of the intracellular C-terminus of NR2A (and perhaps NR2B). Protein kinase C also has been found to enhance NMDA receptor function, and to disrupt the clustering of NMDA receptors, perhaps by interfering with the interaction between cytoskeletal elements and the C-terminus of NR1. Protein kinase A, on the other hand, can affect the Ca^{2+} permeability of NMDA receptors.

$GABA_A$ receptors are phosphorylated by at least two different protein serine–threonine kinases: protein kinase C and protein kinase A. In most studies, protein kinase C inhibits $GABA_A$ receptor function, in part by phosphorylating serine residues on β_1 and γ_2 subunits. The effects of protein kinase A on $GABA_A$ receptors are more variable. Protein kinase A can phosphorylate the same serine on the β_1 subunit as protein kinase C and thereby attenuate $GABA_A$ receptor-mediated currents; however, the biophysical consequences of protein kinase A phosphorylation depend on the exact subunit composition of the $GABA_A$ receptor. In certain cell types, such as cerebellar Purkinje and retinal bipolar cells, the activation of protein kinase A potentiates GABA-mediated responses, although the molecular mechanisms responsible for these effects remain to be determined.

Because G protein-coupled receptors are linked to the activation or inhibition of protein kinases, many types of neurotransmitters, such as the monoamines, acetylcholine, and several neuropeptides, can modulate glutamate and GABA receptor function. Similarly, changes in the amount of intracellular Ca^{2+} can regulate protein phosphorylation cascades and thereby modify receptor function. Furthermore, the phosphorylation states of these receptors are controlled by protein phosphatases, the inhibition of which often mimics the effects of increased protein kinase activity. An important goal of current research is to determine how phosphorylation and dephosphorylation of glutamate and GABA receptor subunits regulates the functioning of neural circuits and in turn the complex behaviors they underlie.

which is deficient in Fragile X syndrome due to abnormal methylation of the FMRP gene promoter, normally opposes group I mGluR-mediated induction of local protein synthesis in dendrites and the resulting LTD. Accordingly, it is proposed that Fragile X symptoms arise in part through excessive dendritic protein synthesis and LTD. Consistent with this hypothesis are the recent findings that many of the Fragile X-like symptoms exhibited in mouse models can be reversed by **MPEP**, a group I mGluR antagonist. This raises the possibility of novel treatments for Fragile X syndrome in humans.

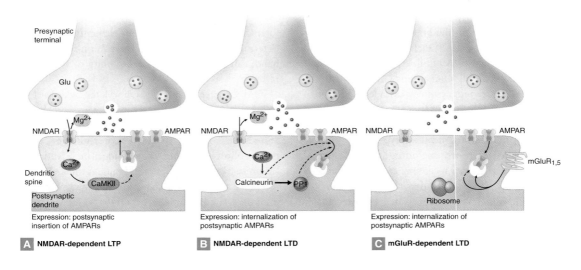

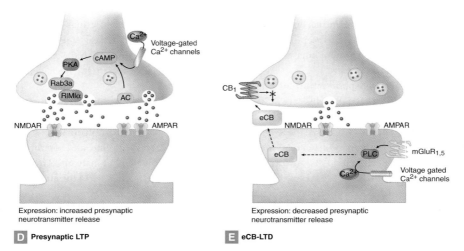

5-8 **Major forms of LTP and LTD**. Highly simplified diagrams of the induction and expression mechanisms thought to underlie some major forms of LTP and LTD. **A.** NMDA receptor–dependent LTP is dependent on post-synaptic NMDA receptor activation leading to a rise in Ca^{2+} and activation of CaM-kinase II (CaMKII) for its initiation. AMPA receptor insertion into the postsynaptic membrane is a major mechanism underlying LTP expression. **B.** NMDA receptor–dependent LTD is triggered by a modest Ca^{2+} entry through postsynaptic NMDA receptor channels leading to increases in the activity of the protein phosphatases calcineurin and protein phosphatase 1 (PP1). The primary expression mechanism involves internalization of postsynaptic AMPARs. **C.** mGluR-dependent LTD is due to activation of postsynaptic mGluR1/5 leading to the internalization of postsynaptic AMPARs, a process that under some conditions appears to require protein synthesis. **D.** Presynaptic LTP is triggered by a large rise in presynaptic Ca^{2+}, which activates Ca^{2+}-sensitive adenylyl cyclases (AC) leading to a rise in cAMP and activation of PKA. This in turn modifies the functions of Rab3a and RIM1α causing a long-lasting increase in glutamate release. **E.** Endocannabinoid (eCB) LTD is commonly triggered by increases in intracellular Ca^{2+} levels, either by mGluR1/5-mediated activation of phospholipase C (PLC) or by activation of voltage-gated Ca^{2+} channels, in the postsynaptic neuron. This triggers the synthesis and release of an eCB that travels retrogradely to bind to presynaptic cannabinoid 1 receptors (CB_1). This prolonged activation of CB_1 depresses neurotransmitter release via unknown mechanisms (Chapter 8). (Adapted from Kauer JA, Malenka RC. Synaptic plasticity and addiction. *Nature Rev Neurosci.* 2007;8:844–858.)

The aforementioned forms of synaptic plasticity are all triggered by activation of postsynaptic glutamate receptors and involve changes in the number of AMPA receptors at synapses. In contrast, there are also forms of LTP and LTD that involve long-lasting presynaptic changes in the release of glutamate. A presynaptic form of LTP was first described in the CA3 region of the hippocampus and is now known to occur in the striatum and cerebellum as well. This form of LTP does not require NMDA receptors and appears to be initiated by an activity-dependent rise in intracellular Ca^{2+} within the presynaptic terminals **5–8D**. The Ca^{2+} rise activates particular isoforms of adenylyl cyclases to produce cAMP, with subsequent activation of cAMP-dependent protein kinase (PKA) (Chapter 4). This in turn leads to a persistent increase in the amount of glutamate released each time an action potential enters the nerve terminal. Playing an essential role in the increased release are Rab3A and RIM1α, proteins that act to coordinate synaptic vesicle interactions with the presynaptic active zone (Chapter 3).

A potentially important form of presynaptic LTD may also occur at certain glutamatergic as well as at some inhibitory GABAergic synapses. This is commonly due to postsynaptic activation of mGluRs or voltage-gated Ca^{2+} channels, which triggers the synthesis of *endocannabinoids*, lipophilic molecules that are released by postsynaptic cells and can travel retrogradely across the synapse to bind to presynaptic cannabinoid receptors (discussed further in Chapter 8). Depending on the specific synapse, these endocannabinoids can either transiently depress neurotransmitter release for a period of many seconds or cause an LTD mediated by a long-lasting depression of transmitter release **5–8E**. Why endocannabinoid release produces only a transient synaptic depression at some synapses, but more persistent LTD at others, is not fully understood.

GABA

The Major Inhibitory Neurotransmitter in the Brain

GABA is present in highly diverse inhibitory interneurons and projection neurons throughout the brain. In the past, the action of GABA on its receptors was considered to be solely inhibitory, based on the observation that GABA receptor activation moves the membrane potential of a cell away from action potential threshold. However, recent evidence suggests that the role of GABA is more complex. During brain development, GABA also may function as an excitatory neurotransmitter because in certain circumstances GABA transmission can depolarize neurons. In addition, GABA released from local-circuit inhibitory interneurons assists in generating membrane oscillations such as the theta rhythm (Chapter 12).

The wide-ranging and ubiquitous role of GABA as an inhibitory transmitter means that enhancement of GABAergic function is a highly effective approach for the treatment of some forms of anxiety, insomnia, and epilepsy. GABA may play a role in diverse neuropsychiatric disorders, including **epilepsy, Huntington disease, tardive dyskinesia, alcoholism** and other **addictions,** and **sleep disorders.** Animal models of epilepsy have been generated by use of agents that compromise GABAergic transmission; such interference results in an imbalance of excitation and inhibition and leads to hyperexcitability and various forms of epileptiform activity.

Synthetic and Degradative Pathways

The portion of cellular GABA that functions as a neurotransmitter is formed by a metabolic pathway commonly referred to as the GABA shunt **5–9**. As with glutamate synthesis, the most common precursor of GABA is glucose; pyruvate also can act as a precursor. The first step in the GABA shunt is the conversion of α-ketoglutarate into glutamate by the action of α-oxoglutarate transaminase (GABA transaminase or GABA-T). Glutamic acid decarboxylase (GAD) then catalyzes the decarboxylation of glutamic acid to produce GABA.

Like most neurotransmitters, GABA is packaged into small synaptic vesicles in presynaptic terminals for release into the synaptic cleft. Like the vesicular glutamate transporter, the vesicular GABA transporter is highly dependent on the electrical potential across the vesicle membrane. The vesicular GABA and glutamate transporters differ from the vesicular transporters for monoamines and acetylcholine in terms of this bioenergetic dependence. Specific inhibitors of vesicular GABA transport have not yet been identified.

After it is released, GABA is removed from the synaptic cleft by the actions of several types of plasma membrane GABA transporters. Through this action GABA can be returned to GABAergic nerve terminals where it is repackaged for release; it can also be taken up by glial cells. In glia, GABA is metabolized into succinic semialdehyde by the action of GABA-T. To conserve the available supply of GABA, this transamination step occurs only when the precursor α-ketoglutarate is also present to accept the amino group removed from GABA. GABA is then converted back into glutamic acid, which is transferred back

5-9 **The GABA shunt.** This metabolic pathway traces the synthesis and degradation of the neurotransmitter pool of GABA. GAD, glutamic acid decarboxylase; GABA-T, GABA transaminase; SSADH, succinic semialdehyde dehydrogenase.

to the neuron. GABA-T inhibitors are being developed for use as **anticonvulsant** agents. One such drug, **vigabatrin,** has shown promise in clinical trials and is approved in several countries but not yet in the United States. A model GABAergic synapse is depicted in **5-10**.

Release and Reuptake

Once released, free synaptic GABA is taken back into the presynaptic terminal or into glial cells by plasma membrane GABA transporters. This is the major mechanism for terminating the synaptic actions of GABA. Such transport requires extracellular Na^+ and Cl^-; two Na^+ ions and one Cl^- ion are transported for each GABA molecule. Molecular cloning has revealed the genes for four distinct GABA transporters (GAT-1, GAT-2, GAT-3, and the low affinity transporter BGT-1). GABA transporters are expressed on nerve terminals and glial cell membranes throughout the nervous system.

Hydroxynipecotic acid, a rigid GABA analogue, has been used as an inhibitor of GABA transport. Its selectivity for glial transporters is approximately 20-fold greater than its selectivity for GABA transporters on nerve terminals. Related inhibitors **nipecotic acid** and **guvacine** block nerve terminal and glial transporters with similar potency. The cloning of GABA transporters led to a clearer understanding of their pharmacology. **Guvacine**, nipecotic acid, and hydroxynipecotic acid are equipotent blockers of the GAT-1 transporter, with IC_{50}s between 20 and 40 μM. **L-DABA** (2,4-diaminobutyric acid) and **ACHC** are approximately four times less potent, and β-**alanine, hypotaurine,** and **taurine** all have a low potency at GAT-1. One of the most potent compounds at this transporter is **NNC-711,** a lipophilic derivative of guvacine with an IC_{50} of less than 400 nM. NNC-711 is 40,000 times more selective for GAT-1 than for GAT-3. The **anticonvulsant** drug **tiagabine** and the lipophilic inhibitors **Cl-966** and **SKF89976** also act at the GAT-1 transporter. By inhibiting GABA transport, these drugs act to potentiate the inhibitory effects of GABA on CNS function.

GABA Receptors

Like glutamate receptors, GABA receptors are divided into two main functional groups. The ionotropic $GABA_A$ receptor is a heterooligomeric protein complex that consists of a GABA binding site coupled to an integral Cl^- channel **5-11**. This receptor is the site of action for **anxiolytic benzodiazepines** and other **sedative-hypnotics**. $GABA_A$ receptors are blocked by the convulsant **bicuculline**, a competitive antagonist at the GABA binding site.

$GABA_B$ receptors belong to the superfamily of G protein-coupled receptors. Thus they are considered to be metabotropic: their ligand-binding domain is not directly associated with an ion channel effector.

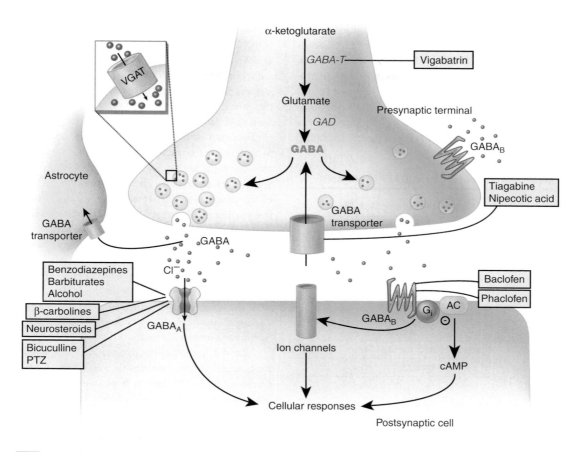

5-10 Typical GABAergic synapse.

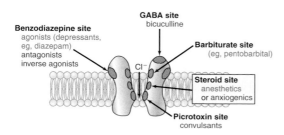

5-11 **Pharmacologic binding sites of the GABA_A receptor.** Drugs that promote receptor function appear in green, and drugs that inhibit receptor function appear in red. Only drugs that interact with the GABA binding site are considered competitive agonists or antagonists; all other drugs are considered noncompetitive agonists or antagonists.

These receptors, which are resistant to bicuculline, are activated by **baclofen,** a competitive agonist, and inhibited by **phaclofen,** a competitive antagonist.

Recent evidence supports the existence of an ionotropic $GABA_C$ receptor that is distinct from $GABA_A$ and $GABA_B$ receptors and resistant to the actions of both bicuculline and baclofen. These receptors are found in many CNS locations, primarily the retina, but also including the cerebellum, hippocampus, optic tectum, and spinal cord. It has been hypothesized that the more complex $GABA_A$ receptor evolved from the simpler, possibly homomeric, $GABA_C$ receptor. However, little is known about the functional significance of the $GABA_C$ receptor, and it is likely just a subclass of $GABA_A$ receptors.

Molecular composition of GABA_A receptors The cloning of the first $GABA_A$ receptor subunits occurred in 1987. Since then, 19 different subunits have been identified and placed into eight functionally distinct families. The α subfamily comprises six known subunits, the β subfamily four, the ρ subfamily three, and the γ subfamily three; the δ, ε, θ, and π subfamilies each have one member **5-2**. GABA$_A$ subunits are approximately 50 kDa in size. All possess a similar putative membrane topology, comprising a long N-terminal extracellular domain, four α-helical transmembrane spanning segments (M1–M4), a long intracellular sequence between M3 and M4, and a short extracellular

5-2 γ-Aminobutyric Acid (GABA) Receptors

Ionotropic GABA$_A$ Receptor	Metabotropic GABA$_B$ Receptor
Gene Families	
α_1-α_6	GABA$_B$R$_{1a}$
β_1-β_4	GABA$_B$R$_{1b}$
γ_1-γ_2	
δ	GABA$_B$R$_2$
$\rho1$-$\rho3$	
ε	
π	
Agents That Bind to the GABA Site	
Agonists	**Agonists**
GABA	L-Baclofen
Isoguvacine	CGP27492
Muscimol	
THIP	
Piperidine 4-sulphonic acid	
Antagonists	**Antagonists**
Bicuculline	2-OH-s-saclofen
	CGP35348
	CGP55845
	CGP64213
Agents That Bind to the Benzodiazepine Site	
Agonists	
Flunitrazepam	
Zolpidem	
Abecarnil	
Inverse agonists	
DMCM	
RoI94603	
Antagonists	
Flumazenil	
ZK93426	
Antagonists That Bind to Other Sites	
Picrotoxin	
Zn^{2+}	

C-terminal loop (see **5-4**). In the rat, a high degree of conservation exists among members of a subfamily, with 70% to 80% sequence homology at the amino acid level. Although GABA$_A$ subunits exhibit a low sequence homology (approximately 10%–25%) with glycine, 5HT$_3$, and nicotinic acetylcholine receptors, they are distantly related and are placed within the same superfamily of ionotropic receptors.

The heterogeneity of GABA$_A$ receptors is partly due to the existence of multiple splice variants. Alternative exon splicing generates, for example, two versions of the γ_2 and of the β_2 subunits. These isoforms differ in terms of the presence of a short peptide sequence between transmembrane domains M3 and M4, which carries a protein kinase C phosphorylation site (see **5-2**).

Heteromeric subunit assembly can occur among members of the α, β, γ, δ, and ε subfamilies; members of the ρ subfamily, which are predominently expressed in the retina, are believed to form the GABA$_C$ receptors. The π subfamily is expressed primarily in reproductive tissues and also is believed to exist only in homomeric form.

Like the homologous glycine, 5HT$_3$, and nicotinic acetylcholine ionotropic receptors, GABA$_A$ receptors probably exist as a pentameric complex positioned around a water-filled ion-conducting pore. The size of a GABA$_A$ receptor complex (approximately 275 kDa) is estimated to be five times that of its individual subunits. Within most receptor complexes, members of α, β, and γ subunit families are believed to be identical; that is, a given receptor is not expected to contain two different forms of an α (or β or γ) subunit. However, a minority of receptors may contain more than one form. Based on the large number of receptor subunits and their potential combinations, calculations indicate that more than 2000 distinct GABA$_A$ receptors may be formed. However, evidence suggests that less than 20 different GABA$_A$ receptors are widely expressed, and a relatively few subtypes predominate.

The composition of GABA$_A$ receptors in vivo is ultimately influenced by the relative levels of expression of subunits in a given cell type. The most prevalent subunit in the brain is α_1, with the major GABA$_A$ receptor subtype in brain having a stoichiometry of $\alpha_1\beta_2\gamma_2$. Receptors containing the α_2 subunit are most abundant in regions where the α_1 subunit is absent or expressed at low levels, such as the hippocampus, striatum, and olfactory bulb. Similarly, the α_3 subunit is expressed in regions complementary to the α_1 subunit, including the lateral septum, reticular nucleus of the thalamus, and brainstem nuclei. Notably, the α_6 subunit is expressed almost exclusively in cerebellum.

Surprisingly, the molecular composition of $GABA_A$ receptors at different subcellular locations within a single cell may differ. The mechanisms responsible for this targeting remain unknown but likely involve anchoring proteins, based on analogy with mechanisms responsible for glutamate receptor clustering at synapses (see **5–1**). *Gephyrin* is one protein that has been established to be important for the trafficking and clustering of $GABA_A$ receptors as well as glycine receptors.

$GABA_A$ receptor subunit expression changes during brain development and it is likely that such plasticity is maintained throughout adult life. Indeed $GABA_A$ receptor expression is altered during diseases such as **Huntington disease, epilepsy,** and **alcoholism,** and such changes may contribute to their pathophysiology and also offer clues for the development of novel treatments.

$GABA_A$ receptor pharmacology $GABA_A$ receptor pharmacology originated in the 1970s, when researchers discovered that the convulsant alkaloid **bicuculline** antagonizes certain inhibitory actions of GABA. This observation paved the way for the discovery of GABA's role as the principal inhibitory neurotransmitter in the brain. Other antagonists of $GABA_A$ receptors include **pitrazepin**, the convulsant **securinine**, the aminidine steroid analogue **RU5135**, and the pyridazinyl derivative **SR95531 (gabazine)**. In addition to GABA, selective agonists at this site include **muscimol**, **isoguvacine**, **THIP** (4,5,6,7-tetrahydroisoxazolo[5,4-*c*]-pyridone), and **piperidine-4- sulphonic acid** (see **5–2**). Competitive agonists and competitive antagonists of $GABA_A$ receptors interact with the GABA binding site (see **5–11**), which for most receptor complexes is located on the β subunit. However, the affinity of GABA for the receptor can be modulated by other subunits in the heteromeric complex. For example, GABA receptors whose subunit composition is $\alpha_1, \beta_1, \gamma_2$ have an EC_{50} for GABA of 41 μM, whereas $\alpha_3, \beta_1, \gamma_2$ receptors have an EC_{50} of approximately 100 μM. In addition to the previously mentioned competitive $GABA_A$ receptor antagonists are antagonists that do not bind to the GABA binding site. The best known are the potent convulsants **pentylenetetrazol** and **picrotoxin** (and the related **picrotoxinin**), which appear to bind at or near the Cl^- channel pore and occlude ion flow.

In the early 1970s, **benzodiazepines** were proven to potentiate the effects of GABA. Shortly thereafter, investigators discovered that benzodiazepines potentiate GABAergic inhibitory synaptic transmission by binding directly to the $GABA_A$ receptor. The benzodiazepine site, which is clearly distinct from the GABA-binding site, is an allosteric modulatory site on the $GABA_A$ receptor pentamer (see **5–11**). Recent evidence indicates that the site is formed by the apposition of α and β subunits but also requires the presence of a γ subunit, which itself is not part of the benzodiazepine binding site.

Drugs targeted at the benzodiazepine site exist on a continuum that ranges from full agonist to full inverse agonist. Indeed, $GABA_A$ receptor pharmacology played an important role in the development of the concept of inverse agonists (Chapter 1). Agonists at the benzodiazepine site, including anxiolytic benzodiazepines such as **diazepam, chlordiazepoxide, lorazepam, alprazolam,** and **clonazepam**, to name a few, act to increase the receptor's affinity for GABA at its own binding site and consequently increase the frequency of channel openings. Such drugs, in addition to being anxiolytic, are anticonvulsant and sedative and sometimes function as muscle relaxants. Partial agonists increase the frequency with which channels open but exert a milder effect on $GABA_A$ receptor functioning. Conversely, inverse agonists such as β-**carboline,** or β-**CCE,** decrease both the frequency of channel openings and the efficacy of GABA binding, and thereby antagonize $GABA_A$ receptor function. Such inverse agonists tend to be **convulsant** and **anxiogenic,** although a weak partial inverse agonist may exert less of an activational effect. Antagonists such as **flumazenil** typically bind to and occlude the benzodiazepine-binding site, but do not affect channel function; they can be used to reverse the actions of an agonist or inverse agonist, as in the treatment of an overdose with a benzodiazepine agonist.

The responsiveness of $GABA_A$ receptors to drugs targeted at the benzodiazepine site varies considerably. Although the γ_2 subunit appears necessary for benzodiazepine binding, the presence of a γ_1 subunit may exert the opposite effect. Of particular interest are the findings that numerous benzodiazepine site agonists and inverse agonists exert α subunit-selective effects on $GABA_A$ receptors. For example, α_4 and α_6 subunits have a low affinity for classical benzodiazepines, particularly when combined with the δ subunit. These discoveries have important clinical ramifications, as discussed later in this chapter.

$GABA_A$ receptors also are the site of action for a large number of **sedative–hypnotic** and **anesthetic** agents, including **barbiturates** and related drugs, **ethanol** and other alcohols, **volatile anesthetics,** and **neurosteroids**. Barbiturates and other sedative-hypnotics, such as **methaqualone** and **chloral hydrate,** exert a modulatory effect on the $GABA_A$ receptor similar to the effect produced by benzodiazepine agonists, but do so by binding to a distinctly separate location, most likely near the Cl^- channel pore (see **5–11**). Barbiturates increase the duration of channel openings without affecting the frequency with which channels open. They can exert this effect even in the absence of GABA, which makes barbiturates more potent and potentially dangerous than benzodiazepines. **Pentobarbital** and **phenobarbital** are the most commonly used barbiturates; phenobarbital, because of its long-duration of action, has been in use as an anticonvulsant since the early part of the 20th century. Variation in the subunit composition of GABA$_A$ receptors does not seem to alter their sensitivity to barbiturates.

The effects that **ethanol** exerts on the GABA$_A$ receptor complex are similar to those produced by benzodiazepines and barbiturates: it facilitates GABA's ability to activate the receptor and prolongs the time that the Cl$^-$ channel remains open. Interestingly, the alternatively spliced forms of the γ_2 subunit include a short form (γ_{2S}) and a long form (γ_{2L}), and ethanol potentiates GABA$_A$ responses only in receptors containing γ_{2L}. This splice variant also contains a consensus sequence for protein kinase C phosphorylation; when this sequence is mutated, the receptor's sensitivity to ethanol is lost.

Volatile anesthetics such as **enflurane** represent another class of drugs that prolong channel opening of GABA$_A$ receptors. Molecular mutagenesis has been used to identify sites in most GABA$_A$ receptor subunits that are responsible for the potentiating effects of both ethanol and volatile anesthetics. Given their location, typically near the extracellular regions of transmembrane domains M2 and M3, these sites may be part of the protein pocket that binds both ethanol and the volatile anesthetics, although this hypothesis remains unproven.

Neurosteroids, such as 3α,5α-THPROG (3,5-tetrahydroprogesterone), similarly promote channel opening of the GABA$_A$ receptor. Receptors containing the δ subunit are particularly sensitive, although most subtypes have some sensitivity to neurosteroids. GABA acts as only a partial agonist at δ subunit containing receptors, and neurosteroids can serve to promote it into a full agonist. α_1 and α_3 subunits are more susceptible than other α subunits, while γ_1-containing receptors are relatively resistent compared to receptors expressing γ_2 or γ_3. Neurosteroids are produced by neurons from progesterone, and steroid levels are altered by stress, aging, and pregnancy, and also by **ethanol**, **γ-hydroxybutyrate** (**GHB**; often referred to as a date-rape drug; see Chapter 12), and some antidepressants such as **fluoxetine**. Neurosteroids can produce anxiolytic, analgesic, sedative, hypotonic, anticonvulsant, and anesthetic effects. Curiously, the neurosteroid antagonist **17PA** (1717-phenylandrost-16-en-3-0l) blocks the effects of 3α,5α-THPROG and related

steroids, but does not inhibit the action of 3α,5β-THPROG and other 5β steriods, suggesting that there might be alternate binding sites for these steroids. See Chapter 10 for further discussion of neurosteroids.

Because barbiturates, benzodiazepines, and ethanol have related actions on a shared receptor substrate, the use of these agents can result in clinical complications. Their pharmacologic synergy increases the dangers associated with overdose and can lead to the development of cross-dependence. In fact, such cross-dependence often is exploited in **alcohol detoxification: benzodiazepines** are the treatment of choice and are used to prevent the emergence of alcohol withdrawal symptoms such as hallucinosis, delirium tremens, and seizures, which are potentially fatal.

Prolonged exposure to benzodiazepines results in tolerance to some of their pharmacologic actions, particularly to their sedative and anticonvulsant effects. Their effectiveness in the prolonged treatment of chronic insomnia or long-term treatment of epilepsy is therefore limited. Surprisingly, tolerance to the anxiolytic effects of benzodiazepines may not develop; patients often benefit from these effects for many years. In addition to tolerance, benzodiazepines and related sedative–hypnotics can produce profound dependence, which is manifested by rebound withdrawal symptoms that appear when drug administration ceases.

Both tolerance and dependence are characterized by a down-regulation of GABAergic transmission and by a reduction in the benzodiazepine modulation of GABA$_A$ currents. Despite considerable research, little consensus exists as to the mechanisms that underlie tolerance caused by prolonged exposure to benzodiazepines. Several reports have suggested that tolerance is caused by the down-regulation of the benzodiazepine recognition site on GABA$_A$ receptor complexes, indicating that distinct receptor subunits that lack such sites may be expressed in response to continued exposure to benzodiazepines.

The extensive heterogeneity of GABA$_A$ receptors, and the broad array of pharmacologic agents that are currently known to modulate these receptors, offer hope for more specific therapeutic agents. Such optimism has been bolstered by the hypothesis that GABA$_A$ receptors responsible for mediating the disparate effects of benzodiazepine agonists are located in distinct brain regions and are composed of distinct α subunits. Receptors containing the α_1 subunit appear to mediate the sedative actions of benzodiazepines, while α_2- or α_3-containing receptors primarily mediate the anxiolytic effects and α_5-containing receptors may be particularly important for the cognitive effects of these drugs. For example,

zolpidem, **eszopiclone**, and **zaleplon**, nonbenzodiazepine sedative-hypnotics that bind at the benzodiazepine site of the $GABA_A$ receptor, are somewhat selective for $GABA_A$ receptors that possess the α_1 subunit. Another endorsement of this hypothesis was the development of **RO 15-4513**, a benzodiazepine site antagonist that acts selectively on $GABA_A$ receptors that contain the α_6 subunit, which is concentrated in the cerebellum. This drug reduces the ataxia produced by **ethanol** without altering ethanol's other actions. Thus researchers have been encouraged in their attempts to develop drugs that selectively inhibit the anxiolytic, sedative, or anticonvulsant actions of nonselective agents such as diazepam.

Drug research is also aimed at developing agents that target $GABA_A$ receptors without producing tolerance or dependence, or triggering abuse. One strategy may involve the development of partial agonists that are sufficiently efficacious but less likely than full agonists to elicit compensatory adaptations. A related approach may involve the development of partial inverse agonists that are selective for $GABA_A$ receptors associated with cognitive function and attentional states. Although a full inverse agonist is convulsant and anxiogenic, a weak partial inverse agonist with the right α subunit selectivity may effectively enhance cognition. Indeed, it is conceivable that a single agent might reduce anxiety and enhance cognitive function simultaneously by acting as a partial agonist at anxiolytic $GABA_A$ receptors, and as a weak inverse partial agonist at cognitive $GABA_A$ receptors. However, it is important to note that drugs with these various mechanisms of action have not yet been developed.

$GABA_B$ receptors $GABA_B$ receptors were initially recognized because of their insensitivity to bicuculline and other $GABA_A$ ligands. Subsequently, the GABA analog and muscle relaxant known as **baclofen** proved to be a potent agonist at $GABA_B$ receptors. The physiologic roles of $GABA_B$ receptors were further elucidated after the development and analysis of specific antagonists such as **phaclofen, CGP 35348,** and **2-OH-s-(2)-saclofen.**

Molecular cloning techniques revealed that $GABA_B$ receptors are members of the G protein-coupled receptor superfamily and contain seven transmembrane domains (see 5-6). $GABA_B$ receptors, which are larger than most G protein-coupled receptors, are composed of 850 to 960 amino acids and are structurally similar to mGluRs. The receptors are $G_{i/o}$ coupled and are a heterodimer of two major $GABA_B$ subunits, $GABA_BR_1$ and $GABA_BR_2$. $GABA_BR_1$ binds ligand and has two isoforms: $GABA_BR_{1a}$ and R_{1b}, while

$GABA_BR_2$ subunit couples to $G_{i/o}$. The $GABA_B$ receptors were the first G protein-coupled receptors known to function as multimeric complexes, although many more have been identified (for example, opioid receptors; see Chapter 7).

$GABA_B$ receptors are expressed on both presynaptic and postsynaptic membranes and, like other $G_{i/o}$-linked receptors, have been found to open K^+ channels, decrease Ca^{2+} conductances, and inhibit adenylyl cyclase. Compared with $GABA_A$ receptors, postsynaptic $GABA_B$ receptors produce a slower but longer lasting form of inhibition, an effect largely ascribed to the opening of inwardly rectifying K^+ channels (GIRKs). In the hippocampus, thalamus, and cortex, low-intensity stimulation of inhibitory interneurons evokes inhibitory postsynaptic potentials (IPSPs) mediated entirely by $GABA_A$ receptors; IPSPs mediated by $GABA_B$ receptors require much stronger stimulation or stimuli of longer duration and higher frequency. These findings have led to the conclusion that the synaptic location of these receptor subtypes may differ. $GABA_A$ receptors are believed to localize at the synapse proper, directly opposite the site of GABA release, and can therefore be activated by the release of a single quantum of neurotransmitter. In contrast, $GABA_B$ receptors may be extrasynaptic. An extrasynaptic location would explain their need for high-intensity stimulation or for prolonged, high-frequency stimuli, either of which would increase GABA release and make it possible for GABA to diffuse out of the synaptic cleft.

On the presynaptic side, $GABA_B$ receptors can function as autoreceptors and inhibit further GABA release from GABAergic nerve terminals. Other $GABA_B$ receptors are located on excitatory presynaptic terminals, where their activation inhibits the release of glutamate. Receptors at this location are activated by synaptically released GABA that has, in a paracrine fashion, spilled out from an inhibitory synapse and diffused to adjacent excitatory synapses 5-12 . The activation of presynaptic $GABA_B$ receptors can also inhibit the release of several other neurotransmitters, including norepinephrine, dopamine, serotonin, and substance P. $GABA_B$-mediated inhibition of transmitter release occurs, at least in part, through the inhibition of Ca^{2+} channels and the consequent decreases in Ca^{2+} influx in response to action potentials. Such inhibition also may involve K^+ conductances, or direct modulation of the release machinery in the terminal via regulation of cAMP signaling cascades.

The only major drug in clinical use that interacts with $GABA_B$ receptors is **baclofen**, which acts as a

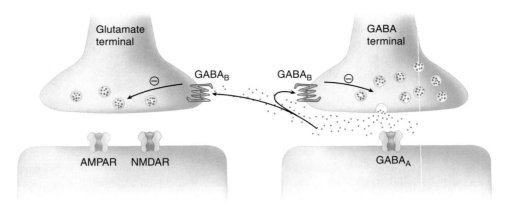

5-12 **Presynaptic actions of GABA_B receptors.** An excitatory, glutamatergic synapse (*left*) is compared with an inhibitory, GABAergic synapse (*right*). In the latter, synaptically released GABA activates presynaptic GABA_B autoreceptors located on the same inhibitory nerve terminal. Under certain conditions, GABA can also diffuse out of the synaptic cleft and activate GABA_B receptors on adjacent excitatory nerve terminals. At both types of nerve terminals, GABA_B receptors inhibit transmitter release.

muscle relaxant and is used to decrease spasticity in a variety of neurologic disorders. It is used less frequently for the treatment of **trigeminal neuralgia**. Inhibition of glutamate release is believed to underlie its clinical efficacy. Other applications for GABA_B receptor agonists are currently under investigation and may include their use in the treatment of **seizure disorders, anxiety,** and **depression**. GABA_B antagonists may also be used in the future to enhance cognition.

GLYCINE

Synthetic and Degradative Pathways

Most of the glycine in the mammalian CNS is synthesized de novo from glucose through serine. Serine is converted to glycine by serine hydroxymethyltransferase (SMHT), a pyridoxal phosphate-dependent enzyme. Pyridoxal phosphate is a derivative of **vitamin B_6**. It is believed that this conversion occurs in the mitochondrial compartment because the distribution of mitochondrial SMHT mirrors the distribution of glycine **5-13**.

Glycine is an amino acid primarily used for the synthesis of proteins. Only a small fraction of the cellular pool of glycine in a small subset of neurons is packaged into small synaptic vesicles for release as neurotransmitter. This packaging is mediated by a vesicular transport system identical to that previously described for GABA. Glycine acts as a neurotransmitter predominantly in the brainstem and spinal cord, where, like GABA, it is a principal mediator of inhibitory neurotransmission.

The degradation of glycine occurs mainly by means of the glycine cleavage system (GCS), which has four protein components (see **5-13**). A defect in the GCS, which is located in the inner mitochondrial membrane, causes a group of metabolic disorders termed **nonketotic hyperglycinemias**, which are characterized by high concentrations of glycine in the cerebrospinal fluid **5-3**.

Glycine Release and Reuptake

As with the release of other neurotransmitters, the arrival of an action potential in the presynaptic terminal of a glycinergic neuron initiates a cascade involving vesicular fusion and the release of glycine into the synaptic cleft. Glycine thus released is free to diffuse and bind with its receptors clustered on the postsynaptic face of adjacent cells.

Glycine is removed from the synaptic cleft by reuptake transporters located on the plasma membranes of glial cells and of presynaptic nerve terminals (see **5-13**). The electrochemical gradients of Na^+ and Cl^- assist in transporting glycine against its concentration gradient. This uptake mechanism is electrogenic and results in a net movement of positive charge. Two glycine transporters have been cloned thus far: GLYT1 and GLYT2. GLYT1 exists in three isoforms, which

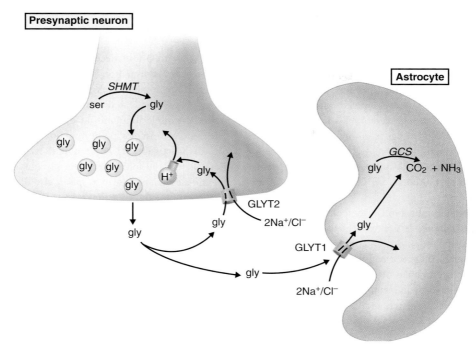

5-13 **Synthesis and metabolism of the neurotransmitter pool of glycine.** Serine (ser) is converted to glycine (gly) by the enzyme serine hydroxymethyltransferase (SHMT) in the mitochondrial compartment of a presynaptic neuron. Glycine is packaged into vesicles for release as neurotransmitter by a vesicular transport system identical to that used for GABA. Subsequently, glycine is removed from the synaptic cleft by uptake transporters located on glial cells (GLYT1) and on presynaptic nerve terminals (GLYT2). The transport of glycine against its concentration gradient and along the electrochemical gradients of Na^+ and Cl^- produces a net movement of positive charge. The degradation of glycine occurs mainly by means of the glycine cleavage system (GCS) in the inner mitochondrial membrane.

most likely are generated by alternative splicing; these exhibit no known variation in their uptake properties but possess distinct patterns of expression in the CNS.

Because only GLYT1 isoforms are sensitive to **sarcosine** (*N*-methylglycine), GLYT1 and GLYT2 can be differentiated pharmacologically. Both GLYT1 and GLYT2 are expressed in caudal regions of the CNS, a location consistent with their role in terminating glycinergic neurotransmission. In addition, GLYT1 is expressed in several forebrain regions that are devoid of glycinergic transmission. This forebrain GLYT1 might regulate NMDA glutamate receptor function in these areas by controlling levels of glycine in the extracellular fluid available to allosterically modulate these receptors (see earlier sections of this chapter). This would suggest the **GLYT1 inhibitors** may be useful clinically in promoting NMDA receptor function. GLYT1 is expressed in both astrocytes and neurons, whereas GLYT2 is localized on axons and terminal boutons of neurons that contain vesicular glycine.

Glycine Receptors

Glycine receptors are primarily restricted to the brainstem and spinal cord. Like $GABA_A$ receptors, the glycine receptor is a receptor ionophore that contains a Cl^- channel. It is also similar in size to the $GABA_A$ receptor and is believed to possess a quasisymmetrical pentameric structure that surrounds a water-filled ion conduction pore. Glycine receptors, which are unrelated to the glycine binding sites present on NMDA glutamate receptors, are defined pharmacologically by **strychnine,** a selective antagonist and a potent **convulsant.** Agonists at these receptors, which are competitive and limited to a few ligands, are ranked according to potency as follows: glycine > β-alanine > taurine > L- and D-alanine > L-serine >> D-serine. The potent convulsants **picrotoxin** and **picrotoxinin** are noncompetitive inhibitors of some of these receptors and are believed to interact directly with the receptor's ion channel to block Cl^- permeation.

One disease clearly associated with glutamate receptor dysfunction is **Rasmussen encephalitis,** a childhood autoimmune disorder characterized by epileptic seizures and associated with progressive destruction of a single cerebral hemisphere. One of the targeted autoantigens is the AMPA glutamate receptor subunit GluR3. Presumably, the disease is caused by anti-GluR3 antibodies entering the brain, where they precipitate an immune response that destroys nervous tissue.

Mutations in the protein components of the GCS, which is responsible for the degradation of glycine, cause metabolic disorders known as **nonketotic hyperglycinemias**. These diseases, which are characterized by high concentrations of glycine in the cerebrospinal fluid, develop early in infancy and are associated with severe neurologic defects such as lethargy, hypotonia, myoclonus, and generalized seizures.

Mutations in glycine receptor subunits contribute to abnormalities in two mouse mutants and also underlie a hereditary disease in humans. The mouse mutant known as *spasmodic* contains a recessive missense mutation in the α_1 subunit that causes a 2- to 3-fold decrease in its affinity for glycine. A similar mutation is responsible for **hyperekplexia,** a relatively rare dominant hereditary disorder in humans. This disease is characterized by increased muscle tone and an exaggerated startle reflex, and is caused by point mutations at position 271 of the α subunit. These mutations result in more than a 100-fold decrease in glycine affinity. The mouse mutant known as *spastic* also displays a complex motor disorder that is caused by reduced expression of the adult form of glycine receptor, due to a reduction in correctly spliced β subunit mRNA.

Inactivation of the GABA$_A$ β_3 subunit in mice causes developmental abnormalities that include **cleft palate**. Moreover, the **ataxia** characteristic of the mutant mouse known as *lurcher* results from a loss of cerebellar Purkinje cells during development, recently attributed to a missense mutation in the *GRID2* homolog. This gene encodes the orphan glutamate receptor subunit δ_2, the normal function of which is unknown. Current research is examining whether similar mutations occur in humans.

Glycine receptors are composed of 2 types of glycosylated integral transmembrane proteins: 48-kDa α subunits and 58-kDa β subunits, which are closely associated with gephyrin, a large (93 kDa) cytoplasmic protein. The α and β subunits possess similar sequence homologies (see **5-4**), which in turn are similar to those of other receptor ionophores; thus glycine receptors belong to the same superfamily as nicotinic cholinergic, GABA$_A$, and 5HT$_3$ receptors. Like other members of this superfamily, glycine receptors possess a large N-terminal extracellular domain and four transmembrane spanning regions. The glycine receptor pentamer is formed by α subunits either alone or in association with a β subunit; only the α subunit contains the functional glycine binding site. Four α subunits and a single β subunit have been cloned, and each of these is known to have several splice variants. Gephyrin associates with the intracellular region of the β subunit and links the receptor to cytoplasmic tubulin; it thereby functions as an anchoring protein for glycine receptors and controls receptor clustering.

The composition of the glycine receptor is developmentally regulated. In rat embryonic tissue, these receptors are exclusively composed of α_2 subunits; however, in the adult they typically are composed of $3\alpha_1$ and 2β subunits **5-14**. The transient expression of α_2 subunits during development occurs in most regions of the CNS. In mature animals, only a few neurons in the spinal cord exhibit persistent expression of α_2. In adults, the distribution of α_1 corresponds closely to the distribution of strychnine binding sites throughout the spinal cord, in brainstem nuclei, and in the reticular, auditory, and vestibular systems. An increase in α_3 transcription during development is restricted to the infralimbic system; in the adult such transcription is restricted to the hippocampal complex and cerebellar granule cell layer. Interestingly, β mRNA transcripts are found throughout the mammalian adult CNS, although β subunits alone are incapable of forming functional glycine receptors.

The pharmacology of glycine receptors remains limited. Among the known antagonists of these receptors, **strychnine** is the most commonly used experimentally

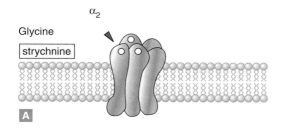

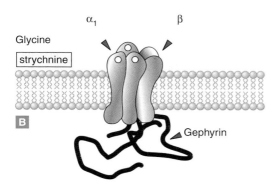

5-14 **Developmental differences in the molecular composition of glycine receptors. A.** In embryonic tissue, glycine receptors comprise only α_2 subunits. **B.** Adult receptors typically comprise $3\alpha_1$ and 2β subunits. The β subunit allows the glycine receptor to interact with gephyrin, which links it to cytoplasmic tubulin. Strychnine antagonizes both forms of glycine receptors.

because it blocks receptors composed of all α subunits. The binding pocket of the glycine receptor binds both strychnine and glycine agonists and is composed of several discontinuous domains of the α subunit. Interestingly, the residues important for ligand binding are homologous to amino acid positions that determine the ligand-binding affinities of nicotinic cholinergic and GABA$_A$ receptors; thus it appears that the ligand-binding pockets of all members of this receptor superfamily may share a common architecture. Other glycine receptor antagonists include **cyanotriphenylborate** (CTB), which preferentially binds to receptors containing the α_1 subunit; **picrotoxin,** which most effectively blocks recombinant α_2 homomeric receptors; and **picrotoxinin,** which most effectively blocks α_1 homomeric receptors. The presence of the β subunit enables glycine receptors to resist antagonism by picrotoxinin.

The glycine receptor is also modulated by Zn^{2+} ions. Low concentrations of Zn^{2+} enhance glycinergic transmission by increasing agonist affinity, while high Zn^{2+} concentrations inhibit transmission by reducing channel opening. Zn^{2+} mediates these effects through two distinct binding sites on the extracellular N-terminals of the α subunits.

SELECTED READING

Alexander SPH, Peters JA. Receptor and ion channel nomenclature supplement. *Trends Pharmacol Sci.* 2000 (suppl).

Bear MF, Dolen G, Osterweil E, Nagarajan N. Fragile X: Translation in action. *Neuropsychopharmacology* 2008; 33:84–87.

Belelli D, Lambert JJ. Neurosteroids: endogenous regulators of the GABA-A receptor. *Nature Rev Neurosci.* 2005;6:565–575.

Bettler B, Tiao JY. Molecular diversity, trafficking and subcellular localization of GABA$_B$ receptors. *Pharmacol Ther.* 2006;110:533–543.

Betz H, Laube B. Glycine receptors: recent insights into their structural organization and functional diversity. *J Neurochem.* 2006;97:1600–1610.

Borden LA. GABA transporter heterogeneity: pharmacology and cellular localization. *Neurochem Int.* 1996;29:335–356.

Bowery NG. GABA$_B$ receptor: a site of therapeutic benefit. *Curr Opin Pharmacol.* 2006;6:37–43.

Conn PJ, Pin J-P. Pharmacology and functions of metabotropic glutamate receptors. *Annu Rev Pharmacol Toxicol.* 1997;37:205–237.

Derkach VA, Oh MC, Guire ES, Soderling TR. Regulatory mechanisms of AMPA receptors in synaptic plasticity. *Nature Rev Neurosci.* 2007;8:101–113.

Dingledine R, Borges K, Bowie D, Traynelis SF. The glutamate receptor ion channels. *Pharmacol Rev.* 1999;51:7–61.

Huang YH, Bergles DE. Glutamate transporters bring competition to the synapse. *Curr Opin Neurobiol.* 2004;14:346–352.

Kauer JA, Malenka RC. Synaptic plasticity and addiction. *Nature Rev Neurosci.* 2007;8:844–858.

Kew JN, Kemp JA. Ionotropic and metabotropic glutamate receptor structure and pharmacology. *Psychopharmacology* 2005;179:4–29.

Kittler JT, Moss SJ. Modulation of GABA$_A$ receptor activity by phosphorylation and receptor trafficking: implications for the efficacy of synaptic inhibition. *Curr Opin Neurobiol.* 2003;13:341–347.

Knuessel M, Betz H. Clustering of inhibitory neurotransmitter receptors at developing postsynaptic sites: the membrane activation model. *Trends Neurosci.* 2000;23:429–435.

Kornau HC. GABA(B) receptors and synaptic modulation. *Cell Tissue Res.* 2006;326:517–533.

Lechner SM. Glutamate based therapeutic approaches: inhibitors of glycine transport. *Curr Opin Pharmacol.* 2006;6:75–81.

Lerma J. Roles and rules of kainate receptors in synaptic transmission. *Nature Rev Neurosci.* 2003;4:481–495.

Lynch G, Gall CM. Ampakines and the threefold path to cognitive enhancement. *Trends Neurosci.* 2006;29:554–562.

Madden DR. The structure and function of glutamate receptor ion channels. *Nature Rev Neurosci.* 2002;3:91–101.

Mayer ML. Glutamate receptor ion channels. *Curr Opin Neurobiol.* 2005;15:282–288.

Mohler H. GABA(A) receptor diversity and pharmacology. *Cell Tissue Res.* 2006;326:505–516.

Patel ST, Zhang L, Martenyi F, et al. Activation of mGluR2/3 receptors as a new approach to treat schizophrenia: a randomized phase II clinical trial. *Nature Med.* 2007;13:1102–1106.

Pinheiro P, Mulle C. Kainate receptors. *Cell Tissue Res.* 2006;326:457–482.

Schoepp DD, Jane DE, Monn JA. Pharmacological agents acting at subtypes of metabotropic glutamate receptors. *Neuropharmacology.* 1999;38:1431–1476.

Swanson CJ, Bures M, Johnson MP, Linden AM, Monn JA, Schoepp DD. Metabotropic glutamate receptors as novel targets fo anxiety and stress disorders. *Nature Rev Drug Discov.* 2005;4:131–144.

Vannier C, Triller A. Biology of the postsynaptic glycine receptor. *Int Rev Cytol.* 1997;176:201–244.

Wolosker H. D-Serine regulation of NMDA receptor activity. *Sci. STKE.* 2006;356:pe41.

CHAPTER 6

Widely Projecting Systems: Monoamines, Acetylcholine, and Orexin

- The monoamine neurotransmitters (dopamine, norepinephrine, epinephrine, serotonin, and histamine), the related small molecule neurotransmitter, acetylcholine, and the neuropeptides, orexin A and B, have an unusual but functionally significant organization in the brain. Their cell bodies are restricted to a small number of nuclei in the brainstem, hypothalamus, and basal forebrain, but their axons project widely throughout the nervous system. This widely projecting organization permits each of these neurotransmitters to modulate activity in diverse circuits, sometimes in a coordinated fashion.

- For example, these systems play critical roles in sleep, arousal, and attention, and in survival responses to relevant stimuli.

- Widely projecting dopamine (DA) neurons have their cell bodies in the midbrain, within the substantia nigra pars compacta and the ventral tegmental area. DA is also produced by neurons in the arcuate nucleus of the hypothalamus; and by local circuit neurons in the retina. Midbrain dopamine neurons project widely to the forebrain and influence motivation, motor behavior, and multiple forms of memory. Dopamine released from the hypothalamus suppresses synthesis and release of prolactin by the anterior pituitary.

- Norepinephrine (NE) is synthesized in nuclei within the medulla and pons, the most prominent of which is the locus ceruleus (LC). The LC provides virtually all of the NE to the cerebral cortex. Norepinephrine regulates arousal, attention, vigilance, and memory. Descending NE fibers modulate afferent pain signals.

- Serotonin (5HT or 5-hydroxytryptamine) is synthesized by neurons within the raphe nuclei of the midbrain. Their axons project very widely in the brain to influence diverse circuits involved in arousal, sensory processing, mood and different forms of emotion.

- Acetylcholine (ACh) is the neurotransmitter at nerve-muscle synapses. In the brain it is produced by widely projecting neurons with cell bodies in the brainstem and in the basal forebrain that project to the cerebral cortex and hippocampus. It is also produced by interneurons in the striatum. ACh in the forebrain influences many processes including motivation, learning, and memory.

- Histamine is produced by neurons in the tuberomammillary nucleus that lies within the posterior hypothalamus. These neurons project throughout the brain to regulate arousal. Inactivity of histamine neurons promotes sleep. Peripherally, histamine in the stomach promotes secretion of gastric acid via H_2 receptors; histamine released from mast cells is involved in allergic responses mediated via H_1 receptors.

- Orexin A and B (also known as hypocretins 1 and 2) are related neuropeptides that regulate sleep and wakefulness by interacting with monoaminergic and cholinergic neurons which in turn regulate emotion, motivation, and feeding. Orexin neurons have cell bodies in the lateral hypothalamus, and project widely throughout the brain. Among the major recipients of orexinergic projections are the locus ceruleus, a source of NE, and the tuberomammillary nucleus of the hypothalamus, the source of histamine.

- All receptors for DA, NE, and histamine and 12 of the 13 5HT receptors are G protein–coupled receptors. The $5HT_3$ receptor is a ligand–gated ion channel. Acetylcholine receptors are divided into two major classes; nicotinic receptors, which are ligand-gated ion channels, and muscarinic receptors, which are G protein–coupled receptors. Like most neuropeptide receptors, both orexin receptors, OX_1 and OX_2 receptors, are G protein–coupled receptors.

- The monoamines, DA, NE, and 5HT, share a common vesicular monoamine transporter (VMAT) which loads them into vesicles to be stored for release. DA, NE, and 5HT each has a specific plasma membrane transporter in their respective presynaptic terminals which terminates their synaptic actions after release by reuptake into the terminals. The monoamines are metabolized by monoamine oxidase (MAO), which exists in two forms, MAO_A and MAO_B. The catecholamines, norepinephrine and dopamine, are also metabolized by catechol-O-methyltransferase.

- Degeneration of dopaminergic neurons in the substantia nigra causes Parkinson disease; dopaminergic ventral tegmental area neurons play a central role in normal reward-related behavior and in addiction and also in attention and working memory.

- Dopamine acts on two related families of G protein–linked receptors, the D_2 family (D_2, D_3, and D_4 receptors), that are coupled to G_i/G_o and the D_1 family (D_1 and D_5 receptors) that are coupled to G_s and the closely related G_{olf}.

- Proteins within dopaminergic synapses are targets for several significant classes of drugs. The psychostimulants, cocaine, amphetamine, and methylphenidate, are indirect dopamine agonists that interact with DA transporters. Parkinson disease is treated with the dopamine precursor L-dopa, D_2 receptor agonists, and monoamine oxidase inhibitors (MAOIs). All currently used antipsychotics are D_2 receptor antagonists.

- Norepinephrine interacts with α- and β-adrenergic receptors. Many antidepressants (which are also anxiolytic) increase synaptic NE or 5HT levels by blocking their plasma membrane transporters; others increase synaptic NE or 5HT by blocking metabolism (MAOIs). β-Adrenergic antagonists may dampen memories encoded under strong emotion including trauma.

- Proteins within 5HT synapses are targets for the treatment of depression and anxiety. Drugs that block the serotonin transporter are efficacious in obsessive-compulsive disorder (OCD). Many second generation antipsychotic drugs, such as clozapine and many others, block the $5HT_{2A}$ receptor, which may help limit Parkinson-like side effects due to concomitant blockade of D_2 dopamine receptors. Hallucinogens, such as LSD, are partial agonists at $5HT_{2A}$ receptors.

- The five different muscarinic ACh receptors can be divided into two families based on the subtype of G protein to which they couple.

- Nicotinic ACh receptors (nAChRs) are pentamers constructed of subsets of 12 different subunits. Stimulation of nAChRs at the neuromuscular junction triggers muscle contractions. nAChRs are also found in the brain, where, among other roles, they are targets of the addictive drug, nicotine.

The survival and reproduction of free-living animals requires that they obtain nutrition and hydration, find safety, succeed in mating, and avoid predators and other dangers. Such behaviors require regulation of sleep-wake cycles in response, eg, to the waking times of predators or prey and the predominant environment (such as dark-light cycles and diurnal temperature variation). Successful survival also requires that arousal, vigilance, and attention be regulated appropriately in response to salient stimuli, and that behaviors be selected and executed in accordance with adaptive goals. Likewise, success demands that an organism engage in goal-directed behaviors when the risks and costs warrant it and disengage when the costs are too high. An organism must be able to record in memory the circumstances under which significant threats or rewards are found and learn motor programs that will maximize the speed and efficiency of escape from threats or the attainment of rewarding goals. Many circuits and neurotransmitters are involved in such behaviors, but the neurotransmitters discussed in this chapter play the central coordinating roles. Chapters on arousal and sleep (Chapter 12), higher cognitive function (Chapter 13), mood and emotion (Chapter 14), and reinforcement and addiction (Chapter 15) will develop these topics in greater detail, but will refer to the basic information presented in this chapter.

Most excitatory synaptic transmission in the brain is dedicated to precise point-to-point communication. Much inhibitory neurotransmission is based on local factors, such as the need for feedback control, although there are also inhibitory long projection neurons. Together these form precise information-rich circuits largely served by excitatory and inhibitory amino acids that activate rapidly and transiently responsive ligand-gated channels (Chapter 5). Such circuits are involved in the kind of highly specific information processing that permits the brain to create detailed sensory representations of the world and to plan and execute precise motor movements. Overlaying such circuits are diverse neurotransmitter systems that "fine-tune" or modulate their activity in response to salient stimuli, homeostatic needs, and emotional states. These neurotransmitters generally, but not exclusively, produce slower forms of synaptic transmission acting via G protein–linked receptors.

Neurotransmitters exerting such modulatory functions may act at varying distances from their targets. They may act locally, as in the case of cannabinoids and purines (Chapter 8); they may act at intermediate or longer distances, as is the case for some neuropeptides (Chapter 7). A small number of neurotransmitters exhibit a striking organization: they are synthesized by a very small number of neurons located within the brainstem, hypothalamus, or basal forebrain. These neurons project very widely throughout the brain, and in some cases descend also into the spinal cord, with some individual axons innervating an astoundingly large number of targets. Such architecture is clearly not consistent with precise information transfer, but rather with the ability to coordinate the responses of many neurons in response to global state changes or significant stimuli. Neurotransmitters with such widely projecting organization include the *monoamines* (so-called because they contain a single amine group; **6-1**), the functionally closely related neurotransmitter *acetylcholine*, and the peptide *orexin* (also called *hypocretin*). The monoamines include three *catecholamines*: *dopamine* (DA), *norepinephrine* (NE), and *epinephrine* (E), which are produced in a single biosynthetic pathway, as well as *serotonin* (5-hydroxytryptamine or 5HT), and *histamine*. These neurotransmitters have sometimes been referred to as *neuromodulators* because their actions via G protein–linked receptors alter the responses of neurons to excitatory and inhibitory amino acids carrying fine-grained information. We do not encourage the use of the term neuromodulator because many neurotransmitters, including acetylcholine, glutamate, and GABA, have both G protein–linked receptors and receptors that are ion channels. Function is determined by the receptor and its associated effector molecules rather than by the neurotransmitter.

DA illustrates the remarkable organization of widely projecting neurotransmitter systems in the brain: of the approximately 100 billion neurons in the human brain, only about 500 000 produce DA. Most of these neurons have their cell bodies in two contiguous regions of the midbrain, the substantia nigra pars compacta (SNc) and the ventral tegmental area (VTA). This small number of midbrain DA neurons innervates extensive terminal fields within the forebrain. Neurons from the SNc densely innervate the dorsal striatum where they play a critical role in the learning and execution of motor programs. Neurons from the VTA innervate the ventral striatum (nucleus accumbens), olfactory bulb, amygdala, hippocampus, orbital and medial prefrontal cortex, and cingulate cortex **6-1**. VTA DA neurons play a critical role in motivation, reward-related behavior (Chapter 15), attention, and multiple forms of memory. This organization of the DA system, wide projection from a limited number of cell bodies, permits coordinated responses to potent new rewards. Thus, acting in diverse terminal fields, dopamine confers motivational salience ("wanting") on the reward itself or associated cues (nucleus

[1] Melatonin (discussed in greater detail in Chapter 12) is another indoleamine neurotransmitter, but acts only in the pineal gland, and is not used by widely projecting systems.

accumbens shell region), updates the value placed on different goals in light of this new experience (orbital prefrontal cortex), helps consolidate multiple forms of memory (amygdala and hippocampus), and encodes new motor programs that will facilitate obtaining this reward in the future (nucleus accumbens core region and dorsal striatum). In this example, dopamine modulates the processing of sensorimotor information in diverse neural circuits to maximize the ability of the organism to obtain future rewards.

CATECHOLAMINES AND SEROTONIN

Synthetic and Degradative Pathways

Catecholamine biosynthesis   Catecholamines are molecules that contain a catechol nucleus with an ethylamine group attached at the 1 position **6–2**.

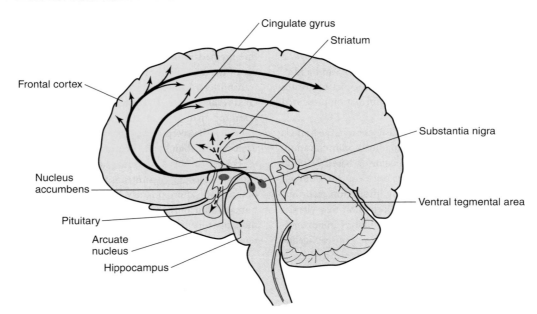

6–1   **The three major dopaminergic projections in the CNS.** (1) The mesostriatal (or nigrostriatal) pathway: the substantia nigra pars compacta (SNc) projects to the dorsal striatum (*upward dashed arrows*); this is the pathway that degenerates in Parkinson disease. (2) The ventral tegmental area (VTA) projects to the ventral striatum (nucleus accumbens), olfactory bulb, amygdala, hippocampus, orbital and medial prefrontal cortex and cingulate gyrus (*solid arrows*). The terms "mesoaccumbens" and "mesocortical" are sometimes used to describe components of the VTA projection. (3) The arcuate nucleus of the hypothalamus projects via the tuberoinfundibular pathway in the hypothalamus, from which dopamine is delivered to the anterior pituitary (*downward dashed arrow*). In rat brain, the SNc is often still designated as area A9 and the VTA as A10 based historically on maps generated by Dahlstrom and Fuxe using the Falck-Hillarp method, the earliest method to detect monoamine neurotransmitters in the brain. This method is based on autofluorescence of monoaminergic neurons after exposure of brain sections to formaldehyde.

6-2 **Chemical structure of catecholamines.** An ethylamine group is attached to a catechol nucleus at the 1 position.

5HT is an indolamine with a hydroxy group at the 5 position and a terminal amine group on the carbon chain **6-3**. The catecholamine neurotransmitters, NE, DA, and E, are sequential products of a single biosynthetic pathway that originates with the amino acid tyrosine **6-4**. 5HT and melatonin are synthesized from the amino acid tryptophan **6-5**. The catecholamine neurotransmitters and serotonin are discussed together because they have closely related functions, closely related mechanisms of clearance from synapses, some shared pathways of metabolism, and, perhaps most importantly, are jointly targeted by several important classes of drugs, including **psychostimulants** (DA, NE, and 5HT), **tricyclic antidepressants** (NE and 5HT), **monoamine oxidase inhibitors** (DA, NE, and 5HT), and **serotonin- norepinephrine selective reuptake inhibitors** (NE and 5HT).

Catecholamine biosynthesis begins with dietary tyrosine, which is actively transported into the brain (or peripheral sympathetic neurons). It is hydroxylated within neurons at the 3 position by the enzyme

6-3 **Chemical structure of indolamines.** Serotonin is an indolamine where R_1 and R_2 are hydrogen atoms, and a hydroxy group is substituted at the 5 position.

tyrosine hydroxylase (TH) to form dihydroxyphenylalanine (**dopa**). TH requires Fe^{2+} as a cofactor, as well as molecular oxygen and tetrahydrobiopterin (a hydrogen donor). An inhibitor of TH, α-**methylparatyrosine** (**AMPT**) has been used historically as an experimental tool to study catecholamine function; more recent alternatives include mice genetically engineered to lack TH or other enzymes in the biosynthetic pathway.

In dopaminergic neurons, one additional enzyme in this pathway is expressed, L-aromatic amino acid decarboxylase (AADC), which converts dopa to DA. AADC is a cytoplasmic enzyme that requires pyridoxal phosphate, a cofactor derived from **vitamin B$_6$**. AADC was originally known as dopa decarboxylase until it was recognized that it decarboxylates other substrates, including 5-HT, the precursor of serotonin **6-5**.

In noradrenergic neurons, an additional enzyme, dopamine-β-hydroxylase (DBH), is expressed that catalyzes the conversion of DA to NE. DBH requires Cu^{2+} and ascorbic acid (**vitamin C**) as cofactors. DBH is associated with synaptic vesicles that store NE.

In the adrenal medulla and in brainstem neurons that produce epinephrine, a still additional enzyme, phenylethanolamine-N-methyltransferase (PNMT), is expressed that converts NE to E. S-adenosyl- l-methionine (SAM), a methyl donor, is a required cofactor for this step.

TH, the rate-limiting enzyme in catecholamine synthesis, is regulated by multiple mechanisms. Increased catecholamine release leads to increased TH activity that results from regulation at the transcriptional, translational, and posttranslational levels. Rapid activation of TH activity occurs via its phosphorylation at 4 serine residues in the N terminus of the protein by several protein kinases, including protein kinase A, Ca^{2+}/calmodulin-dependent protein kinase II (CaM-kinase II), and protein kinase C. It is believed that such phosphorylation induces a conformational change in the protein that results in a higher affinity for its tetrahydrobiopterin cofactor and a lower affinity for catecholamines that trigger end-product inhibition of TH. The end result is an increase in the catalytic activity of TH. Longer term changes in TH activity can occur through transcriptional regulation of the TH gene by extracellular stimuli. Stimuli that up-regulate TH expression include chronic environmental stress and drugs such as **caffeine, nicotine,** and **morphine;** drugs that down-regulate TH expression include many antidepressants.

The ability of tyrosine to penetrate the blood–brain barrier depends on an active transport process. With normal dietary consumption of tyrosine, both active

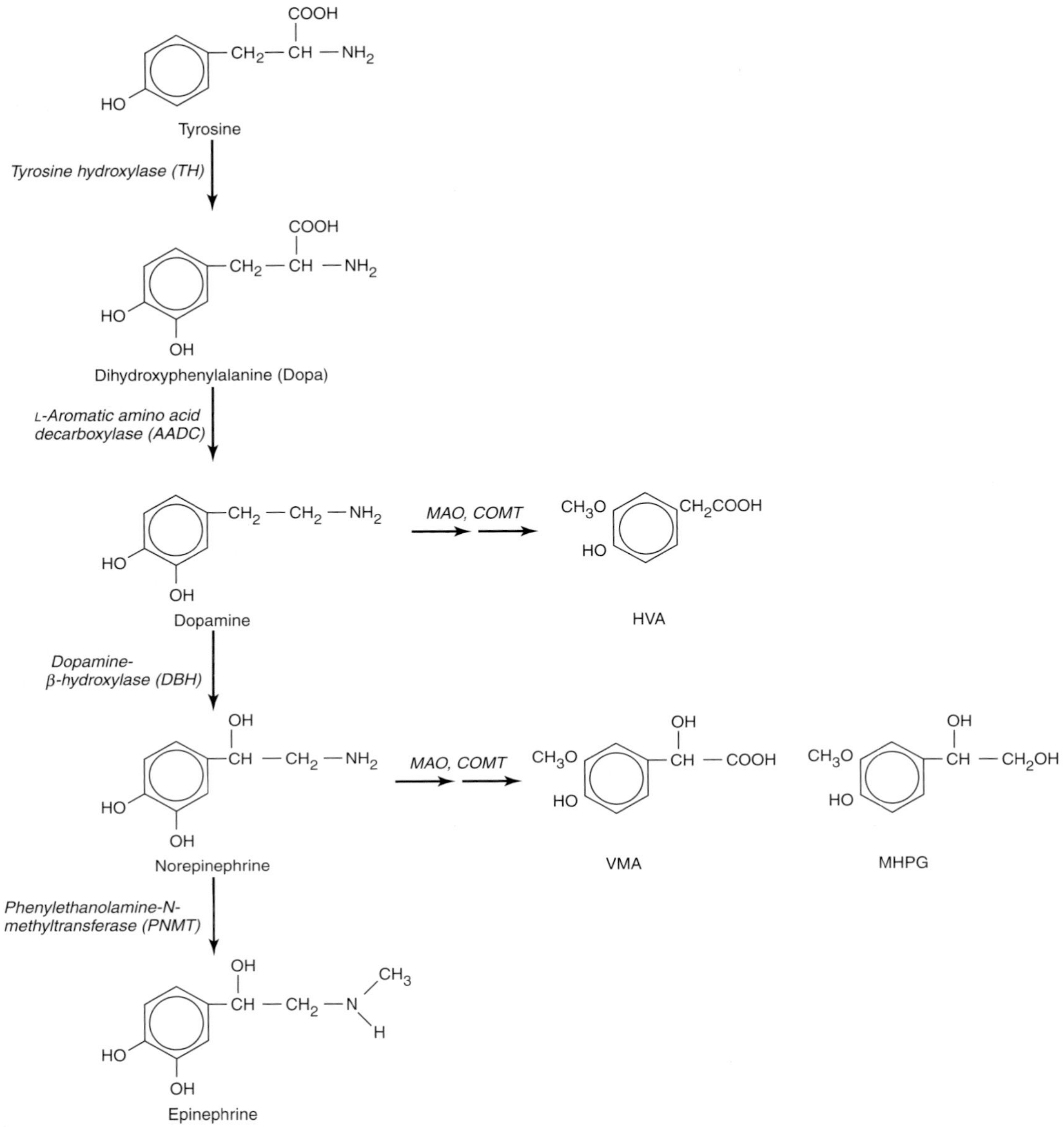

6-4 Biosynthetic pathway of catecholamines. Dopamine, norepinephrine, and epinephrine are derived from the multistep processing of tyrosine, a dietary amino acid that is actively transported across the blood–brain barrier and concentrated in catecholaminergic neurons. Region-specific expression of the enzymes shown here determine which neurotransmitters are expressed in a given cell; for example, both dopaminergic and noradrenergic cells express tyrosine hydroxylase (TH) and L-amino acid decarboxylase (AADC), but only noradrenergic cells express dopamine-β-hydroxylase (DBH). The principal metabolites of dopamine and norepinephrine are HVA, VMA, and MHPG. MAO, monoamine oxidase; COMT, catechol-O-methyl transferase; HVA, homovanillic acid; VMA, 3-methoxy-4-hydroxy-mandelic acid (also known as vanillylmandelic acid); MHPG, 3-methoxy-4-hydroxy-phenylglycol.

6-5 **Biosynthetic pathway of serotonin and melatonin.** Serotonin, also known as 5-hydroxytryptamine or 5HT, and melatonin are both derived from the multistep processing of the dietary amino acid tryptophan. Serotonin is synthesized neuronally in various brainstem nuclei and is converted by monoamine oxidase and aldehyde dehydrogenase into its primary metabolite, 5-HIAA. Serotonin is also produced in cells of the pineal gland, which contain two enzymes—5HT *N*-acetylase and 5-hydroxyindole-*O*-methyltransferase—not expressed in serotonergic cells. These enzymes rapidly convert serotonin to melatonin.

transport and TH activity are fully saturated. Thus, the administration of supplemental tyrosine cannot produce significant increases in catecholamine synthesis in the CNS. However, increased catecholamine synthesis can be achieved by peripheral administration of L-dopa (**levodopa**), which bypasses this rate-limiting enzymatic step and penetrates the **blood-brain** barrier, so long as its peripheral metabolism is blocked. For this reason, L-dopa is used in the treatment of **Parkinson disease** (Chapter 17).

Serotonin biosynthesis 5HT is synthesized from the amino acid tryptophan 6-5 , which is actively transported across the blood-brain barrier and hydroxylated by tryptophan hydroxylase (TPH) to produce 5HT. This product is then decarboxylated to form serotonin by AADC, the same enzyme involved in the biosynthesis of catecholamines. In the pineal gland, additional enzymatic steps convert serotonin to *melatonin*, which is discussed further in Chapter 12.

TPH is the rate-limiting enzyme for 5HT biosynthesis. There are two closely related genes, TPH1, predominantly expressed in the periphery, and TPH2, expressed preferentially in the brain. TPH is subject to short-term and long-term regulatory processes similar to those described for TH, a related amino acid hydroxylase. Like TH, TPH requires molecular oxygen and tetrahydrobiopterin as cofactors, and can be activated by protein kinase A and CaM-kinase II.

An additional member of the amino acid hydroxylase family is phenylalanine hydroxylase, which converts phenylalanine to tyrosine. Mutations of this enzyme that decrease its catalytic activity result in **phenylalaninemias** (eg, **phenylketonuria**) which, if untreated, can cause severe mental retardation. Interference with the metabolism of phenylalanine causes the buildup of oxidized derivatives such as phenylketones, which exert toxic effects on neurons. Individuals with such mutations can avoid symptoms of phenylketonuria by eliminating phenylalanine from the diet, a remarkable example of preventing a genetic disease with an environmental intervention.

Levels of 5HT in the brain can be altered by several means. Drugs such as *p*-**chlorophenylalanine** (PCPA), for example, can irreversibly inhibit TPH to produce a long-lasting depletion of 5HT. Experimental manipulation of tryptophan intake also can reduce levels of 5HT in the brain. Individuals who are asked to follow a low-tryptophan diet and subsequently are challenged with a beverage containing other amino acids but lacking tryptophan typically experience not only a dramatic reduction in blood tryptophan levels but also a substantial reduction of 5HT in the brain. In nonhuman primates, where direct measures are possible, a 90% reduction can be achieved. Among patients who have recovered from **depression**, tryptophan depletion induces a return of depressive symptoms in those who were successfully treated with a **selective serotonin reuptake inhibitor** (**SSRI**); however, depressive symptoms do not occur in healthy individuals or in those who were treated with antidepressants that influence NE reuptake. Thus, depletion of 5HT most likely does not cause depression; instead, patients treated with SSRIs may experience withdrawal symptoms upon tryptophan depletion that include transient return of depressive symptoms.

Degradation of catecholamines and serotonin

The most significant mechanism by which the synaptic actions of catecholamines, 5HT, and histamine are terminated is by *reuptake* into the nerve terminal via neurotransmitter-specific transporters expressed on the membranes of presynaptic terminals. In addition, these monoamines are enzymatically catabolized by *monoamine oxidase* (*MAO*). The catecholamines, but not 5HT or histamine, are also metabolized by *catechol-O-methyltransferase* (*COMT*).

MAO has both intracellular and extracellular forms. The intracellular form is associated with the outer membrane of mitochondria; given that mitochondria are plentiful in presynaptic terminals the primary action of MAO is to metabolize catecholamines, 5HT, and histamine after they are taken up into presynaptic terminals. However, the extracellular form may also act to metabolize neurotransmitter while in the synapse. Two major forms of MAO have been described: MAO_A and MAO_B. These forms are derived from distinct genes on the X chromosome and differ with regard to several biochemical properties, including their substrate specificity, cellular localization, and regulation by pharmacologic agents. MAO_A mRNA is expressed almost exclusively in noradrenergic neurons, such as those in sympathetic ganglia and *locus ceruleus* (described below and shown in 6-7). MAO_B mRNA is detected predominantly in serotonergic and histaminergic neurons. There are conflicting reports about the expression of MAO genes and protein in dopaminergic neurons, although the evidence favors expression of MAO_A.

Both enzymes oxidize monoamines but differ somewhat in their affinity for substrates. MAO_A displays a strong affinity for NE and 5HT, even though it is not expressed in serotonergic neurons. The function of MAO_B may be not to oxidize 5HT, but rather to metabolize *trace amines* that might act as false neurotransmitters, such as β-phenylethylamine, for which it has highest affinity. Extracellular 5HT appears to be oxidized by MAO_A derived from sources other than 5HT neurons.

The MAO loci on the X chromosome have preliminarily been linked to risk of **antisocial behavior** in several studies. In one Dutch family, an X chromosome deletion that spanned both MAO genes correlated with multiple severely violent individuals. Despite numerous human genetic and animal studies, the influence of developmental inactivation of MAO on human behavior is not yet clear. Certainly the inhibition of MAO pharmacologically in adults does not produce antisocial behavior and, to the contrary, may produce improvement in symptoms of anger and irritability associated with mood disorders.

MAOIs, such as **phenelzine** and **tranylcypromine,** are used to treat **depression** and **anxiety disorders;** the MAOI **selegiline** is used to treat **Parkinson disease** (Chapters 14 and 17). However, clinical use of MAOIs

as antidepressants and antianxiety agents has been limited by their side effects   6–1 .

Catecholamines are also catabolized by COMT. Peripherally the major isoform is soluble, but, in the brain, a longer, membrane-bound isoform predominates, which is found in catecholamine synapses.

6–1   Monoamine Oxidase Inhibitors

Most MAOIs, such as **phenelzine, tranylcypromine,** and **isocarboxazid,** that have been used clinically are nonselective, blocking both MAO_A and MAO_B. The first MAOI used in the clinic, **iproniazid,** was tested in the 1950s as a treatment for tuberculosis. Although it was ineffective against mycobacteria, it relieved the depression that was common among patients hospitalized with TB. Its actions on MAO were only subsequently recognized. Iproniazid is no longer used clinically because it is hepatotoxic, but the other MAOIs proved highly efficacious in the treatment of depression and diverse anxiety disorders. They were shown to be more effective than tricyclic antidepressants in the treatment of so-called **atypical depression,** which is characterized by a reversal of the usual neurovegetative symptoms of depression (eg, hypersomnia instead of insomnia, and hyperphagia instead of anorexia). Today, **SSRIs** are far more widely used for this clinical syndrome because of their superior tolerability.

MAOs are expressed not only in brain but also in peripheral tissues. MAO_A, found in gut and liver, catabolizes biogenic amines present in foods. Some aged or fermented foods, including many wines and cheeses, have particularly high levels of biogenic amines such as tyramine. When MAO_A is inhibited, as in response to the therapeutic use of nonselective MAOIs, biogenic amines in foods can enter the general circulation and can be taken up into sympathetic nerve terminals by norepinephrine transporters. This process can lead to the displacement and release of norepinephrine from sympathetic nerve terminals and the release of epinephrine from the adrenal medulla. Such release can produce a hyperadrenergic crisis, which is characterized by headache, hypertension that can be severe, and chest pain. To prevent a potentially dangerous hyperadrenergic syndrome, individuals who take nonselective MAOIs must eliminate tyramine-containing

foods from their diet. Despite their efficacy, it is this complexity of use that has relegated MAOIs to rare clinical use.

Because the inhibition of MAO_A appears to be required for antidepressant action and also necessitates dietary restrictions, there has been considerable interest in the development of reversible inhibitors of MAO_A (so-called **RIMAs** such as **meclobemide**). Unfortunately, RIMAs may be less efficacious than other antidepressants.

MAOIs also have been used to treat **Parkinson disease.** They were initially tested for this purpose after investigators discovered that the dopamine neurotoxin, **1-methyl-4-phenyl-1,2,3,6-tetrahydropyridine (MPTP),** which can cause Parkinson disease, must be converted to MPP^+ by MAO_B before it can exert its toxic effects. MPTP was discovered when an illicit drug laboratory, attempting to make the opiate **meperidine,** left MPTP as a contaminant. The individuals who injected it became acutely and severely Parkinsonian and were found to have destroyed their SNc dopamine neurons, likely by extreme oxidative damage. As a result, the MAO_B-selective inhibitor **selegiline** (also known as **deprenyl**) was administered to patients with early Parkinson disease in clinical trials as a putative neuroprotective agent (presumably preventing the activation of endogenous or exogenous MPTP-like neurotoxins). Although selegiline is efficacious, its mechanism of action remains unclear; it is more likely that its modest benefits are related to its ability to increase levels of synaptic dopamine rather than to any putative neuroprotective effect. At low doses selegiline does not affect MAO_A and thus does not require alterations in diet. However, at the high doses required for antidepressant effects, the drug becomes a nonselective MAOI and its use requires precautions against dietary tyramine.

COMT methylates catecholamines using *S*-adenosyl-methionine as a methyl donor. COMT inhibitors, such as **entacapone** and **tolcapone,** increase levels of catecholaminergic neurotransmitter in synapses and prolong receptor activation. In general, COMT appears to play a far smaller role in terminating the synaptic action of DA and NE than their specific membrane transporters, but in the prefrontal cortex, where the **dopamine transporter** (**DAT**) is expressed at relatively low levels, COMT may exert a more significant effect. Recent interest in COMT has been spurred by the possible association of genetic variants within the COMT gene with cognitive phenotypes, and perhaps with risk of psychiatric disorders 6-2 .

The major products that emerge from the enzymatic breakdown of catecholamines by MAO and COMT are shown in 6-4 . Historically, these metabolites were investigated as indirect measures of brain catecholaminergic function in depression and schizophrenia. They were measured in cerebrospinal fluid, blood, and urine; however, interpretation of metabolite levels was significantly confounded by activity of the sympathetic nervous system and adrenal medulla and by many other factors. Thus, their usefulness as markers of CNS catecholamine function proved quite limited. 5HT metabolites were also historically investigated. After serotonin is oxidized by MAO, aldehyde dehydrogenase acts to produce 5-hydroxyindoleacetic acid (5-HIAA) as an end product 6-5 . Reduction of 5-HIAA in cerebrospinal fluid has been reported to correlate with impulsive violence in

some circumstances, most notably among individuals who have attempted suicide by violent means. Despite considerable research, the significance of these findings remains unclear. Overall, it may have been naïve to believe that major neuropsychiatric disorders reflected global abnormalities in levels of one neurotransmitter, rather than disorders of more specific neural circuits that could be influenced by DA, NE, or 5HT.

Functional Anatomy

Dopamine   The overall anatomy of DA in the brain is described above and shown in 6-1 . Much of the function of DA projections was initially inferred from disease processes or from the actions of pharmacologic agents that act at DA synapses 6-6 . Historically, the first recognition of the importance of DA systems in the brain came from the investigation of **Parkinson disease**, which results from degeneration of SNc DA neurons. Death of these neurons results in denervation of the neostriatum (comprised of the caudate and putamen in the human brain and the dorsal striatum in the rat and mouse brains) resulting in a movement disorder that includes difficulty in initiating movement. Parkinson disease may result from rare Mendelian dominant or recessive mutations or more commonly from the interaction of multiple as yet unknown genetic and environmental factors (Chapter 17). DA itself cannot penetrate the blood-brain barrier. Thus, L-**dopa** is the mainstay in the treatment of Parkinson disease. It is transported across the

---

6-2   **COMT and Neuropsychiatric Disorders**

A common genetic variant in the COMT gene produces a valine (Val) to methionine (Met) substitution at amino acid 158. The Met allele confers lower activity on the enzyme, suggesting that individuals with the Met/Met variant would have slower termination of DA action in their prefrontal cortices (and thus more dopamine) than individuals with Val/Met or Val/Val proteins. Linkage studies have produced variable support for COMT as a risk locus for **schizophrenia**, **bipolar disorder**, and **schizoaffective disorder**. Association studies focused on the region of the COMT gene that produces the Val-Met substitution have failed to establish a convincing association with schizophrenia. Several association studies examining

frontal lobe–dependent cognitive performance have found poorer performance in healthy subjects, schizophrenics, and unaffected siblings of schizophrenics who have the Val allele. Other studies fail to replicate such findings on some or all cognitive tests or else find complex relationships between dosage of these Val or Met variants and performance in both healthy and ill subjects. Given the possible biologic effect of COMT on DA in the prefrontal cortex, this gene has also been examined in **attention deficit hyperactivity disorder** (**ADHD**) and **addictive disorders**. To date, however, no definitive phenotypic associations have been made.

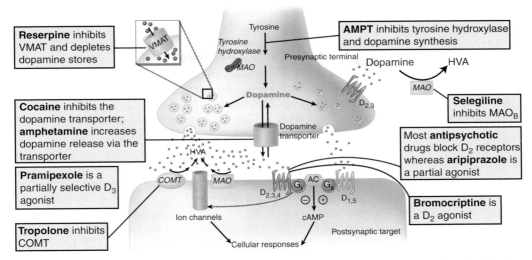

6-6 **Model of a dopaminergic synapse.** Presynaptic and postsynaptic molecular entities involved in the synthesis, release, signaling, and reuptake of dopamine are shown. Although MAO is shown extracellularly, it also exists in glia proximate to DA synapses and possibly in mitochondria within dopaminergic nerve terminals. VMAT, vesicular monoamine transporter; G_i and G_s, inhibitory and stimulatory guanine nucleotide–binding proteins; MAO, monoamine oxidase; COMT, catechol-*O*-methyltransferase; HVA, homovanillic acid; AC, adenylyl cyclase.

blood-brain barrier to dopaminergic nerve terminals where it is taken up by DAT and converted into dopamine by AADC. However, because AADC also resides in peripheral tissues, a significant fraction of L-dopa is decarboxylated into dopamine before it can be transported into the brain. Among other side effects, this produces nausea because there are dopamine receptors in the *area postrema* of the medulla, an area of the brain that controls nausea and vomiting, and which lies outside the blood-brain barrier so that it can sample the systemic environment (Chapter 2). L-dopa is thus coadministered with an AADC inhibitor such as **carbidopa** that cannot penetrate into the brain.

Given the role of DA receptors in vomiting, D_2 antagonists are effective **antiemetic** medications. However, due to their risk of causing Parkinson-like side effects, alternatives have been sought. $5HT_3$ antagonists such as **odansetron** and **neurokinin 1** (NK_1) **receptor antagonists** (the NK_1 receptor recognizes the neuropeptide, substance P; Chapter 7) are both highly effective antiemetics as a result of receptors in the area postrema that are free of the side effects of D_2 receptor antagonists.

VTA projections to the limbic forebrain, including the nucleus accumbens, and to the prefrontal cortex

are required for most reward-related behaviors. VTA DA projections also form the substrate upon which certain drugs produce **addiction**, which is described in detail in Chapter 15. Under normal circumstances VTA dopamine neurons fire prior to behaviors that are elicited by cues predictive of reward. In order to coordinate responses to such cues, the VTA receives inputs from diverse brain regions. These include reciprocal inputs with regions involved in valuation of rewards and also inputs from other widely projecting systems involved in arousal, attention, and memory. Different subregions of the VTA receive glutamatergic inputs from the prefrontal cortex, orexinergic inputs from the lateral hypothalamus (see 6-25), cholinergic and also glutamatergic and GABAergic inputs from the laterodorsal tegmental nucleus and pedunculopontine nucleus 6-18, noradrenergic inputs from the locus ceruleus 6-7, serotonergic inputs from the raphe nuclei 6-10, and GABAergic inputs from the nucleus accumbens and ventral pallidum.

DA has multiple actions in the prefrontal cortex. It promotes the "cognitive control" of behavior: the selection and successful monitoring of behavior to facilitate attainment of chosen goals. Aspects of cognitive control in which DA plays a role include **working memory**, the ability to hold information "on line" in order to guide actions, suppression of prepotent behaviors that compete with goal-directed actions, and control of attention and thus the ability to overcome distractions (Chapter 13). Cognitive control is impaired in several disorders, including **attention deficit hyperactivity disorder (ADHD)**, which is treated with **psychostimulants**, a term used to describe **indirect dopamine agonists** such as **methylphenidate** and **amphetamines** that block DAT or cause reverse transport of DA into synapses. Cognitive control is also deficient in **addiction** and **impulse control disorders**. Working memory is defective in **schizophrenia** and to a lesser degree in some nonpsychotic relatives of individuals with schizophrenia (Chapter 16). Current **antipsychotic drugs** do not have a therapeutic benefit for working memory.

Antipsychotic drugs produce their main therapeutic effects (diminishing psychotic symptoms, eg, delusions and hallucinations) by blocking D_2 receptors in the terminal fields of VTA DA neurons in subcortical structures in the limbic forebrain. The mechanism by which excessive dopaminergic stimulation of these structures might produce psychotic symptoms is unclear. Because antipsychotic drugs block D_2 receptors in the caudate and putamen as well as in desired limbic targets, these drugs produce side effects that are similar to the symptoms of **Parkinson disease**. (These are often called extrapyramidal side effects to distinguish striatally based motor systems from the corticospinal motor system, the fibers of which descend in a brainstem structure called the "pyramids".) Antipsychotic drug–induced Parkinson-like effects are not treated with L-dopa or indirect DA agonists because these drugs might worsen psychotic symptoms. Instead they are treated with **anticholinergic** drugs (ie, drugs that block muscarinic cholinergic receptors) or by the choice of antipsychotic drugs such as **clozapine** that have less tendency to produce these side effects by virtue of their combination of receptor binding properties including a lower affinity for D_2 receptors, antagonism of $5HT_{2A}$ receptors, antagonism of muscarinic cholinergic receptors, or some combination (Chapter 16).

The tuberoinfundibular DA system inhibits prolactin synthesis and release from the anterior pituitary. **Antipsychotic** drugs, which antagonize D_2 receptors, elevate levels of **prolactin**. Conversely, D_2 receptor agonists, such as **bromocriptine,** can be used to suppress hyperprolactemia, which is most commonly caused by prolactin-secreting **pituitary adenomas** (Chapter 10).

Norepinephrine   NE is produced by neurons contained within multiple nuclei of the pons and medulla 6-7. The *locus ceruleus* (*LC*), which is located on the

floor of the fourth ventricle in the rostral pons, contains more than 50% of all noradrenergic neurons in the brain; it innervates both the forebrain (eg, it provides virtually all of the NE to the cerebral cortex) and regions of the brainstem and spinal cord. Yet in the human brain, the LC contains only about 12,500 neurons per side, illustrating its remarkably wide projections. The other noradrenergic neurons in the brain occur in loose collections of cells in the brainstem, including the lateral tegmental regions. These neurons project largely within the brainstem and spinal cord.

NE, along with 5HT, ACh, histamine, and orexin, is a critical regulator of the sleep–wake cycle and of levels of arousal (Chapter 12). Not surprisingly, the LC receives significant input from other widely projecting systems involved in regulating sleep and arousal, such as orexin-containing neurons 6-25. LC neurons fire at a basal (tonic) rate during the waking state; the firing rate decreases during slow-wave sleep, and the LC does not fire during paradoxical sleep, the rodent equivalent of *rapid eye movement* (REM) sleep in humans. Transient increases in LC firing (phasic firing) are correlated with the onset of sensory stimulation; the highest rates of firing are associated with stimuli that portend threat. In addition to increasing arousal, the LC influences diverse aspects of attention and vigilance. In response to threat, LC firing may also increase anxiety, by releasing NE in the *amygdala* and other regions of the limbic forebrain. Stimulation of β-adrenergic receptors in the amygdala results in enhanced memory for stimuli encoded under strong negative emotion, facilitating the recall of stimuli that predict danger. However, this mechanism may contribute to **posttraumatic stress disorder (PTSD)** in humans; thus β-adrenergic receptor antagonists (eg, **propranolol**) are being investigated as interventions to decrease the intensity of traumatic memories (Chapter 14). In the laboratory, administration of $α_2$-adrenergic receptor antagonists, such as **yohimbine**, which increase firing of LC neurons by blocking inhibitory autoreceptors 6-9, induces fear and anxiety in laboratory animals and in humans. **Opiates**, which bind to μ opioid receptors, inhibit LC firing and are thus anxiolytic, among the many other actions of these drugs. With chronic administration, cellular adaptations within LC neurons lead to tolerance and dependence. With cessation of opiate administration, very high rates of LC firing contribute to the opiate physical withdrawal syndrome. These mechanisms are discussed fully in Chapter 15.

Recent electrophysiological studies in monkeys suggest that the LC may have relatively specific roles in arousal and attention-related behaviors, that is, survival-related

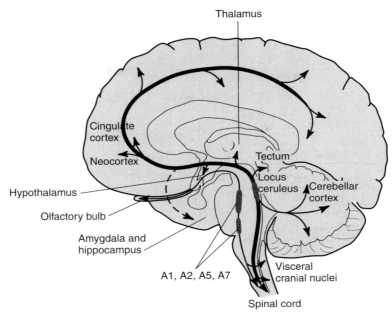

6-7 **Noradrenergic projections in the CNS.** The locus ceruleus (LC), which lies in the rostral pons, is the largest noradrenergic nucleus. It provides virtually all norepinephrine (NE) to the cerebral cortex and innervates many other forebrain areas (*thick arrows*). Other sources of NE come from clusters of cells within other brainstem nuclei. In the rat, the LC is often designated as area A6 and the other noradrenergic brainstem nuclei as A1, A2, A5, and A7, based on the Falck–Hillarp method of mapping (see **6-1**).

behaviors, including exploring the environment for sources of reward (eg, food, water, or safety), exploiting these resources, and disengaging with satiety or when the source of reward is depleted or otherwise becomes problematic. The LC receives inputs from the orbitofrontal cortex, which is involved in valuation of rewards, and which responds both to anticipation of rewards and to satiety. It also receives inputs from the anterior cingulate cortex, which is involved in monitoring task performance, and providing information as to whether performance is successfully approaching the selected goal. It has been argued that phasic LC firing optimizes task performance (exploitation), while tonic firing returns when task utility wanes and correlates with disengagement from the task and a search for alternative behaviors (exploration). In response to these altered firing patterns, NE released in the prefrontal cortex and other brain regions would modulate task-related behaviors. If correct, this model of LC function would contribute to our understanding of **ADHD** and other disorders of "top-down" cognitive control. In ADHD, there is impaired control of engagement and disengagement with tasks, as well as impaired ability to resist distractions. Noradrenergic projections from the LC thus interact with

dopaminergic projections from the VTA to regulate cognitive control. Drugs that increase synaptic NE **6-8** by blocking the **NE transporter (NET)**, such as the antidepressant **despiramine** or **atomoxetine**, exhibit some efficacy in treating ADHD. Psychostimulants have greater efficacy in most patients, however, probably because they increase DA as well as NE. Indeed stimulants act not only on DAT and NET, but also on the **serotonin transporter (SERT)**, although it has not been shown that 5HT makes a therapeutic contribution to treatment of ADHD. This model also suggests limits to current selective NE reuptake inhibitor or stimulant treatment because these produce sustained elevations in synaptic NE and DA, rather than optimizing the phasic and tonic firing patterns of monoamine neurons.

Epinephrine   Epinephrine occurs in only a small number of central neurons, all located in the medulla. Epinephrine is involved in visceral functions, such as the control of respiration. It is also produced by the adrenal medulla.

Serotonin   It has been estimated that there are several hundred thousand serotonergic neurons in the human brain. These neurons are confined almost

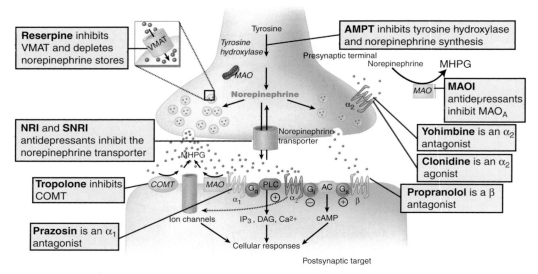

Model of a noradrenergic synapse. Presynaptic and postsynaptic molecular entities involved in the synthesis, release, signaling, and reuptake of norepinephrine are shown. MAO is shown extracellularly and in mitochondria within noradrenergic nerve terminals. MHPG, 3-methoxy-4-hydroxyphenylglycol; PLC, phospholipase Cβ; IP₃, inositol triphosphate; DAG, diacylglycerol. See **6-6** for other abbreviations.

exclusively to discrete nuclei in the brainstem raphe (raphe refers to their midline location; **6-10**). The most caudal clusters of the raphe innervate the medulla as well as the spinal cord. The dorsal and median raphe are located in the midbrain and innervate much of the rest of the CNS by means of numerous and sometimes diffuse projection pathways. The dorsal raphe forms the ventral-most portion of the periaqueductal gray matter. The median raphe is located ventral to the dorsal raphe in roughly the same anterior–posterior position of the midbrain. Although these two nuclei have overlapping terminal fields, the dorsal raphe preferentially innervates the cerebral cortex, thalamus, striatal regions (caudate-putamen and nucleus accumbens), and dopaminergic nuclei of the midbrain (eg, the substantia nigra and ventral tegmental area), while the median raphe innervates the hippocampus, septum, and other structures of the limbic forebrain. Projections from these and other raphe nuclei are so extensive that virtually every neuron in the brain may be contacted by a serotonergic fiber.

The function of serotonergic projections has been challenging to study partly because of their remarkably extensive nature, partly because the raphe nuclei contain a mixed population of neurons of which only a minority produce 5HT (making physiological recordings difficult), and partly because of the large number of 5HT receptors for which selective antagonists have only recently become available or are still not available. Well-formulated, testable hypotheses on the overall effects of 5HT on the cerebral cortex or limbic forebrain have not been developed. Yet, at a more granular level, it is clear that 5HT influences sleep, arousal, attention, processing of sensory information in the cerebral cortex, and important aspects of emotion (likely including aggression) and mood regulation.

Storage, Release, and Reuptake

Most biosynthesis of catecholamines and 5HT does not occur in the cell bodies of their neurons; rather, the synthetic enzymes are transported to nerve terminals, where transmitter synthesis predominantly takes place (**6-6**, **6-8**, and **6-11**). DA is synthesized in the cytoplasm and is packaged in storage vesicles by means of the vesicular monoamine transporter protein (VMAT). In noradrenergic terminals, DA is converted to NE by DBH, which also is located in storage vesicles. Thus NE may be synthesized both in the cytoplasm and in vesicles. DA, NE, and 5HT are all transported by the same VMAT protein, which spans the vesicle membrane. Vesicular storage not only permits rapid release of neurotransmitter in response to

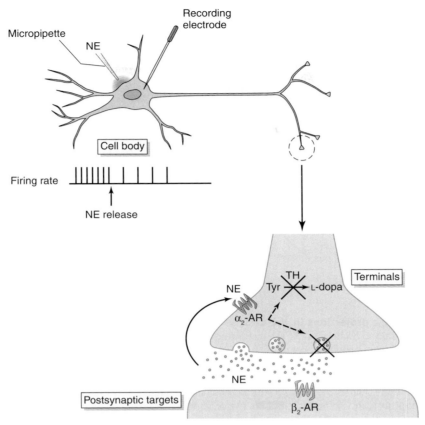

6-9 **Autoreceptors.** Autoreceptors typically function to inhibit activity in cell bodies and in synaptic terminals. Activation of α_2-adrenergic receptors (α_2-ARs) in a noradrenergic cell body, illustrated by the micropipette release of norepinephrine (NE), leads to a decrease in the firing rate of the cell, which can be recorded experimentally with an extracellular electrode. In the synaptic terminal, release of NE into the synaptic cleft allows for the diffusion of transmitter and the activation of presynaptic α_2-ARs. Such activation can inhibit further synthesis of NE and block the release of more transmitter. Thus autoreceptors function in negative feedback loops to modulate signaling between neurons. Tyr, tyrosine; TH, tyrosine hydroxylase.

action potentials, but also protects a reservoir of neurotransmitter from metabolism by MAO.

Reserpine, a compound initially derived from rauwolfia, a plant used in Indian herbal medicine, disrupts catecholamine and 5HT reuptake into storage vesicles by blocking VMAT; the monoamine transmitters are then subject to metabolism by MAO. Based on its ability to deplete NE, reserpine was once used as an antihypertensive agent. Based on its ability to deplete DA, it can act as an antipsychotic drug. Indeed, it was used empirically for this purpose in the 1950s. Clinical use of reserpine was abandoned, however, because of its side effects. Perhaps 15% of individuals treated with this drug experience serious depression. This side effect may result from the depletion of catecholamines and serotonin.

Plasma membrane transporters   As mentioned above, the DA, NE, and 5HT transporters (DAT, NET, and SERT, respectively) are related transmembrane proteins that move neurotransmitter from the synapse into the cytoplasm of the presynaptic terminal, where it is either reloaded into vesicles by VMAT or degraded by MAO. Each of the plasma membrane transporters has 12 hydrophobic membrane-spanning domains **6-12**. The rapid reuptake of synaptic transmitter by these transporters has several consequences that are vitally important to signaling among neurons. First, reuptake limits the duration of presynaptic and postsynaptic

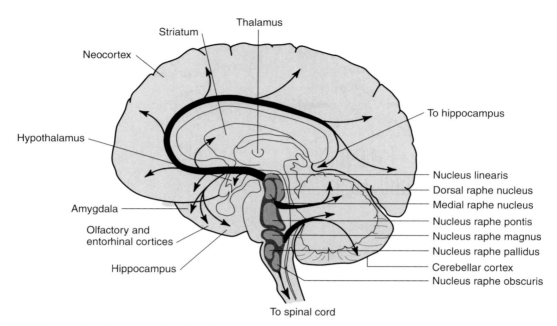

6–10 **Serotoninergic projections in the CNS.** Serotonin is produced by several discrete brainstem nuclei, shown here in rostral and caudal clusters. The rostral nuclei, which include the nucleus linearis, dorsal raphe, medial raphe, and raphe pontis, innervate most of the brain, including the cerebellum. The caudal nuclei, which comprise the raphe magnus, raphe pallidus, and raphe obscuris, have more limited projections that terminate in the cerebellum, brainstem, and spinal cord. Together, the rostral and caudal nuclei innervate most of the CNS. In the rat, the raphe nuclei are termed areas B1–B9 based on the original histochemical studies conducted by Dahlstrom and Fuxe using the Falck-Hillarp method (see **6–1**). The large dorsal raphe nucleus is designated as area B7 and the median raphe nucleus as area B8.

receptor activation. Second, it limits the diffusion of transmitter molecules to other synapses. Third, it permits recycling and reuse of unmetabolized transmitter. The critical role played by these transporters (compared with the action of MAO or COMT) is illustrated by DAT knockout mice. These mice exhibit extreme hyperactivity, and exhibit other evidence of a hyperdopaminergic state, despite multiple compensatory adaptations in enzyme and receptor function that help to counter the elevated synaptic levels of DA.

NET, DAT, and SERT are targets for two major classes of psychotropic drugs, antidepressants and psychostimulants **6–2**. The **tricyclic antidepressants (TCAs)** and newer **serotonin-norepinephrine reuptake inhibitors (SNRIs)** block NET, SERT, or both with differing selectivity. The **norepinephrine reuptake inhibitors (NRIs)** and **SSRIs** are selective for NET or SERT, respectively. Less commonly, antidepressants such as **bupropion** may also block DAT (Chapter 15). The most significant clinical difference

between SSRIs, SNRIs, and NRIs versus TCAs is that the TCAs are also antagonists of α_1 adrenergic receptors, H_1 histamine receptors, and muscarinic cholinergic receptors resulting in postural hypotension (due to α_1 receptor blockade), sedation (due to H_1, α_1, and muscarinic cholinergic receptor blockade), and dry mouth, failure of pupillary accommodation, constipation, and urinary retention (due to muscarinic antagonism) (Chapter 9). While the newer antidepressants also have significant side effects (eg, sexual dysfunction), they tend to be better tolerated by most people. The clinical utility of these antidepressants is discussed further in Chapters 11 and 14.

Psychostimulants interact with DAT, NET, and SERT. **Cocaine** blocks these three transporters and thereby blocks reuptake of all three neurotransmitters after normal vesicular release. **Amphetamines** are a family of related drugs that have a more complex mode of action. They enter monoaminergic nerve terminals via DAT, NET, and SERT, and disrupt the action

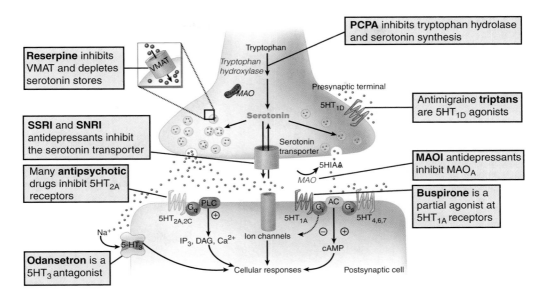

6-11 **Model of a serotonergic synapse.** Presynaptic and postsynaptic molecular entities involved in the synthesis, release, signaling, and reuptake of serotonin are shown. MAO is shown extracellularly and in mitochondria within serotonergic nerve terminals. 5HIAA, 5-hydroxyindoleacetic acid. See **6-6** for other abbreviations.

of VMAT to cause leakage of neurotransmitter out of synaptic vesicles. This causes cytoplasmic levels of the neurotransmitters to rise, which triggers the "reverse transport" of the neurotransmitters by DAT, NET, and SERT into the synapse. The rewarding and addictive actions of the psychostimulants result primarily from their actions on DAT (Chapter 15).

Halogenated amphetamines such as **fenfluramine** are selective for SERT, and stimulate rapid "reverse-transport" of 5HT into the synapse. Fenfluramine was prescribed as an appetite suppressant, but was removed from the market because it was associated with cardiac valvular disease and primary pulmonary hypertension that appear to be related to its peripheral effects on 5HT and the activation of $5HT_{2B}$ receptors. (In blood, platelets are a significant source of serotonin.) Fenfluramine had been prescribed either alone or in combination with **phentermine** (so-called "fen-phen"), a sympathomimetic drug with amphetamine-like actions. There is evidence that the weight loss caused by these agents is mediated via activation of $5HT_{2C}$ receptors in the medial hypothalamus (Chapter 10).

The brain expresses low levels of additional types of plasma membrane transporters, which may also contribute to the removal of monoamines from the synapse, although this remains speculative. There is evidence that certain members of the SLC29 (equilibrative nucleoside transporter) family, discussed in Chapter 8, can transport dopamine and serotonin nearly as effectively as DAT and SERT. Organic cation transporters (OCTs), which are expressed in discrete brain areas, are reported to transport E and histamine. While the physiologic role of OCTs requires further investigation, they may be involved in maintenance of salt and fluid homeostasis.

Receptors

Catecholamine receptors All receptors for DA and NE belong to the G protein–coupled receptor (GPCR) superfamily. E does not have its own receptors, but utilizes the same receptors as NE. As described in Chapter 4, binding of neurotransmitters to GPCRs initiates a conformational change in the receptor such that it activates a G protein, which in turn is coupled to regulation of an ion channel or second messenger-generating enzyme. Although DA and NE each have only one membrane transporter, each has numerous receptors encoded by different genes. Each of these receptors has unique pharmacologic properties and localization, features that can be exploited in the

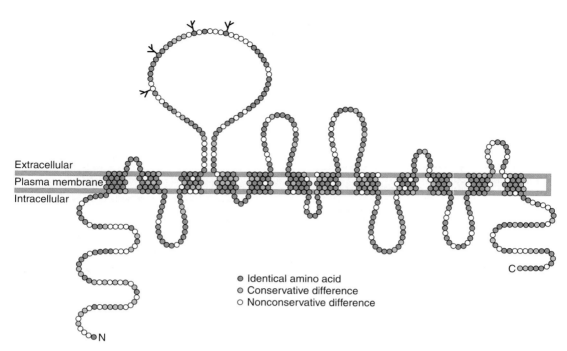

Extracellular
Plasma membrane
Intracellular

- Identical amino acid
- Conservative difference
- Nonconservative difference

6-12 **Two-dimensional model of a monoamine transporter.** This beads-on-a-string model illustrates several features of these proteins. Both the N terminus (N) and C terminus (C) reside intracellularly. Second, the protein possesses 12 hydrophobic, membrane-spanning domains with intervening extracellular and intracellular loops. The second extracellular loop is the largest and contains several potential glycosylation sites (indicated with tree-like symbols). Third, the color coding of the beads reveals the similarity between norepinephrine and dopamine transporters in terms of constituent amino acids. The most highly conserved regions of these transporters are located in transmembrane domains; the most divergent areas occur in N and C termini. (Adapted with permission from Buck KJ, Amara S. *Mol Pharmacol*. 1995;48:1035.)

design of drugs. There are more receptors than G proteins, thus there is some convergence of actions at the level of intracellular signaling (eg, D_1 DA receptors, β_1 and β_2 adrenergic receptors, and $5HT_4$ serotonin receptors activate the stimulatory G protein G_s), but specificity of action is maintained by the cell types on which these receptors are expressed, the location of the receptors on these cells (eg, distal or proximal dendrites, dendritic spines or shafts, perikarya, or presynaptic terminals), and their interactions with other receptor-activated signaling systems in the cells expressing them.

Dopamine receptors **6-3** are divided into the D_1 family (D_1 and D_5 receptors, coupled to G_s or the related G_{olf}) and the D_2 family (D_2, D_3, and D_4, coupled to G_i/G_o). D_2 and D_3 receptors function as inhibitory presynaptic autoreceptors and as postsynaptic receptors (ie, heteroreceptors expressed on noncatecholamine neurons). D_2 receptors have two splice

variants, D_{2short} and D_{2long}; however, functional differences between these isoforms have not been identified. Numerous medications produce their clinical effects via actions on dopamine receptors. All **antipsychotic drugs** are antagonists of D_2 receptors (Chapter 16). By contrast, D_2 agonists (eg, **bromocriptine**) are useful in the treatment of **Parkinson disease** and **hyperprolactinemia** (Chapters 10 and 17). **Pramipexole** and **ropinirole** are agonists at D_2-like receptors, with some selectivity toward D_3 receptors, and show some promise in the treatment of Parkinson disease and **restless leg syndrome**.

Adrenergic receptors are divided into α and β families, both of which have multiple receptor subtypes **6-4**. Each subtype responds in varying degrees to both NE and E. All β receptors are G_s coupled, and most α_1 receptors are G_q coupled; α_2 receptors, which are generally G_i coupled, function as inhibitory autoreceptors and as postsynaptic receptors. Many medications

6-2 **Binding Properties of Monoamine Plasma Membrane Transporters**

Norepinephrine (NET)		Dopamine (DAT)		Serotonin (SERT)	
Drug	K_i or K_m nM	Drug	K_i or K_m nM	Drug	K_i or K_m nM
Mazindol	1.4	Mazindol	11	Clomipramine	0.3
Desipramine	4.0	Nomifensine	17	Imipramine	2.1
Imipramine	6.5	Benztropine	55	Fluoxetine	2.1
Amitriptyline	100	GBR12783	13	Amitriptyline	15
Nortriptyline	16.5	GBR 12209	17	Mazindol	100
Cocaine	140	Cocaine	58	Cocaine	4200
D-Amphetamine	55	D-Amphetamine	2260	Amphetamine	>10,000

on the market act via adrenergic receptors; most of their actions are in the autonomic nervous system, as discussed in Chapter 9.

The physiologic responses elicited by receptor stimulation vary not only among receptors but also for any given receptor, depending on the neuronal cell type involved. The latter phenomenon occurs because the ion channels regulated by GPCRs are separate molecules (as described in Chapters 2 through 4), unlike the situation for receptors that are ligand-gated channels, and different signaling molecules and ion channels are found in different cells types. For example, an ion channel that is inhibited by protein kinase A phosphorylation may predominate in one cell type, but a channel activated by protein kinase A phosphorylation might predominate in another, leading to very different responses to activation of the same receptor. Because the physiologic responses elicited by catecholamine

6-3 **The Dopaminergic Receptor Family**

Receptor	Agonists[1]	Antagonists[1]	G Protein Coupling	Areas of Localization[2]
D_1	SKF82958*; SKF81297*	SCH23390;* SKF83566; haloperidol	G_s	Neostriatum; cerebral cortex; olfactory tubercle; nucleus accumbens
D_2	Bromocriptine*	Raclopride; sulpiride; haloperidol	$G_{i/o}$	Neostriatum; olfactory tubercle; nucleus accumbens[3]
D_3	Quinpirole*; 7-OH-DPAT	Raclopride	$G_{i/o}$	Nucleus accumbens; islands of Calleja
D_4		Clozapine	$G_{i/o}$	Midbrain; amygdala
D_5	SKF38393	SCH23390	G_s	Hippocampus; hypothalamus

[1]Asterisks indicate selective agonists and antagonists.
[2]mRNA expression has been determined predominantly in rat brain and may differ from the expression patterns found in human brain.
[3]D_2 long and D_2 short forms, which differ in the length of the third cytoplasmic loop, have been cloned. Although they are expressed in different brain regions, the funtional significance of these splice variants is not known.

6-4 **The Adrenergic Receptor Family**

Receptor	Agonists[1]	Antagonists[1]	G Protein Coupling	Areas of Localization in Brain
α_{1A}	A61603* Phenylephrine Methoxamine	Nigulpidine* Prazosin Indoramin	$G_{q/11}$	Cortex Hippocampus
α_{1B}	Phenylephrine Methoxamine	Spiperone* Prazosin Indoramin	$G_{q/11}$	Cortex Brainstem
α_{1D}	Phenylephrine Methoxamine	Prazosin Indoramin	$G_{q/11}$	
α_{2A}	Oxymetazoline*; clonidine	Yohimbine; rauwolscine; prazosin	$G_{i/o}$	Cortex; brainstem; midbrain; spinal cord
α_{2B}	Clonidine	Yohimbine; rauwolscine; prazosin	$G_{i/o}$	Diencephalon
α_{2C}	Clonidine	Yohimbine; rauwolscine; prazosin	$G_{i/o}$	Basal ganglia; cortex; cerebellum; hippocampus
β_1	Isoproterenol; terbutaline*	Alprenolol*; betaxolol*; propranold	G_s	Olfactory nucleus; cortex; cerebellar nuclei; brainstem nuclei; spinal cord
β_2	Procaterol*; zinterol*	Propranolol	G_s	Olfactory bulb; piriform cortex; hippocampus; cerebellar cortex
β_3		Pindolol*; bupranolol*; propranolol	$G_s/G_{i/o}$	

[1]Asterisks indicate selective agonists and antagonists.

receptor activation are numerous and complex, only general themes related to these responses are presented here.

The electrophysiologic consequences of activation of D_1-like receptors have been extremely difficult to pin down because of conflicting reports. Such inconsistencies likely reflect the heterogeneity of the cell types that have been studied, and also the complex cascades of protein kinases and protein phosphatases that are influenced by D_1-like receptors and that regulate many types of ion channels. The consequences of D_2 receptor activation appear to be more uniform, and frequently give rise to inhibitory responses, like most G_i/G_o-linked receptors, caused by the activation of inwardly rectifying K^+ channels (Chapter 4).

β-adrenergic receptors (β-ARs; **6-13**), coupled to G_s, lead to the activation of adenylyl cyclase, the synthesis of cAMP, and the activation of protein kinase A (Chapter 4). Such activation in turn leads to excitatory or inhibitory effects in neurons, depending on the protein kinase A substrates expressed in the particular cell type. In addition, cAMP can, independently of protein kinase A, activate cyclic nucleotide–gated channels called HCN (hyperpolarization and cyclic nucleotide activated) channels (Chapter 2). In the cerebral cortex and hippocampus, β-AR activation facilitates the excitation of pyramidal cells by blocking the activity of a Ca^{2+}-activated K^+ channel. In contrast, in cardiac muscle, β-AR activation leads to the phosphorylation and activation of voltage-gated Ca^{2+} channels, representing the mechanism by which NE released from sympathetic neurons and circulating E released from the adrenal medulla increase the force and rate of cardiac contraction.

The activation of α_1 receptors by means of G_q coupling triggers the phosphatidylinositol cascade, which can have multiple effects on neuronal excitability.

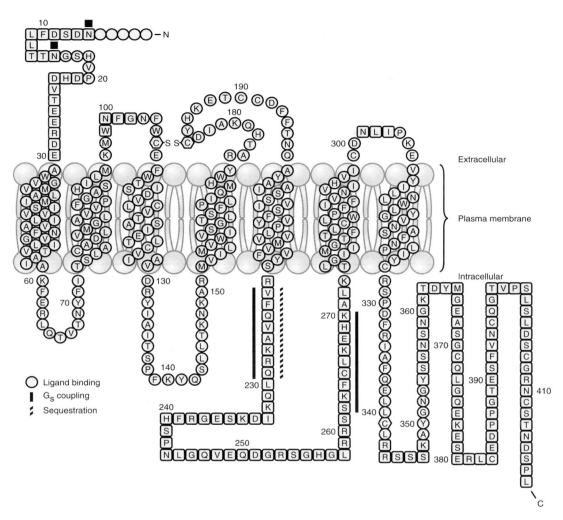

6–13 **Model of a β-adrenergic receptor (β-AR).** This two-dimensional beads-on-a-string model illustrates features common to most catecholamine receptors. The N terminus (N) is extracellular and the C terminus (C) is intracellular; in between are seven hydrophobic membrane-spanning domains and alternating intracellular and extracellular loops. Glycosylation sites (*red boxes*) reside near the N terminus; consensus phosphorylation sites (not shown) reside intracellularly. Amino acid residues that can be deleted from the protein without disrupting ligand binding or receptor insertion into the membrane are indicated with open boxes. Residues that alter ligand binding or protein folding when deleted appear in circles. The amino acids adjacent to the red bars are critical for G protein coupling, and those adjacent to the striped bar are necessary for ligand-mediated internalization. (Reproduced with permission from Strader CD, Sigal IS, Dixon RA. *FASEB J.* 1989;3:1826.)

In contrast, the activation of α_2 receptors, typically through G_i coupling, causes inhibitory responses in many cells; indeed α_2 receptors serve as autoreceptors on NE neurons as stated earlier.

The brain and certain peripheral tissues also express receptors for so-called "trace amines," which refer to endogenous amines (eg, tryptamine) that are structurally related to catecholamines and present in mammalian brain at extremely low levels. Trace amines can activate trace amine–associated receptors (TAARs) which are G protein-coupled. There is some evidence that **amphetamine** and related drugs can bind to TAARs, however, the functional importance of trace amines and TAARs remains unknown.

Serotonin receptors   There are 13 known human 5HT receptors **6-5**, 12 of which are GPCRs and 1, the $5HT_3$ receptor, is ionotropic. Activation of the $5HT_3$ receptor by 5HT opens a nonselective cation channel and triggers a rapid, transient depolarizing current that is carried by Na^+ and K^+. Like the nicotinic cholinergic and $GABA_A$ receptors, $5HT_3$ receptors are pentamers with subunits arrayed around a central pore. Unlike other ionotropic receptors, however, for which multiple subunits are known, only a single subunit of the $5HT_3$ receptor has been identified. Moreover, this subunit forms a functional channel when it is expressed in vitro, indicating that additional subunits are not required for $5HT_3$ receptor activity.

$5HT_{1A}$ receptors function as *somatodendritic autoreceptors* because they reside on the cell bodies and dendrites of 5HT neurons; their activation reduces cell firing and inhibits the synthesis and release of 5HT. The activation of serotonergic autoreceptors expressed on presynaptic nerve terminals, $5HT_{1D}$ receptors in humans (and $5HT_{1B}$ receptors in rodents), decreases local synthesis and release of transmitter. $5HT_{1A}$ and $5HT_{1D}$ receptors are highly homologous, and signal by coupling to the inhibitory G protein, G_i. It is believed that their inhibitory effects on serotonergic neurons,

6-5   **The Serotonergic Receptor Family**

Receptor[1]	Agonists	Antagonists	G protein	Localization[2]
$5HT_{1A}$	8-OH-DPAT; buspirone, gepirone	WAY 100135	$G_{i/o}$	Hippocampus; septum; amygdala; dorsal raphe; cortex
$5HT_{1B}$	Sumatriptan and related triptans		$G_{i/o}$	Substantia nigra; basal ganglia
$5HT_{1D}$	Sumatriptan and related triptans	GR 127935	$G_{i/o}$	Substantia nigra; striatum nucleus; accumbens; hippocampus
$5HT_{1E}$			$G_{i/o}$	
$5HT_{1F}$			$G_{i/o}$	Dorsal raphe; hippocampus; cortex
$5HT_{2A}$	DMT and related psychedelics[3]	Ketanserin; cinanserin; MDL900239	$G_{q/11}$	Cortex; olfactory tubercle; claustrum
$5HT_{2B}$	DMT		$G_{q/11}$	Not located in brain
$5HT_{2C}$	DMT; MCPP	Mesulergine; fluoxetine	$G_{q/11}$	Basal ganglia; choroid plexus; substantia nigra
$5HT_3$		Ondansetron; granisetron	Ligand-gated channel	Spinal cord; cortex; hippocampus; brainstem nuclei
$5HT_4$	Metoclopramide	GR 113808	G_s	Hippocampus; nucleus accumbens; striatum substantia nigra
$5HT_{5A}$		Methiothepin	G_s	Cortex; hippocampus; cerebellum
$5HT_{5B}$		Methiothepin	Unknown	Habenula; hippocampal CA1
$5HT_6$		Methiothepin; clozapine; amitriptyline	G_s	Striatum; olfactory tubercle; cortex; hippocampus
$5HT_7$		Methiothepin; clozapine; amitriptyline	G_s	Hypothalamus; thalamus; cortex; suprachiasmatic nucleus

[1]The nomenclature of 5-HT receptors is extremely complicated because so many subtypes have been cloned. Some require further characterization before definitive classifications may be made. Represented in the table is the nomenclature recently approved by the International Union of Pharmacology Classification of Receptors Subcommittee on 5-HT Receptors.
[2]mRNA expression has been determined for some subtypes in rat brain and may differ from patterns of expression in human brain.
[3]Other examples include lysergic acid (LSD), psilocybin, and mescaline.
DMT, *N,N*-dimethylamine; MCPP, metachlorophenylpiperazine

like those of other G_i-linked receptors, are mediated by the activation of inwardly rectifying K^+ channels, the inhibition of voltage-gated Ca^{2+} channels, and the inhibition of adenylyl cyclase. The actions of both types of autoreceptor are represented in **6-14**. These various 5HT receptors are also expressed on nonserotonergic neurons where they mediate the postsynaptic actions of the neurotransmitter.

Pharmacology of serotonin receptors   The development of agents that selectively target individual 5HT receptors either as probes of neural function or as drugs remains in its early stages. Many genetic knockout mice lack the targeted receptor throughout development, with significant biological consequences. Thus, much remains to be learned about the function of individual 5HT receptors. Nonetheless, several drugs that act on 5HT receptors have had clinical applications. Partial $5HT_{1A}$ receptor agonists, eg, **buspirone** and **gepirone**, have been used to

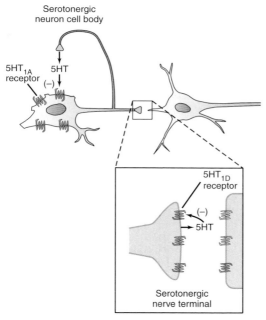

6-14 **Serotonergic autoreceptors.** The $5HT_{1A}$ receptor is a somatodendritic autoreceptor. As such it resides on cell bodies and dendrites; it regulates not only cell firing and therefore release of serotonin, but also serotonin synthesis, by influencing second messenger systems that regulate tryptophan hydroxylase. The $5HT_{1D}$ receptor is localized in presynaptic terminals and also regulates the synthesis and release of serotonin. The $5HT_{1B}$ receptor, not shown, is the rodent homolog of the human $5HT_{1D}$ receptor.

treat generalized anxiety disorder (GAD). They lack the risks of dependence, sedation, or abuse that characterize benzodiazepines, but exhibit only modest efficacy (Chapter 14). **Sumatriptan** and a large number of related **triptan** drugs, which activate $5HT_{1D}$ receptors, are important treatments for migraine headaches (Chapter 11). **Clozapine**, and many second generation antipsychotic drugs, such as **risperidone** and **olanzapine,** are antagonists at $5HT_{2A}$ receptors in addition to their D_2 antagonist properties. $5HT_{2A}$ receptor antagonism appears to counteract some of the risk of Parkinson-like side effects caused by D_2 receptor antagonism which is required for their therapeutic effects. Hopes that $5HT_{2A}$ receptor antagonism also contributes to the therapeutic effects of antipsychotic drugs have not been borne out. The idea that $5HT_{2A}$ receptor blockade might be antipsychotic derived partly from the observation that the **hallucinogens**, sometimes also described as "**psychedelic drugs**," are partial agonists at $5HT_{2A}$ receptors **6-3**. As was mentioned above, $5HT_3$ antagonists, such as **ondansetron** and **granisetron,** are effective **antiemetics** that lack the Parkinson-like side effects of D_2 receptor antagonists. There is great interest in the therapeutic potential of drugs that activate or inhibit the other 5HT receptor subtypes, eg, $5HT_{2C}$ agonists as antiobesity drugs (Chapter 10) or $5HT_4$ agonists as antidepressants (Chapter 14), but their clinical utility remains unproven.

Receptor desensitization   To prevent excessive stimulation, GPCRs undergo short- or long-term desensitization (loss of responsiveness to agonist). As discussed in Chapter 4, 2 main mechanisms govern GPCR desensitization. GPCRs can be phosphorylated and desensitized by second messenger–activated protein kinases (eg, protein kinase A). They also undergo phosphorylation by G protein receptor kinases (GRKs) when occupied by their ligand. GRK phosphorylation triggers receptor internalization and in some cases degradation by stimulating receptor binding to another protein, arrestin, and subsequent clathrin-mediated endocytosis **6-15**.

ACETYLCHOLINE

Synthetic and Degradative Pathways

Acetylcholine (ACh) is synthesized in a reversible reaction in which an acetyl group is transferred from acetyl coenzyme A (CoA) to choline by the enzyme *choline acetyltransferase (ChAT)* **6-16**. Its synthesis is regulated by the rate-limiting availability of choline. Choline is transported into neuronal terminals, either in its free form or bound to membrane phospholipids,

6-3   Hallucinogens

The indolamine **d-lysergic acid diethylamide** (**LSD**, "acid"; see figure) was first synthesized in 1943 by Albert Hoffman, who accidentally ingested a small dose and discovered that it produced sensory distortions (eg, visual illusions), hallucinations (most commonly visual, in contrast with schizophrenia in which hallucinations are more commonly auditory), and emotional changes. These can include elevated emotion or, alternatively, anxiety that may be severe. LSD was tested for use in the treatment of a variety of disorders including schizophrenia and alcoholism without convincing benefit. LSD was widely used as a recreational drug (to produce acid "trips") in the 1960s and 1970s; its use has waxed and waned since.

Although LSD is a nonselective serotonin receptor agonist, its effects on sensory perception are mediated through partial agonist effects on $5HT_{2A}$ receptors. This is a shared property of other psychedelic agents, including other indolamine hallucinogens (eg, **N,N-dimethylamine** [**DMT**] and **psilocybin**) and the phenethylamine psychodelics (eg, **mescaline** and **dimethoxymethylamphetamine** [**DOM**]) (see figure). Selective $5HT_{2A}$ receptor antagonists can block these actions in animal models. The distorting effects of these drugs on sensory perception and their capacity to produce hallucinations presumably reflect the dense innervation of the cerebral cortex by serotonin fibers 6-10. Under normal circumstances serotonin acts within sensory regions of cerebral cortex to modulate sensory processing and attention in response to changes in levels of arousal and in response to the onset of significant environmental stimuli.

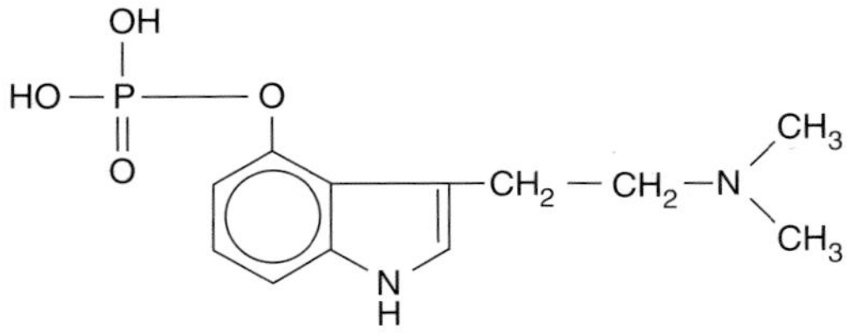

Psilocybin

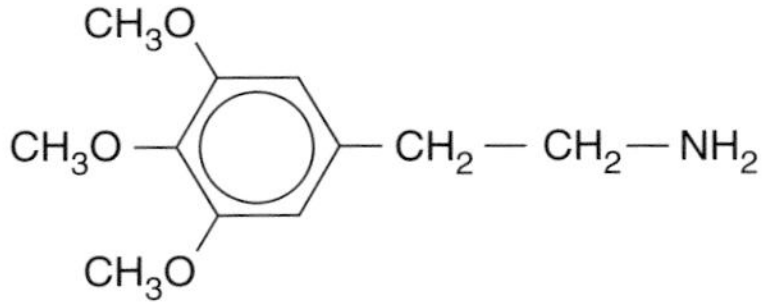

Mescaline

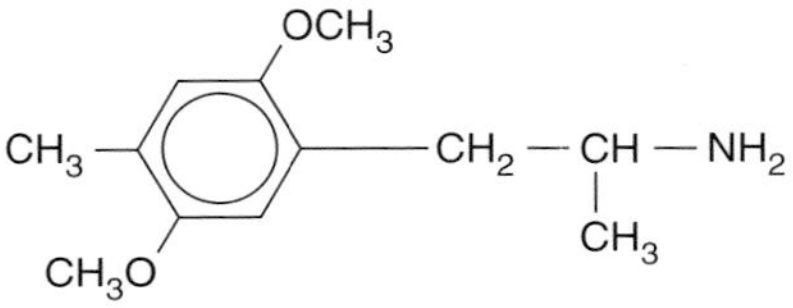

2,5-Dimethoxy-4-methylamphetamine (DOM, STP)

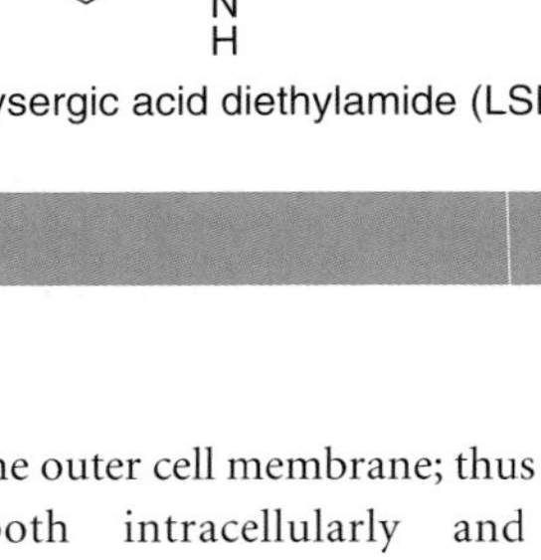

Lysergic acid diethylamide (LSD)

by distinct high-affinity and low-affinity transport mechanisms 6-17. Most ACh is synthesized in terminals, which are rich in ChAT and also in mitochondria, which are the site of acetyl CoA synthesis.

The synaptic actions of ACh are terminated by the enzyme *acetylcholinesterase (AChE)*, which hydrolyzes ACh into acetate and choline 6-17. AChE is an extraordinarily efficient enzyme that is capable of hydrolyzing 1000 ACh molecules per second per molecule of enzyme. This enzyme occurs in the cytoplasm and in the outer cell membrane; thus it can metabolize ACh both intracellularly and extracellularly. **Anticholinesterases,** which inhibit AChE, cause released ACh to accumulate extracellularly, producing excessive stimulation of ACh receptors throughout the nervous system. Reversible inhibitors, such as **physostigmine** and **neostigmine,** inactivate AChE for as many as 4 hours and are used clinically to treat **glaucoma, myasthenia gravis,** and **smooth muscle dysfunction** of the bladder and intestines. Unlike

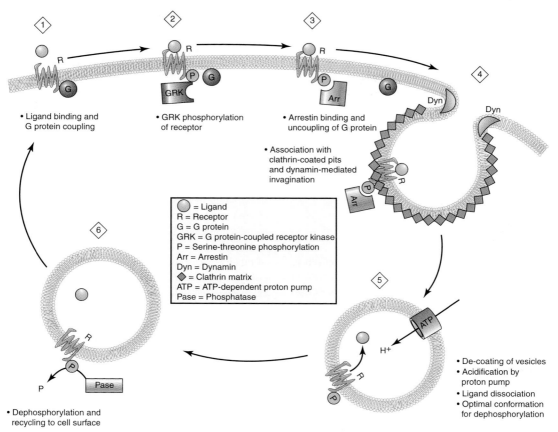

6-15 **Receptor trafficking.** G protein–coupled receptor trafficking involves a series of molecular events after ligand binding takes place (step **1**). Phosphorylation of the ligand-bound receptor occurs (step **2**); arrestin then binds to the phosphorylated receptor–ligand complex (step **3**). Bound arrestin complexes with clathrin lattices to bring about receptor sequestration in clathrin-coated pits and internalization by means of a dynamin-mediated process (step **4**). After the receptor is internalized in a vesicle, acidification alters its conformation and triggers the release of the ligand (step **5**). The receptor is dephosphorylated before it is recycled to the cell membrane (step **6**).

physostigmine, neostigmine cannot enter the brain because it is a quaternary ammonium compound and thus is too highly charged to cross the blood–brain barrier (Chapter 2). Centrally acting anticholinesterases, such as **tacrine** and **donepezil,** are used to increase central ACh concentrations in patients with **Alzheimer disease** (see below). Irreversible anticholinesterases completely inhibit ACh breakdown. Restoration of AChE activity requires new AChE synthesis. These irreversible inhibitors are used as insecticides, and are highly toxic if ingested by humans. These agents were a major class of **nerve gases**. Just before World War II, first German and then Allied scientists began to explore potential uses for organophosphate agents in chemical warfare. Their

efforts resulted in the development of several lethal compounds, including **sarin, soman,** and **tabun**, which can cause death within five minutes of exposure. The primary cause of death is respiratory failure, which typically is preceded by cognitive impairment and severe autonomic symptoms. Treatment for exposure to these toxins involves combined administration of a muscarinic receptor antagonist, such as **atropine,** with the AChE antagonist, **pralidoxime**, which paradoxically restores AChE function.

Functional Anatomy

ACh is synthesized by widely projecting neurons with cell bodies in the basal forebrain and brainstem **6-18** and by interneurons in striatum.

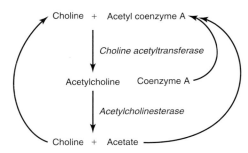

Choline $(CH_3)_3N^+ — CH_2 — CH_2 — OH$

Acetylcholine $(CH_3)_3N^+ — CH_2 — CH_2 — O — \overset{\overset{O}{\|}}{C} — CH_3$

6–16 Biosynthetic pathway of acetylcholine.
Choline and acetyl coenzyme A produce acetylcholine in a reversible reaction catalyzed by choline acetyltransferase (ChAT). After it is synthesized, acetylcholine is rapidly metabolized by acetylcholinesterase into choline and free acetate. Subsequently both metabolites may be recycled to produce more acetylcholine.

Widely projecting cholinergic neurons arise from eight nuclei that are clustered in two areas, the basal forebrain and the upper brainstem. The basal forebrain cholinergic nuclei are comprised of the *medial septal nucleus*, the *diagonal band*, and the *nucleus basalis of Meynert*. The dense innervation of the sensory and limbic cortices arising predominantly from the diagonal band and nucleus basalis is thought to influence arousal, cortical responsiveness to sensory input, and emotional states. Cholinergic neurons of the diagonal band and the nucleus basalis also innervate regions of the hippocampus and cerebral cortex involved in learning and memory. Because these basal forebrain cholinergic neurons tend to undergo early and severe degeneration in **Alzheimer disease**, likely contributing to cognitive impairment, they have been investigated as therapeutic targets. These neurons are dependent on *nerve growth factor (NGF)* for trophic support (Chapter 8); accordingly, NGF and drugs aimed at NGF signaling pathways have been tested as treatments but have not proven successful. It is because of the loss of ACh in the hippocampus and cerebral cortex that acetylcholinesterase inhibitors have been used in Alzheimer disease. Unfortunately, they are only modestly efficacious; at best they delay symptomatic deterioration for a few months, but do not slow neurodegeneration and do not produce dramatic clinical improvement (Chapter 17).

The pedunculopontine nucleus and the laterodorsal tegmental nucleus within the brainstem innervate dopaminergic neurons of the VTA and play a role in reward. While these nuclei, as well as the nucleus basalis, innervate the basal ganglia, the most significant cholinergic innervation of striatum comes from large cholinergic interneurons intrinsic to this region. These interneurons are critical components of the complex circuitry that underlies motor learning and motor control. As mentioned above, loss of dopaminergic input to the striatum in **Parkinson disease** leads to a profound motor disorder that can be partly counteracted by muscarinic cholinergic antagonists such as **trihexyphenidyl** and **benztropine**. These can be used in the early stages of the disease, or to supplement other drugs, such as L-dopa. Antimuscarinic agents also are used to treat the extrapyramidal side effects of antipsychotic drugs. Muscarinic cholinergic antagonists are believed to act at muscarinic receptors on striatal medium spiny neurons, where they partially compensate for the decreased dopaminergic signaling in striatal circuits (Chapter 17).

Storage and Release

The cholinergic nerve-muscle synapse is the best studied synapse in neurobiology and has taught us an enormous amount about synaptic transmission as well as the mechanisms of synaptogenesis in both development and repair. Central cholinergic synapses differ in important regards, most significantly by being nerve–nerve synapses. In presynaptic terminals, ACh is concentrated in storage vesicles by a vesicular transporter **6–18** that can be inhibited by **vesamicol**, resulting in depletion of ACh from vesicles. Vesicles fuse with the presynaptic terminal membrane in response to depolarization, releasing ACh into the synapse. Several toxins interfere selectively with this vesicular release of ACh. **Botulinum toxin A** and **tetanus toxin,** which prevent ACh release from cholinergic motor neuron terminals, cause paralysis. Small injections of botulinum toxin (**Botox**) are used therapeutically to treat dystonias (by causing profound muscle relaxation) and also cosmetically to inhibit the movement of facial muscles that cause wrinkles. **Black widow spider venom,** which contains α-**latrotoxin,** promotes massive vesicular release of ACh and a subsequent overstimulation of postsynaptic neurons. It exerts its effects in part by uncoupling Ca^{2+} signals from the release process. α-Latrotoxin stimulates exocytosis by binding to neurexins and latrophilins, critical components of nerve terminals (Chapter 3).

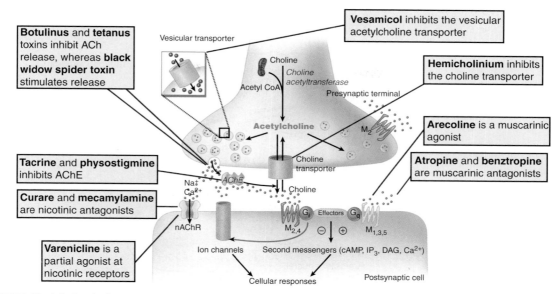

Botulinus and **tetanus** toxins inhibit ACh release, whereas **black widow spider toxin** stimulates release

Vesamicol inhibits the vesicular acetylcholine transporter

Hemicholinium inhibits the choline transporter

Tacrine and **physostigmine** inhibits AChE

Curare and **mecamylamine** are nicotinic antagonists

Varenicline is a partial agonist at nicotinic receptors

Arecoline is a muscarinic agonist

Atropine and **benztropine** are muscarinic antagonists

Vesicular transporter
Choline
Choline acetyltransferase
Acetyl CoA
Presynaptic terminal
Acetylcholine
M₂
Choline transporter
Na⁺ Ca²⁺
AChE
Choline
nAChR
Gᵢ Effectors Gq
M₂,₄ ⊖ ⊕ M₁,₃,₅
Ion channels
Second messengers (cAMP, IP₃, DAG, Ca²⁺)
Cellular responses
Postsynaptic cell

6-17   Model of a cholinergic synapse. Several interesting features of this synapse distinguish it from monoamine synapses. First, the most significant mechanism by which the action of acetylcholine is terminated is not by a (reuptake) transporter, but by a highly active enzyme, acetylcholinersterase (AChE). Second, the vesicular transporter for acetylcholine is distinct from the vesicular monoamine transporter (VMAT). Third, the membrane transporter does not return neurotransmitter to the presynaptic neuron but rather transports its metabolite (choline). Fourth, the presence of mitochondria is especially important because these organelles supply the acetyl coenzyme A necessary for acetylcholine synthesis. Finally, both G protein–coupled receptors, such as muscarinic subtypes M_1–M_5, and ligand-gated ion channels, such as nicotinic receptors (nAChRs), may be present.

Because ACh is not returned to the presynaptic terminal by a membrane transporter, it cannot be recycled like the monoamines. Instead, choline, released by the action of AChE on ACh, is returned to cholinergic terminals by a high-affinity choline transporter, where it is used to synthesize new transmitter. Choline transport is the primary mechanism regulating ACh concentrations in nerve terminals. **Hemicholinium** is a high-affinity inhibitor of the choline transporter.

Acetylcholine Receptors

ACh acts on two major types of receptors named for naturally occurring agonists: (1) muscarinic receptors, which are members of the GPCR superfamily, and (2) nicotinic receptors, which are members of the ligand-gated ion channel superfamily. Other members of this latter family include $5HT_3$ receptors, the ionotropic glutamate receptors, $GABA_A$ receptors, and glycine receptors. Structural similarities among these ligand-gated channels are represented in **6-19** .

Muscarinic receptors   Muscarinic receptors were named for their ability to bind muscarine, a compound

derived from the poisonous mushroom *Amanita muscaria*. They are located peripherally in the autonomic nervous system (Chapter 9) and in the CNS. There are five subtypes, all expressed in brain, each with the canonical seven membrane–spanning domains that characterize GPCRs. Muscarinic receptors can be subgrouped based on their patterns of G protein coupling: M_1, M_3, and M_5 receptors couple to G_q, and M_2 and M_4 receptors couple to G_i **6-6** . Electrophysiologic responses elicited by the activation of any given subtype can vary from one cell to another, depending on the second messenger systems and ion channels expressed in the cell. M_1, M_3, and M_5 receptors produce their effects by stimulating the phosphatidylinositol system. As with most other G_i-linked receptors, M_2 and M_4 receptors elicit mostly inhibitory responses; they act by activating inwardly rectifying K^+ channels, inhibiting voltage-gated Ca^{2+} channels, and inhibiting adenylyl cyclase.

M_1, M_3, and M_4 receptors are primarily located in the cerebral cortex and hippocampus, where their activity may mediate some of the effects of ACh on

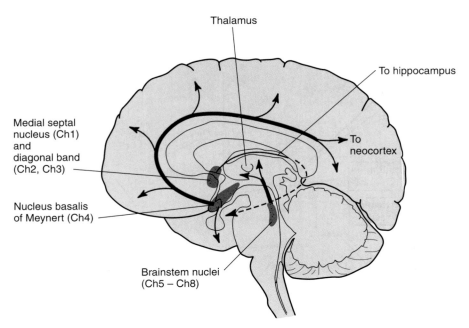

6-18 **Cholinergic projections in the CNS.** Eight small nuclei in the basal forebrain and brainstem, designated Ch1–8 (for cholinergic nucleus 1-8) in the rat, supply the cholinergic innervation in the brain. The basal forebrain cholinergic nuclei are comprised of the medial septal nucleus (Ch1), the vertical nucleus of the diagonal band (Ch2), the horizontal limb of the diagonal band (Ch3), and the nucleus basalis of Meynert (Ch4). Brainstem cholinergic nuclei include the pedunculopontine nucleus (Ch5), the laterodorsal tegmental nucleus (Ch6), the medial habenula (Ch7), and the parabigeminal nucleus (Ch8).

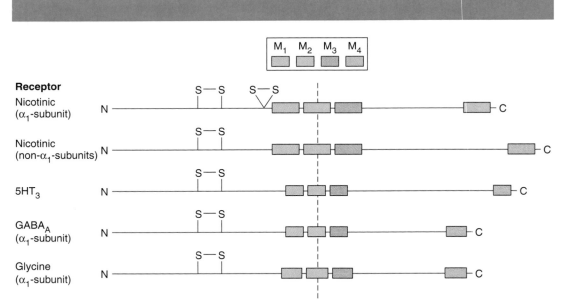

6-19 **Ligand-gated ion channels.** Considerable structural similarity characterizes the neurotransmitter receptors in this superfamily. Each receptor subunit has an extracellular N terminus, four membrane-spanning domains (M_1–M_4), and a short extracellular C terminus. A single disulfide bond is conserved among all members of this family, with the exception of nicotinic α_1 subunits, which possess two disulfide bonds.

6–6   Muscarinic Cholinergic Receptors

Receptor	Agonists[1] (carbachol, arecoline, pilocarpine, oxotremorine)	Antagonists[1] (atropine, scopolamine)	G Protein	Localization[2]
M_1	McN-A-343	Pirenzepine telenzepine	$G_{q/11}$	Cortex; hippocampus; striatum
M_2	—	AF-DX-116	$G_{i/o}$	Basal forebrain; thalamus
M_3	—	Hexhydrosiladifenidol	$G_{q/11}$	Cortex; hippocampus; thalamus
M_4	—	Himbacine; tropicamide	$G_{i/o}$	Cortex; striatum; hippocampus
M_5	—	4-DAMP	$G_{q/11}$	Substantia nigra

[1]Very few selective agonists and antagonists are available for muscarinic receptor subtypes. Some nonspecific or general agents are given in parentheses.
[2]mRNA expression for these receptors has been determined in rat brain, the distribution of each subtype may differ in human tissue.
4-DAMP, 4-diphenylacetoxy-N-methylpiperidine; McN-A-343, 4-(3-chlorophenylcarbamoyl-oxy)2-butynyltrimethylammonium chloride

learning and memory. In the striatum, M_1 and M_4 subtypes occur in abundance and mediate cholinergic signaling in extrapyramidal motor circuits and in responses to rewards. M_2 receptors are concentrated in the basal forebrain, the site of several cholinergic nuclei, where they act as autoreceptors to control ACh synthesis and release. The M_5 receptor is the least abundant of the muscarinic receptors and is expressed at low levels throughout brain.

Few muscarinic receptor agonists and antagonists are subtype selective, and none of the selective agents are used clinically. General muscarinic agonists include several alkaloids, such as **muscarine, pilocarpine**, and **arecoline**, and many synthetic compounds, such as **carbachol** and **oxotremorine**. Centrally acting agonists produce arousal as well as peripheral effects such as excessive salivation and sweating. Arecoline is an ingredient of **betel leaves**, which are chewed in some Asian cultures to produce mild increases in arousal. Muscarinic cholinergic agonists are used clinically to treat glaucoma and urinary retention, and to ameliorate the dry mouth that characterizes **Sjögren syndrome**, a disorder of autoimmune degeneration of the salivary glands.

Prototypical muscarinic antagonists include **atropine** and **scopolamine**. Neither of these is subtype selective. Atropine is a derivative of **belladonna**, whose name (beautiful woman) reflects its historical cosmetic use as a pupillary dilator. Belladonna is produced by the deadly nightshade plant, named because ingestion of excessive amounts are dangerous. Indeed, any excess use of antimuscarinic drugs produces cognitive

impairment, and at higher doses delirium, along with tachycardia and other dangerous autonomic symptoms. As stated earlier, muscarinic antagonists, such as **benztropine,** are commonly used to treat parkinsonian symptoms induced by first-generation antipsychotic drugs. Many psychotropic drugs, including **tricyclic antidepressants** and low-potency **antipsychotic drugs** (eg, **chlorpromazine** and **thioridazine**), have muscarinic antagonist properties, as do many first generation histamine H_1 antagonists (**antihistamines**) used to treat allergies and as over the counter hypnotic agents. In addition to expected autonomic effects, such as dry mouth, constipation, and urinary retention, these drugs can cause delirium. The latter is seen most commonly in geriatric patients treated with high doses of these agents or when combinations of drugs that share anticholinergic properties are used.

Nicotinic receptors Nicotinic ACh receptors (nAChRs) are located at the neuromuscular junction, autonomic ganglia, adrenal medulla, and CNS. These ligand-gated ion channels were first characterized based on their ability to bind nicotine isolated from the tobacco plant *Nicotiana tabacum.* Their activation by ACh leads to the rapid influx of Na^+ and Ca^+ and subsequent cellular depolarization. A prominent feature of nAChRs is their very rapid desensitization. Unlike desensitization of GPCRs, which requires the actions of other proteins (Chapter 4), desensitization of nAChRs is an intrinsic property of the receptors themselves. The same may hold true for other ionotropic receptors. This latter type of desensitization

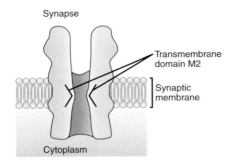

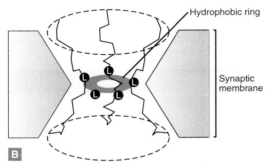

6-20 **Model of the nicotinic acetylcholine receptor.**
Crystallized synaptic membranes were examined with
an electron microscope to predict the three-dimensional structure of this receptor. **A.** A cylindrical membrane-embedded structure with a central pore is
shown. The second transmembrane domain (M2) of
each subunit lines the pore and bends inward to block
ion flow through the channel. **B.** A highly conserved
leucine residue (L) in the M2 bend of each subunit is
believed to protrude into the pore to form a tight
hydrophobic ring, which may act as a barrier to the
flow of hydrated ions across the channel. (Adapted
with permission from Unwin N. *J Mol Biol.*
1993;229:1118–1120.)

may be similar to inactivation of voltage-gated Na^+
channels (Chapter 2). However, the rate of desensitization of nAChRs can be regulated by the phosphorylation of receptor subunits.

nAChRs expressed in neurons and those expressed
in muscle differ in their subunit composition. nAChRs
are composed of five subunits organized around a central pore **6-20**. Most receptors are composed of heterologous subunits, of which at least twelve have been
identified to date. Eight are classified as alpha subunits
(α_2–α_9) and three as beta subunits (β_2–β_4); α_1 and β_1
subunits are expressed in muscle. Like other members

of the ligand-gated ion channel family, each subunit
has four membrane-spanning domains and disulfide
loops **6-20**. The second transmembrane (M2) region
of each subunit in each pentameric receptor lines the
pore of the channel to regulate its gating properties.

Most neuronal nAChRs contain both α and β subunits, and their stoichiometry is such that the ratio of
these subunits typically is two to three. However, some
nAChRs are homomeric; α_7 subunits, for example, are
capable of forming functional channels in vitro without
the presence of other subunits. Several major types of
nAChR complexes have been identified based on their
affinities for certain toxins; for example, one population
of receptors (ie, α_7 homomeric receptors) binds α-
bungarotoxin with high affinity and nicotine with low
affinity, whereas most other populations bind nicotine
with high affinity and are insensitive to bungarotoxin.

Research using mice with genetically engineered
nicotinic receptor subunits (knockout and knockin
mice) indicates that the predominant nAChR in most
brain regions contains a β_2 subunit coupled with any
of several α subunits, in many regions the α_4 subunit.
Homomeric α_7 receptors have been implicated in the
effects of nicotine on sensory gating, whereas receptors
containing the α_4/β_2 subunits partly mediate nicotine's
reinforcing, cognitive-enhancing, and analgesic effects.

Only a small number of ligands bind at nAChRs.
Curare blocks muscular and, to a lesser extent, neuronal nAChRs. **Succinylcholine**, a paralytic agent that
is used clinically during anesthesia, acts as a weak partial agonist; it mildly activates nAChRs and subsequently induces their prolonged desensitization.
Several blocking agents, including **hexamethonium**
and **mecamylamine**, inhibit nAChRs that mediate
neurotransmission in both sympathetic and parasympathetic ganglia (Chapter 9). Very few antagonists that
are selective for subtypes of neuronal nAChRs have
been developed. Perhaps the most selective antagonist
available is **methyl-lycaconitine**, which preferentially
antagonizes α_7 homomeric receptor complexes.
Recently, **varenicline**, a parital agonist at α_4/β_2
nAChRs, has been introduced to promote smoking
cessation; its clinical efficacy is not yet established. The
selective agonist **epibatidine** binds with high affinity
at nicotinic receptors but has been used only for experimental purposes (eg, as an antinociceptive agent).

As their name implies, nAChRs bind nicotine, which
is a highly addictive substance (Chapter 15). The normal role of nicotinic receptors, however, appears to lie in
arousal, attention, and memory. The widespread use of
tobacco by people with **schizophrenia** has raised the
questions of whether nicotine is being used to self-medicate cognitive impairments. Some epidemiologic studies

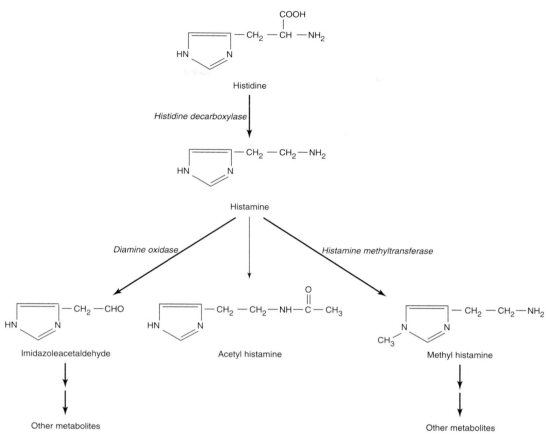

6-21 **Biosynthetic pathway of histamine.** Histamine is produced from the decarboxylation of the amino acid histidine and is subsequently metabolized into one of three products. Diamine oxidase converts histamine into imidazoleacetaldehyde, and histamine methyltransferase converts the neurotransmitter into its other major metabolite, methyl histamine. Acetyl histamine is a minor metabolite.

indicate that smoking reduces the likelihood of developing two neurodegenerative diseases, **Alzheimer disease** and **Parkinson disease**. Unfortunately, the use of nicotine or tobacco products is fraught with complications, most notably addiction and the diverse ill effects of inhaling or chewing tobacco (including cardiovascular disease, respiratory disease, and diverse cancers). Nevertheless, interest remains high in the pharmaceutical industry to develop more selective nicotinic agents for a range of medicinal purposes.

HISTAMINE

Synthetic and Degradative Pathways

Histamine is produced in one-step by decarboxylation of the amino acid histidine by histidine decarboxylase

6-21. Histidine also can be decarboxylated by L-aromatic amino acid decarboxylase (AADC), which, as previously discussed, is involved in the synthesis of DA, NE, and 5HT. Histamine is metabolized into methyl histidine by histamine methyltransferase. Alternatively, diamine oxidase may convert the neurotransmitter into imidazoleacetaldehyde.

Functional Anatomy

Within the brain, histamine is synthesized exclusively by neurons with their cell bodies in the tuberomammillary nucleus (TMN) that lies within the posterior hypothalamus **6-22**. There are approximately 64000 histaminergic neurons per side in humans. These cells project throughout the brain and spinal cord. Areas that receive especially dense projections include the

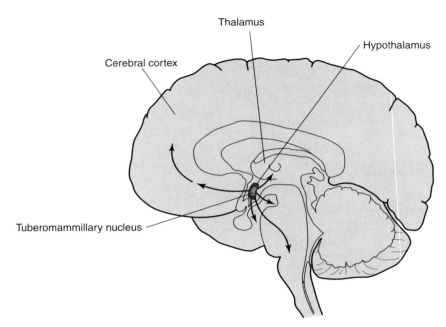

6-22 **Histaminergic projections in the CNS.** Histaminergic neurons are located solely in the tuberomammillary nucleus of the hypothalamus and give rise to widespread projections.

cerebral cortex, hippocampus, neostriatum, nucleus accumbens, amygdala, and hypothalamus.

The TMN is innervated by other widely projecting systems including monoaminergic and orexinergic neurons. Histaminergic neurons project back, in turn, to monoamine and cholinergic neurons involved in arousal, attention, learning, and memory **6-23**. While the best characterized function of the histamine system in the brain is regulation of sleep and arousal, histamine is also involved in learning and memory through its direct actions on the cerebral cortex, hippocampus, and amygdala, and indirectly by its effects on cholinergic and monoamine neurons. It also appears that histamine is involved in the regulation of feeding and energy balance. The firing rate of histaminergic neurons in the TMN is strongly correlated with states of arousal. Firing is fastest during periods of wakefulness and slower during sleep; indeed, these cells fall silent during slow-wave sleep (Chapter 12).

In the periphery, histamine is released from mast cells, where it plays a role in inflammatory, allergic, pruritic, and algesic responses. Histamine released in the stomach activates H_2 receptors to cause release of acid.

Storage, Release, and Reuptake

The mechanisms underlying the storage, release, and reuptake of histamine remain poorly defined **6-24**. It is presumed that histamine is concentrated in synaptic vesicles, yet the vesicular transporter responsible for such localization has not been determined. When histamine is released from nerve terminals in response to electrical stimulation, it acts on presynaptic and postsynaptic histamine receptors. Histamine is metabolized by the cytoplasmic enzyme, histamine N-methyltransferase. It is not clear how released histamine might be transported into neurons if this is, indeed, the major mechanism of inactivation. The organic cation transporter (OCT)-2 and -3 can transport histamine when expressed in cell culture. Whether it functions as a significant histamine transporter in the brain is not yet established.

Histamine Receptors

Four histamine receptors (H_1 to H_4) have been identified; all are members of the GPCR superfamily **6-7**. H_1 receptors couple to G_q and H_2 receptors couple to G_s. The H_3 receptor is thought to couple to G_i and to act both as an inhibitory autoreceptor and as a heteroreceptor that regulates the release of other neurotransmitters from nerve terminals. H_3 receptors have their highest distribution in the striatum, nucleus accumbens, and cerebral cortex. Antagonists are being explored as potential therapeutic agents to increase

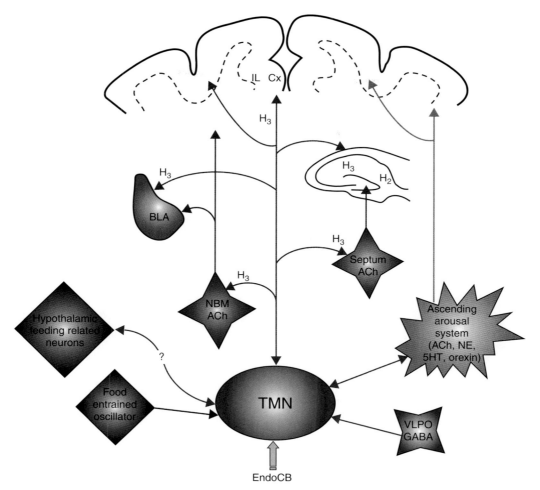

6-23 **Afferent and efferent connections of the tuberomammillary nucleus.** The diagram shows possible connections of histamine neurons involved in sleep and arousal, feeding, and cognition. All histamine in the brain and spinal cord is produced by the tuberomammillary nucleus (TMN) of the hypothalamus (see **6-22**). The TMN is under inhibitory control of GABAergic neurons from the ventrolateral peroptic area (VLPO). There is evidence that endocannabinoids activate TMN neurons. Histaminergic neurons influence learning and memory both by direct projections to the cerebral cortex and hippocampus and also by stimulating the cholinergic basal forebrain, which innervates these structures. Histaminergic neurons also project to regions of the brain involved in feeding. BLA, basolateral amygdala; NBM, nucleus basalis of Meynert (From Passani MB, Giannoni P, Bucherelli C, Baldi E, Blandina P. Histamine in the brain: beyond sleep and memory. *Biochem Pharmacol.* 2007;73(8):1113–1122.)

alertness, and also to enhance cognition. H_4 receptors appear to play a role in inflammation in peripheral tissues. They are expressed at low levels in the brain.

Many drugs block H_1 receptors, either as an unwanted side effect (eg, the tricyclic antidepressant **doxepin** and the antipsychotic drug **clozapine**), or as a desired mechanism as in the case of many allergy medications such as **diphenhydramine**. CNS penetrant H_1 receptor antagonists are sedating. Newer antihistamines used as allergy medications, such as **loratadine** and **terfenadine**, are nonsedating because they do not cross the blood–brain barrier. Centrally acting antihistamines are the active ingredient in many over-the-counter sleep aids. Most agents that are selective for the histamine H_2 receptor do not cross the blood–brain barrier. These agents such as **cimetidine** and **ranitidine** inhibit the secretion of gastric acid.

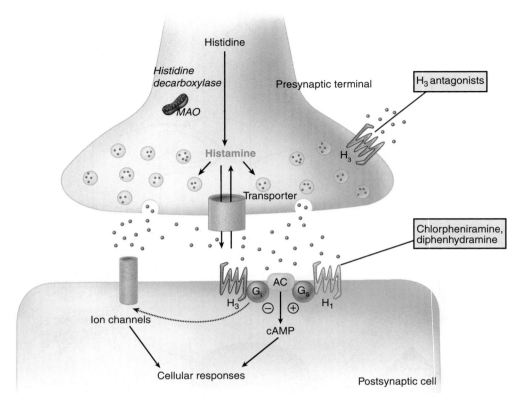

6–24 **Model of a histaminergic synapse.** Presynaptic and postsynaptic molecular entities involved in the synthesis, release, signaling, and reuptake of histamine are shown. Histamine can be metabolized by MAO (shown intracellularly) as well as by histamine methyltransferase and diamine oxidase (not shown). The transporter responsible for the reuptake of histamine has not yet been identified with certainty. See **6–6** for abbreviations.

6–7 **The Histamine Receptor Family**

Receptor	Agonists	Antagonists	G Protein	Localization
H_1		Mepyramine[1]; triprolidine; diphenhydramine; dimenhydrinate	$G_{q/11}$	Cortex; hippocampus; nucleus accumbens; thalamus
H_2	Dimaprit[1]	Ranitidine[1]; cimetidine[1]	G_s	Basal ganglia; hippocampus; amygdala; cortex
H_3	R-α-methylhistamine[1]; imetit[1]	Thioperamide[1]	$G_{i/o}$	Basal ganglia; hippocampus; cortex

[1]Selective agonists or antagonists.

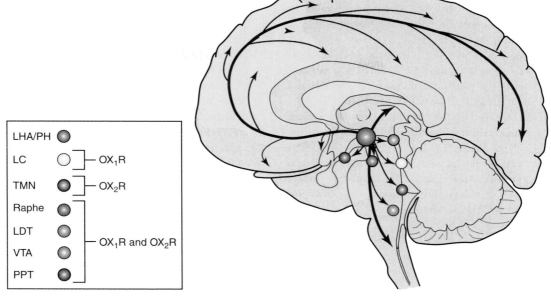

6–25 **Orexinergic projections in the CNS.** Orexin neurons with cell bodies in the lateral hypothalamic area (LHA) and posterior hypothalamus (PH) project throughout the brain (excluding the cerebellum) with dense projections to the noradrenergic locus ceruleus (LC), histaminergic tuberomamillary nucleus (TMN), serotonergic raphe nuclei, cholinergic laterodorsal and pedunculopontine nuclei (LDT and PPT), and the dopaminergic ventral tegmental area (VTA). (Adapted from Sakuri, using the underlying anatomic diagram from Martin JH, *Neuroanatomy.* Appleton & Lange, 1996.)

OREXINS (HYPOCRETINS)

Unlike the other neurotransmitters released by widely projecting systems in the brain, the orexins (also known as hypocretins) are peptides. Orexin A and orexin B (or hypocretin 1 and hypocretin 2) are produced in the lateral hypothalamic area (LHA) and posterior hypothalamus (PH) **6–25** and bind to two receptors which, like nearly all neuropeptide receptors, are G protein-linked: orexin receptors 1 and 2 (OX_1 and OX_2). Like all neuropeptides (Chapter 7), the orexins are synthesized by transcription and translation and packaged in dense core vesicles for release. Differences in vesicles and release mechanisms between small molecule and peptide neurotransmitters are discussed in Chapter 7.

Orexin neurons project to and activate monoaminergic and cholinergic neurons involved in the maintenance of a long "awake" period. Lack of orexin produces **narcolepsy** (Chapter 12). Orexin neurons are regulated by peripheral mediators that carry information about energy balance, including glucose, leptin, and ghrelin. They also receive inputs from limbic structures. Orexin neurons are, therefore, in a position not only to regulate sleep-wake cycles, but also to respond to significant environmental and metabolic signals. Accordingly, orexin plays a role in the regulation of energy homeostasis, reward, and perhaps more generally in emotion. There is a great deal of interest in generating orexin receptor agonists to promote wakefulness and perhaps improve mood, although such agents await definitive clinical trials.

SELECTED READING

Amara SG, Sonders MS, Zahniser NR, et al. Molecular physiology and regulation of catecholamine transporters. *Adv Pharmacol.* 1998;42:164–168.

Aston-Jones G, Cohen JD. An integrative theory of locus coeruleus-norepinephrine function: adaptive gain and optimal performance. *Annu Rev Neurosci.* 2005;28:403–450

Bayer HM, Glimcher PW. Midbrain dopamine neurons encode a quantitative reward prediction error signal. *Neuron.* 2005;47(1):129–141.

Brunner HG, Nelen M, Breakefield XO, et al. Abnormal behavior associated with a point mutation in the structural gene for monoamine oxidase A. *Science*. 1993;262(5133):578–580.

Craddock N, Owen MJ, O'Donovan MC. The catechol-*O*-methyl transferase (COMT) gene as a candidate for psychiatric phenotypes: evidence and lessons. *Mol Psychiatry*. 2006;11(5):446–458

Dani JA. Overview of nicotinic receptors and their roles in the central nervous system. *Biol Psychiatry*. 2001;49(3):166–174.

Fields HL, Hjelmstad GO, Margolis EB, et al. Ventral tegmental area neurons in learned appetitive behavior and positive reinforcement. *Annu Rev Neurosci*. 2007;30:289–316

Gainetdinov RR, Premont RT, Bohn LM, et al. Desensitization of G protein-coupled receptors and neuronal functions. *Annu Rev Neurosci*. 2004;27:107–144.

Haas H, Panula P. The role of histamine and the tuberomamillary nucleus in the nervous system. *Nat Rev Neurosci*. 2003;4(2):121–130.

Hill SJ, Ganellin CR, Timmerman H, et al. Classification of histamine receptors. *Pharmacol Rev*. 1997;49:253–278.

Hurlemann R, Hawellek B, Matusch A, et al. Noradrenergic modulation of emotion-induced forgetting and remembering. *J Neurosci*. 2005;25(27):6343–6349.

Mesulam MM. The systems-level organization of cholinergic innervation in the human cerebral cortex and its alterations in Alzheimer's disease. *Prog Brain Res*. 1996;109:285–297.

Missale C, Nash SR, Robinson SW, et al. Dopamine receptors: from structure to function. *Physiol Rev*. 1998;78:189–225.

Ordway GA, Stockmeier CA, Cason GW, et al. Pharmacology and distribution of norepinephrine transporters in the human locus ceruleus and raphe nuclei. *J Neurosci*. 1997;17:1710–1719.

Passani MB, Giannoni P, Bucherelli C, et al. Histamine in the brain: beyond sleep and memory. *Biochem Pharmacol*. 2007;73(8):1113–1122.

Prado VF, Martins-Silva C, de Castro BM, et al. Mice deficient for the vesicular acetylcholine transporter are myasthenic and have deficits in object and social recognition. *Neuron*. 2006;51:601–612.

Sakurai T. The neural circuit of orexin (hypocretin): maintaining sleep and wakefulness. *Nat Rev Neurosci*. 2007;8(3):171–181.

Schultz W. Multiple dopamine functions at different time courses. *Annu Rev Neurosci*. 2007;30:259–288.

Strader CD, Sigal IS, Dixon RA. Structural basis of β-adrenergic receptor function. *FASEB J*. 1989;3:1825–1832.

Tapper AR, McKinney SL, Nashmi R, et al. Nicotine activation of alpha4* receptors: sufficient for reward, tolerance, and sensitization. *Science*. 2004;306:129–132

Unwin N. Nicotinic acetylcholine receptor at 9 Angstrom resolution. *J Mol Biol*. 1993;229:1118–1120.

Vialou V, Amphoux A, Zwart R, et al. Organic cation transporter 3 (Slc22a3) is implicated in salt-intake regulation. *J Neurosci*. 2004;24:2846–2851.

Wess J. Muscarinic acetylcholine receptor knockout mice: novel phenotypes and clinical implications. *Annu Rev Pharmacol Toxicol*. 2004;44:423–450.

CHAPTER 7

Neuropeptides

- Neuropeptides are small proteins or polypeptides that serve as neurotransmitters in the nervous system generally acting via G protein–linked receptors. Other signaling peptides such as growth factors and cytokines are considered to be distinct even though they may have some overlapping functions.

- Like the monoamines and acetylcholine, neuropeptide transmitters serve primarily modulatory roles in the nervous system.

- The synthesis of neuropeptides, like that of all proteins, requires the transcription of DNA and translation of the resulting mRNA into protein.

- Neuropeptides are synthesized as large precursor prepropeptides that undergo extensive posttranslational processing, which includes cleavages into smaller peptides and enzymatic modification. The "pre" refers to an N-terminal signal sequence that directs newly synthesized peptides into the regulated secretory pathway.

- As a result of alternative RNA splicing and differential cleavage of propeptides in different tissues, a single gene can give rise to diverse signaling peptides with distinct functions.

- Unlike small-molecule neurotransmitters, which are packaged in small synaptic vesicles, neuropeptides are generally packaged in large dense core vesicles; both types of vesicles may be found in the same neuron.

- Neuropeptides may diffuse for long distances within the extracellular space before binding to their specific receptors.

Neuropeptides are short proteins or polypeptides that serve as neurotransmitters. Neuropeptides generally bind to G protein–linked receptors; there are rare exceptions in which peptides, such as insulin, have receptors that are enzymes (eg, protein tyrosine kinases) and act in a neurotransmitter-like fashion. Stimulation of G protein–linked receptors produces slower responses than stimulation of ligand-gated channels (Chapter 4). Moreover, many of the actions mediated by G proteins and second messengers alter the response properties of neurons resulting in "modulation" rather than simple excitation or inhibition. More than 100 neuropeptide transmitters are known; they play diverse roles in the nervous system, including regulation of sleep and arousal, emotion, reward, feeding and energy balance, pain and analgesia, and learning and memory. However, much remains to be discovered about neuropeptide function because selective antagonists are still lacking for many neuropeptide receptors.

This chapter focuses on general aspects of neuropeptide synthesis, release, and action, and describes several neuropeptides in more detail to illustrate these concepts. Several neuropeptides are discussed at greater length in other chapters; for example, hypothalamic peptides are considered in conjunction with the regulation of neuroendocrine function, stress responses, and feeding behavior (Chapter 10), and opioid peptides and substance P are considered in connection with pain (Chapter 11). Orexin (hypocretin) peptides are described in Chapter 6 because of their widely projecting organization in the nervous system and in Chapter 12 in relation to sleep and arousal.

CHARACTERISTICS OF NEUROPEPTIDES

Peptides are small proteins or polypeptides and thus composed of amino acids covalently linked by peptide bonds **7-1**. The term *neuropeptide* is reserved for small proteins or polypeptides that act as neurotransmitters in the nervous system. Other signaling peptides in the nervous system, such as growth factors and cytokines (Chapter 8), are generally distinguished from the neuropeptides even though they may have overlapping functions. Neuropeptides are found within the central nervous system and in the periphery, including both the sympathetic and parasympathetic nervous systems (Chapter 9). In addition to their neurotransmitter functions, some neuropeptides (eg, oxytocin and vasopressin) are released directly into the blood by neurons and act as hormones

(Chapter 10); others (eg, luteinizing hormone) act as hormones secreted by endocrine glands; yet others (eg, cholecystokinin) act within peripheral organs such as the digestive system. A sampling of neuropeptides is listed in **7-1**.

Neuropeptide Synthesis

In contrast to small molecule neurotransmitters, the synthesis of neuropeptides, like that of all proteins, requires the transcription of DNA into messenger RNA (mRNA) and translation of mRNA into protein **7-2**. A striking aspect of neuropeptide synthesis is that many steps can be regulated so that a single gene can give rise to diverse neuropeptides in a tissue-specific manner.

Diversity can be generated by alternative splicing of primary RNA transcripts to produce different mRNAs (Chapter 4). Thus, for example, calcitonin and calcitonin gene–related peptide (CGRP) are generated in a tissue-specific fashion by alternative splicing of a single primary transcript to yield peptides with very different biological actions. Calcitonin is produced in the parafollicular "C" cells of the thyroid gland and plays a central role in Ca^{2+} and phosphorus metabolism. CGRP is produced in neurons and, among its other actions, is a potent vasodilator, which has made its receptor a potential target for treating **migraine**. The tachykinin family (the members of which share a C-terminal sequence) provides another example of alternative splicing of neuropeptide-encoding mRNAs. There are two genes that encode tachykinins in humans, preprotachykinin (PPT) A and B. PPT-A is alternatively spliced and, as a result, encodes three distinct prepropeptides that give rise to multiple peptides, including substance P and neurokinin A **7-3**. PPT-B gives rise to neurokinin B.

Following splicing, the mature mRNA is exported to the cytoplasm for translation. The initial protein product translated on the ribosome is not an active signaling molecule, but a precursor polypeptide (a *prepropeptide*) that undergoes processing that converts it into one or more neuropeptides. Prepropeptides contain an N-terminal signal sequence (or "pre" sequence) that directs the newly synthesized protein into the lumen of the rough endoplasmic reticulum (ER) and thus into the proper, regulated secretory pathway **7-2**. The signal sequence is cleaved by a signal peptidase even before translation is completed, described as *cotranslational processing*. The removal of the signal sequence results in a *propeptide* that is released from the ribosome after translation is complete, transferred to the Golgi complex, and subsequently packaged within large dense core vesicles (LDCVs). Within the

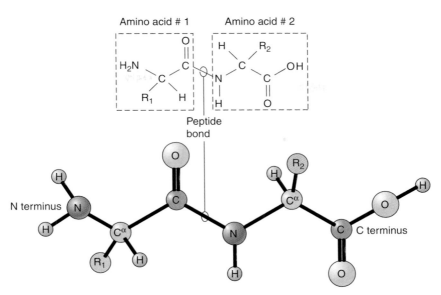

7-1 **Peptide bond.** Peptides are linear polymers composed of amino acids. The amino acids are joined by peptide bonds that result from the free carboxy group (C terminus) of one amino acid forming an amidoester bond with the free amino group (N terminus) of an adjacent amino acid. The 20 amino acids that form proteins differ from each other based on their side chains (denoted R_1 and R_2 in the figure). See Chapter 4 for further information.

Golgi complex and within LDCVs, the propeptide undergoes additional *posttranslational processing*, which involves additional cleavages and covalent modifications.

Propeptide Processing

Different patterns of tissue-specific cleavage is another step by which a diversity of signaling peptides can be generated. Posttranslational processing can be illustrated by the cleavage and modification of proopiomelanocortin (POMC; **7-4**), the precursor of several peptides with distinct biological actions, including adrenocorticotropic hormone (ACTH), α-melanocyte-stimulating hormone (α-MSH; also called melanocortin), and β-endorphin.

The endoproteases, prohormone convertases 1 and 2 (PC1 and PC2), which make the initial cleavages within propeptides, do so at dibasic amino acid pairs (Lys–Arg, Lys–Lys, Arg–Arg, or Arg–Lys). The resulting peptides are further modified by exopeptidases, which remove the free N- and C-terminal Lys or Arg **7-2** . In addition to the action of proteases, many neuropeptides are further modified. N-terminal acetylation of α-MSH significantly enhances its biologic activity; conversely, acetylation of β-endorphin reduces its activity. Peptides with a C-terminal glycine, such as α-MSH, may also undergo α-amidation.

There is an interesting and successful example of a peptide processing enzyme serving as a drug target: inhibitors of angiotensin converting enzyme (ACE), also known as peptidyl dipeptidase A, such as **captopril**, **enalapril**, and **lisinopril**, are widely used to treat **hypertension**. ACE cleaves the decapeptide angiotensin I to yield the far more active octapeptide, angiotensin II. ACE is also involved in inactivation of an additional neuropeptide, bradykinin. Because angiotensin II is a potent vasoconstrictor and bradykinin is a vasodilator, ACE inhibitors decrease blood pressure. This example may not be generalizable to enzymes such as PC1 and PC2, because they act on a very large number of neuropeptides and would thus lack specificity.

Storage and Release

Neuropeptides are processed and stored in LDCVs, which are assembled in the Golgi apparatus and transported to the synapse. In contrast, glutamate, γ-aminobutyric acid (GABA), and other small molecule neurotransmitters are stored in small clear synaptic vesicles (SSVs), which can be assembled in synaptic terminals. In central neurons, monoamines (eg, norepinephrine, dopamine, and serotonin) are largely stored in SSVs, although they are stored in LDCVs in adrenal chromaffin cells and various cultured cell

7-1 **Examples of Neuropeptides**

Calcitonin Family

Calcitonin
Calcitonin gene-related peptide

Hypothalamic Hormones

Oxytocin
Vasopressin

Hypothalamic Releasing and Inhibitory Hormones

Corticotropin-releasing factor (CRF or CRH)
Gonadotropin-releasing hormone (GnRH)
Growth hormone–releasing hormone (GHRH)
Somatostatin
Thyrotropin-releasing hormone (TRH)

Neuropeptide Y Family

Neuropeptide Y (NPY)
Neuropeptide YY (PYY)
Pancreatic polypeptide (PP)

Opioid Peptides

β-Endorphin (also a pituitary hormone)
Dynorphin peptides
Leu-enkephalin
Met-enkephalin

Pituitary Hormones

Adrenocorticotropic hormone (ACTH)
α-Melanocyte-stimulating hormone (α-MSH)
Growth hormone (GH)
Follicle-stimulating hormone (FSH)
Luteinizing hormone (LH)

Tachykinins

Neurokinin A (substance K)
Neurokinin B
Neuropeptide K
Substance P

VIP-Glucagon Family

Glucagon
Glucagon-like peptide-1 (GLP-1)
Pituitary adenylate cylase–activating peptide (PACAP)
Vasoactive intestinal polypeptide (VIP)

Some Other Peptides

Agouti-related peptide (ARP)
Bradykinin
Cholecystokinin (CCK; multiple forms)
Cocaine- and amphetamine-regulated transcript (CART)
Galanin
Ghrelin
Melanin-concentrating hormone (MCH)
Neurotensin
Orexins (or Hypocretins)
Orphanin FQ (or Nociceptin)
  (also grouped with opioids)

The traditional families of peptides listed here are based partly on other functions of the peptides (eg, hypothalamic releasing and inhibitory hormones), partly on amino acid sequence (eg, NPY family), and partly on pharmacology (opioids peptides), and must be considered at best a rough and incomplete guide to relationships among peptides. For example, β-endorphin is traditionally counted among the opioid peptides, and ACTH and α-MSH as pituitary hormones, but all 3 are derived from the same gene, proopiomelanocortin (POMC) **7-4**.

lines. LDCVs containing peptides commonly coexist with SSVs containing small molecule neurotransmitters. A few examples of neuropeptides and small molecule neurotransmitters that are colocalized to the same terminals are given in **7-3**. There are also examples of multiple peptides being colocalized within the same neurons. One striking example are some neurons of the supraoptic nucleus of the hypothalamus that may contain oxytocin, enkephalin, dynorphin, cholecystokinin, and cocaine- and amphetamine-regulated transcript (CART).

Although LDCVs and SSVs can be colocalized to the same terminals, their contents are released by different mechanisms, and indeed in response to different types of stimulation. SSVs are clustered in active zones abutting the synaptic cleft (Chapter 3). LDCVs appear to be excluded from these zones and are found at greater distances from the synapse **7-5**. The exocytosis of SSVs

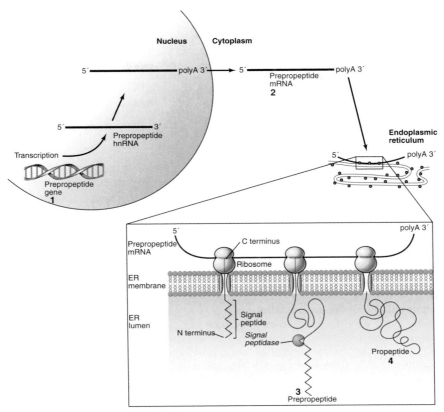

7-2 **Synthesis of a neuropeptide.** Neuropeptide synthesis is a multistep process that begins with (1) nuclear transcription of the gene that encodes one or more prepropeptides in the nucleus, splicing of the resulting primary RNA transcript to produce a messenger RNA (mRNA; described in detail in **7-5**), and (2) transport of the mRNA into the cytoplasm where it is translated by ribosomes in the rough (ribosome studded) endoplasmic reticulum (ER). (3) The N terminus of the growing prepropeptide is translated first, and contains a signal sequence that targets the growing peptide to the lumen of the ER and thence to the regulated secretory compartment. The signal sequence is cleaved by a signal peptidase even before the entire peptide is translated to yield (4) a propeptide that must undergo further enzymatic modification as required to produce active peptides.

occurs in response to large, transient increases in intracellular Ca^{2+}, whereas the exocytosis of large dense core vesicles requires increases in Ca^{2+} of lesser magnitude but longer duration, so that the Ca^{2+} can diffuse in adequate concentrations to reach these vesicles. Typically, a single action potential can cause SSVs to fuse with the cell membrane, but a rapid train of action potentials may be required to trigger release of neuropeptides from LDCVs. Thus, specific patterns of electrical activity in a neuron may lead to the preferential release of a neuropeptide or a small-molecule neurotransmitter, or may prompt the release of both. Because neuropeptides tend to be released under conditions of

sustained activity, they may regulate strongly stimulated synapses by providing positive or negative feedback.

Long-Distance Signaling by Neuropeptides

Another difference between neuropeptide signaling and small molecule neurotransmitters relates to the diffusion distances after release. When most small-molecule neurotransmitters are released into a synapse, molecules that do not bind a receptor are rapidly cleared by a transporter or, in the case of acetylcholine rapidly metabolized by a highly active enzyme, acetylcholinesterase. Neuropeptides are not rapidly

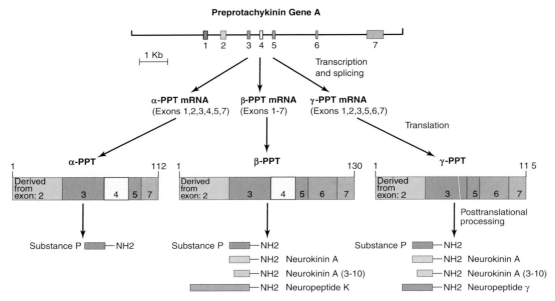

7–3 **Alternative splicing of the preprotachykinin-A (PPT-A) gene.** This gene, also called PPT-I gene or substance P–neurokinin A gene, contains seven exons (numbered boxes), which are alternatively spliced into three prepropeptides (α, β, and γ PPT). The number shown above each PPT splice variant represents its amino acid length after translation. After translation and proteolytic processing, all three PPT splice variants liberate substance P, which is encoded in exon 3. Neuropeptide K is encoded in exons 3–6 and thus is derived only from β-PPT. Neuropeptide γ is encoded in exons 3, 5, and 6, which occur together only in γ-PPT. Neurokinin A and the neurokinin A fragment (3-10) can be synthesized from either β- or γ-PPT. (Adapted with permission from Helke CJ, Krause JE, Mantyh PW, et al. *FASEB J.* 1990;4:1608.)

cleared from the synapse. Their action is terminated by endopeptidases and exopeptidases (different from those involved in synthesis) that cleave peptide bonds. These peptidases reside on extracellular membranes and, in contrast to acetylcholinesterase, their concentration and activity is such that peptides can diffuse relatively large distances in the nervous system. In fact, some neuropeptide receptors are found at significant distances from release sites.

As noted, most neuropeptide receptors belong to the superfamily of G protein–coupled receptors. Like small-molecule neurotransmitters, a given neuropeptide may have several receptor subtypes, as indicated in **7–4**. However, in cases that have been studied, receptors for neuropeptides bind their ligands with greater affinities than do the receptors for small-molecule transmitters; for example, acetylcholine binds to its receptors in the 100 μM to 1 mM range, whereas some neuropeptides can bind with nanomolar affinity. This high affinity means that neuropeptides can act at low concentrations, which is what would be expected if they often diffuse for great distances.

Neuropeptide Receptor Types and Subtypes

The interactions between neuropeptides and their receptors are quite complex. Imagine a small molecule such as norepinephrine interacting with the binding pocket of its receptor. Only so many atoms of the norepinephrine molecule can possibly interact ionically or sterically with the receptor; thus the molecular modeling of feasible interactions is relatively straightforward. Now envision a peptide such as neuropeptide Y (NPY), which is 36 amino acids in length. How does such a large molecule fit into the binding pocket of a G protein–coupled receptor? Which conformation has the highest affinity for the receptor, and which amino acid residues are critical for binding? Most importantly from a pharmacologic point of view, how might nonpeptide analogs be developed to mimic or antagonize NPY binding? All of these questions are difficult to answer and currently are the focus of investigation. Many, perhaps most, available ligands for neuropeptide receptors are modified peptide analogs, and

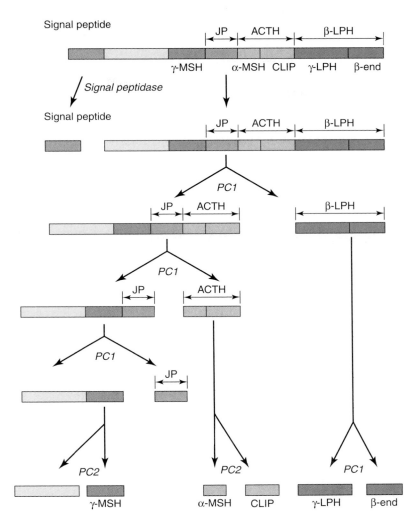

7–4 **Proteolytic processing of proopiomelanocortin (POMC).** After the signal peptide is removed from pre-POMC, the remaining propeptide undergoes an ordered process of endoproteolysis by prohormone convertases 1 and 2 (PC1 and PC2) at dibasic residues. PC1 is involved in the early steps of POMC processing and liberates the bioactive peptides adrenocorticotropic hormone (ACTH), β-endorphin (β-End), and γ-lipotropic hormone (γ-LPH). PC2 cleaves ACTH into corticotropin-like intermediate lobe peptide (CLIP) and α-melanocyte stimulating hormone (α-MSH) and also releases γ-MSH from the N-terminal portion of the propeptide. The joining peptide (JP) is the region of the precursor between ACTH and γ-MSH. Some of the resulting peptides are amidated or acetylated before they become fully active (see also **7-2**).

peptides are far from ideal as potential drugs. Synthetic peptides are subject to proteolysis by ubiquitous peptidases and, more importantly, they generally cannot cross the blood–brain barrier. Hence, nonpeptide agents are essential if neuropeptide systems are to be exploited for the treatment of central nervous system disorders.

Like small molecule neurotransmitters, neuropeptides may have multiple receptor subtypes **7-4** with distinct patterns of expression. In rare cases, such as norepinephrine and epinephrine, small-molecule neurotransmitters can share receptors. This is more often the case for neuropeptides, such as the receptors of corticotrophin-releasing factor (CRF; also known as

7-2 **Enzymes Involved in Posttranslational Processing of Neuropeptides**

Enzyme	Function
Prohormone convertases 1 and 2 (PC1, 2)	Endoproteolysis between dibasic amino acid residues (Lys and/or Arg)
Carboxypeptidase E	Removes carboxyterminal basic residues exposed by cleavages
Aminopeptidases	Removes N-terminal basic residues exposed by cleavages
Peptidyl glycine α-amidating monooxygenase (PAM)	Amidates C-terminal glycine residues
N-Acetyltransferases	Acetylates N-terminal amino acids of some peptides
Signal peptidase	Cleaves N-terminal signal sequence

See also **7-4**.

corticotrophin-releasing hormone, or CRH). The CRF$_1$ receptor shows high affinity for both CRF and a related peptide urocortin, whereas the CRF$_2$ receptor binds preferentially to urocortin. Each of the melanocortin receptor family members, termed MC$_{1-5}$, is activated by different peptides derived from POMC, with ACTH, α-MSH, and γ-MSH displaying varying degrees of potency. MC$_4$ receptors also can be antagonized by a distinct peptide called agouti–related peptide (ARP); indeed, MC$_4$ was the first receptor determined to have both endogenous agonists and an antagonist. These MC$_4$ ligands are involved in the regulation of feeding behavior (Chapter 10)

Although neuropeptide receptors tend to be localized in synapses, they also have been detected on the plasma membranes of axons, cell bodies, and dendrites. In fact, some of these receptor subtypes are hypothesized to reside primarily in extrasynaptic locations. This situation has been described for certain other G protein–coupled receptors, including those for some small-molecule neurotransmitters, such as dopamine. In contrast, the ligand-gated channels that subserve fast excitatory and inhibitory neurotransmission are expressed solely at synapses.

Neuropeptide receptors, like most G protein–coupled receptors, undergo internalization after sustained binding to a ligand; subsequently, the internalized receptors are either recycled to the plasma membrane or degraded (Chapters 4 and 6). For several neuropeptide receptors, such as neurotensin receptors, internalization may lead to transport from the synapse to the cell body. Interestingly, neuropeptide-receptor complexes have been detected near the cell nucleus.

7-3 **Examples of Neuropeptides and Small-Molecule Neurotransmitters Colocalized in the Same Nerve Terminals**

Neuropeptides	Small Molecule	Sites of Colocalization
Neuropeptide Y (NPY)	Norepinephrine	Locus ceruleus neurons; sympathetic preganglionic neurons
VIP	Acetylcholine	Parasympathetic preganglionic neurons
CGRP	Acetylcholine	Spinal motor neurons
Neurotensin, cholecystokinin	Dopamine	Substantia nigra neurons
TRH, substance P, enkephalin	Serotonin	Raphe nuclei neurons
Enkephalin	GABA	Striatal neurons projecting to the globus pallidus
Dynorphin, substance P	GABA	Striatal neurons projecting to the substantia nigra pars reticulata

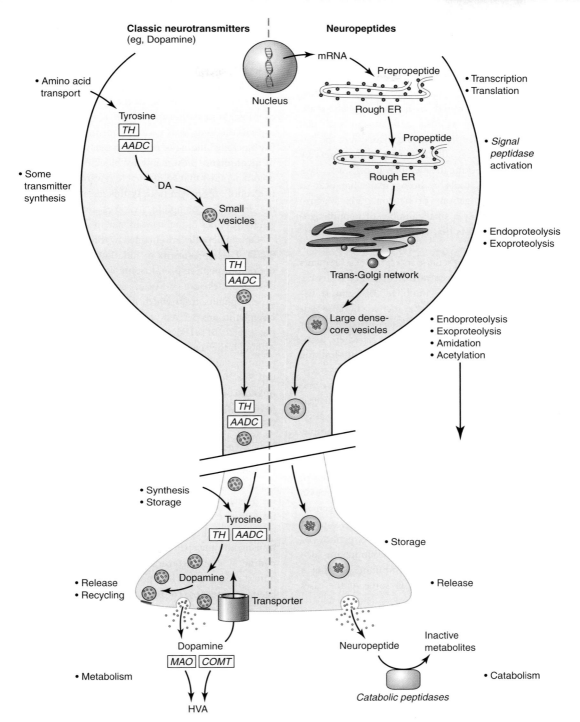

7-5 **Comparison between classic neurotransmitter and neuropeptide systems.** Dopamine is used here to represent a classic neurotransmitter. A principal difference between these two systems is the cellular location of their synthesis. Although some dopamine is synthesized in the cell body, most is produced in nerve terminals. In contrast, neuropeptide synthesis begins in the cell body and continues as it is transported down the axon. Unlike dopamine, which is stored in small clear synaptic vesicles, neuropeptides are stored in large dense core vesicles. Both dopamine and the neuropeptide are enzymatically degraded, but only dopamine is transported back into the nerve terminal, where it is repackaged for subsequent release. ER, endoplasmic reticulum; TH, tyrosine hydroxylase; AADC, aromatic amino acid decarboxylase; DA, dopamine; MAO, monoamine oxidase; COMT, catechol-*O*-methyltransferase; HVA, homovanillic acid.

Neuropeptide Functions

The functions of most small-molecule neurotransmitters have been discovered partly because of the availability of selective agonists and antagonists. Such agents have enabled investigators to ascertain the cellular and behavioral effects of these transmitters by mimicking or blocking their actions. In contrast, a lack of pharmacologic tools has been a major handicap in functional investigations of neuropeptide systems. Unfortunately, only a small number of peptide agonists and antagonists that cross the blood–brain barrier are known.

It has also been difficult to interpret measurements of neuropeptide concentration in nervous tissue. When neuronal activity is inhibited, for example, tissue levels of a neuropeptide may increase because synthesis may not be inhibited. This is in contrast, for example, to catecholamine biosynthesis where accumulation of end products inhibits the rate-limiting enzyme, tyrosine hydroxylase (Chapter 6). Conversely, sustained neuronal activation can lead to release and thus depletion of peptide stores. In vivo microdialysis has been used to overcome this challenge by measuring extracellular levels of a neuropeptide, for example, CRF and substance P, following some stimulation.

Because of the limited pharmacologic tools and the obstacles to neuropeptide measurement, studies of neuropeptide function have relied to a great degree on the construction of gene knockouts and other genetically engineered mice. While often difficult to interpret, especially, in mouse lines lacking the peptides or receptors of interest throughout development, such tools have significantly advanced our understanding of function, as will be illustrated in some of the cases described below.

EXAMPLES OF NEUROPEPTIDES

Opioid Peptides

Primarily because of their potent analgesic properties, but also because of their antitussive and antidiarrheal effects, **opiates** have long ranked among the most important drugs in the pharmacopoeia. Indeed, of the drugs commonly used today, **morphine** is one of a small number that were available in the 19th century. The medical importance of opiate analgesics (Chapter 11), combined with their addictive liabilities (Chapter 15), has produced much research in an unsuccessful attempt to develop potent opiate analgesics that are also nonaddictive. Products of this research include the discovery of lipophilic, small-molecule opioid receptor antagonists, such as **naloxone** and **naltrexone**, which have been critical tools for investigating the physiology and behavioral actions of opiates. In addition, naloxone is effective in the treatment of opiate overdoses and naltrexone, which is longer acting, is used in the long-term treatment of **opiate addiction** (by blocking binding of opiates to their receptors) and of **alcoholism** (presumably by blocking endogenous opioid peptides that contribute to rewarding responses to alcohol). More significantly, this research motivated the discoveries of opioid receptors and endogenous opioid peptides in the nervous system **7–1**.

Opioid peptides are encoded by three distinct genes **7–6**. These precursors include POMC, from which the opioid peptide β-endorphin and several nonopioid peptides are derived, as discussed earlier; proenkephalin, from which met-enkephalin and leu-enkephalin are derived; and prodynorphin, which is the precursor of dynorphin and related peptides. Although they come from different precursors, opioid peptides share significant amino acid sequence identity. Specifically, all of the well-validated endogenous opioids contain the same four N-terminal amino acids (Tyr-Gly-Gly-Phe), followed by either Met or Leu (see **7–6**).

There are three opioid receptors, μ, κ, and δ **7–4**, and a fourth related receptor (ORL-1 which binds nociceptin; see below). However, there is growing evidence that heterodimers form (eg, μ-δ dimers), yielding a receptor with distinct properties. As well, several isoforms of the μ receptor, generated by alternative splicing, have been reported. The σ receptor, a single transmembrane spanning protein that binds **phencyclidine**, was once considered to be a possible fourth opioid receptor, but it is now considered to be unrelated (Chapter 16). The μ, κ, and δ opioid receptors are all linked to the $G_{i/o}$ family of G proteins (Chapter 4). Among endogenous opioid peptides, β-endorphin binds preferentially to μ receptors. Two other brain peptides, endomorphin-1 and -2, which lack the signature opioid peptide sequence shown in **7–6** (Tyr-Gly-Gly-Phe), bind selectively and with high affinity to μ receptors as well. Enkephalins bind with high affinity to δ receptors and dynorphin peptides to κ receptors. However, opioid peptides do not bind exclusively to the receptors for which they have highest affinity; in vivo binding is also likely to be influenced by relative locations of released peptides and opioid receptors. Moreover, the complex pharmacology of opiate drugs suggests that posttranslational modifications and the aforementioned heterodimerization of μ and δ receptors create a far richer possibility for opiate drug and peptide binding than the three cloned receptors would initially suggest.

7–1 ▪ The Body's Own Opiates

Historically, three types of observations suggested the presence of specific opioid receptors in the human body. (The term *opioid* refers to endogenous peptides with opiate-like pharmacology, whereas opiate refers to morphine and related nonpeptide analogs.) (1) Opiate analgesics such as morphine produce effects at extremely low concentrations; for example, a few milligrams of morphine can produce clinically significant analgesia. This suggested action at a small number of high-affinity receptors rather than "mass action." (2) Opiate drugs exhibit stereoselectivity, suggesting a receptor that could only bind a drug with a specific conformation. (3) A competitive antagonist of opiate action (**naloxone**) had been identified in early studies. In the 1970s, several independent laboratories used radiolabeled ligand binding methods in preparations of synaptic membranes to produce convincing evidence of opioid receptors in neural tissues.

The discovery of opioid receptors raised the question of whether the body contained endogenous opioids. A more convincing indicator of endogenous opiate-like activity came from physiologic experiments. Under certain conditions of stress, animals can exhibit markedly elevated pain thresholds (stress-induced analgesia). The injection of naloxone can prevent the development of this stress effect, which suggested the involvement of an endogenous substance that bound to opioid receptors. Using a sensitive bioassay–contraction of guinea pig ileum (opiates are clinically constipating), and extracts of porcine brain, it was possible to identify opiate-like activity in brain tissue. These early studies discovered two pentapeptides with opioid activity, which were named enkephalins (Greek for *in the head*). Subsequently, it has been determined that three separate genes encode at least 18 endogenous peptides with opiate-like activity.

Morphine-like opiate drugs preferentially bind to μ receptors, which are concentrated in regions associated with descending analgesic pathways, such as the periaqueductal gray matter, rostroventral medulla, medial thalamus, and dorsal horn of the spinal cord (Chapter 11). Significantly, these receptors also reside in reward-related regions including the ventral tegmental area (VTA) of the midbrain and the nucleus accumbens, where they are responsible for the addictive effects of opiates (Chapter 15) and may play a more general role in the hedonic effects of natural rewards, such as food. In addition, μ receptors are expressed in the dorsal striatum and in the locus ceruleus (LC). In the LC, μ receptors mediate important aspects of opiate physical dependence and withdrawal (Chapter 15).

Enkephalins, rather than any clinically available drugs, are the molecules with the greatest affinity for δ opioid receptors. δ receptors are expressed not only in the dorsal horn of the spinal cord where they play a role in analgesia, but in many brain regions as well.

Some κ receptor agonists such as **nalbuphine** and **butorphanol** exert clinically useful analgesic effects acting via κ receptors (Chapter 11), but are also potent μ receptor antagonists. **Pentazocine**, also used as an analgesic, is a κ receptor agonist and a partial μ receptor agonist or weak antagonist. As such these drugs may precipitate withdrawal if used as analgesics in individuals who are dependent on morphine or heroin. κ receptors are found in the dorsal horn of the spinal cord, in the dorsal striatum and nucleus accumbens, in deep cortical layers, and in many other brain regions. Even though they are analgesic, κ receptor agonists and dynorphin peptides may produce dysphoria rather than euphoria because they are expressed on the presynaptic terminals of dopamine neurons that project from the VTA to the nucleus accumbens and other forebrain regions. Because κ receptors are coupled via $G_{i/o}$ to a K^+ conductance that hyperpolarizes dopamine terminals, κ agonists decrease dopamine release. In contrast, μ receptors are expressed on inhibitory interneurons in the VTA that suppress firing of dopamine neurons. Morphine-like opiates acting via μ receptors thereby disinhibit dopamine neurons and stimulate dopamine release, an effect opposite to κ agonists.

Another peptide, alternatively termed **nociceptin** or **orphanin FQ**, binds to a G protein–coupled receptor termed the *nociceptin receptor*, also known as ORL1. The terminology derives from ORL1 having been an *orphan receptor* because it did not have a known ligand (hence the term orphanin). Nociceptin/orphanin F/Q is a

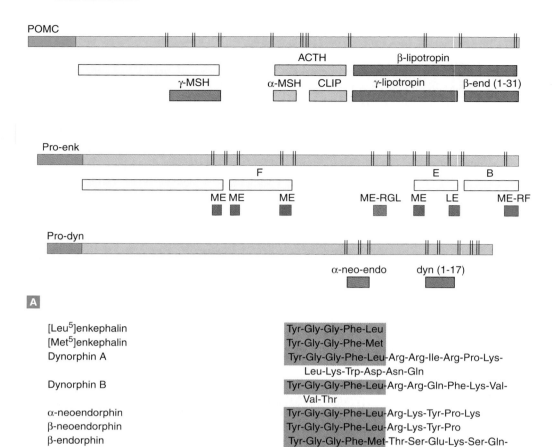

POMC

ACTH | β-lipotropin

γ-MSH | α-MSH | CLIP | γ-lipotropin | β-end (1-31)

Pro-enk

F | E | B

ME ME | ME | ME-RGL | ME | LE | ME-RF

Pro-dyn

α-neo-endo | dyn (1-17)

A

[Leu⁵]enkephalin	Tyr-Gly-Gly-Phe-Leu
[Met⁵]enkephalin	Tyr-Gly-Gly-Phe-Met
Dynorphin A	Tyr-Gly-Gly-Phe-Leu-Arg-Arg-Ile-Arg-Pro-Lys-Leu-Lys-Trp-Asp-Asn-Gln
Dynorphin B	Tyr-Gly-Gly-Phe-Leu-Arg-Arg-Gln-Phe-Lys-Val-Val-Thr
α-neoendorphin	Tyr-Gly-Gly-Phe-Leu-Arg-Lys-Tyr-Pro-Lys
β-neoendorphin	Tyr-Gly-Gly-Phe-Leu-Arg-Lys-Tyr-Pro
β-endorphin	Tyr-Gly-Gly-Phe-Met-Thr-Ser-Glu-Lys-Ser-Gln-Thr-Pro-Leu-Val-Thr-Leu-Phe-Lys-Asn-Ala-Ile-Ile-Lys-Asn-Ala-Tyr-Lys-Lys-Gly-Glu

B

7–6 Opioid peptides. A. Structures of the three opioid precursors. Proopiomelanocortin (POMC) gives rise to the opioid β-endorphin and other nonopioid peptides, including melanocyte-stimulating hormones (MSH), adreno-corticotropin (ACTH), and corticotropin-like intermediate lobe peptide (CLIP). Proenkephalin (Pro-enk) gives rise to multiple copies of the pentapeptide met-enkephalin (ME), one copy of the pentapeptide leu-enkephalin (LE), and several extended enkephalin-containing peptides, including two extended versions of met-enkephalin, ME-Arg-Gly-Leu (ME-RGL) and ME-Arg-Phe (ME-RF). Other large enkephalin fragments are designated peptides E, F, and B. Prodynorphin (Pro-dyn) gives rise to dynorphin and α-neo-endorphin. **B.** Shared opioid peptide sequences. Although they vary in length from as few as five amino acids (enkephalins) to as many as 31 (β-endorphin), the endogenous opioid peptides shown here contain a shared N-terminal sequence followed by either Met or Leu.

hectadecapeptide closely related to dynorphin A. It is derived from the pronociceptin/orphanin FQ gene. Nociceptin/orphanin F/Q has been reported to have antiopioid effects, and thus pro-nociceptive functions at least in some experimental paradigms, raising the possibility that ORL1 antagonists may be analgesic. However, possible antinociceptive effects of Nociceptin/orphanin F/Q are also under investigation.

Corticotropin-Releasing Factor

CRF (also called CRH) is a 41-amino-acid peptide that was first isolated in the search for a hypothalamic releasing factor that causes ACTH secretion from the anterior lobe of the pituitary gland. CRF shares this capability with vasopressin in many species, including humans (see below). CRF is synthesized by a subset of

7–4 Neuropeptide Receptors and Their G Protein Coupling

Neuropeptide					
Bradykinin	B_1 $G_{q/11}$	B_2 $G_{q/11}$			
Cholecystokinin	CCK_1 (or A) $G_{q/11}$, G_s	CCK_2 (or B) $G_{q/11}$			
CRH	CRF_1 G_s	CRF_2 G_s			
Galanin	Gal_1 $G_{i/o}$	Gal_2 $G_{i/o}$, $G_{q/11}$	Gal_3 $G_{i/o}$		
MCH	MCH_1 $G_{i/o}$	MCH_2[1] $G_{q/qq}$			
MSH	MC_1 G_s	MC_2 G_s	MC_3 G_s	MC_4 G_s (antagonized by ARP)	MC_5 G_s
NPY	Y_1 $G_{i/o}$	Y_2 $G_{i/o}$	Y_4 $G_{i/o}$	Y_5 $G_{i/o}$	Y_6 $G_{i/o}$
Neurotensin	NT_1 $G_{q/11}$	NT_2 $G_{q/11}$	NT_3 Single transmembrane		
Opioid peptides	μ $G_{i/o}$	δ $G_{i/o}$	κ $G_{i/o}$	ORL-1[2] $G_{i/o}$	
Orexin	OX_1 $G_{q/11}$	OX_2 $G_{i/o}$			
Oxytocin	OT $G_{q/11}$				
Somatostatin	SST_1 $G_{i/o}$	SST_2 $G_{i/o}$	SST_3 $G_{i/o}$	SST_4 $G_{i/o}$	SST_5 $G_{i/o}$
Tachykinins	NK_1 $G_{q/11}$	NK_2 $G_{q/11}$	NK_3 $G_{q/11}$		
TRH	TRHR $G_{q/11}$				
VIP, PACAP[3]	$VPAC_1$ G_s	$VPAC_2$ G_s	PAC_1 G_s		
Vasopressin	V_{1a} $G_{q/11}$	V_{1b} $G_{q/11}$	V_2 G_s		

[1]The MCH_2 receptor, expressed in human brain, is not present in rodents.
[2]ORL-1 is not always included with the other opioid receptors since its ligand, nociceptin/orphanin FQ, does not derive from the three "classic" opioid peptide encoding genes.
[3]Pituitary adenylyl cyclase–activating peptide.
See further discussion of several of these neuropeptides in later chapters.

neurons in the paraventricular nucleus (PVN) of the hypothalamus. A subset of these neurons project to the median eminence from which CRF is released into the portal–hypophyseal circulation, from which it acts on pituitary corticotrophs (these neuroendocrine functions are described in Chapter 10). CRF is not only delivered into the portal circulation, however; PVN neurons and other neurons, located elsewhere in brain, synthesize CRF and release it synaptically in the brainstem, cerebral cortex, central nucleus of the amygdala, and the bed nucleus of the stria terminalis (BNST), among other regions. CRF localized within the amygdala and BNST appears to play a role in **anxiety** and fear-related behavior (Chapter 14). Amygdala CRF is also important in mediating the negative emotional symptoms of withdrawal from most, and possibly all, addictive drugs (Chapter 15).

Two CRF receptors have been identified and cloned. CRF_1 receptors are expressed widely in the brain, while CRF_2 receptors exhibit a much narrower distribution. They are concentrated in the lateral septal nuclei of the forebrain. The endogenous ligand for CRF_2 is not CRF, but a related 40 amino acid peptide, urocortin. Urocortin can exert potent hypotensive and anorexigenic effects. Other members of the CRF family are urocortin II and III, urotensin I (isolated from certain fish), and sauvagine (isolated from frog skin).

CRF_1 receptor antagonists are being studied for use as potential **anxiolytic** and **antidepressant** drugs (Chapter 14), as well as for the treatment of drug withdrawal states (Chapter 15). While none have yet been approved, several have shown promise in small clinical trials. There is a growing consensus that these drugs exert their major anxiolytic and antidepressant effects within the amygdala and BNST rather than in the pituitary. Indeed, these drugs are probably safe because vasopressin has an independent ability to release ACTH. Otherwise, CRF antagonists might produce a dangerous syndrome of cortisol deficiency (Chapter 10).

Oxytocin and Vasopressin

These closely related nonapeptides  have both neuroendocrine and more purely neural functions. Oxytocin and vasopressin are synthesized in the PVN and supraoptic nucleus of the hypothalamus and transported within the long axons of these neurons for storage and ultimately release into the blood as neurohormones. Axons of the magnocellular (large) neurons of these two hypothalamic nuclei project to the posterior pituitary (neurohypophysis) where the two peptides are stored in presynaptic terminals and released into the systemic circulation. Vasopressin acts

Vasopressin

Cys-Tyr-Phe-<u>Gln-Asn-Cys-Pro</u>-Arg-<u>Gly</u>

Oxytocin

Cys-Tyr-Ile,-<u>Gln-Asn-Cys-Pro</u>-Leu-<u>Gly</u>

A

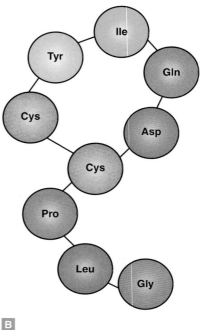

B

7–7 Vasopressin and oxytocin. **A.** Sequence comparison of vasopressin and oxytocin. These are closely related nonapeptides (ie, comprised of nine amino acids) that differ by only two amino acids. Shared amino acids are underlined. **B.** Both peptides also share the feature of an internal disulfide bond between the two cysteine residues. The structure of oxytocin is shown.

in the distal tubules of the kidney to facilitate water reabsorption (it is also called antidiuretic hormone, or ADH), and oxytocin stimulates uterine contraction at parturition and milk letdown during nursing. Axons from the parvocellular (small) neurons of the PVN and supraotpic nucleus also project to the portal hypophyseal vessels. Vasopressin can act in the anterior pituitary, like CRF, to stimulate synthesis and release of ACTH. The neuroendocrine functions of these peptides are described in Chapter 10; however, they also act within the brain.

Vasopressin has three receptors **7–4** , V_{1a} and V_{1b} (once called V_3), and V_2. All are G protein-linked, V_{1a}

and V_{1b} to $G_{q/11}$ and thus to the phosphatidylinositol second messenger system, and V_2 to G_s and to adenylyl cyclase (Chapter 4). A large body of research has implicated vasopressin and its V_{1a} receptor in the regulation of affiliative behavior 7-2. The V_{1b} receptor is located in the anterior pituitary where it stimulates ACTH secretion in concert with CRF. It is also expressed in the brain. V_{1b} knockout mice exhibit reduced aggression. Oxytocin has a single receptor which is linked to $G_{q/11}$.

Overall vasopressin and oxytocin play important roles in the ability of rodents to recognize previously encountered individuals of the same species and regulate social behavior through actions in diverse regions of the brain. Oxytocin appears to increase male–female bonding after mating and mother–infant bonding. In the amygdala, vasopressin acting via V_{1a} receptors may increase **anxiety**. Acting in a different region of the amygdala, oxytocin may decrease fear and anxiety and may promote prosocial behaviors by inhibiting avoidance and decreasing aggression. Is there any relevance for humans? Oxytocin can be delivered to humans via nasal spray following which it crosses the blood–brain barrier. In a functional MRI experiment, oxytocin decreased amygdala activation in human volunteers in response to fearful faces or scenes 7-8. In a double-blind experiment, oxytocin spray increased trusting behavior compared to a placebo spray in a monetary trust game with real money at stake. These results in humans are quite early, but suggest an important role for these peptides in regulating social interactions.

Tachykinins

Substance P, neurokinin A (NKA; previously known as substance K), neurokinin B (NKB), and neuropeptide K are members of the tachykinin family, all of which share the C-terminal sequence Phe-X-Gly-Leu-Met-NH$_2$. Substance P, NKA, and neuropeptide K are encoded by the preprotachykinin-A gene, and are produced by alternative splicing 7-3. The preprotachykinin-B gene encodes NKB. The three known tachykinin receptors, all of which are $G_{q/11}$-coupled, are designated NK$_1$, NK$_2$, and NK$_3$ 7-4. Substance P binds with highest affinity to the NK$_1$ receptor, NKA preferentially binds to the NK$_2$ receptor, and NKB binds somewhat selectively to the NK$_3$ receptor.

Of the tachykinins, substance P has gained the most attention. It was first discovered in 1931 in extracts of brain and gut. It is expressed in the dorsal horn of the spinal cord, amygdala, medulla, hypothalamus, substantia nigra, cerebral cortex, and striatum. In the latter region, it is colocalized with GABA and dynorphin in the striatonigral neurons that make up the "direct" striato-thalamo-cortical pathway of great interest in **Parkinson disease** (Chapters 13 and 17).

Substance P was long thought to be a critically important neurotransmitter carrying **pain** signals. Primary afferent nociceptors that synapse in the dorsal horn of the spinal cord (Chapter 11) express a complex array of neuropeptides, of which the most abundant include substance P, NKA, and CGRP. Substance P is colocalized with glutamate in the synaptic terminals of a class of nociceptors called C fibers. NK$_1$

7-2 **Vasopressin and Affiliative Behavior**

Species differences in the promoter of the V_{1a} receptor gene result in markedly different patterns of receptor expression in the brain, which in turn lead to variations in behavioral responses to vasopressin. V_{1a} receptor expression patterns influence male reproductive and social behavior in several rodent species, most notably in two types of voles. The male montane vole, which has a V_{1a} receptor pattern similar to that found in mice, tends to be asocial and promiscuous. In contrast, the male prairie vole, which exhibits more extensive V_{1a} receptor expression in the brain, is highly social and monogamous. Studies of mice have provided direct evidence that such differences in V_{1a} receptor expression affect affiliative behavior. Transgenic mice that express the prairie vole V_{1a} receptor gene show prairie vole-like patterns of V_{1a} receptor distribution superimposed on their normal, endogenous expression of V_{1a} receptors. Such mice respond to vasopressin administration with an increase in affiliative behavior, whereas control mice do not exhibit this response. These experiments not only show significant effects of vasopressin on social behavior, but also underscore the importance of patterns of receptor expression, and thus neural circuit activation, on the actions of any neurotransmitter.

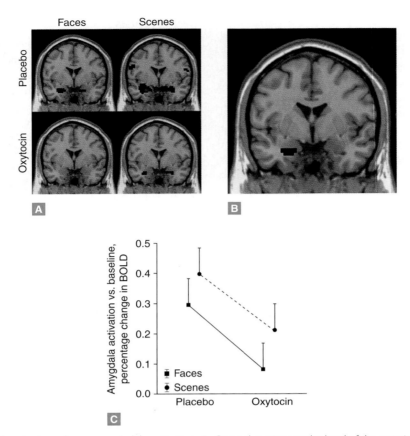

7-8 Effect of oxytocin on human amygdala activation. **A.** Coronal sections at the level of the anterior commissure. The response to fearful or angry faces is on the left and to fearful or threatening scenes is on the right. The effect of oxytocin is greater for faces, a social stimulus. **B.** Compared with placebo, oxytocin suppresses amygdala activation, predominantly on the left. **C.** This result is shown quantitatively as a function of BOLD functional MRI signal. (From Kirsch P, Esslinger C, Chen Q, et al. Oxytocin modulates neural circuitry for social cognition and fear in humans. *J Neurosci.* 2005;25:11489–11493.)

receptors are found in abundance in the dorsal horn. Accordingly, NK_1 receptors were considered an important target for the development of nonopioid analgesics. The first clues that this strategy might not succeed came from mice in which the prepro-tachykinin-A or NK_1 receptor gene had been knocked out; the phenotypes did not show substantial alterations in pain threshold. More definitively, potent and selective NK_1 antagonist drugs did not have significant effects in clinical tests on humans. Based on NK_1 receptor expression in the amygdala and on animal models of distress, NK_1 antagonists have also been studied as possible **antidepressants**. To date, most clinical trials have shown no efficacy. The main clinical use of NK_1 antagonists has been in blocking the nausea and vomiting caused by cancer chemotherapy.

These drugs, such as **aprepitant**, are likely exerting their actions in the medullary vomiting centers.

Substance P is released not only in the dorsal horn but also in retrograde fashion from the free nerve endings of nociceptive neurons. This retrograde release contributes to the phenomenon of **neurogenic inflammation**; other peptides such as bradykinin also contribute (Chapter 11).

Neurotensin

Neurotensin is a 13-amino-acid peptide derived from a larger precursor that also contains neuromedin N, a related 6-amino-acid peptide. Neurotensin is expressed in the brain, adrenal gland, and gut in slightly different forms that illustrate tissue-specific posttranslational processing. Its C terminus contains one of three different Lys–Arg sequences, which are differentially cleaved depending on the tissue in which neurotensin is processed. In the brain, the precursor gives rise to both neurotensin and neuromedin N, whereas in the adrenal gland, neurotensin, a larger form of neuromedin N, and a larger form of neurotensin sequence are produced. In the gut, the most common products are neurotensin and large neuromedin N. Central administration of neurotensin produces hypothermia and analgesia.

There are three neurotensin receptors **7-4**. Two of these, NTS_1 and NTS_2, are G protein–coupled receptors **7-4**. NTS_3 is a single membrane–spanning receptor analogous to type I amino acid receptors, exceptional for neuropeptide signaling. Neurotensin mRNA is induced in striatopallidal neurons of the striatum by D_2 receptor antagonists, including **antipsychotic** drugs, and in striatonigral neurons by psychostimulant drugs such as **cocaine** and **amphetamine**. Therefore, it has been hypothesized that neurotensin influences dopamine signaling and perhaps contributes to the plasticity induced by drugs that act on dopamine systems in the brain. These observations, however, have not yet led to new treatments for psychotic disorders or drug addiction.

Orexins (Hypocretins)

Orexin A and B (also referred to as hypocretin 1 and 2), products of a single gene, were discovered by convergent approaches in rat brain. One group of investigators found a peptide that stimulated feeding (thus the name "orexin") and the other group was searching for ligands for "orphan" hypothalamic G protein–linked receptors (thus the alternative name, hypocretin). The two known orexin receptors, OX_1 and OX_2, are coupled via G_q and $G_{i/o}$, respectively. Soon after the peptides were discovered, a loss of function mutation in the OX_2 receptor was found to be the cause of canine **narcolepsy** (Chapter 12), and orexin peptide knockout mice were shown to exhibit a narcolepsy-like syndrome. Subsequently, humans with the most common form of narcolepsy were found to have a depletion of orexin from cerebrospinal fluid and from the hypothalamic neurons where the peptide is normally synthesized. These discoveries have stimulated great interest in the development of orexin receptor ligands to modulate sleep and alertness. The diverse functions of orexin peptides, which in addition to sleep and arousal include feeding and reward, result from an anatomic organization that is reminiscent of monoamine neurotransmitters (Chapter 6). Orexin peptides are synthesized solely by neurons in the lateral and posterior hypothalamus and project to and activate monoaminergic and cholinergic neurons, among many other neuronal types **6-25**. Orexins are discussed further in Chapters 6 and 12.

Neuropeptide Y

NPY is the best known of a related peptide family that also includes peptide YY (PYY) and pancreatic polypeptide (PP). NPY gains its name for its N- and C-terminal tyrosines ("Y" is the single letter symbol for tyrosine). NPY is the most abundant neuropeptide in cerebral cortex. It also is concentrated in the dorsal horn of the spinal cord and arcute nucleus of hypothalamus. It is colocalized with norepinephrine in both the locus ceruleus and sympathetic nervous system **7-3**. NPY is a potent stimulator of feeding. Leptin, which inhibits feeding, acts partly by inhibiting the synthesis and release of hypothalamic NPY. Nonetheless, mice lacking NPY continue to feed normally, underscoring the complex interactions of hypothalamic systems that control feeding and energy balance (Chapter 10). In the periphery, NPY sensitizes smooth muscle to the effects of norepinephrine, resulting in a potent vasoconstrictor effect.

NPY, PYY, and PP bind to a group of 6 G protein–linked receptors, designated Y_1 to Y_6 **7-4** with varying selectivity; all couple to $G_{i/o}$. These receptors display marked region-specific distributions in brain and are located on both postsynaptic and presynaptic sites. Activation of the Y_1 receptor is thought to cause a decrease in anxiety-like behavior, acting, perhaps, in the amygdala. This hypothesis has generated interest in exploring the use of Y_1 agonists for the treatment of **anxiety disorders**. In contrast, activation of the Y_5 receptor has been proven to stimulate feeding, acting presumably within the hypothalamus; accordingly, Y_5 antagonists may be useful medications for the treatment of **obesity**. Applications of NPY pharmacology have not yet borne fruit in the clinic.

SUMMARY

Although less is known about neuropeptides than about many small molecule neurotransmitters, our understanding of the former is expanding rapidly based on the use of genetically engineered mice and the slowly growing catalog of selective agonists and antagonists. Given the modulatory influences of many peptides on functions such as sleep, arousal, feeding, anxiety, stress responses, reward, social interactions, and learning and memory, peptides and their receptors remain a potential storehouse of therapeutic targets that remain largely unexploited.

SELECTED READING

Bale TL, Vale WW. CRF and CRF receptors: role in stress responsivity and other behaviors. *Annu Rev Pharmacol Toxicol.* 2004;44:525–557.

Binder EB, Kinkead, B, Owens MJ, Nemeroff CG. Neurotensin and dopamine interactions. *Pharmacol Rev.* 2001;53:453–486.

Castro MG, Morrison E. Posttranslational processing of proopiomelanocortin in the pituitary and in the brain. *Crit Rev Neurobiol.* 1997;11:35–57.

Dumont Y, Quirion R. An overview of neuropeptide Y: pharmacology to molecular biology and receptor localization. *EXS.* 2006;95:7–33.

Gupta A, Decaillot FM, Devi LA. Targeting opioid receptor heterodimers: strategies for screening and drug development. *AAPS J.* 2006;8:E153–E159.

Hauger RL, Risbrough V, Brauns O, Dautzenberg FM. Corticotropin releasing factor (CRF) receptor signaling in the central nervous system: new molecular targets. *CNS Neurol Dis Drug Targets.* 2006;5:453–479.

Hokfelt T, Broberger C, Xu ZQ, et al. Neuropeptides—an overview. *Neuropharmacology.* 2000;39:1337–1356.

Kirsch P, Esslinger C, Chen Q, et al. 2005. Oxytocin modulates neural circuitry for social cognition and fear in humans. *J Neurosci.* 2005;25:11489–11493.

Kosfeld M, Heinrichs M, Zak PH, Fischbacher U, Fehr E. Oxytocin increases trust in humans. *Nature* 2005;435:673–676.

Seidah NG, Chretien M. Proprotein and prohormone convertases: a family of subtilases generating diverse bioactive peptides. *Brain Res.* 2000;848:45–62.

Storm EE, Tecott LH. Social circuits: peptidergic regulation of mammalian social behavior. *Neuron.* 2005;47:483–486.

Waldhoer M, Bartlett, SE, Whistler JL. Opioid receptors. *Annu Rev Biochem.* 2004;73:953–990

CHAPTER 8

Atypical Neurotransmitters

KEY CONCEPTS

- The common designation of a group of neurotransmitters as purines is a misnomer; what are called purinergic signaling molecules are the nucleoside and nucleotide derivatives of purine and perhaps pyrimidine bases.

- The two principal purinergic signaling molecules are adenosine and ATP. ATP is stored in small synaptic vesicles and released in a Ca^{2+}-dependent fashion, whereas adenosine is released from nonvesicular cytoplasmic stores, likely via bidirectional nucleoside transporters.

- Purine receptors form a relatively large and diverse group and have been categorized as P1 and P2 receptors.

- P1 receptors, also called adenosine receptors, bind adenosine and its analogs and are G protein-coupled. Stimulant drugs of the methylxanthine family, including caffeine, are antagonists of adenosine receptors. P2 receptors consist of both ligand-gated ion channels termed P2X receptors and G protein-coupled receptors termed P2Y receptors. P2X receptors play an important role in pain processing.

- Cannabinoids, the principal active ingredients of marijuana, primarily act in the brain on the CB_1 receptor, a G protein-coupled receptor found on presynaptic terminals in the CNS.

- Anandamide and 2-arachidonylglycerol are endogenous cannabinoids (endocannabinoids), which are released from postsynaptic cells and activate presynaptic CB_1 receptors.

- Nitric oxide (NO) is generated from arginine by nitric oxide synthase, which is stimulated by activation of postsynaptic NMDA receptors and increases in cellular Ca^{2+} levels. It diffuses out of cells and activates soluble guanylyl cyclase leading to the production of cGMP in adjacent cells and nerve terminals.

- Carbon monoxide (CO) is produced by the breakdown of heme by heme oxygenase-2 and also may function as an atypical, diffusible messenger.

- Neurotrophic factors are polypeptides or small proteins that support the growth, differentiation, and survival of neurons. They produce their effects by activation of tyrosine kinases.

- The neurotrophins, which comprise nerve growth factor (NGF), brain-derived neurotrophic factor (BDNF), and neurotrophins-3 (NT-3), and (NT-4), act by binding to a family of Trk receptors, TrkA, TrkB, and TrkC, with intrinsic tyrosine kinase activity.

- Several cytokine-like factors, including ciliary neurotrophic factor (CNTF), leukemia inhibitory factor (LIF), and interleukin-6 (IL-6), are characterized by binding to receptors that activate a family of protein tyrosine kinases called Janus kinases (JAKs), which in turn activate transcription factors called signal transducers and activators of transcription (STATs).

- Chemokines are small proteins involved in immune responses; in the brain, chemokines are expressed predominately by microglia.

Atypical neurotransmitters include a host of intercellular signaling molecules that have unusual properties or more recent dates of discovery compared to better known small-molecule and neuropeptide neurotransmitters that were reviewed in Chapters 5, 6, and 7. The atypical neurotransmitters include the *purinergic neurotransmitters adenosine* and *adenosine triphosphate* (*ATP*); *endogneous cannabinoids* (*endocannabinoids*); the gases *nitric oxide* and *carbon monoxide*, and families of *neurotrophic factors* and *cytokines*. Each of these neurotransmitters is found in specific subsets of neurons (and in some cases glia), has specific biochemic machinery for their synthesis, and exerts its biological effects via activation of specific receptors or enzymes. Because of their discrete anatomical distributions and, in many cases, modulatory functions, these atypical neurotransmitters, their receptors, and the proteins involved in their production and degradation are potentially significant targets for drug development.

PURINES

The purinergic neurotransmitters, adenosine and ATP, were long considered improbable mediators of neurotransmission because of their roles in intermediary metabolism and as building blocks of RNA and DNA. However, we now know that they are concentrated at certain synapses, they are released in response to synaptic stimulation, and they activate specific receptors to produce significant responses in target neurons. It is also established that purinergic receptors mediate the actions of several pharmacologic agents, most notably **caffeine** and related stimulants.

Biochemistry

The practice of referring to these signaling molecules as purines is to some degree a misnomer. Purines are ring-structured basic compounds that include adenine and guanine. These molecules do not function as neurotransmitters; nor do the pyrimidines, which include uracil, thymidine, and cytosine. So-called purinergic signaling molecules are in fact the nucleoside and nucleotide derivatives of purine bases 8–1A . The two principal neurotransmitters in this family are adenosine and ATP. Related to these are the adenine dinucleotides, which consist of two adenosine molecules covalently linked by a chain of two to six phosphate groups. Adenine dinucleotides are represented by the abbreviation ApnA, wherein *n* equals the number of phosphates between the two adenosines 8–1B . ApnA molecules are released by neurons and thus may

be considered part of the purinergic signaling family. There is also some evidence that nucleoside and nucleotide derivatives of pyrimidine bases may serve as neurotransmitters, although this possibility remains poorly characterized.

Storage and Release

Despite their similarities, adenosine and ATP have distinct properties. ATP and ApnA are stored in small synaptic vesicles and are released in response to action potentials in a Ca^{2+}-dependent process similar to the release process for classic neurotransmitters (Chapter 3). Indeed, ATP and classic neurotransmitters often can be detected in the same synapses and even in the same synaptic vesicles indicating that they can be coreleased. Release of ATP from sympathetic nerve terminals as well as vascular endothelial cells and tumor cells may play a particularly important role in various pain states. In contrast, adenosine is released from nonvesicular cytoplasmic stores and most likely reaches the extracellular space by one of two means. First, any of several bidirectional nucleoside transporters can secrete adenosine into the extracellular space, including the synapse. Second, ATP is very rapidly metabolized into adenosine once it is released from a cell. A membrane-bound ectodiphosphohydrolase converts ATP into ADP and AMP, and subsequently a membrane-associated or soluble ecto-5′-nucleotidase converts AMP into adenosine. Because the conversion of ATP to adenosine takes place in less than a second, the synaptic release of ATP should be regarded as an important source of extracellular adenosine.

The schematic representation of the purinergic cascade in 8–2 shows that the release of ATP can lead to the production of other purinergic compounds and to the subsequent activation of several different receptors. It should be noted that ApnA is hydrolyzed much more slowly than ATP and can reside in the synaptic cleft for longer periods of time.

Transporters

Nucleoside transporters are membrane-bound proteins that shuttle purine and pyrimidine nucleosides into and out of many cells, including neurons. The transporters are purine selective or pyrimidine selective. Some act to concentrate the nucleosides in a cell in a Na^+-dependent fashion. Others transport nucleosides down their concentration gradients. Pharmacologic and genetic studies indicate that there are at least seven nucleoside transporters, which belong to two gene families. The so-called equilibrative nucleoside transporter gene family (Slc29A1-A4 or

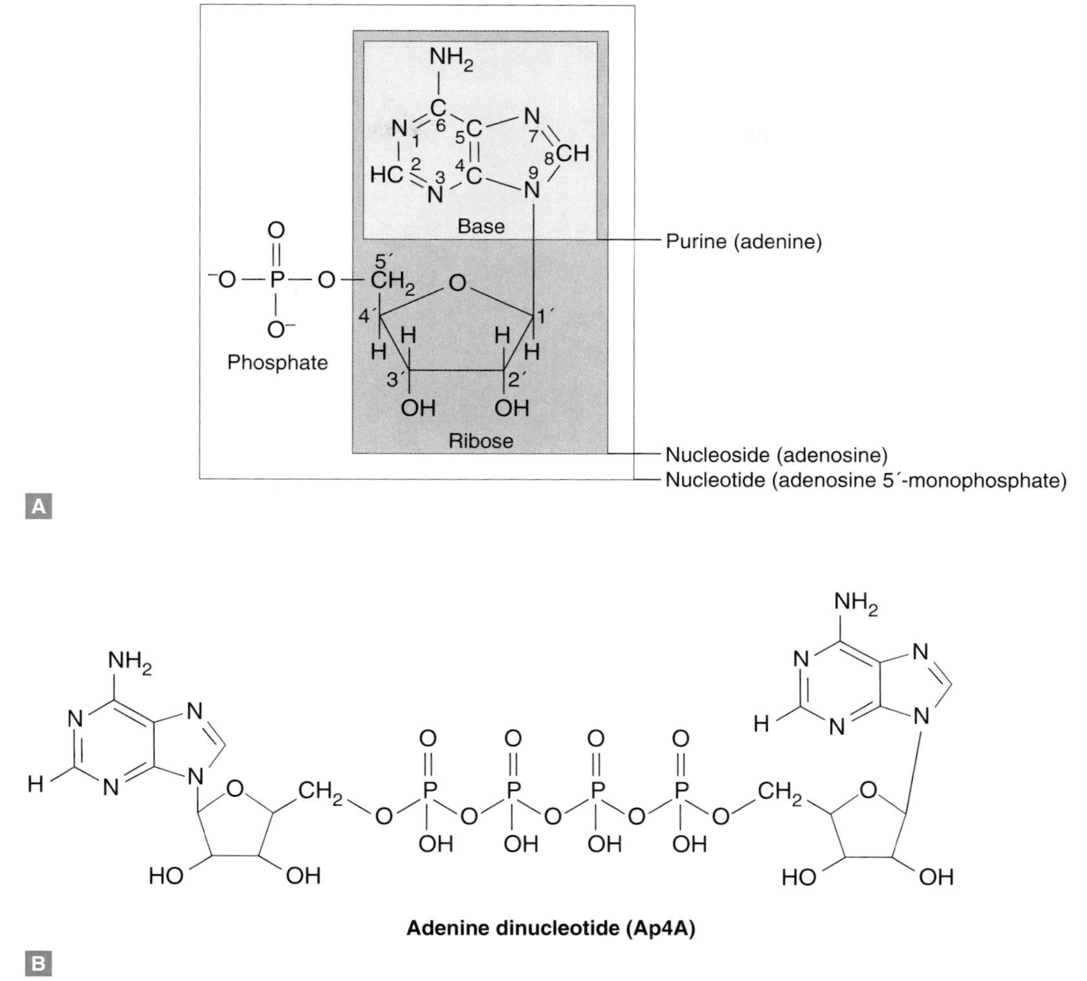

A

Adenine dinucleotide (Ap4A)

B

8-1 **Structures of purinergic compounds. A.** Purines, such as adenine, are basic ring-structured molecules, often referred to as bases. Nucleosides are molecules composed of a pentose sugar, such as ribose, covalently linked to a nitrogen atom in the base. Nucleotides are nucleosides whose mono-, di-, or triphosphate groups are linked to the 5′ carbon of a pentose sugar. Adenine's nucleosides and nucleotides are neurotransmitters, but adenine is not involved in neurotransmission. **B.** Adenine dinucleotides are two nucleosides linked by 2 to 6 phosphate groups. For example, Ap4A signifies a diadenosine molecule with four intervening phosphate groups.

ENT1-4), which consists of four subtypes (Slc29A1 or ENT1-4), mediates both efflux and influx of nucleosides; the concentrative nucleoside transporter family, which has three members (Slc28A1-A3 or CNT1-3), mediates Na$^+$-dependent influx of nucleosides. Although much remains to be learned about the structure and function of these proteins, they have been exploited in the development of powerful therapeutic agents. A number of cancer chemotherapeutic drugs, such as **gemcitabine**, and several potent antiviral compounds, such as **zidovudine (AZT)**, which are used in the treatment of **AIDS**, are nucleoside analogs that enter target cells by means of nucleoside transporters. Given the powerful effects that adenosine exerts on brain function, it is possible that drugs that regulate nucleoside transporters might eventually prove useful in the treatment of neuropsychiatric disorders.

Receptors

Purine receptors form a relatively large and diverse group of proteins that comprise two main subgroups,

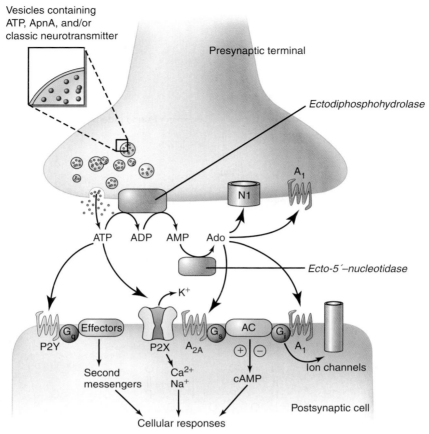

8–2 **A purinergic synapse.** Adenosine triphosphate (ATP) and ApnA typically are colocalized with a classic neurotransmitter and are released into the synaptic cleft in a Ca^{2+}-dependent fashion. After it is released, ATP can directly activate P2Y and P2X receptors. P2Y receptors are coupled to G proteins and activate second messenger systems. Most are coupled to $G_{q/11}$ and activate phospholipase C (PLC) and the phosphatidylinositol pathway. P2X receptors are ligand-gated channels that depolarize the postsynaptic membrane. ATP remaining in the synapse is rapidly converted into adenosine (Ado) by the actions of an ectodiphosphohydrolase and an ecto-5'-nucleotidase. Subsequently Ado is able to activate presynaptic and postsynaptic G protein-coupled P1 receptors (A_1 and A_2) and regulate adenylyl cyclase (AC) and the cAMP pathway, and in turn can be recycled into the presynaptic cell by means of a Na^+-dependent transporter (N1).

referred to as P1 and P2 receptors. Characteristics of both of these receptor families are discussed here and are summarized in **8-1**. P1 receptors, also known as adenosine receptors (A_1 and A_2), bind adenosine and its analogs and are coupled to G proteins. Four subtypes have been cloned and characterized (A_1, A_{2A}, A_{2B}, A_3) and each displays the canonical seven-transmembrane domains found in other members of the G protein-coupled receptor superfamily. The A_1 receptor subtype is the most widely expressed in the brain and spinal cord and has the highest affinity for adenosine. Its activation has been implicated in the putative anxiolytic,

anticonvulsant, analgesic, and sedative properties of adenosine. Conversely, antagonism of A_1 receptors by **methylxanthines** such as **caffeine** and similar drugs results in stimulatory effects, including increased alertness at low doses and anxiety and irritability at much higher doses (**8-1**; see also Chapter 12).

The two subtypes of the A_2 receptor, A_{2A} and A_{2B}, have a somewhat lower affinity for adenosine than do A_1 receptors. The A_{2B} receptor is ubiquitous in the human body yet is expressed only at very low levels in the brain and spinal cord. In contrast, the A_{2A} receptor is highly concentrated in the dorsal striatum, nucleus

8–1 **Purine Receptor Families**

	Receptor Subtype				
P1 (Adenosine) Receptor G protein coupling	A_1 $G_{i/o}$	A_{2A} G_s	A_{2B} G_s	A_3 $G_{i/o}$	
P2Y Receptor G protein coupling Substrate specificity	$P2Y_1$ $G_{q/11}$ ADP, ATP, ApnA	$P2Y_2$ $G_{q/11}, G_{i/o}$ ATP = UTP	$P2Y_4$ $G_{q/11}, G_i$ UTP > ATP	$P2Y_6$ $G_{q/11}$ UDP	$P2Y_{11}$? ATP > ADP
P2X Receptor (ionotropic) Substrate specificity	$P2X_1$ ATP > ADP	$P2X_2$ ATP	$P2X_3$ ATP	$P2X_4$ ATP > CTP	$P2X_5$ ATP
Substrate specificity	$P2X_6$ Unknown	$P2X_7$ ATP			

Purine receptors are divided into P1 and P2 subfamilies. P2 receptors can be further divided into P2X ligand-gated channels and P2Y G protein-coupled receptors. Jumps in the numbering of receptors, eg, no $P2Y_5$ receptor is listed, stem from the incorrect initial identification of cloned proteins as purine receptor subtypes. These incorrectly identified entities subsequently have been withdrawn. For some subtypes, such as the $P2X_6$ receptor, no information is provided because the human variant remains incompletely characterized.

accumbens, and olfactory tubercle—three brain regions that receive rich dopaminergic innervation (Chapters 6, 15–17). Indeed, the actions of adenosine and dopamine are interrelated in these regions. In the striatum, A_{2A} receptor agonists inhibit dopamine D_2 receptor–mediated behaviors, and A_{2A} antagonists mimic D_2 receptor agonists. This latter action likely contributes to the locomotor-activating properties of

---

8–1 **Java Nation**

Although most people have never heard of the term **methylxanthines,** almost everyone is familiar with several of these drugs and their behavioral effects. One of these agents, 1,3,7-trimethylxanthine, is better known to most of us as **caffeine,** arguably the world's most widely used psychoactive substance as it and its derivatives—including **theophylline** (found in tea) and **theobromine** (found in cocoa)—are found in coffee, tea, cocoa, chocolate, and many soft drinks. The stimulatory properties of these drugs are caused primarily by the antagonism of the adenosine A_1 receptor, but also to some degree the A_{2A} receptor (Chapter 12). The average daily dose of caffeine in the United States is approximately 200 mg, which is equivalent to two cups of coffee or approximately four cans of cola. At such doses in most individuals, it decreases fatigue, can enhance cognition, and does not produce significant side effects. However, prolonged use of products containing methylxanthines can lead to tolerance to the stimulatory properties of the drug and to physical dependence—which is not synonymous with addiction (Chapter 15). As anyone who habitually consumes large volumes of coffee knows, quitting the habit suddenly can lead to withdrawal symptoms that include headaches, drowsiness, and nausea. In addition, consuming high doses of caffeine (400 mg or more per day) can lead to anxiety and nervousness and can trigger panic symptoms in vulnerable individuals.

methylxanthines. The inverse relationship between adenosine and dopamine has led to speculation that selective A_{2A} antagonists might be useful in the treatment of **Parkinson disease,** as discussed in the next section of this chapter.

The A_3 receptor is expressed at low levels in the brain, and its function is not yet known. It is distinguished from the other subtypes in that it has a much lower affinity for adenosine. Whereas A_1 and A_2 receptors bind adenosine with nanomolar affinity, micromolar concentrations are necessary to activate A_3 receptors.

The P2 receptor family is intriguing because it comprises both G protein-coupled receptors (the P2Y family) and ligand-gated ion channels (the P2X family). Eight human P2Y receptor subtypes have been cloned and characterized. These receptors display unique pharmacologic profiles, and bind purine and pyrimidine nucleotide diphosphates and triphosphates, as well as ApnA molecules, with varying affinities (see **8-1**). The $P2Y_1$ receptor, for example, binds ATP and ADP but not UTP or UDP. In contrast, the $P2Y_2$ receptor is activated by ATP and UTP with equal affinity. Both $P2Y_1$ and $P2Y_2$ subtypes have been detected in the brain, but the regional distribution and functional significance of P2Y receptors in the central nervous system (CNS) are still being characterized.

Seven P2X receptor subtypes have been cloned and characterized. Each is an ATP- or ApnA-gated cation channel composed of multiple subunits. Although the exact stoichiometry of P2X receptors is unknown, functional homomeric receptors have been constituted in vitro, and there is evidence for heteromeric $P2X_{2/3}$ receptors. Because these receptors have multiple subunits, each of the cloned proteins in **8-1** should be regarded as a subunit rather than as a complete receptor. P2X receptor activation leads to rapid Na^+, K^+, and Ca^{2+} flux and subsequent membrane depolarization. These fast-acting channels have been detected in the peripheral nervous system, neuromuscular junction, spinal cord, and many brain regions. When on postsynaptic cells, their activation leads to membrane depolarization. They are also found on many presynaptic nerve terminals throughout the CNS and their activation routinely leads to enhancement of transmitter release. Via their actions in both the periphery and the spinal cord, they appear to play important roles in mediating a variety of different forms of pain and thus are important targets for the development of novel analgesic medications (Chapter 11).

Purine Functions

The cloning of the P1 and P2 receptor families opened up numerous avenues for investigating purine function

in the nervous system. Receptor-selective agonists and antagonists are being developed, and transgenic animals that underexpress or overexpress individual receptor subtypes have been generated. Although many putative roles for nucleosides and nucleotides have been hypothesized, only a handful have been clearly established.

Adenosine has both anxiolytic and hypnotic properties, and the administration of adenosine receptor antagonists confirms these observations. As described in **8-1**, **caffeine** and other methylxanthine compounds, by blocking endogenous adenosine action, increase alertness and improve cognitive performance. The cognition-enhancing properties of these drugs are particularly interesting, partly because of the wide use of caffeine, and partly because adenosine receptor antagonists may prove useful as symptomatic treatments for the cognitive deficits associated with **Alzheimer disease** and other forms of dementia (Chapter 17).

Adenosine also is being investigated for its neuroprotective effects; it is hoped that these properties might be exploited in the treatment of **stroke**. Stroke is characterized, in part, by an ischemia-induced increase in glutamate levels followed by an overstimulation of glutamate receptors and massive influx of Ca^{2+} into neurons, which unleashes a cascade of cytotoxic events (Chapter 19). Thus, an ideal neuroprotective agent would inhibit glutamate release presynaptically and prevent postsynaptic membrane depolarization and subsequent Ca^{2+} influx. Adenosine can accomplish both feats. Adenosine activation of presynaptic A_1 receptors inhibits the release of glutamate and other neurotransmitters at many synapses throughout the brain. Activation of postsynaptic A_1 receptors opens K^+ channels, and thereby hyperpolarizes neurons and counters the excitatory effects of glutamate. The net result is believed to be decreased Ca^{2+} influx and decreased neuronal death. Experiments in animal models support this hypothesis. The administration of selective A_1 agonists just before or during an ischemic event in animals significantly reduces neuronal loss. Conversely, the administration of A_1 antagonists augments ischemic brain damage. It is important to note that ischemia dramatically increases adenosine levels in the brain which will likely influence the net effects of drugs that target adenosine receptors.

Although activation of A_1 receptors may provide some measure of neuroprotection, the actions of adenosine at other receptor subtypes may exert the opposite effect. Activation of A_2 receptors, for example, has had deleterious effects on animals in models of stroke. Conversely, A_2-selective antagonists can produce neuroprotective effects. Acute activation of A_3 receptors with selective agonists also profoundly increases brain damage and mortality in animal models. In contrast, chronic administration of these adenosine agonists improves survival. Adenosine's actions on vascular tone and platelet function likely contribute to these various observations. The interplay that occurs among adenosine receptor subtypes during ischemia clearly requires further investigation.

Adenosine systems also may prove to be promising targets for drugs designed to treat **Parkinson disease**. As discussed in Chapter 17, this disease is caused by a loss of dopaminergic innervation to the striatum, which leads to rigidity, tremor, and slowness of movement. The striatum, as previously mentioned, expresses high levels of adenosine A_{2A} receptors. A_{2A} receptor agonists produce biochemical and behavioral effects (decreased motor activity) that mimic those associated with Parkinson disease because they decrease dopamine neurotransmission in the striatum. Accordingly, blocking A_{2A} receptors might have the opposite effect; that is, dopamine function in the striatum and motor activity might be expected to increase.

Several orally active compounds that selectively block A_{2A} receptors have been described. When used in animal models of Parkinson disease, these drugs significantly reverse motor deficits while inducing little if any dyskinesia, a side effect associated with L-**dopa** therapy (Chapter 17). Moreover, when coadministered with L-dopa, A_{2A} antagonists diminish L-dopa-induced dyskinesia. Currently, A_{2A} receptor antagonists are in development for the treatment of Parkinson disease.

Adenosine also has been reported to exhibit anticonvulsant, anxiolytic, and antidepressant activity, as well as both analgesic and pain-enhancing properties. Although these purported functions require further investigation, they point to the therapeutic potential of selective adenosine receptor agonists and antagonists.

Over the last decade, a role for ATP and P2X receptors in **pain** has become apparent. Application of ATP to human skin elicits acute pain. Several different subtypes of P2X receptors are found in sensory neurons in dorsal root ganglia and other sensory ganglia with $P2X_3$ and $P2X_{2/3}$ receptors generally having the highest levels of expression. These receptors are also found at nociceptive nerve terminals in the periphery where they can respond to the release of ATP from various sources including tumors and vascular endothelium 8-3 .

Molecular and pharmacologic studies of P2X receptors, in particular $P2X_3$ and $P2X_{2/3}$ receptors, suggest that while they may not be critically involved in acute pain sensation, changes in their levels and functions importantly contribute to the development and maintenance of various forms of **neuropathic** and **inflammatory pain**. As these pain states are common, and among the most resistant to treatment, P2X receptors appear to be important targets for potential novel analgesic medications (Chapter 11).

ENDOGENOUS CANNABINOIDS

In 1964, identification of the psychoactive ingredient in marijuana as Δ^9-tetrahydrocannabinol (THC) led to the synthesis of related compounds that displayed saturable binding and pharmacology consistent with the existence of a so-called cannabinoid receptor. Some of these agents 8-4 were found to cause a GTP-dependent inhibition of adenylyl cyclase, which suggested that the receptor for cannabinoids is a member of the large superfamily of G protein-coupled receptors. These observations led to the eventual cloning of two cannabinoid receptors known as the CB_1 and CB_2 receptor. CB_1 receptors are found at very high concentrations throughout the brain including the cerebellum, hippocampus, basal ganglia, cortex, brainstem, thalamus, and hypothalamus. This broad anatomic distribution of the CB_1 receptor helps to explain the diverse effects elicited by **marijuana** 8-2 . The CB_2 receptor has low overall homology with CB_1 and is found primarily in immune cells with some limited expression in the brainstem.

CB_1 and CB_2 receptors couple to effectors by means of $G_{i/o}$ proteins. Like other receptors that couple with these G proteins, CB_1 receptors inhibit adenylyl cyclase and, depending on the cell type, inhibit voltage-gated Ca^{2+} channels or stimulate inwardly rectifying K^+ channels. As they are primarily found on presynaptic terminals of both excitatory and inhibitory neurons, activation of CB_1 receptors inhibits transmitter release and thereby synaptic transmission in a wide range of brain regions.

The identification of cannabinoid receptors led to the speculation that an endogenous cannabinoid-like substance might exist; such speculation was partly based on the discovery of endogenous opioid peptides soon after the detection of opioid receptors (Chapter 7). Because cannabinoids are highly lipophilic, the search for an endogenous substance focused on membrane extracts from the brain. This led to the identification of two substances, *anandamide* and *2-arachidonylglycerol (2-AG)*, which function as endogenous cannabinoids or *endocannabinoids*: they are released in response to neural activity and activate CB_1 receptors. As shown in 8-5A , both anandamide and 2-AG are thought to be synthesized from membrane-derived

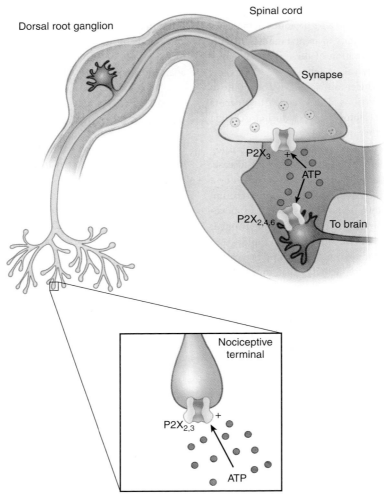

8-3 **Role of P2X receptors in pain processing.** Hypothetical scheme of the actions of purine nucleotides and nucleosides in pain pathways. At sensory nerve terminals in the periphery, $P2X_3$ homomeric and $P2X_{2/3}$ heteromeric receptors have been identified as the principal P2X receptors present, although recent studies have also shown expression of $P2Y_1$ and possibly $P2Y_2$ receptors on a subpopulation of $P2X_3$ receptor-immunopositive fibers. Other known P2X receptor subtypes (1–7) are also expressed at low levels in dorsal root ganglia. Although less potent than ATP, adenosine appears to act on sensory terminals, probably directly via $P1(A_2)$ receptors; however, it also acts synergistically to potentiate $P2X_{2/3}$ receptor activation, which may be true for serotonin, capsaicin, and protons as well. At synapses in sensory pathways in the CNS, ATP acts postsynaptically via $P2X_2$, $P2X_4$, and/or $P2X_6$ receptor subtypes, perhaps as heteromultimers. As well, after release, ATP is rapidly degraded into adenosine, which acts as a prejunctional inhibitor of neurotransmission via $P1(A_2)$ receptors. $P2X_3$ receptors on the central projections of primary afferent neurons in lamina II of the dorsal horn mediate facilitation of glutamate and probably also ATP release. Sources of ATP acting on $P2X_3$ and $P2X_{2/3}$ receptors on sensory terminals include sympathetic nerves, endothelial, Merkel, and tumor cells. Yellow dots, molecules of ATP.

lipid precursors. Abundant evidence suggests that their release from postsynaptic neurons is coupled to their synthesis. Specifically, in a variety of cell types, strong depolarization leads to Ca^{2+} influx via voltage-dependent Ca^{2+} channels and this in turn causes activation of the enzymes responsible for generating anandamide or

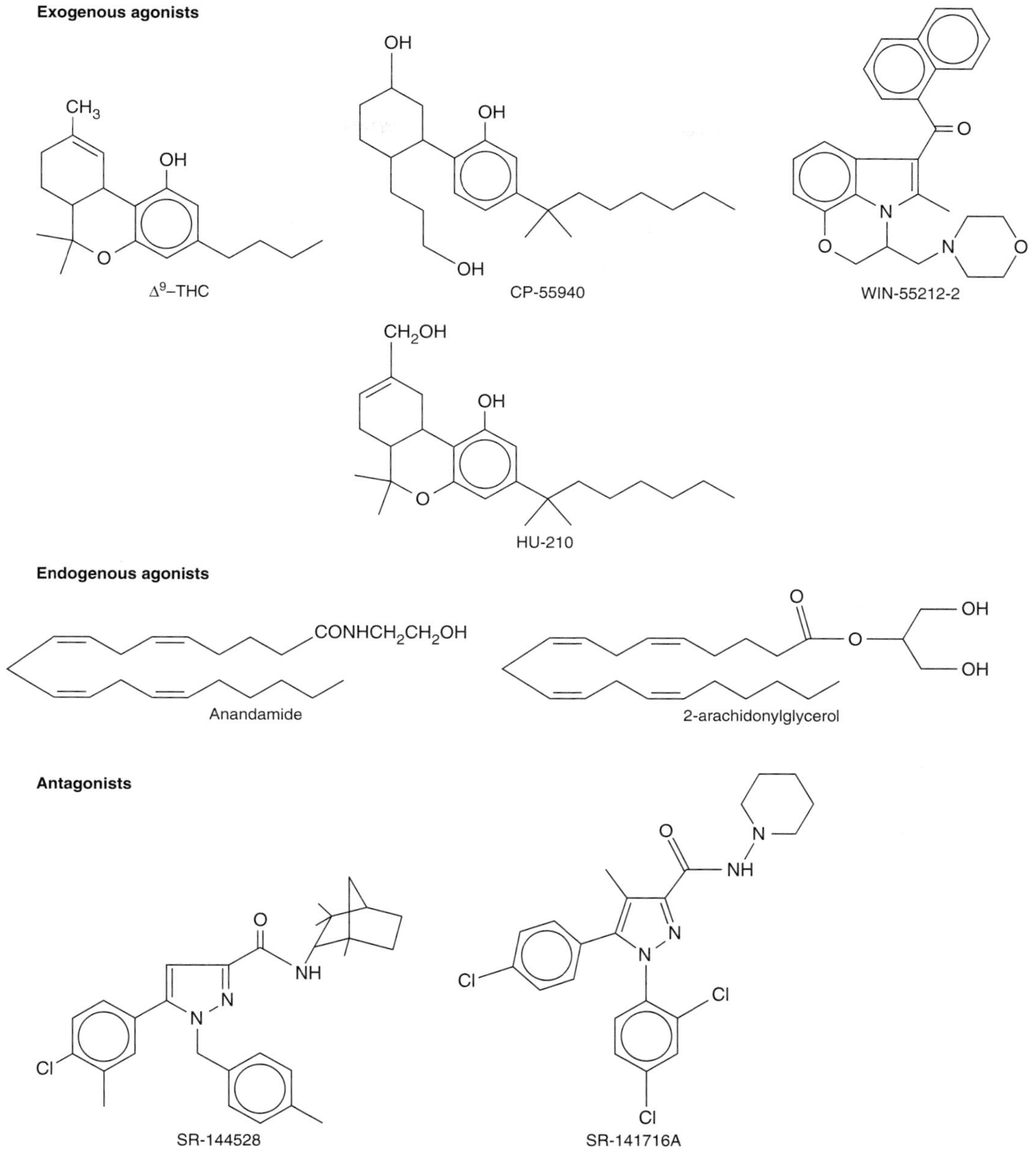

Exogenous agonists

Δ^9–THC   CP-55940   WIN-55212-2

HU-210

Endogenous agonists

CONHCH$_2$CH$_2$OH

Anandamide   2-arachidonylglycerol

Antagonists

SR-144528   SR-141716A

8-4 **Chemical structures of representative agonists and antagonists of cannabinoid receptors.**

2-AG **8-6**. In certain cell types, the generation of these endocannabinoids can also be stimulated by activation of postsynaptic G protein-coupled receptors, specifically metabotropic glutamate receptors or muscarinic receptors **8-6**.

There is extensive evidence that anandamide and 2-AG can function as true **retrograde messengers** in that they can escape from postsynaptic cells and bind

to adjacent presynaptic CB$_1$ receptors to inhibit transmitter release **8-6**. Depending on the cell types being examined, this endocannabinoid-mediated depression of synaptic transmission can last for seconds, minutes, or even hours. This action of endocannabinoids has been shown to greatly influence neural circuit function. Endocannabinoids are not stored in vesicles like classic neurotransmitters and it remains unclear

8–2 Marijuana

Marijuana is the most commonly used illegal drug in the United States and in many other countries throughout the world. The term marijuana refers to a preparation that is typically smoked and made from the dried leaves of the hemp plant *Cannabis sativa* (hence the name cannabinoids). Several other preparations are commonly used, including hashish, which consists of the psychoactive resin pressed into blocks, and bhang, a liquid distillate used in India. Throughout much of its history, cannabis has been known as much for its analgesic properties as its psychoactive effects. However, controversy continues to surround its use as an analgesic and for other medical indications. Although it has been used experimentally to stimulate appetite in patients with **AIDS**, to reduce intraocular pressure in patients with **glaucoma**, and to treat the **nausea** caused by cancer chemotherapy, little formal research has focused on these actions because of concerns about its abuse potential.

The marijuana intoxication syndrome varies greatly. Some individuals become giddy and others become morose and depressed. Use of the drug also may be accompanied by introspection and a sense of time moving slowly. In many ways, marijuana intoxication is similar to intoxication produced by hallucinogens; indeed cannabinoids often are considered "minor hallucinogens." Distortions of sensory perceptions are fairly common during marijuana intoxication and hallucinations may occur, albeit rarely. Potential adverse effects include an impairment in short-term and perhaps long-term memory, and impaired motor coordination. The addicting properties of marijuana are covered in Chapter 15.

---

whether they passively diffuse through the postsynaptic plasma membrane or are transported by a specific transporter protein. The physiologic actions of anadamide and 2-AG are terminated by their transport into cells followed by intracellular hydrolysis. There is strong evidence for a specific transporter process, likely involving facilitated diffusion, although the key transporter protein has not yet been identified. Nevertheless, selective inhibitors of this transport activity have been developed 8–5B . Two specific intracellular enzymes, *fatty acid amide hydrolase* (FAAH) and *monoacylglycerol lipase* (MGL), breakdown anandamide and 2-AG, respectively 8–5 . Inhibitors of these enzymes increase levels of the endocannabinoids 8–5B , which likely accounts for the broad behavioral effects of this class of compounds.

There is great interest in the possible therapeutic potential of drugs that target individual components of the endocannabinoid signaling pathways. Given the strong stimulatory effects on appetite of CB_1 agonists such as marijuana, it may not be surprising that one of the first clinically available cannabinoid drugs is the CB_1 antagonist **rimonabant**, which is available in Europe for the treatment of **obesity**. It is thought that the key site of action of rimonabant that leads to weight loss is in areas of the hypothalamus that are involved in the control of food intake and energy expenditure (Chapter 10). As of the writing of this section, the FDA has not yet approved the use of rimonabant in the United States, likely because its maintained efficacy over the long term has not been proven and there is some evidence that it can cause depressive and anxiety symptoms.

A CB_1 agonist, **dronabinol**, is currently available for the treatment of the nausea and vomiting associated with cancer chemotherapy and for stimulating appetite in people with advanced **HIV/AIDS**. Because activation of CB_1 receptors has significant analgesic effects in models of **neuropathic** and **inflammatory pain**, likely because of actions on periphal nerve endings, there are efforts to develop CB_1 agonists that do not cross the blood-brain barrier and therefore will not have CNS effects.

Compounds that inhibit the degradative enzymes for anandamide and 2-AG (FAAH and MGL, 8–5) also may have therapeutic potential. In animal models, these compounds affect behavior in a manner suggesting that they may have **analgesic** and **anxiolytic** as well as **antidepressant** activities. Furthermore, when combined with dopamine receptor agonists, they improve motor perfomance in **Parkinson disease** models. These drugs may exert effects different from CB_1 receptor agonists because, unlike the agonists, which indiscriminantly activate all CB_1 receptors in the brain, inhibition

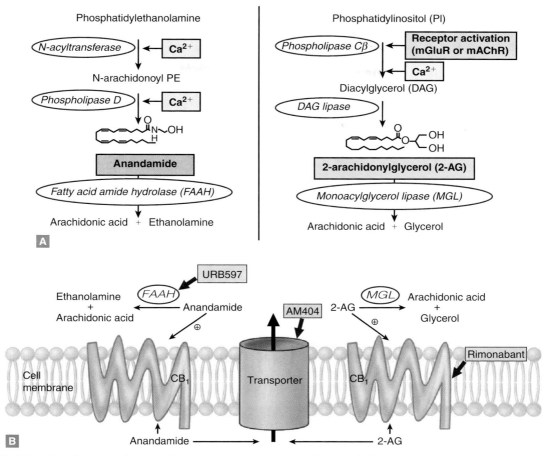

8-5 **A. Synthesis and degradation of anandamide and 2-arachidonylglycerol.** *N*-Arachidonyl PE, *N*-arachidonyl phosphatidylethanolamine. **B. Site of action of representative drugs that target endocannabinoid systems**.

of degradative enzymes should enhance only the specific actions of endogenously released cannabinoids.

GASES

Nitric Oxide

Nitric oxide (NO) was first identified as a cellular messenger when it was established to be the much sought endothelial-derived relaxing factor that is released from vascular endothelial cells and causes vasodilation. Soon thereafter it was found that NO is released from neurons by stimulation of **nitric oxide synthase (NOS)** in response to NMDA receptor activation. Three different isoforms of NOS exist, each the product of a distinct gene. Neuronal NOS (nNOS) is expressed exclusively in neurons, endothelial NOS (eNOS) originally was identified in endothelial cells, and inducible NOS (iNOS) originally was identified in

certain immune system cells. Some neurons may express eNOS and iNOS in addition to nNOS. NO is synthesized from arginine by nNOS, which is activated on binding to Ca^{2+}–calmodulin complexes. nNOS is ideally positioned to respond to the rise in intracellular Ca^{2+} elicited by activation of NMDA receptors since it directly binds to PSD-95, a key synaptic scaffold protein that also binds to NMDA receptors **8-7**. Because NO is a soluble gas, it is not stored in vesicles but rather freely diffuses out of the neurons in which it is generated. Its major action is to stimulate cytosolic guanylyl cyclase, which catalyzes the formation of cGMP (Chapter 4) in neighboring cells. Thus, NO can function as a retrograde messenger to activate guanylyl cyclase in adjacent presynaptic terminals, an action that at some synapses can influence neurotransmitter release. Another important action of NO is selective and reversible *S*-nitrosylation of cysteine residues in a

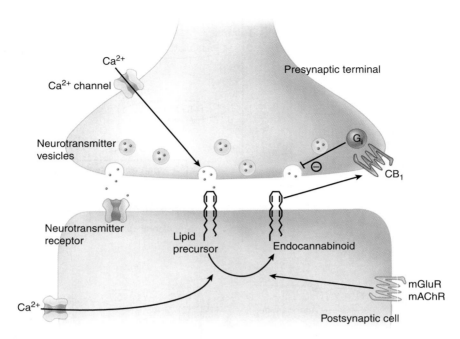

8-6 **Endocannabinoids function as retrograde messengers to inhibit the presynaptic release of neurotransmitter.** Strong activation of voltage-dependent Ca^{2+} channels, metabotropic glutamate receptors (mGluR), or muscarinic acetylcholine receptors (mAChR) in the postsynaptic cell can cause the production of endocannabinoids. These can escape from the postsynaptic cell and activate presynaptic CB_1 receptors, which inhibit neurotransmitter release.

wide variety of proteins including intracellular signaling enzymes, pumps, G proteins, and ion channels. Like phosphorylation, S-nitrosylation is a posttranslational modification that can either increase or decrease the target protein's activity. NO also can inhibit cellular enzymes containing iron–sulfur complexes, such as mitochondrial NADH–ubiquitone oxidoreductase and NADH–succinate oxidoreductase, which are crucial to metabolism. Finally, NO can react with oxygen and other free radicals to yield reactive NO species such as peroxynitrite. This is particularly important in mediating the neurotoxic effects of excessive NO production, which likely contributes to the neural damage caused by **strokes** (Chapter 19).

Carbon Monoxide

Carbon monoxide (CO), best known as a highly toxic gas when breathed in large amounts, also may function

as a neurotransmitter although its roles in the brain are still being elucidated. It is generated in neurons by **heme oxygenase (HO)**, an enzyme that degrades heme to generate biliverdin, iron, and CO. There are three isoforms of HO (HO1-3) with HO2 being selectively enriched in neurons. Like NO, CO stimulates soluble guanylyl cyclase, a finding that is consistent with the observation that the expression of HO2 and guanylyl cyclase overlap in many brain regions. The regulation of HO2 activity in neurons is not as well understood as that of NOS. One potentially important mechanism for increasing HO2 activity involves activation of protein kinase C by metabotropic glutamate receptors or phorbol esters, which in turn leads to the direct phosphorylation of HO2 by CK2 (casein kinase 2) **8-8**. Like NOS, there is also evidence that HO2 can be directly activated by Ca^{2+}-calmodulin.

Evidence for a role for CO as a neurotransmitter is strongest for the enteric nervous system and olfactory

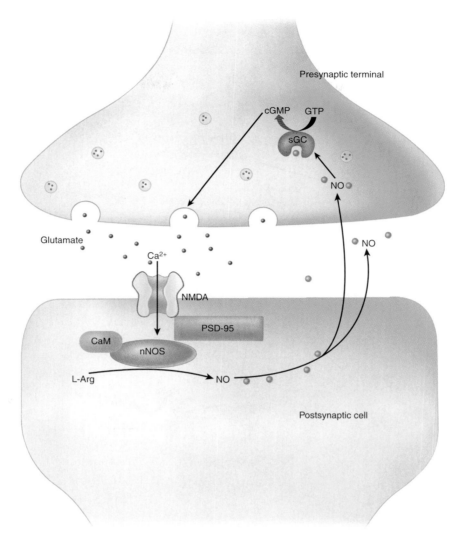

8-7 **Activation of NMDA receptors leads to the production of nitric oxide (NO) which can function as a retrograde messenger.** The entry of Ca^{2+} via NMDA glutamate receptors activates neuronal nitrix oxide synthase (nNOS) which converts L-arginine to NO. nNOS is positioned next to NMDA receptors by the scaffolding protein PSD-95. NO can escape from the postsynaptic cell and activate presynaptic soluble guanylyl cyclase (sGC) which produces cGMP and regulates functioning of the presynaptic terminal.

receptor neurons. HO2 as well as nNOS are enriched in neurons of the myenteric plexus, and genetic deletion or pharmacologic inhibition of HO2 significantly reduces noradrenergic, neurotransmission in the gut. Similarly, HO inhibition can reduce the generation of cGMP in olfactory neurons which normally generate sufficient CO to activate guanylyl cyclase. CO production also has been suggested to play a role in the regulation of circadian rhythms by influencing the DNA binding activity of key circadian transcription factors.

NEUROTROPHIC FACTORS

The belief that extracellular signals can promote the growth and differentiation of nerve cells is more than a half century old, yet the molecular diversity of neurotrophic factors and of their intracellular

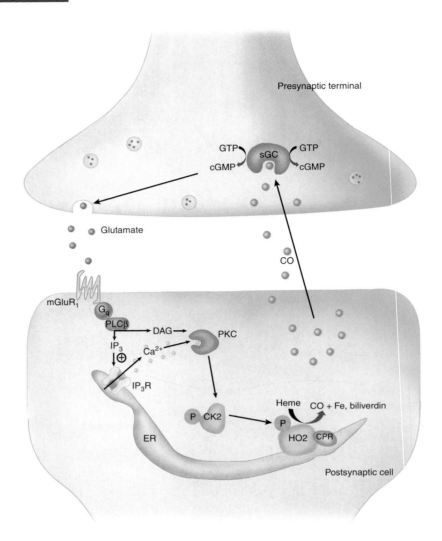

8-8 **Activation of metabotropic glutamate receptors (mGluR) can lead to the production of carbon monoxide (CO) which may function as a retrograde messenger.** Activation of group I mGluRs (eg, mGluR$_1$), which are G$_q$-linked, leads to a protein kinase cascade involving protein kinase C (PKC) and casein kinase 2 (CK2), which then phosphorylates and activates heme oxygenase 2 (HO2) leading to the generation of CO from heme. Like NO, CO may function as a retrograde messenger by activating soluble guanylyl cyclase (sGC) in presynaptic terminals.

signaling cascades did not become apparent until the past decade. Knowledge of neurotrophic factor signaling has dramatically enhanced our understanding of the ways in which the nervous system evolves during development and adapts throughout the adult life of an organism. Such knowledge also has provided insight into mechanisms responsible for neuronal survival, whose failure may underlie neurodegenerative disorders such as **Alzheimer disease, Parkinson disease, Huntington disease,** and **amyotropic lateral sclerosis (ALS)** (Chapter 17).

Moreover, neurotrophic factors and their signaling proteins represent a large number of potential targets for the pharmacotherapeutic treatment of these and other neuropsychiatric disorders.

A discussion of neurotrophic factors requires the definition of several terms. *Neurotrophic factors* themselves are peptide growth factors for nerve cells: they influence the cell cycle, growth, differentiation, and survival of neurons. Due to overlap among growth factors for neurons and glia, we also apply the term neurotrophic factor to any molecule that produces trophic effects on the nervous system by influencing glia. To add to the confusion, the term *neurotrophin* applies to only one family of neurotrophic factors. A broader term is *cytokine*, which is borrowed from the field of immunology and refers to molecules released by one cell to modulate the activity of other cells. The term cytokine therefore applies to all growth factors, including neurotrophic factors. The term neurotrophic factor is restricted to proteins and excludes the many non-peptide molecules—for example, steroid hormones, retinoic acid, and many small-molecule neurotransmitters—that also can influence the growth and integrity of the nervous system.

Although neurotrophic factors originally were distinguished from neurotransmitters based on their role in nervous system development, as opposed to synaptic transmission in the adult, we now know that there is considerable overlap in the actions of these molecules. Like neurotransmitters, many neurotrophic factors are synthesized by neurons and alter the functioning of other neurons; under some circumstances, they may even be released as a result of neuronal activity. Moreover, some neurotrophic factors, such as *brain-derived neurotrophic factor (BDNF)*, may produce rapid changes in target neurons that are indistinguishable from those elicited by conventional neurotransmitters. Likewise, many small-molecule neurotransmitters not only elicit the rapid changes associated with synaptic transmission but also affect the growth, differentiation, and survival of neurons during development and in adulthood.

Certain key features of neurotrophic factors distinguish them from peptide neurotransmitters. Notably, neurotrophic factors tend to be larger proteins, whereas peptide neurotransmitters typically are very small peptides (Chapter 7). In addition, most neurotrophic factors produce their biologic effects through the regulation of protein tyrosine kinases, whereas most peptide neurotransmitters signal through G protein-coupled receptors and classic second messenger cascades.

Functional Characteristics of Neurotrophic Factors

We know much less about the synthesis, action, and degradation of most neurotrophic factors than we know about the neurotransmitters discussed in previous chapters. Neurotrophic factors are synthesized by transcription and translation in the cell bodies of particular neurons and glia. Some are stored in these cells, perhaps in large dense core vesicles (Chapter 3), and are transported either to nerve terminals or to dendrites. The mechanisms controlling the release of

neurotrophic factors are poorly understood. Many factors, such as *interleukin-1 (IL-1)*, BDNF, and *glial cell line–derived neurotrophic factor (GDNF)* are encoded by immediate early genes (Chapter 4); consequently, activity-dependent transcription may be the major determinant of release of these factors. The release of many neurotrophic factors can be triggered by depolarization. The major mechanism responsible for the termination of neurotrophic factor signals appears to be proteolytic degradation. However, some factors, such as BDNF, are sequestered by a functionally inactive, truncated receptor that limits their diffusion and thereby perhaps the duration of their action.

According to the *neurotrophic hypothesis*, neurotrophic factors are indispensable in the establishment of suitable nerve–target connections during development. While the sites of action of many neurotrophic factors are unclear, the case of NGF in the peripheral nervous system is well understood. The first growth factor to be identified, *nerve growth factor (NGF)* was discovered more than 50 years ago when certain sympathetic and sensory neurons were shown to require this protein for their survival 8-9. NGF was subsequently demonstrated to be synthesized by the target organs of these nerve cells and required to maintain the sympathetic and sensory neurons that innervate the organs. Because the supply of NGF is limited, competition for the factor exists among growing nerve fibers. Growing neurons that do not receive the NGF signal from their target do not survive. Likewise, only neurons that successfully respond to NGF survive and make appropriate connections with their targets. These findings demonstrate that NGF is required for proper nerve–target connections during development 8-10.

Although this pattern of NGF synthesis and action predominates in the peripheral nervous system,

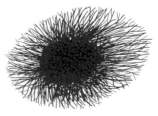

8-9 **The effect of nerve growth factor (NGF) on cultured spinal neurons.** (Adapted with permission from Levi-Montalcini R. The nerve growth factor 35 years later. *Science.* 1987;237:1157.)

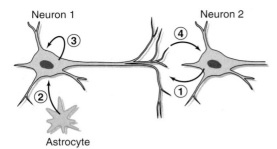

Neuron 1   Neuron 2

Astrocyte

8-10 **Modes of intercellular communication subserved by neurotrophic factors. 1.** In this classic model, a target-derived neurotrophic factor acts on an innervating nerve terminal. **2.** Paracrine transmission. A neurotrophic factor released from a neighboring cell (neuron or glial cell, such as astrocyte) acts on many nearby neurons in the absence of formal synaptic connections. **3.** Autocrine transmission. A neurotrophic factor acts on the neurons that release it. **4.** Anterograde transmission. A neurotrophic factor released from the terminals of a nerve cell acts on the synaptic targets of these terminals. The mode of transmission that predominates in the adult brain and spinal cord has yet to be determined.

different patterns emerge in the brain and spinal cord (see **8-10**). In the CNS, a target neuron may supply neurotrophic factor for an innervating neuron, but may also synthesize many other neurotrophic factors and receptors. Thus, factors in the brain and spinal cord may serve additional autoregulatory, or autocrine, functions. Furthermore, certain neurotrophic factors can be transported in an anterograde fashion to axon terminals where, after release, they act on the cell bodies or nerve terminals of other nerve cells. As well, neurotrophic factor–receptor complexes, formed on the plasma membrane of nerve terminals, can be retrogradely transported back to cell bodies, where they exert some of their biologic effects.

Glia further complicate our understanding of the production of neurotrophic factors. Some factors are synthesized by both neurons and glia and act on receptors expressed by both cell types. Such patterns of synthesis and activity result in highly complex forms of intercellular communication among neurons and glia that investigators have yet to disentangle.

Families of Neurotrophic Factors

The classification of neurotrophic factors is complicated by the history of their discovery: the names of many factors were based on the actions with which they were originally associated. Interleukins were given their name because they were identified as proteins that mediate communication among white blood cells, even though they are also produced by glia. GDNF was named for its original source, even though it is also made by many types of neurons and other cells in the body. *Fibroblast growth factor (FGF)* was regarded as a growth factor for fibroblasts, even though it is also produced by glia. *Ciliary neurotrophic factor (CNTF)* was named for its contribution to the growth and maintenance of ciliary ganglion neurons in the eye, even though it is also generated by glia and is important for the survival of many types of neurons, notably motor neurons.

Currently, neurotrophic factors can be categorized based on their homologies and on the shared signal transduction mechanisms through which they produce their biologic effects **8-2** . This chapter focuses primarily on the neurotrophins, which are among the best characterized in the nervous system. The chapter also provides brief discussions of GDNF, CNTF, some neurotrophic factors better known for their role as immune-response cytokines or chemokines, as well as *vascular endothelial growth factor (VEGF)*.

Neurotrophins

The neurotrophin family comprises NGF and subsequently identified factors that employ similar signaling mechanisms, including BDNF, *neurotrophin-3 (NT-3)*, and *neurotrophin-4 (NT-4*; also known as *neurotrophin-4/5)*. All neurotrophins are small peptides. BDNF, for example, has a molecular mass of approximately 14 kDa. Another common feature of neurotrophins is that they produce their physiologic effects by means of the *tropomyosin receptor kinase (Trk)* receptor family (also known as the *tryosine receptor kinase* family).

Neurotrophins produce effects on a wide range of neurons. As previously mentioned in connection with NGF, their role in ensuring the survival of neurons in the peripheral nervous system is well established. NGF, for example, is present in target fields of small sympathetic and sensory neurons that have nociceptive and temperature-sensing functions, and the NGF receptor is expressed in these neurons. BDNF is produced in skeletal muscle (innervated by motor neurons). BDNF, NT-4, and NT-3 each support the survival of a subset of peripheral sensory neurons.

Neurotrophins may similarly affect the survival and maintenance of some neurons in the CNS, although their precise roles are less clear. In different

8-2   Examples of Neurotrophic Factors and Their Receptors

Neurotrophic Factor Family and Representative Examples	Receptor Family and Representative Examples

Neurotrophins
  NGF, BDNF, NT-3, NT-4
	Trk (R-PTKs)
	  TrkA, TrkB, TrkC[1]

GDNF family
  GDNF, neurturin, persephin
	Coupled to Ret
	  GFRα1, GFRα2, unknown

CNTF family
  CNTF, LIF, IL-6
	Coupled to Janus kinase (JAK)
	  GP130, CNTFRα, LIFRα

Ephrins	Eph (R-PTKs)
EGF family EGF, TGFα, neuregulins[2]	ErbB (R-PTKs)
VEGF	VEGFR1, VEGFR2
Other growth factors Insulin, IGF, FGF, PDGF	R-PTKs

Interleukins and related
  cytokines
    Interleukin-1 (IL-1)
    IL-2
    IL-3, IL-5
    TNFα, TNFβ
	
	IL-1R coupled to PS/TK
	R-PTK
	Coupled to JAK
	Related to p75[3]

TGF family TGFβ	R-PS/TKs

Other cytokines
  Interferons (IFNα, β, γ)
  m-CSF
  gm-CSF
	
	Coupled to JAK
	R-PTKs
	Coupled to JAK

Chemokines
  CC chemokines (IL-8)
  CXC chemokines (MIP, MCP)
  CX_3C chemokines
    (neurotactin)
	G protein-coupled receptors
	  CC_1-CC_8R
	  CXC_1-CXC_4R
	  CX_3C_1R

[1]Specificity of neurotrophins for the various Trk receptors is shown in **8-11**.
[2]Neuregulins are also referred to as ARIA, heregulin, or neu differentiation factor.
[3]TNF receptors couple to so-called "death receptors" of the TRADD and related families (Chapter 17).
BDNF, brain-derived neurotrophic factor; NT-3 and -4, neurotrophin-3 and -4; GDNF, glial cell line-derived neurotrophic factor; GFR, GDNF-neurturin receptor; CNTF, ciliary neurotrophic factor; LIF, leukemia inhibitory factor; VEGF1, vascular endothermal growth factor; VEGFR1 and R2, VEGF receptors 1 and 2; EGF, epidermal growth factor; R-PTK, receptor-associated protein tyrosine kinase; IGF, insulin-like growth factor; FGF, fibroblast growth factor; PDGF, platelet-derived growth factor; TNF, tumor necrosis factor; IL, interleukin; R-PS/TK, receptor-associated protein serine/threonine kinase; TGF, transforming growth factor; IFN, interferon; m-CSF, macrophage colony stimulating factor; gm-CSF, granulocyte-monocyte CSF; MIP, macrophage inflammatory protein; MCP, monocyte chemoattractant protein.

circumstances their primary function might be target-derived support of afferent neurons, the support of efferent neurons, or the generation and maintenance of differentiated neurons. For example, NGF promotes the survival of cholinergic neurons in the septal nuclei of the basal forebrain, and BDNF, NT-3, and NT-4 promote the survival of some cortical motor and hippocampal neurons, and of noradrenergic, dopaminergic, and serotoninergic neurons located in the brainstem. Because cholinergic neurons are affected early in **Alzheimer disease** (Chapter 17), NGF has been proposed as a potential treatment; the use of other neurotrophins has been proposed for the treatment of **Parkinson disease**. Unfortunately, clinical trials have not shown significant efficacy as shown later in this chapter. To complicate matters further, recent work has shown that precursors of mature neurotrophins (eg, pro-NGF or pro-BDNF) are themselves released from neurons and antagonize the actions of mature neurotrophins. These proneurotrophins may, therefore, also be important for regulating cell death during development and after injury.

We now know that neurotrophins continue to play a role in the adult brain, where evidence has suggested that they support the survival and plasticity of fully differentiated neurons and may even contribute to synaptic transmission. BDNF, in particular, is important for some forms of long-term potentiation (LTP) as well as certain types of learning and memory. BDNF also has been implicated in regulation of adult hippocampal neurogenesis, epilepsies, and animal models of several psychiatric disorders, as will be discussed in later chapters of this book.

Trk receptors All neurotrophins bind to a class of highly homologous receptor tyrosine kinases known as Trk receptors, of which three types are known: TrkA, TrkB, and TrkC. These transmembrane receptors are glycoproteins whose molecular masses range from 140 to 145 kDa. Each type of Trk receptor tends to bind specific neurotrophins: TrkA is the receptor for NGF, TrkB the receptor for BDNF and NT-4, and TrkC the receptor for NT-3. However, some overlap in the specificity of these receptors has been noted **8-11**.

The characteristic structural domains of the Trk receptor are represented in **8-12**. The binding of a neurotrophin to its Trk receptor causes activation of the receptor's catalytic domain. Neurotrophins bind as dimers, and in turn cause the dimerization of Trk molecules, which results in the autophosphorylation of Trk on several key cytoplasmic tyrosine residues. Such autophosphorylation initiates intracellular signaling cascades that lead to many of the biologic effects of

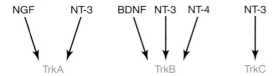

8–11 Specificity of various Trk receptors for members of the neurotrophin family. NGF, nerve growth factor; NT, neurotrophin; BDNF, brain-derived neurotrophic factor.

receptor activation (Chapter 4). Intracellular signaling occurs by way of phosphorylated tyrosine residues that form a recognition sequence for the SH2 domains that are present on several types of cellular proteins. SH2 domains on Shc and Grb2, for example, eventually link Trk receptors to the activation of the small G protein Ras, which in turn triggers the activation of the microtubule-associated protein (MAP)-kinase cascade. Genetic abnormalities in Ras-related proteins cause **neurofibromatosis** in humans, which involves excessive growth and occasionally cancerous degeneration of Schwann cells (Chapter 4).

Other biologic effects of Trk receptor activation result from the phosphorylation of different signaling proteins on tyrosine residues. The most important of these are phospholipase Cγ (PLCγ), which triggers the

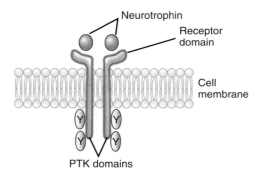

8–12 Structure of the Trk tyrosine kinase receptor. This receptor contains two major domains: an extracellular neurotrophin-binding domain and an intracellular protein tyrosine kinase (PTK) domain. Here, a neurotrophin dimer binds to a Trk receptor dimer. Receptor dimerization is required for autophosphorylation of the receptor at specific tyrosine residues (Y). Such autophosphorylation (1) enables phosphorylation of other substrates, such as PLCγ, and (2) forms docking sites, or SH2 domains, for other signaling proteins such as Shc and Grb2 (Chapter 4).

phosphatidylinositol cascade, and insulin receptor substrate (IRS), which leads to activation of the phosphatidylinositol-3-kinase cascade. Mutations in the ATM gene, which encodes 1 subtype of phosphatidylinositol-3-kinase, have been shown to cause **ataxia-telangiectasia,** a disease characterized by progressive degeneration and atrophy of several brain regions, particularly that of the cerebellum. The various intracellular signaling cascades activated by the neurotrophins and their Trk receptors are discussed in greater detail in Chapter 4.

Trk receptors display multiple splice variants. The best understood are the TrkB and TrkC isoforms that contain normal extracellular ligand-binding domains but lack the catalytic tyrosine kinase domain. As previously discussed, truncated Trk receptors limit the scope and duration of neurotrophin activity, either by heterodimerizing with full-length Trk receptors and preventing their phosphorylation or by sequestering extracellular neurotrophins and preventing their activation of full-length Trk receptors.

p75 receptor The first neurotrophin receptor to be cloned was not a Trk receptor, but p75, a 75-kDa protein that is currently described as the low-affinity neurotrophin receptor. The p75 receptor binds to all neurotrophins with roughly equal affinity. It also appears to modulate Trk signaling, perhaps by allowing Trk receptors to respond to lower concentrations of NGF and other neurotrophins—a highly desirable trait in a receptor that competes for limited quantities of growth factor. In addition, p75 may make TrkA and TrkB more selective for their respective primary ligands, NGF and BDNF. While the mechanism by which p75 exerts these effects is not well understood, it is hypothesized that p75, Trk, and a neurotrophin form a stable trimolecular complex. Importantly, however, Trk receptors are fully capable of mediating functional responses to neurotrophins in the absence of p75.

Despite evidence that p75 can enhance neurotrophin and Trk function and promote cell survival under some conditions, p75 has been implicated in cell death pathways, which are described in greater detail in Chapter 17. p75 has a so-called "death domain," analogous to similar domains in the *tumor necrosis factor-α (TNFα)* receptor, through which it activates programmed cell death or **apoptosis** (Chapter 17). Recent discoveries suggest that the opposing actions of p75 may depend on the presence of the coreceptor sortilin, a member of the Vps10p-receptor family. The p75-sortilin complex has high affinity for the proneurotrophins (eg, pro-BDNF and pro-NGF), which have strong proapoptotic activity. Studies to determine the functional implications of proneurotrophin action as well as that of p75 and sortillin are ongoing.

Neurotrophins and Synaptic Plasticity Studies of developing visual cortex have confirmed that neurotrophins play a role in some forms of synaptic plasticity. As axons from the lateral geniculate nucleus (LGN) of the thalamus grow into the primary visual cortex and form synapses, they segregate into eye-specific, alternating patches known as ocular dominance columns. Monocular deprivation experiments have revealed that LGN neurons that receive inputs from the deprived eye exhibit weakened synaptic connections. NT-4 can rescue these neurons from such plastic changes. It is possible that LGN neurons might compete for TrkB ligands and that this competition might be crucial for the formation of ocular dominance columns. In support of this hypothesis, both infusion of excess BDNF or NT-4 and infusion of a neurotrophin antagonist into the visual cortex are sufficient to block formation of ocular dominance columns.

Evidence suggests that neurotrophins also are involved in regulating synaptic plasticity in the adult brain. Neuronal activity dramatically and rapidly regulates the expression of certain neurotrophins and their Trk receptors in adult neurons. The induction of BDNF and TrkB, for example, has been observed in neurons of the hippocampus in response to trains of synaptic stimuli (including those associated with the formation of LTP; Chapter 5). The rapidity of BDNF induction is consistent with that of other immediate early genes, such as c-fos (Chapter 4) and induction of BDNF is mediated by the activation of preexisting transcription factors such as CREB.

Increasing evidence suggests that neurotrophins can modulate synaptic transmission and regulate the formation and strengthening of synapses. Such actions may be mediated by cross-talk between neurotrophin and neurotransmitter signaling pathways. For instance, NT-3, via its Trk receptor, rapidly enhances synaptic transmission at the neuromuscular junction by increasing the probability of acetylcholine release from the presynaptic neuron. BDNF and NT-3 are reported to increase the size of excitatory postsynaptic potentials at the Schaeffer collateral–CA1 synapse in the hippocampus. Accordingly, BDNF knockout mice exhibit reduced basal synaptic transmission at this synapse, and hippocampal slices from these mice are reportedly deficient in LTP. Although these data clearly implicate the involvement of BDNF in hippocampal function in the adult, some of these results have proved difficult to replicate. Thus further research is needed to support these findings.

GDNF Family

GDNF, a glycosylated protein of approximately 18 kDa, was first isolated from a glial cell line that supports the survival of dopaminergic neurons from the midbrain. Because **Parkinson disease** is caused by the degeneration of dopaminergic neurons in the midbrain (Chapter 17), GDNF has received considerable attention as a potential therapeutic agent for this disease, although obstacles remain as will be discussed at the end of this chapter.

More recently, GDNF has been proven to support the survival of many other neuronal cells, including those of the myenteric plexus within the gut. However, the most profound abnormality observed in GDNF knockout mice is maldevelopment of the kidney, which causes death shortly after birth. This finding demonstrates that GDNF plays a critical role outside of the nervous system.

Like the neurotrophins, GDNF produces its biologic effects through the activation of a protein tyrosine kinase, but such activation is achieved indirectly through an intervening receptor protein **8-13**. This receptor, termed GFRα1, binds to and activates Ret, a transmembrane protein tyrosine kinase of about 150 kDa, which then mediates GDNF action. Loss-of-function mutations in Ret are associated with **Hirschsprung disease** in humans, a disorder characterized by abnormal gut motility, consistent with Hirschsprung-like abnormalities in GDNF knockout mice. In contrast, gain-of-function mutations in Ret are associated with neural crest malignancies in

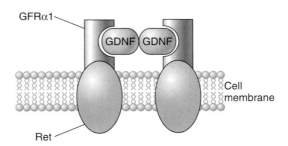

8-13 **GDNF receptor complex**. A GDNF dimer binds to GFRα₁, which subsequently associates with the tyrosine kinase Ret, a transmembrane protein. This association triggers Ret activation and the phosphorylation of specific substrates, which in turn produce the biologic effects of GDNF. Most of the specific substrates involved in this process remain unknown. GDNF, glial cell line-derived neurotrophic factor.

humans, such as **multiple endocrine neoplasias** and **medullary thyroid carcinoma**.

Other members of the GDNF family of neurotrophic factors include neurturin, artemin, and persephin, which also signal by means of Ret. Like GDNF, each binds to a specific Rα subunit, which subsequently converges on Ret. Also like GDNF, neurturin can support the survival of dopaminergic neurons in the midbrain, which raises its potential utility for **Parkinson disease**.

CNTF Family

CNTF belongs to a family of growth factors whose members also include *leukemia inhibitory factor (LIF)*, *interleukin-6 (IL-6)*, *prolactin*, *growth hormone*, *leptin*, *interferons*, and *oncostatin-M*, among others (see **8–2**). This family is defined by the shared signaling mechanisms described below. Many members of the CNTF family are best known for their roles outside of the nervous system. Yet several of these factors, including CNTF, LIF, and IL-6, have been associated with the dramatic regulation of neuronal survival or differentiation and thus can be considered neurotrophic factors.

The actions of CNTF, a protein approximately 24 kDa in size, are best characterized for neuronal cells. As previously mentioned, CNTF initially was studied as a survival factor for chick ciliary ganglion neurons and was known to up-regulate choline acetyltransferase (Chapter 6) in these cells. More recently, CNTF has been proven to regulate the survival or differentiation of many other neuronal cells, including motor neurons, hippocampal neurons, and midbrain dopaminergic neurons. Its effects on motor neurons are perhaps the most dramatic: CNTF prevents their

degeneration after axotomy and improves some motor defects in murine models of motor neuron disease. Consequently, CNTF has been tested as a therapeutic agent in the treatment of the motor neuron disease **ALS.** However, clinical trials were abandoned due to toxic side effects. Attempts to overcome these side effects have been unsuccessful (see below), but there is still promise for CNTF in the treatment of **Huntington Disease** as well as in recovery from spinal cord injury. LIF and IL-6 are believed to similarly regulate neuronal growth, differentiation, and lineage commitment, although the mechanisms by which they achieve such regulation are not as well established.

CNTF and related family members exert their effects through a characteristic signaling pathway **8–14**. Each ligand binds a unique receptor-α (Rα) subunit, which is tethered to the plasma membrane by glycophosphatidylinositol (GPI). Upon ligand binding, the receptor complexes with LIF receptor (LIFR) and glycoprotein of 130 kDa (gp130). The formation of this tripartite receptor complex triggers activation of Janus kinase (JAK) and of related protein tyrosine kinases, such as Tyk, which subsequently mediate biologic effects such as activation of the signal transducers and activation of transcription (STAT) family of transcription factors (Chapter 4).

Surprisingly, CNTF knockout mice develop normally and exhibit only mild motor neuron defects during adulthood. Also surprising is a related finding in humans: approximately 2.5% of the Japanese population are homozygous for inactivating mutations of CNTF and thus are, in a sense, human CNTF "knockouts"; these individuals develop without obvious deficits. In contrast, mice lacking the CNTF receptor CNTFRα lose almost all of their motor neurons and die within

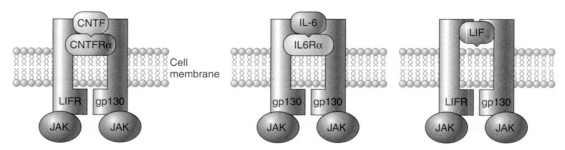

8–14 **Receptor complexes formed by the CNTF family of neurotrophic factors.** CNTF binds to CNTFRα, which in turn forms a tripartite complex with gp130 and LIFR. The resulting trimer induces the biologic effects of CNTF by binding to the protein tyrosine kinase JAK. Interleukin-6 (IL-6) binds to IL-6Rα, which subsequently associates with two gp130 molecules; the resulting trimer associates with JAK. LIF associates with JAK by binding to a gp130-LIFR dimer. CNTF, ciliary neurotrophic factor; LIFR, leukemia inhibitory factor receptor; JAK, Janus kinase.

24 hours of birth. The striking discrepancies between CNTF and CNTFRα knockout mice suggest the existence of another endogenous ligand for CNTFRα that has yet to be discovered.

Glial cells are generally believed to be the primary or sole source of CNTF, LIF, and IL-6 in the brain, although neural expression of these factors has not been ruled out. However, the receptor signaling mechanisms for these factors are clearly expressed by both neuronal and glial cell types. Thus, these factors may mediate critical effects of glial cells on their neighboring neurons, particularly after injury. The details of such involvement in cell–cell communication remain largely unknown.

Immune-Response Cytokines and the CNS

As alluded to previously, the best studied effects of many cytokines are their actions on the immune system. Only recently has it emerged that some of these factors, particularly IL-1 and IL-6, TNFα, and *transforming growth factor-β (TGFβ)*, also mediate CNS responses to immunologic challenges.

Cytokines implicated in immune function appear to be critical for systemic homeostasis. Serious stressors or illness elicit a defense response that aids in the body's recovery. This response involves processes that are mediated in part by the CNS, such as fever, reduced appetite, cardiovascular changes, sleep disturbances, and malaise. A more detailed discussion of these processes is provided in Chapters 10 and 11; the section that follows is devoted to the general schemes by which cytokines affect brain function, whether they are generated in the CNS or peripherally.

The impact that immune-response cytokines can have on the brain is exemplified by the **fever**—which is mediated by the brain—that occurs in animals and humans in response to the peripheral injection of IL-1. Although the blood-brain barrier is believed to limit cytokine entry to most of the brain, some cytokines may enter at sites where the blood-brain barrier is incomplete, such as certain periventricular areas. Cytokines also may act by inducing lipophilic signals, such as prostaglandins, within endothelial cells, which can diffuse into the brain parenchyma.

Interestingly, the brain itself can synthesize many of these immune-response cytokines. Such cytokines are believed to be synthesized primarily in glia—particularly in microglia, the CNS equivalent of macrophages—and in astrocytes. Receptors for these cytokines are also expressed primarily in glia, although expression in at least some neuronal cell types appears likely. After almost

any dramatic perturbation, such as brain infection or injury, activated microglia and astrocytes produce cytokines, including IL-1, IL-6, TNFα, and TGFβ. These factors may further activate glial cells and in turn stimulate *gliosis*—the generation of new astrocytes and microglia. The activated glia presumably help the brain recover by restoring normal homeostasis.

However, excessive levels of these cytokines can contribute to neural injury. This phenomenon is demonstrated dramatically in mutant mice that overexpress specific factors such as IL-1 or IL-6; such mice exhibit significant neurodegeneration in the vicinities of cytokine overexpression. Moreover, elevated levels of immune-response cytokines have been associated with several neurodegenerative disorders, including **Alzheimer disease**. Elevated cytokine levels are also observed in individuals with **multiple sclerosis,** an autoimmune disease that results in the degeneration of myelin sheaths around axons. The immune-response cytokine known as *interferon-β (IFN-β)* has shown promise as a treatment for this disease, although its precise mechanism of action remains obscure 8-3 .

In some cases, immune-response cytokines produce effects similar to those produced by CNTF and related proteins. IL-1, like IL-6, enhances survival of several types of central neurons. TGF-β, like CNTF, is important for neural crest cell differentiation during development. On the other hand, TNF-α released from macrophages contributes to the waves of programmed cell death of motor neurons required for proper development. Like other neurotrophic factors, these cytokines may also directly affect neurons in the adult brain. Receptors for IL-1, TNF-α, and TGF-β are most densely concentrated in the hippocampus and hypothalamus, where some of their corresponding factors have been proven to influence synaptic plasticity. For example, IL-1 is reported to attenuate the generation of hippocampal LTP while TNF-α may directly influence synaptic properties in developing neural circuits. Immune-response cytokines also may influence the rate of neurogenesis and the survival of newly formed neurons in the dentate gyrus of the adult hippocampus. More research will be required to better characterize the direct effects of these cytokines on neurons, and to explore their possible role in the regulation of nervous system function under normal and pathologic conditions.

CHEMOKINES

Chemokines are a family of small (8–10 kDa) proteins originally characterized for their involvement in immune responses. Recent studies have revealed that many chemokines and their receptors are expressed in

Like many neurotrophic factors, interferons first received attention outside the nervous system, principally for their role in immunity. Among other functions, interferons help the body respond to viral infection by activating natural killer cells and macrophages. In recent years, attention has shifted to interferon function in the nervous system, in part due to the promise of interferon as a treatment for multiple sclerosis (MS).

MS is a devastating inflammatory demyelinating syndrome of the CNS. It is caused by the deterioration of the myelin that surrounds nerve fibers and is required for the efficient transduction of nerve impulses along most axons. MS is believed to be an autoimmune illness. Patients with MS show autoimmunity to some myelin proteins. Immune responses to such antigens appear to be both humoral and cellular. MS is associated with genes that encode human leukocyte antigens (HLAs). According to one hypothesis, the autoimmune response can be attributed to molecular mimicry; that is, an immune response mounted toward bacterial or viral pathogens cross-reacts with an endogenous protein, leading to autoimmunity.

There has been considerable interest in determining whether some cytokines play a role in the etiology of MS, and in turn whether other cytokines might be used to treat the illness. Interferon-γ (INF-γ) and TNF-α are two cytokines that have been implicated in the pathophysiology of MS. Both are secreted by peripheral lymphocytes or macrophages as well as by central microglia. Moreover, both INF-γ and TNF-α have been detected in MS plaques but not in healthy white matter. Cytokines may contribute to the pathophysiology of MS by (1) activating central microglia, which may enhance the immune response to central antigens such as myelin-associated proteins, or (2) exerting direct toxic effects on oligodendrocytes.

The treatment of MS has depended primarily on the use of anti-inflammatory agents, yet clinical trials involving the use of interferon-β (INF-β) have been promising. INF-β ameliorates clinical symptoms of the illness, reduces the number and size of plaques detectable by magnetic resonance imaging (MRI), and appears to decrease the rate at which relapses recur. INF-β is more effective for earlier stages of MS and less effective for more severe stages. Although the mechanism by which INF-β exerts these effects is unclear, it likely involves modulation of the immune response. INF-β reduces the production of INF-γ and exerts general anti-inflammatory effects in vitro and in vivo. Such actions may occur both peripherally and centrally. Moreover, INF-β may act to restrict the movement of peripheral lymphocytes across the blood-brain barrier and in turn may further reduce the immune response to myelin-associated proteins. Regardless of the mechanism of action by which INF-β improves the symptoms of MS, its application represents the first widespread use of a neurotrophic factor for the treatment of a neurologic disorder.

---

the brain, predominantly by microglia but also in astrocytes and certain neurons. Chemokines are categorized based on the spacing between two required cysteine residues in their primary structure, with either contiguous (CC) residues, one intervening residue (CXC), or several intervening residues (CX$_3$C). Receptors for these chemokines—all of which belong to the G protein-coupled receptor family—are likewise named according to these categories (see **8–2**).

Chemokines may mediate part of the brain's inflammatory response and they may be involved in several human disorders, including **multiple sclerosis, brain tumors,** and **stroke**. Chemokines also may play a role in regulating the migration of neurons during development and in attracting growing nerve fibers toward target neurons, for example, in axonal guidance. For instance, mice that lack the chemokine receptor CXC$_4$R exhibit abnormal migration of cerebellar granule cells during late stages of development. Investigators have speculated that chemokines may assist in regulating neuron–neuron interactions during adulthood. According to this hypothesis, chemokines may contribute to the formation or retraction of synapses in the context of long-term plasticity.

VEGF

VEGF is a 23-kDa protein that has long been known for its effects in growth and permeability of blood vessels. Only recently has it been recognized for its neurotrophic properties. VEGF exerts its effects through two receptor tyrosine kinases, VEGFR1 (also known as flt-1) and VEGFR2 (or flk-1). VEGF and its receptors are expressed in neurons and glia, and this expression is highly up-regulated by hypoxia.

The neurotrophic properties of VEGF were first identified when mutations in the VEGF promoter of mice resulted in **ALS**-like symptoms. Subsequently, VEGF was found to rescue hypoxia-induced motor neuron death both in vivo and in vitro. Recently, a polymorphism in the VEGF promoter sequence was identified in a subset of ALS patients. It is thought that low VEGF levels may underlie motor neuron degeneration in at least one group of patients, but measurement of VEGF in ALS patients has proven difficult. VEGF may also be important for response to **stroke** and other forms of neural injury.

Therapeutic Agents Directed at Neurotrophic Factors and Their Signal Pathways

Althought this chapter higlights only a few of the many known families of neurotrophic factors, it is clear that certain neurotrophic factors would be ideal candidates for use in the treatment of neurodegenerative disease, given their ability to promote neuronal survival. Yet clinical trials of such agents have been disappointing. Such setbacks can be attributed in part to inadequate animal models of many human neurodegenerative diseases. Moreover, because neurotrophic factors are relatively large proteins, their delivery to the CNS is particularly challenging. This is compounded by the fact that many neurotrophic factors have multiple roles in different parts of the brain and body. The delivery of quantities large enough to ensure bioavailability can therefore result in serious side effects. Neurotrophins have the additional complication of activating p75 in addition to Trk receptors, often with antagonistic effects. Consequently, small-molecule ligands of Trk and other receptors are needed. Another possible avenue for therapies—with its own challenges—involves expression of neurotrophins in situ with viral vectors.

Clinical experience with neurotrophic factors is reviewed only briefly here. As previously mentioned in this chapter, BDNF, CNTF, *insulin-like growth factor-1 (IGF-1)*, and VEGF have been proven to support motor neuron survival in vitro and in vivo. In addition, treatment with BDNF, CNTF, or a combination of these factors has been shown to slow or arrest the progression of motor neuron degeneration in the *wobbler* mouse. VEGF has been found to have similar effects in the superoxide dismutase-1 (SOD1) knockout mouse, another **ALS** model (Chapter 17).

Encouraged by these results, investigators have used BDNF, CNTF, and IGF-1 in clinical trials involving patients with **ALS**. While BDNF has been well tolerated, it has produced only modest clinical effects, a result also obtained with IGF-1. Clinical trials involving CNTF have been even more problematic. Although treatment with CNTF slowed deterioration of muscle strength, it produced severe toxicity in most patients—especially in those receiving higher doses. Yet such high doses are 30 times lower than the effective dose (corrected for body weight) in *wobbler* mice. In addition, patients treated with this neurotrophic factor can develop neutralizing antibodies to CNTF that limit its bioavailability.

The therapeutic use of neurotrophic factors in the treatment of other diseases has been equally disappointing. Because NGF supports the survival of many sensory neurons, investigators have attempted to treat sensory neuropathy with this factor. However, as in studies of motor neuron therapies, humans have not been able to tolerate the highest doses of NGF, although such doses are 10000 times lower than effective doses used in animal models.

Because BDNF, GDNF, and other factors have enhanced the survival of dopaminergic neurons in animal models, the use of neurotrophic factors in the treatment of **Parkinson disease** is a top research priority (Chapter 17). Experiments with GDNF in a nonhuman primate model of Parkinson disease are promising. Clinical trials in humans, however, have demonstrated only modest benefits, and only when GDNF, or a viral vector expressing GDNF, is infused directly into the striatum. Trials with BDNF have been even less successful.

Likewise, because cholinergic afferent systems, whose function appears to be supported by neurotrophic factors such as NGF and BDNF, may be important for memory function, investigators are exploring the use of NGF and BDNF as treatments for **Alzheimer disease** (Chapter 17). Indeed, after treatment with NGF, aged rats improve in their ability to perform memory tasks. A recent small clinical trial in which fibroblasts expressing NGF were implanted into the brains of Alzheimer disease patients yielded moderate reductions in cognitive decline, but larger scale trials are required.

A major challenge in all of these clinical trials is the difficulty in delivering neurotrophic factors directly to targeted neurons of the CNS. Intracranial injection of these factors in slow-release preparations and injection of cultured cells or viral vectors that overexpress these factors are currently under evaluation.

These systems would have the obvious benefit of being able to target neurotrophic factors directly to the affected areas of the brain, thereby avoiding side effects caused by actions on other areas of the brain and periphery. Ideally, it would be useful to develop viral vectors which allow for modification in the quantity of neurotrophic factor produced, but this is not yet feasible.

The challenges associated with administering neurotrophic factors have inspired hopes of developing small molecules that might promote or antagonize neurotrophic factor function. Only recently have such reagents begun to be developed, and it remains to be seen whether they will have clinical utility. The large size of neurotrophic factors, and presumably of their binding sites on their receptors, by comparison to small molecule neurotransmitters, makes this a challenging prospect in drug development. One recent success is the use of *epidermal growth factor (EGF)* receptor antagonists, such as **gefitinib** or **erlotinib**, for the treatment of several types of cancers, including **glioblastomas** (malignancies of astrocytes) (Chapter 1). More creative approaches to such research may be useful as well. For example for BDNF, rather than development of a traditional TrkB agonist, small molecules that promote the dimerization and hence activation of TrkB might be developed. Such strategies are currently underway.

SELECTED READING

Ann Marrie R, Rudick RA. Drug insight: interferon treatment in multiple sclerosis. *Nat Clin Pract Neurol.* 2006;2:34–44.

Asensio VC, Campbell IL. Chemokines in the CNS: plurifunctional mediators in diverse states. *Trends Neurosci.* 1999;22:504–512.

Baloh RH, Enomoto H, Johnson EM Jr, Milbrandt J. The GDNF family ligands and receptors—implications for neural development. *Curr Opin Neurobiol.* 2000;10:103–110.

Boehning D, Snyder SH. Novel neural modulators. *Annu Rev Neurosci.* 2003;26:105–131.

Burnstock G. Purinergic P2 receptors as targets for novel analgesics. *Pharmacol Ther.* 2006;110: 433–453.

Castren E. Neurotrophic effects of antidepressant drugs. *Curr Opin Pharmacol.* 2004;4:58–64.

Di Marzo V, Bifulco M, De Petrocellis L. The endocannabinoid system and its therapeutic exploitation. *Nat Rev Drug Discov.* 2004;3:771–784.

Duman RS, Monteggia LM. A neurotrophic model for stress-related mood disorders. *Biol Psychiatry.* 2006;59:1116–1127.

Dunwiddie TV, Masino SA. The role and regulation of adenosine in the central nervous system. *Annu Rev Neurosci.* 2001;24:31–55.

Esplugues JV. NO as a signalling molecule in the nervous system. *Br J Pharmacol.* 2002;135:1079–1095.

Fredhold BB, Battig K, Holmen J, et al. Actions of caffeine in the brain with specific reference to factors that contribute to its widespread use. *Pharmacol Rev.* 1999;51:83–133.

He XL, Garcia KC. Structure of nerve growth factor complexed with the shared neurotrophin receptor p75. *Science.* 2004;304:870–875.

Howlett AC, Breivogel CS, Childers SR, et al. Cannabinoid physiology and pharmacology. 30 years of progress. *Neuropharmacology.* 2004;47 (Suppl 1): 345–358.

Jacobson KA, Ga Z-G. Adenosine receptors as therapeutic targets. *Nat Rev Drug Discov.* 2006;5:247–264.

Khakh BS, North RA. P2X receptors as cell-surface ATP sensors in health and disease. *Nature.* 2006;442: 527–532.

Lambrechts D, Storkebaum E, Carmeliet P. VEGF: necessary to prevent motoneuron degeneration, sufficient to treat ALS? *Trends Mol Med.* 2004;10:275–282.

Levi-Montalcini R. The nerve growth factor 35 years later. *Science.* 1987;237:1154–1162.

Liu XJ, Salter MW. Purines and pain mechanisms: recent developments. *Curr Opin Invest Drugs.* 2005;6:65–75.

Martino G, Furlan R, Brambilla E, et al. Cytokines and immunity in multiple sclerosis: the dual signal hypothesis. *J Neuroimmunol.* 2000;109:3–9.

Mennicken R, Maki R, de Souza EB, Quirion R. Chemokines and chemokine receptors in the CNS: a possible role in neuroinflammation and patterning. *Trends Pharmacol Sci.* 1999;20:73–78.

Nykjaer A, Willnow TE, Petersen CM. p75NTR—live or let die. *Curr Opin Neurobiol.* 2005;15:49–57.

Pezet S, Malcangio M. Brain-derived neurotrophic factor as a drug target for CNS disorders. *Expert Opin Ther Targets.* 2004;8:391–399.

Piomelli D. The endocannabinoid system: a drug discovery perspective. *Curr Opin Invest Drugs.* 2005;6: 672–679.

Sah DW, Ossipov MH, Rossomando A, Silvian L, Porreca F. New approaches for the treatment of pain: the GDNF family of neurotrophic growth factors. *Curr Top Med Chem.* 2005;5:577–583.

Schweigreiter R. The dual nature of neurotrophins. *Bioessays.* 2006;28:583–594.

Skaper SD, Walsh FS. Neurotrophic molecules: strategies for designing effective therapeutic molecules in neurodegeneration. *Mol Cell Neurosci.* 1998;12:179–193.

Teng HK, Teng KK, Lee R, et al. ProBDNF induces neuronal apoptosis via activation of a receptor complex of p75NTR and sortilin. *J Neurosci.* 2005;25: 5455–5463.

Thoenen H, Sendtner M. Neurotrophins: from enthusiastic expectations through sobering experiences to rational therapeutic approaches. *Nat Neurosci.* 2002;5(suppl):1046–1050.

Tuszynski MH, Thal L, Pay M, et al. A phase 1 clinical trial of nerve growth factor gene therapy for Alzheimer disease. *Nat Med.* 2005;11:551–555.

Williams G, Williams EJ, Maison P, Pangalos MN, Walsh FS, Doherty P. Overcoming the inhibitors of myelin with a novel neurotrophin strategy. *J Biol Chem.* 2005;280:5862–5869.

Williams M, Jarvis MF. Purinergic and pyramidinergic receptors as potential drug targets. *Biochem Pharmacol.* 2000;59:1173–1185.

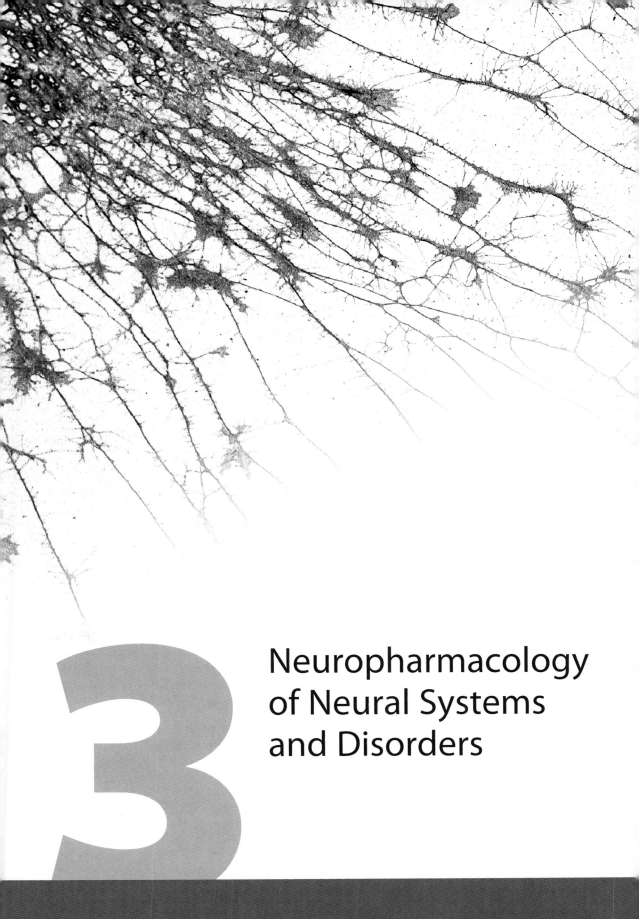

3

Neuropharmacology of Neural Systems and Disorders

CHAPTER 9

Autonomic Nervous System

- The autonomic nervous system plays a central role in maintaining homeostasis and regulates almost every organ system in the body.

- The major functional divisions are the sympathetic and parasympathetic nervous systems. A third division, the enteric nervous system, is an intrinsic neural network that regulates gastrointestinal function.

- In most organs, the sympathetic and parasympathetic nervous systems produce functionally opposite effects and can be viewed in simple terms as physiologic antagonists.

- The sympathetic nervous system is activated in response to changes in the environment and produces a coordinated "fight or flight" response to a threat.

- The parasympathetic nervous system is continuously active, and coordinates the function of multiple organs in accord with the physiologic state of the organism, thereby facilitating such functions as digestion and excretion.

- Because of its importance to the physiology of the organism, the autonomic nervous system is a target for many pharmacologic interventions and is also responsible for the untoward effects of many medications and toxins.

- The peripheral autonomic nervous system (both sympathetic and parasympathetic divisions) consists of a preganglionic neuron in the brainstem or spinal cord which innervates postganglionic neurons in peripheral autonomic ganglia. Synaptic transmission in the autonomic ganglia is mediated by acetylcholine interacting with a nicotinic receptor that is pharmacologically distinct from receptors in the brain or at the neuromuscular junction. The postganglionic neurons innervate target organs throughout the body.

- Acetylcholine is the main neurotransmitter used by parasympathetic postganglionic neurons; its target receptors are muscarinic acetylcholine receptors.

- With a few exceptions, postganglionic sympathetic neurons release norepinephrine, which acts on α- and β-adrenergic receptors located on end organs.

The autonomic nervous system (ANS) is a semiautonomous division of the nervous system that innervates virtually every organ in the body. Central control of autonomic function involves integration of afferent information and cortical input by brainstem centers and the hypothalamus. These structures control the overall activity of the ANS (autonomic tone). The peripheral ANS (or visceral system) serves to distribute autonomic efferents throughout the body and can also mediate simple autonomic reflexes independent of central control.

The overall function of the ANS is to maintain homeostasis in the body (ie, optimize conditions for survival) in the face of constantly changing environmental and activity demands. For example, the ANS adjusts blood pressure and heart rate to meet the circulatory needs of the body which can vary tremendously from supine sleep to vigorous exercise. The ANS also maintains a constant body temperature despite changing environmental conditions and metabolic activity. Under ordinary circumstances, the ANS functions independently of consciousness yet can be influenced to some degree by volition and emotion. Without autonomic innervation, most organ systems continue to function but cannot adapt to changing environmental and emotional conditions.

Because of its anatomic accessibility and its robust regulation of peripheral organ functions, the ANS was among the first components of the mammalian nervous system to be studied. Consequently, many of the principles of neuropharmacology were derived from classic studies of autonomic systems. Such studies enabled investigators to establish the chemical basis of neurotransmission, identify acetylcholine and norepinephrine as neurotransmitters, explore the pharmacology of cholinergic and adrenergic receptors, and discover the role of inhibitory presynaptic autoreceptors in neurotransmission. Indeed, many of the pharmacologic agents studied during the past century originally were characterized according to their actions on the ANS.

ANATOMY OF THE AUTONOMIC NERVOUS SYSTEM

Central autonomic centers are distributed throughout the brain and include limbic cortical areas, amygdala, hypothalamus, and numerous brainstem nuclei `9-1`. Cortical autonomic centers and amygdala are involved with initiating autonomic responses to emotion and pain. Brainstem centers receive visceral information and generate patterns of output through the peripheral autonomic nerves. The hypothalamus has multiple

roles in autonomic regulation and has direct connections to the pituitary, peripheral autonomic neurons, and central autonomic nuclei. The hypothalamus can be considered the main coordinating center of the ANS. It is involved with control of circadian rhythm, temperature regulation, hunger, and thirst and also serves as a relay center for all sympathetic autonomic information descending to the body `9-2`.

Although all parts work together in a coordinated fashion, the ANS can be divided into multiple discrete components. These include the following:

1. Neurohumoral component of the ANS (which is usually considered as part of the endocrine system). This consists of hormones that regulate energy metabolism, blood volume, and other functions (Chapter 10).

2. Intrinsic enteric nervous system. The gut has its own independent nervous system that consists of interconnected neurons in the wall of the bowel from the esophagus to the anus. There are as many neurons in the gut as in the spinal cord. These regulate bowel motility and other functions such that the bowel can operate independent of extrinsic input.

3. Sympathetic nervous system.

4. Parasympathetic nervous system.

The latter two components form the traditional peripheral ANS. The sympathetic and parasympathetic systems usually produce opposite functional effects and thus are viewed as physiologic antagonists. Most organs are innervated by both. Because they also are regulated independently, their combined actions result in an especially fine degree of control `9-3`; `9-1`. The sympathetic nervous system, which is characterized by episodic activity, assists an organism in adjusting to changes in the environment, such as those occurring during periods of danger or stress. It usually discharges as a whole, orchestrating a coordinated, multiorgan response to a threat. Activation of this system is associated with increases in the force and rate of heart contractions, an increase in blood pressure, a shift in blood flow from the skin and viscera to skeletal muscle, an increase in blood glucose, and dilation of the bronchial tree. These responses prepare an organism for fight or flight in response to threatening stimuli. The sympathetic system is also activated in response to emotional stress and anxiety (Chapter 14), exercise, dehydration, and in disease states such as congestive heart failure.

In contrast, the parasympathetic nervous system is characterized by graded activity in anatomically discrete

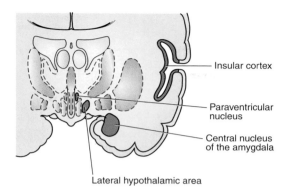

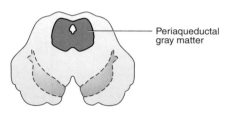

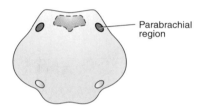

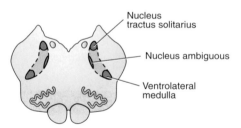

9-1 **Significant areas of the central autonomic network.** (Adapted with permission from Benarroch EE. *Mayo Clin Proc* 1993;68:989–1001.)

branches of the peripheral ANS have several anatomical similarities with the somatic motor system **9-4**. The central (preganglionic) autonomic motor neurons are cholinergic and leave the CNS via cranial nerves and ventral spinal roots **9-5**. The preganglionic autonomic fibers synapse with neurons in autonomic ganglia that are spread throughout the body. The ganglionic neurons then send postganglionic axons to innervate multiple targets throughout the body. Autonomic ganglia are not only relay stations, but they also mediate simple autonomic reflexes and coordinate autonomic function between different organ systems.

Sympathetic Nervous System

Preganglionic sympathetic neurons reside in the intermediolateral cell column of the thoracolumbar (T1 to L2–3) spinal cord **9-3**. Myelinated preganglionic fibers leave the spinal cord and, in most cases, innervate paravertebral sympathetic ganglia connected in a chain by nerve fibers that extend along either side of the vertebral columns from the base of the skull to the coccyx. The postganglionic axons are nonmyelinated and provide sympathetic innervation to most organ systems.

Among cervical sympathetic ganglia, the *superior cervical ganglion* is notable because it gives rise to the carotid plexus, a network of postganglionic fibers that

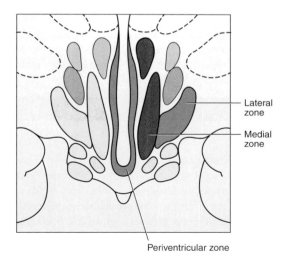

9-2 **Three functional longitudinal zones of the hypothalamus.** The periventricular zone controls biologic rhythms and endocrine and autonomic function. The medial zone initiates responses related to homeostasis and reproduction. The lateral zone controls arousal and motivated behavior. (Adapted with permission from Benarroch EE. *Mayo Clin Proc* 1993;68:989–1001.)

segments that serves to coordinate the functioning of individual organs with the physiologic state of an organism. This system assists in maintaining the organism by facilitating functions such as digestion and excretion. There are many specific functions, including slowing the heart, constricting the pupils, stimulating the gut and salivary glands, stimulating bladder emptying, and sexual function.

It is important to remember that the two branches of the ANS have different neuroanatomy (see **9-3**). Both

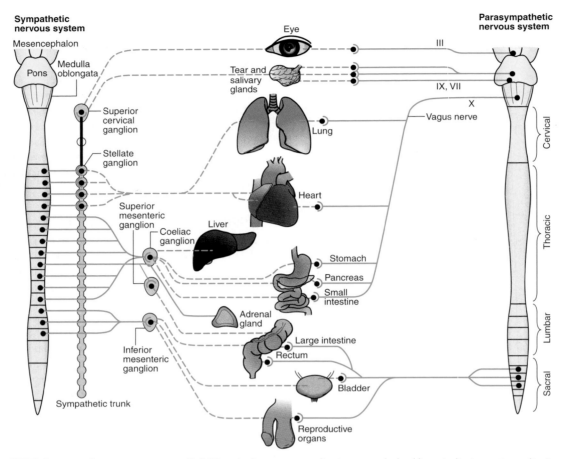

Sympathetic nervous system

Mesencephalon
Pons
Medulla oblongata
Superior cervical ganglion
Stellate ganglion
Superior mesenteric ganglion
Coeliac ganglion
Inferior mesenteric ganglion
Sympathetic trunk

Eye
Tear and salivary glands
Lung
Heart
Liver
Stomach
Pancreas
Small intestine
Adrenal gland
Large intestine
Rectum
Bladder
Reproductive organs

Parasympathetic nervous system

III
IX, VII
X
Vagus nerve

Cervical
Thoracic
Lumbar
Sacral

9-3 **Autonomic nervous system.** Solid lines indicate preganglionic axons; dashed lines indicate postganglionic axons. Sympathetic innervation of blood vessels, sweat glands, and piloerector muscles is not shown. Roman numerals denote cranial nerves. (Adapted with permission from Bannister R, Mathias CJ, eds. *Autonomic Failure.* New York: Oxford University Press; 1992:107.)

follow the ramifications of the carotid arteries and furnish the sympathetic innervation of the entire head. Some fibers end in blood vessels and sweat glands of the head and face; others supply the lacrimal and salivary glands. The eye receives sympathetic fibers that innervate the dilator muscles of the pupil and the smooth muscle fibers that help raise the eyelid. The lower cervical ganglia supply the viscera of the neck.

The heart and lungs receive sympathetic innervation from thoracic sympathetic ganglia. The abdominal and pelvic viscera are supplied by thoracic *splanchnic nerves*, which include the celiac, superior mesenteric, and aorticorenal ganglia. Lumbar splanchnic nerves carry preganglionic fibers to inferior mesenteric and hypogastric ganglia, from which postganglionic fibers reach end organs in the lower abdomen and pelvis.

Parasympathetic Nervous System

Preganglionic fibers of the parasympathetic nervous system originate in the brainstem and in the sacral region of the spinal cord. The brainstem fibers travel in cranial nerves, including the *vagus nerve* (cranial nerve X), which provides parasympathetic input to most of the viscera of the body (from the neck down to the distal one-third of the colon). Sacral preganglionic neurons provide innervation to the rectum, bladder, and reproductive organs via pelvic splanchnic nerves. Parasympathetic preganglionic neurons have relatively long myelinated axons that synapse with postganglionic neurons in the many small ganglia located close to or within target organs (see **9-3**).

9-1 **Prominent Actions of the Autonomic Nervous System**

End Organ	Sympathetic Function[1]	Parasympathetic Function[2]
Eye	Mydriasis (pupillary dilation) (α_1)	Miosis (pupillary constriction) Accommodation (contracts ciliary muscle)
Lacrimal gland	No appreciable effect	Stimulates secretion
Salivary gland	No appreciable effect	Stimulates secretion
Skin		
Sweat glands	Stimulates secretion[3]	Stimulates secretion
Pilomotor muscles	Stimulates piloerection (α_1)	No appreciable effect
Nasopharyngeal glands	Inhibits secretion (α_1)	Stimulates secretion
Heart	Increases heart rate and contractility (β_1)	Decreases heart rate and contractility
Blood vessels	Dilates (β_1) or constricts (α_1) cardiac and skeletal muscle vessels Constricts vessels of the skin and GI tract (α_1)	No appreciable effect
Lung	Dilates bronchial tree (β_2)	Constricts bronchial tree
GI tract		
Gut wall	Decreases motility (β_2)	Increases motility and secretion
Sphincters	Contracts (α_1)	Relaxes
Bladder		
Muscle	Relaxes (β_2)	Contracts
Sphincter	Contracts (α_1)	Relaxes
Penis	Ejaculation (α_1)	Erection
Liver	Increases glycogenolysis (β_2)	No appreciable effect
Skeletal muscle	Increases glycogenolysis (β_2)	No appreciable effect
Fat cells	Increases lipolysis (β_1 and β_3)	No appreciable effect
Pancreatic β-cells	Increases insulin secretion (β_2)	No appreciable effect

[1]The adrenergic receptor that predominantly mediates each effect is shown in parentheses.
[2]All of these actions are mediated by muscarinic ACh receptors. Although five subtypes (M_1–M_5) have been identified, little is known about their selective roles in the responses listed (see Chapter 6).
[3]This effect, mediated by postganglionic sympathetic neurons that are cholinergic, is responsible for sweating at localized sites, such as the palms of the hands.

NEUROTRANSMITTERS OF THE AUTONOMIC NERVOUS SYSTEM

Principal Neurotransmitters

The ANS functions predominantly through the actions of acetylcholine (ACh) and norepinephrine **9-4** . As discussed in Chapter 6, ACh is the neurotransmitter released at the neuromuscular junction. In the ANS, all preganglionic neurons in both the sympathetic and parasympathetic nervous systems are cholinergic. These autonomic neurons are analogous to the anterior horn cells of the somatic motor system. Thus, all of the efferent fibers that leave the CNS are cholinergic. In both sympathetic and parasympathetic ganglia, the synaptic connection between the cholinergic preganglionic neuron and the postganglionic neuron is mediated by nicotinic ACh receptors. These neuronal ACh receptors are structurally similar but pharmacologically different from those at the neuromuscular junction, based on differences in their

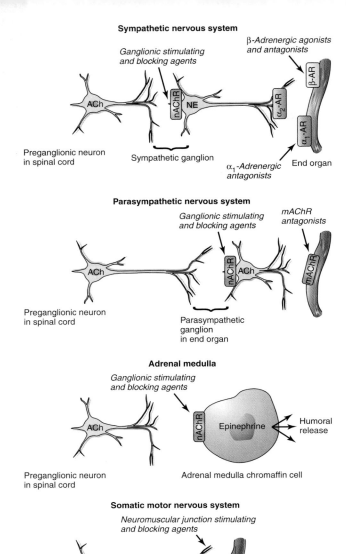

9-4 Patterns of innervation in sympathetic and parasympathetic nervous systems. Both systems comprise preganglionic neurons, which originate in the CNS, and postganglionic neurons, which originate in the peripheral nervous system. Sympathetic ganglia generally are located far from their end organs, whereas parasympathetic ganglia are located in close proximity to their end organs. Preganglionic neurons in both the sympathetic and parasympathetic nervous systems are cholinergic and act by means of nicotinic cholinergic receptors (nAChR) on postganglionic cells. Transmission at these synapses can be modified by nicotinic cholinergic agonists and antagonists (ganglionic stimulating and blocking agents, respectively). With a few exceptions, which are mentioned in this chapter, postganglionic sympathetic neurons are noradrenergic and affect end organ function by means of α_1-, β_1-, and β_2-adrenergic receptors (AR). Presynaptic α_2 receptors generally function as inhibitory autoreceptors. Postganglionic parasympathetic neurons are cholinergic and affect end organ function by means of muscarinic cholinergic receptors (mAChR). Adrenal medulla chromaffin cells may be regarded as an extension of the sympathetic nervous system. These cells are stimulated by preganglionic cholinergic neurons that act on nicotinic receptors and secrete epinephrine into the general circulation. Such activity regulates most of the end organs influenced by postganglionic sympathetic neurons. The somatic motor nervous system is shown for comparison. This system, too, involves central cholinergic neurons (lower motor neurons in the anterior horn of the spinal cord) which innervate skeletal muscle, where transmission is mediated via nicotinic receptors.

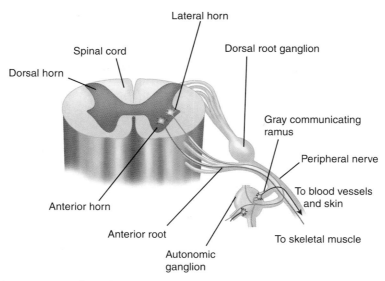

Lateral horn

Spinal cord

Dorsal horn

Dorsal root ganglion

Gray communicating ramus

Peripheral nerve

To blood vessels and skin

Anterior horn

To skeletal muscle

Anterior root

Autonomic ganglion

9–5 **Autonomic neurons reside in the intermediolateral cell column in the spinal cord just lateral to the anterior horn cells of the somatic motor system.** Both neurons are cholinergic and send their axons out via the anterior spinal roots. Unlike the motor nerves, the autonomic nerves make a synapse outside the spinal cord in the autonomic ganglia before going to their targets.

constituent subunits (Chapter 6). ACh is also the main neurotransmitter used by postganglionic neurons in the parasympathetic nervous system **9–4**. The cholinergic signal from postganglionic parasympathetic fibers is transmitted to target organs primarily through muscarinic ACh receptors.

In contrast, norepinephrine is used by most of the postganglionic neurons of the sympathetic nervous system. The norepinephrine signal acts on several α- and β-adrenergic receptors located on target organs. Not all postganglionic sympathetic neurons are adrenergic. Sympathetic neurons that innervate sweat glands and certain blood vessels are cholinergic and act by means of muscarinic ACh receptors. Moreover, chromaffin cells of the adrenal medulla receive innervation from preganglionic sympathetic cholinergic fibers that act through neuronal nicotinic ACh receptors. In response to stimulation, chromaffin cells release epinephrine, which, like norepinephrine, acts on α- and β-adrenergic receptors located on end organs. In this way, adrenal chromaffin cells are functionally analogous to sympathetic postganglionic neurons.

Neuropeptides Most sympathetic and parasympathetic neurons express, in addition to their principal neurotransmitters, a variety of neuropeptides. Neuropeptide Y (NPY) is most often coexpressed with

norepinephrine in postganglionic sympathetic neurons, and vasoactive intestinal peptide (VIP) is typically coexpressed with ACh in postganglionic parasympathetic neurons. Other peptides expressed more sparingly in the ANS include galanin, enkephalin, somatostatin, and substance P. Most evidence suggests that, at least in the ANS, peptide transmitters act synergistically with small-molecule transmitters; for example, VIP promotes salivary gland secretion by itself, and the effect is intensified when VIP is coupled with ACh. Similarly, NPY increases vascular smooth muscle contraction by itself and produces synergistic increases in vascular tone when coupled with norepinephrine. These synergistic actions are significant because, outside of the ANS, peptide cotransmitters sometimes antagonize the actions of small-molecule transmitters (Chapter 7).

PHARMACOLOGY OF THE AUTONOMIC NERVOUS SYSTEM

As previously mentioned, pharmacologic studies of the ANS in many ways defined the field of neuropharmacology during the past 100 years. Indeed, the number and variety of pharmacologic agents that influence autonomic function are vast and well beyond the scope of this book. The sections that follow provide a

9–2 Examples of Drugs That Act on the Autonomic Nervous System

Drug Class	Examples	Examples of Clinical Uses
Adrenergic		
α_1 agonist	Phenylephrine, methoxamine, midodrine	Nasal congestion; orthostatic hypotension
α_1 antagonist	Prazosin, tamsulosin	Hypertension; benign prostatic hypertrophy
α_2 agonist	Clonidine, guanfacine	Hypertension; opiate withdrawal; ADD; Tourette syndrome
α_2 antagonist	Yohimbine	
β agonist (ns[1])	Dobutamine, isoproterenol	Severe cardiac failure
β antagonist (ns[1])	Propranolol, timolol	Heart ischemia; hypertension; social phobia
β_1 antagonist	Atenolol, labetalol	Heart ischemia; hypertension
β_2 agonist	Terbutaline, salbutamol	Chronic obstructive pulmonary disease
Muscarinic cholinergic		
agonist	Bethanechol	Urinary retention
antagonist	Benztropine, scopolamine	Extrapyramidal side effects; motion sickness
Nicotinic cholinergic		
antagonist (ganglionic)	Tetraethylammonium, mecamylamine	Severe hypertension
antagonist (NMJ)	Succinylcholine	Cause paralysis; can aid in anesthesia
Cholinesterase inhibitors		
peripherally acting	Physostigmine, edrophonium, pyridostigmine	Atonic bladder; myasthenia gravis; orthostastic hypotension
centrally acting	Tacrine, donepezil	Dementia

[1]ns, nonspecific, ie, actions at all β-adrenergic receptor subtypes.
ADD, attention deficit disorder; NMJ, neuromuscular junction.

concise summary of the classes of drugs that affect the ANS and an overview of their physiologic actions. Examples of drugs that act on the autonomic nervous system and their clinical uses are summarized in **9–2**.

Ganglionic Stimulating and Blocking Agents

Because cholinergic transmission through sympathetic and parasympathetic ganglia is mediated by nicotinic cholinergic receptors, nicotinic cholinergic agonists and antagonists have profound effects on autonomic function. The best characterized ganglionic stimulating drugs are **nicotine** and **lobeline** **9–6**. Nicotine, also discussed in Chapters 6 and 15, is a natural alkaloid of the tobacco plant. Lobeline is a natural alkaloid of Indian tobacco. Both drugs are agonists at nicotinic cholinergic receptors, although their actions are complicated by the fact that they can rapidly desensitize these receptors. The initial effects of nicotine and lobeline are consistent with the activation of autonomic ganglionic transmission. Such effects include increased heart rate and blood pressure (due to activation of sympathetic neurons and adrenal

medulla); increased salivation (due to activation of the sympathetic and parasympathetic systems); and increased contractile activity of the gut that may lead to nausea, vomiting, and diarrhea (due to activation of enteric and parasympathetic neurons regulating bowel

9–6 **Chemical structures of nicotine and lobeline.**

motility). Prolonged exposure to nicotine leads to desensitization of nicotinic receptors, resulting in sustained inhibition of autonomic activity.

A small number of synthetic nicotinic cholinergic agonists, such as **tetramethylammonium,** have been identified 9–7 . However, the clinical usefulness of such agents is limited. Most efforts in nicotinic cholinergic pharmacology have focused on the use of agonists that selectively activate nicotinic receptors in the brain and spinal cord for cognitive enhancement or analgesia (Chapters 6, 11, and 13). Other efforts have been directed toward the treatment of nicotine addiction (Chapter 15).

Among ganglionic blocking agents, **tetraethylammonium** was the first to be identified; other examples include **trimethaphan, hexamethonium,** and **mecamylamine** 9–7 . The net effect of these agents on end organ function depends on whether sympathetic or parasympathetic regulation of the organ predominates and on the physiologic state of the organism 9–3 . These principles can be illustrated by a consideration of blood pressure, which is regulated by sympathetic tone. Under normal conditions, when an individual is reclining, the maintenance of blood pressure does not require an appreciable level of sympathetic activity. In contrast, when an individual is sitting or standing, the maintenance of blood pressure depends on increased sympathetic tone. Accordingly, ganglionic blocking agents have little effect on supine blood pressure but can cause a precipitous decline in blood pressure when administered to someone sitting or standing.

Ganglionic blocking agents were used clinically to treat hypertension several decades ago but for the most part have been replaced by medications with fewer side

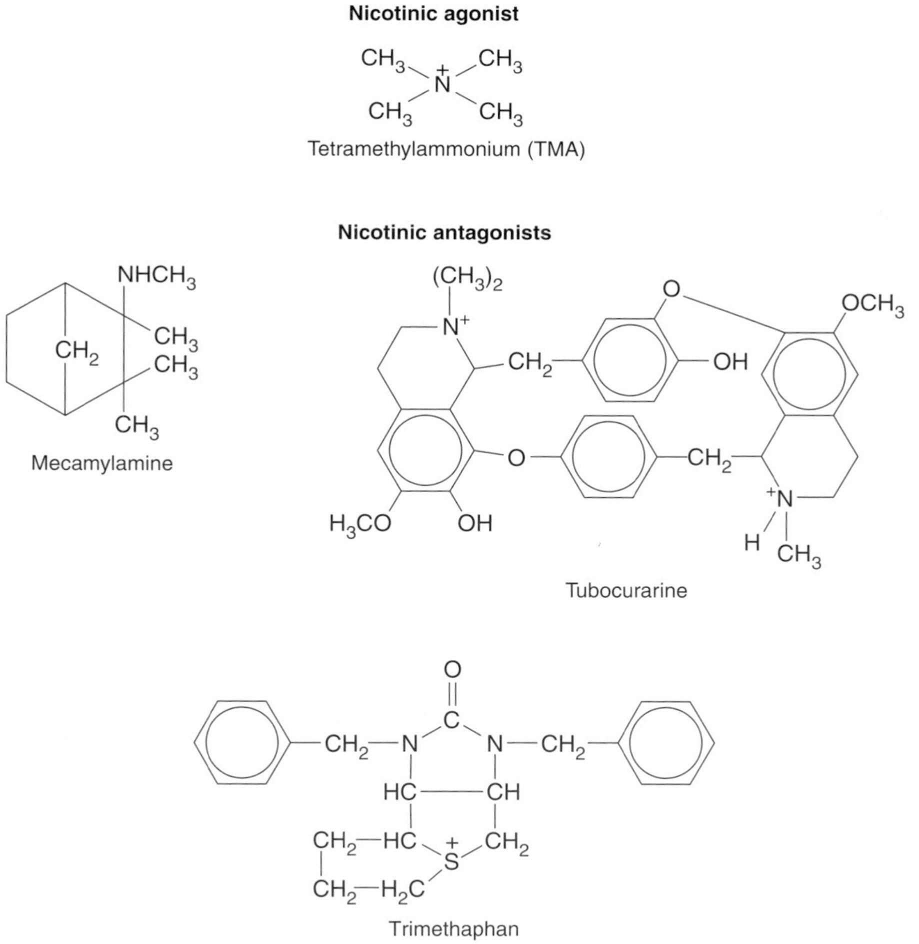

Nicotinic agonist

Tetramethylammonium (TMA)

Nicotinic antagonists

Mecamylamine

Tubocurarine

Trimethaphan

 9–7 **Chemical structures of representative nicotinic cholinergic agonists and antagonists.**

9-3 **Predominance of Sympathetic or Parasympathetic Tone at Various End Organs and Effects of Autonomic Ganglionic Blockade**

Site	Predominant Tone	Effect of Ganglionic Blockage
Arterioles	Sympathetic	Vasodilation; increased peripheral blood flow; hypotension
Veins	Sympathetic	Dilation; peripheral pooling of blood; decreased venous return; decreased cardiac output
Heart	Parasympathetic	Tachycardia
Iris	Parasympathetic	Mydriasis
Ciliary muscle	Parasympathetic	Cycloplegia—loss of accommodation
Gastrointestinal tract	Parasympathetic	Reduced tone and motility; constipation; decreased gastric and pancreatic secretions
Urinary bladder	Parasympathetic	Urinary retention
Salivary glands	Parasympathetic	Xerostomia
Sweat glands	Sympathetic[1]	Anhidrosis

[1]This effect is mediated by cholinergic sympathetic fibers.

effects. Other nicotinic cholinergic antagonists, such as **curare** **9-7** or the snake venom α-**bungarotoxin**, act on nicotinic receptors at both autonomic ganglia and the neuromuscular junction, although actions at the latter site, such as muscular paralysis, predominate. So-called depolarizing agents, such as **succinylcholine,** exert effects primarily on the nicotinic ACh receptors in skeletal muscle. Initially, they activate nicotinic receptors, resulting in muscle contractions, but quickly cause paralysis through sustained depolarization of postsynaptic specializations on muscle cells and subsequent depolarization blockade (Chapter 2).

Adrenergic Receptor Agonists and Antagonists

Agonists and antagonists at various adrenergic receptors exert profound effects on the functioning of many organs by mimicking or antagonizing, respectively, sympathetic innervation. Agonists often are termed **sympathomimetics,** and antagonists are referred to as **sympatholytics.** Further information on adrenergic agonists and antagonists is provided in Chapter 6.

Much of our early knowledge of adrenergic function was obtained from studies of natural plant alkaloids that potently affect sympathetic nervous system activity. A prominent example of such an alkaloid is **reserpine,** which is synthesized from *Rauwolfia serpentina*, a shrub found on the Indian subcontinent **9-8** . Reserpine is a potent sympatholytic agent, which acts by depleting body stores of norepinephrine and other monoamines, including dopamine and serotonin. As discussed in Chapter 6, this effect is mediated through the inhibition of the vesicular monoamine transporter (VMAT), which is responsible for concentrating monoamines into synaptic vesicles. Although reserpine was one of the first **antihypertensive** and **antipsychotic** agents used clinically, its use has been supplanted by that of more specific, and hence safer, medications.

Early information about adrenergic function also was drawn from studies of **ergot** alkaloids, which are produced by *Claviceps purpurea*, a fungus that grows on rye and other grains (see **9-8**). Ergot-containing preparations have been used medicinally for more than two millennia for indications as varied as **uterine bleeding** and **headache.** During the 20th century, a large number of ergot derivatives were prepared; these exerted a variety of effects on the adrenergic system, including receptor agonist and antagonist activity. Such compounds served as invaluable tools in the pharmacologic characterization of different subtypes of adrenergic receptors and in the delineation of their physiologic functions. Some ergot derivatives, such as **lysergic acid diethylamide** (**LSD**), affect the serotonin system (Chapters 6 and 16). Others affect the dopamine system; an example is **bromocriptine,** an agonist at D_2 dopamine receptors that is used in the treatment of **Parkinson disease** (Chapter 17) and **prolactin-secreting pituitary tumors.**

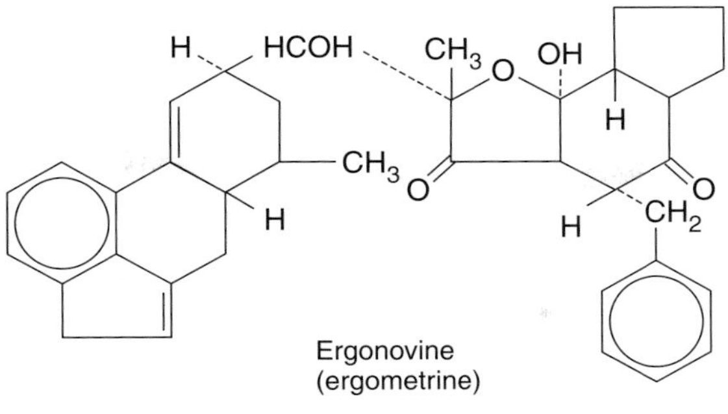

Ergonovine
(ergometrine)

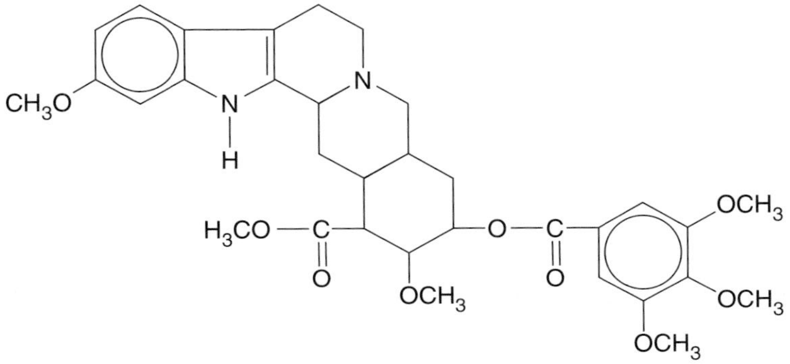

Reserpine

9-8 Chemical structures of ergonovine, an ergot alkaloid, and reserpine.

β-Adrenergic ligands   β-Adrenergic agonists have profound effects on many peripheral organs; clinically, their most important targets are the cardiovascular and pulmonary systems. The activation of β-adrenergic receptors increases the force and rate of heart contractions, and also can lead to the relaxation of vascular smooth muscle. The net effect is a large increase in cardiac output and a relatively modest increase in blood pressure. β-Adrenergic receptor activation causes relaxation of bronchial smooth muscle in the lungs, which increases pulmonary function and facilitates respiration. β-Adrenergic antagonists exert opposite effects. Chemical structures of representative β-adrenergic agonists and antagonists are shown in **9-9**.

In cardiovascular medicine, β-adrenergic agonists such as **dobutamine** are used only under extraordinary circumstances; for instance, they may be used to stimulate a failing heart in an intensive care setting. The prototypical β-adrenergic agonist is **isoproterenol**; it is the agonist most often used in preclinical studies, although it is rarely used clinically. However, β-adrenergic antagonists such as **propranolol** continue to be mainstays in the treatment of **ischemic heart disease** and **hypertension**. In the lungs, β-adrenergic stimulation increases pulmonary function, as previously mentioned. Accordingly, β-adrenergic agonists are one of the primary agents used to treat **asthma** and other **chronic obstructive pulmonary diseases**. The expression of different subtypes of β-adrenergic receptors in the heart (β_1) and lung (β_2) has enabled the development of relatively selective adrenergic agents. Selective β_1-adrenergic antagonists such as **atenolol** can be used to treat ischemic heart disease and hypertension without causing excessive bronchoconstriction; likewise, selective β_2-adrenergic agonists such as **terbutaline** can be used to treat obstructive pulmonary disease without causing excessive tachycardia. β-Adrenergic antagonists are also used clinically to reduce sympathetic activity in individuals with **stage fright**, a type of **social anxiety disorder** (Chapter 14). Interestingly, the attenuation of peripheral symptoms of social anxiety—including increased heart rate, palpitations, sweating, and flushing of skin—that occurs in response to the administration of a β-antagonist is

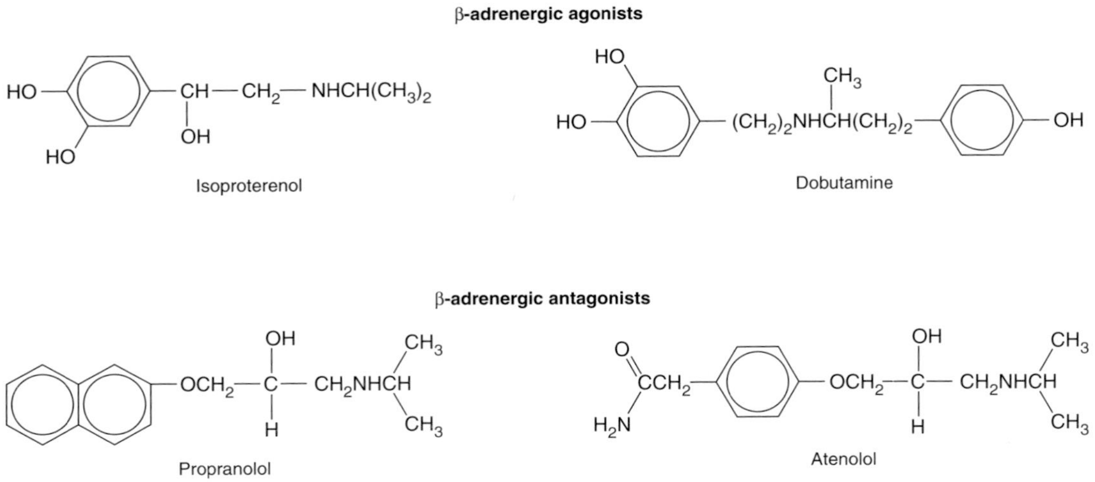

β-adrenergic agonists

Isoproterenol

Dobutamine

β-adrenergic antagonists

Propranolol

Atenolol

9–9 Chemical structures of representative β-adrenergic agonists and antagonists.

often sufficient to improve an individual's performance dramatically.

α-Adrenergic ligands α-Adrenergic agonists and antagonists also are potent modulators of sympathetic nervous system activity. The predominant effect of α_1-adrenergic agonists is the constriction of arterial smooth muscle, which in turn causes an increase in blood pressure. α_1-Adrenergic agonists such as **methoxamine** and **phenylephrine** are used infrequently in clinical practice to increase blood pressure during severe hypotensive episodes. The newer α_1-adrenergic agonist, **midodrine**, is approved to treat severe orthostatic hypotension due to autonomic failure. Although this drug increases standing blood pressure, its limiting side effect is supine hypertension. Phenylephrine and related α_1-adrenergic agonists are widely used as nasal decongestants; their decongestive action may be mediated by the constriction of blood flow to nasal mucosa or by a reduction in airway secretions. α_1-Adrenergic antagonists are used as antihypertensive drugs and to treat benign prostatic hypertrophy. The chemical structures of some of these agents, including the prototypical α_1-adrenergic antagonist **prazosin**, are shown in **9–10**.

α_2-Adrenergic receptors function as inhibitory autoreceptors on noradrenergic neurons (Chapter 6); thus it is not surprising that α_2-adrenergic agonists such as **clonidine** and **guanfacine** reduce sympathetic nervous system activity. Yet it is believed that such agents produce this effect by acting not on nerve terminals of postganglionic sympathetic neurons, but on neurons of the CNS: α_2-adrenergic agonists inhibit

the firing of noradrenergic neurons in the CNS, such as those in the locus ceruleus, which in turn leads to reduced sympathetic activity. Such agonists are commonly used in the treatment of hypertension and of several neuropsychiatric disorders, such as **opiate withdrawal, attention deficit disorder,** and **Tourette syndrome** (Chapters 13 and 15). α_2-Adrenergic antagonists such as **yohimbine** exert opposite effects: they stimulate sympathetic activity by activating noradrenergic neurons of the CNS.

Muscarinic Cholinergic Receptor Agonists and Antagonists

Muscarinic cholinergic agonists and antagonists exert profound effects on the ANS and on many regions of the brain (see Chapter 6 for a more detailed discussion of these compounds). Prototypical muscarinic agonists include synthetic agents such as **carbachol** and **bethanechol,** and natural plant products such as **arecoline, pilocarpine,** and **muscarine** **9–11**. These agents affect the peripheral nervous system by slowing the heart and reducing blood pressure. In the CNS, they exert a characteristic cortical activation. Because they stimulate emptying of the bladder, the major clinical use of muscarinic agonists is in the treatment of **urinary retention**. These drugs are also sometimes used to stimulate motility of the gastrointestinal tract and to stimulate salivary gland secretion. In addition, they have nonmedicinal uses in several Eastern cultures; for example, arecoline is used recreationally on the Indian subcontinent.

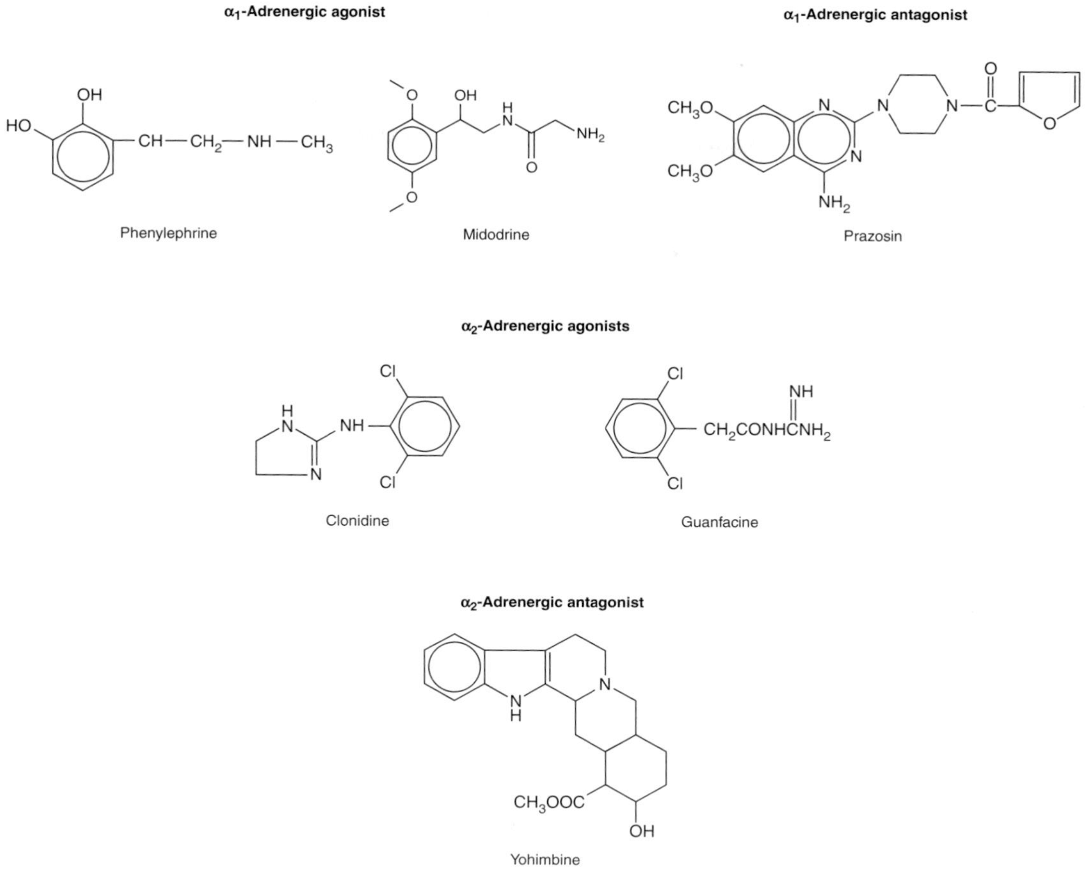

α₁-Adrenergic agonist

Phenylephrine

Midodrine

α₁-Adrenergic antagonist

Prazosin

α₂-Adrenergic agonists

Clonidine

Guanfacine

α₂-Adrenergic antagonist

Yohimbine

9–10 **Chemical structures of representative α-adrenergic agonists and antagonists.**

The effects of muscarinic cholinergic antagonists can be predicted based on their blockade of postganglionic parasympathetic transmission. Muscarinic antagonists decrease the rate and force of cardiac contractions and cause blurred vision, hot and dry skin, pupillary dilation and reduced accommodation, and decreased gastrointestinal motility. Independent of their effects on the ANS, these drugs powerfully affect the CNS and result in pervasive delirium, including confusion, disorientation, and hallucinations. Prototypical muscarinic antagonists include **atropine** and **scopolamine** 9–11. Muscarinic antagonists were once widely used in the treatment of gastrointestinal symptoms (nausea, motion sickness, and diarrhea), but for the most part have been supplanted by newer agents with fewer side effects. Regular clinical use of

muscarinic antagonists occurs in ophthalmology; for example, these drugs are used in routine eye examinations to produce mydriasis. These agents also are used as adjuncts in anesthesia to reduce pharyngeal and bronchial secretions. In emergency situations, intravenous administration of muscarinic antagonists are used to treat severe bradycardia. Another common use of muscarinic cholinergic antagonists is in the treatment of **Parkinson disease** and in the management of parkinsonian side effects associated with D₂ antagonist **antipsychotic** drugs. The use of many psychotropic medications, including **tricyclic antidepressants** and **phenothiazine antipsychotic** agents, is limited by side effects such as blurred vision, dry mouth, constipation, and delirium that are caused by muscarinic cholinergic antagonism.

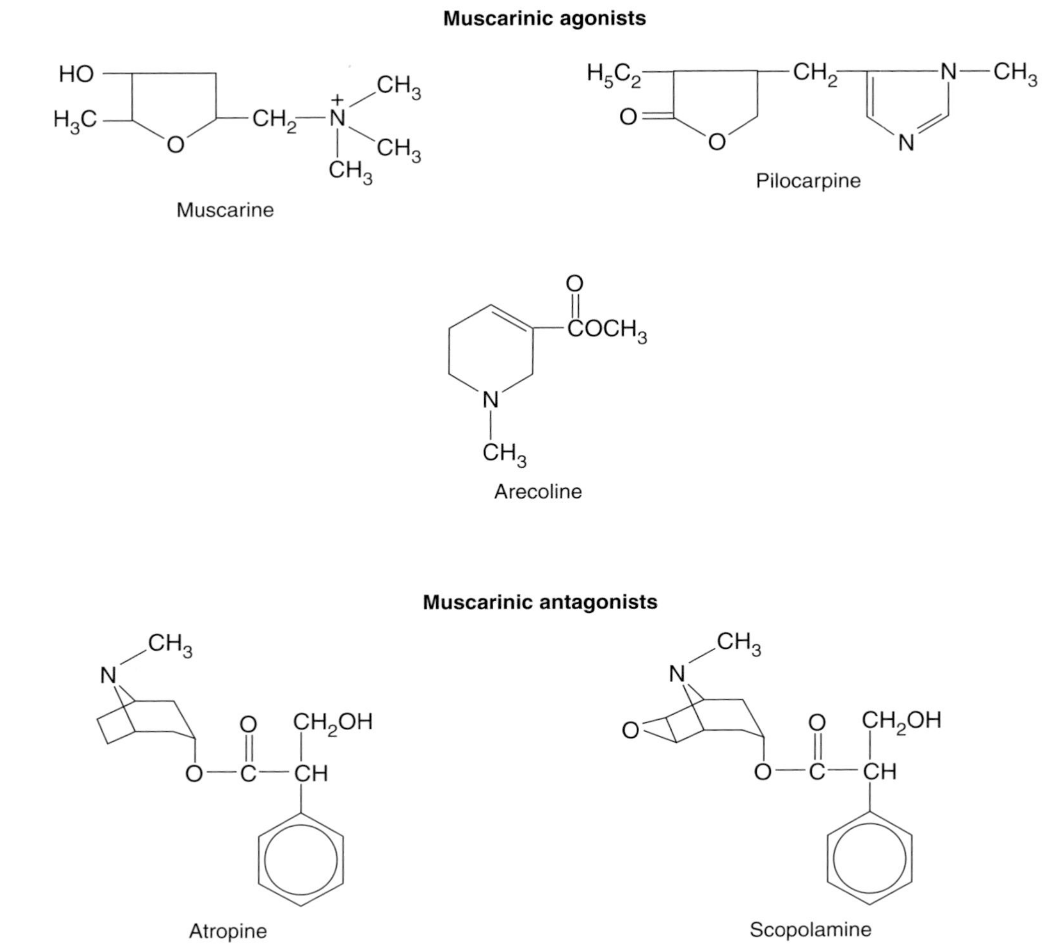

Muscarinic agonists

Muscarine

Pilocarpine

Arecoline

Muscarinic antagonists

Atropine

Scopolamine

9–11 **Chemical structures of representative muscarinic cholinergic agonists and antagonists.**

Acetylcholinesterase Inhibitors

Cholinergic transmission can be enhanced not only by cholinergic receptor agonists, but also by acetylcholinesterase inhibitors. As mentioned in Chapter 6, acetylcholinesterase is the enzyme responsible for the degradation of ACh. Inhibitors of this process in current clinical use include **physostigmine, pyridostigmine, neostigmine,** and **edrophonium** **9–12**. These agents are used for a variety of ophthalmic and gastrointestinal indications as well as for the treatment of **atonic bladder** and **myasthenia gravis**. In patients with orthostatic hypotension due to autonomic insufficiency, recent studies have shown that **pyridostigmine** improves standing blood pressure without causing supine hypertension, presumably by enhancing transmission at sympathetic ganglia. Other acetylcholinesterase inhibitors,

including **tacrine** and **donepezil,** are used to diminish cognitive symptoms of **Alzheimer disease,** although their effectiveness is limited (Chapter 17).

Most of the toxins used in **nerve gas** weapons (including **sarin, soman,** and **Vx**) are potent irreversible acetylcholinesterase inhibitors. They exert their lethal effects on cholinergic synapses in the CNS, ANS, and somatic motor system.

DISORDERS OF THE AUTONOMIC NERVOUS SYSTEM

Autonomic dysfunction, or **dysautonomia,** occurs in a large number of diseases that affect either the central or peripheral nervous systems. **9–4** provides a classification of autonomic disorders. Autonomic

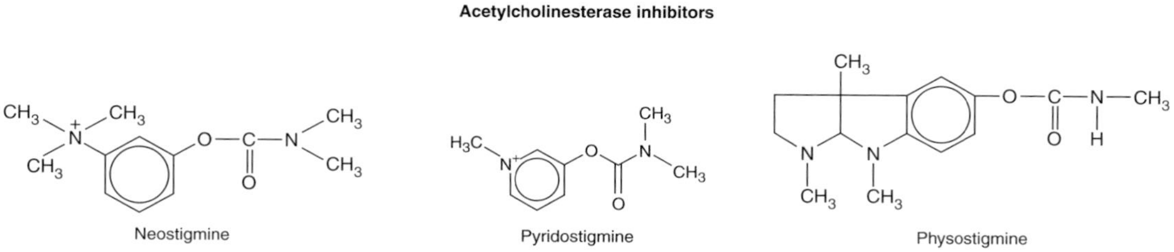

Acetylcholinesterase inhibitors

Neostigmine   Pyridostigmine   Physostigmine

9-12 Chemical structures of representative acetylcholinesterase inhibitors.

dysfunction may involve the sympathetic or parasympathetic nervous system, or both. A disorder that is primarily sympathetic may render the body incapable of dealing appropriately with strenuous physical or emotional stimulation. In contrast, parasympathetic dysfunction may result in more circumscribed symptoms such as bowel or sexual dysfunction. A comprehensive description of autonomic failure is beyond the scope

---

9-4 **Classification of Peripheral Autonomic Disorders**

Acute dysautonomia
 Acute pandysautonomia
 Acute cholinergic dysautonomia
 Acute sympathetic dysautonomia
Hereditary neuropathies
 Familial amyloid polyneuropathy
 Hereditary sensory and autonomic neuropathy, type III (Riley- Day syndrome)
 Hereditary sensory and autonomic neuropathy, type IV (Swanson type)
 Dopamine-β-hydroxylase deficiency
 Hereditary sensory and autonomic neuropathy, types I, II, and V
 Hereditary motor and sensory neuropathy, types I and II
  (Charcot-Marie-Tooth disease)
 Fabry disease
 Multiple endocrine neoplasia, type 2b (MEN 2b)
 Navajo neuropathy, type B
Inflammatory neuropathies
 Acute inflammatory polyneuritis (Guillain-Barré syndrome)
 Chronic inflammatory demyelinative polyradiculoneuropathy (CIDP)
Infections

Leprosy	Diphtheria
Human immuno-	Lyme disease
deficiency virus (HIV)	Botulism
Chagas disease	

Metabolic disorders

Diabetes	Chronic liver disease
Primary amyloidosis	Vitamin B_{12} deficiency
Acute intermittent and	Thiamine deficiency
variegate porphyria	(Wernicke-Korsakoff
Chronic renal failure	syndrome)

Alcohol abuse
Disorders precipitated by cancer

Direct infiltration of nerves	Enteric neuronopathy
Paraneoplastic dysautonomia	Lambert-Eaton myasthenic
Subacute sensory	syndrome
neuronopathy	

Connective tissue disorders

Rheumatoid arthritis	Sjögren syndrome
Systemic lupus erythematosus	Systemic sclerosis
Mixed connective tissue disease	

Inflammatory bowel disease

Crohn disease	Ulcerative colitis

Chronic lung disease
Multiple symmetric lipomatosis (Madelung disease)
Drugs and toxins

Vincristine	Arsenic
Cisplatin	Inorganic mercury
Taxol	Organic solvents
Amiodarone	Hexacarbons
Perhexiline	Acrylamide
Thallium	Vacor

Central nervous system dysfunction

Parkinson disease	Brainstem tumors
Spinal cord lesions	Multiple sclerosis
Wernicke encephalopathy	Adie syndrome
Cerebrovascular disease	Tabes dorsalis

From Bannister R, Mathias CJ, (editors) 1992. *Autonomic Failure*, New York: Oxford University Press, p. 107.

9-5 **Screening Tests for Autonomic Dysfunction**

Heart rate tests
    Response to deep breathing
    Response to standing or tilting
    Response to Valsalva maneuver

Blood pressure tests
    Response to standing or tilting
    Response to sustained hand grip exercise

Sweat tests
    Quantitative sudomotor axon reflex test
    Thermoregulatory sweat test (regional or whole body)
    Sympathetic galvanic skin response

Pupillometry
Plasma catecholamine measurements

of this text; however, a small number of illustrative examples are included in the following sections of this chapter. Autonomic dysfunction also appears to be important in certain pain syndromes, such as **causalgia** and **reflex sympathetic dystrophy,** which are discussed in Chapter 11. Some of the methods used to diagnose and characterize autonomic disorders are listed in **9-5**.

GENETIC CAUSES OF DYSAUTONOMIA

Dopamine β-Hydroxylase Deficiency

Congenital absence of the enzyme dopamine β-hydroxylase (DBH), which converts dopamine into norepinephrine (Chapter 6), results in sympathetic adrenergic failure, with preserved sympathetic cholinergic and parasympathetic function. The clinical syndrome consists of childhood onset of orthostatic hypotension, hypothermia, and hypoglycemia, which progresses in adulthood to marked hypotension, bilateral ptosis, decreased sweating, retrograde ejaculation, reduced vaginal secretions, and hyporeflexia.

Individuals with DBH deficiency have abnormally elevated levels of dopamine but a virtual absence of circulating norepinephrine and epinephrine. Results of parasympathetic tests of heart rate control and sympathetic cholinergic sweat tests are normal. Skin biopsies can be used to demonstrate the absence of the enzyme. D,L-**Dihydroxyphenylserine** (L-DOPS) can dramatically improve the symptoms of this enzyme deficiency; converted by aromatic amino acid decarboxylase directly into norepinephrine, it bypasses the DBH step and thus restores adrenergic function **9-13**. This drug can also be useful in patients with sympathetic failure due to degenerative neurologic disease.

Experimental sympathectomy can be achieved with **6-hydroxydopamine, guanethidine,** or antibodies to nerve growth factor (NGF) or acetylcholinesterase. These agents, administered peripherally, selectively damage sympathetic neurons and exert little or no effect on the parasympathetic nervous system or on enteric or peripheral nerves. Affected animals exhibit a shortened life span, decreased weight gain, low blood pressure, ptosis, and diarrhea.

Familial dysautonomia   Familial dysautonomia, also known as Riley-Day syndrome or type III hereditary sensory and autonomic neuropathy, is an autosomal recessive disease that occurs primarily in children of Jewish descent. The disease is associated with degenerative changes in the CNS and peripheral autonomic system that commence in infancy. The main clinical features are decreased or absent lacrimation, transient skin blotching, hyperhidrosis or erratic sweating, episodes of hypertension and labile blood pressure, episodes of hyperpyrexia and vomiting, impaired taste discrimination, and relative insensitivity to pain. Areflexia, corneal insensitivity and abrasions, loss of fungiform tongue papillae, poor motor coordination, and emotional instability also occur. Poor feeding and recurring aspiration-induced pulmonary infections and dehydration are the usual causes of death during infancy and childhood. During adolescence most autonomic symptoms decrease, with the exception of postural hypotension. Early diagnosis and better management of complications have increased the life expectancy of patients with this disease.

The pathogenesis of familial dysautonomia is believed to involve the abnormal development of neural crest cells. Preganglionic neurons in the intermediolateral columns are reduced in number, as are small myelinated fibers in the ventral roots. Because reduced amounts of NGF have been detected in cultured human fibroblasts and in the serum of patients with familial dysautonomia, investigations have attempted to determine whether the disease is linked to NGF-related defects. Moreover, levels of vanillylmandelic acid (VMA), a urinary norepinephrine and epinephrine metabolite, are decreased in patients with familial dysautonomia, while levels of homovanillic acid (HVA), a dopamine metabolite, are normal; thus an abnormal VMA to HVA ratio may be a sign of this disease.

9-13 **Alternative pathway for the generation of norepinephrine.** Normally, dopa is converted to dopamine by the aromatic amino acid decarboxylase (AADC); subsequently dopamine is converted to norepinephrine by dopamine -β-hydroxylase (DBH) (Chapter 6). In patients with DBH deficiency, this step can be bypassed with the administration of dihydroxyphenylserine, which is converted to norepinephrine by AADC.

SYSTEMIC DISEASES ASSOCIATED WITH AUTONOMIC DYSFUNCTION

Diabetes

Diabetes mellitus is the most common cause of autonomic neuropathy. Most studies indicate that 20% to 70% of individuals with diabetes exhibit abnormal autonomic function; estimates vary depending on the criteria examined. The likelihood of autonomic failure increases with the severity of hyperglycemia, the duration of the diabetes, and the age of the patient. Autonomic dysfunction is seen in animal models of diabetes mellitus, involving genetically diabetic animals or animals treated with pancreatic islet β-cell toxins such as **streptozocin** and **alloxan**.

The precise pathophysiologic mechanisms that underlie changes in the ANS associated with diabetes are unknown. Manifestations of diabetic peripheral neuropathy are heterogeneous, but most commonly include distal sensory and sensorimotor involvement as well as impaired sweating (anhidrosis), pupillary abnormalities, esophageal and gastrointestinal motor abnormalities, atonic bladder, and male impotence.

In patients with diabetes, clinical autonomic neuropathy has been associated with poor long-term prognoses and survival rates. It also is associated with an increased incidence of cardiac arrest and sudden death. A large controlled clinical trial has indicated that long-term diabetic complications, including autonomic dysfunction, are delayed and slowed in response to tight glucose control. In addition, a number of trials have shown that **aldose reductase inhibitors** offer a slight benefit in halting or slowing the progression of neuropathy.

Toxin- or drug-induced neuropathies Autonomic dysfunction occurs in some individuals exposed to environmental and pharmacologic toxins. Such dysfunction is best documented after exposure to organic solvents such as carbon disulfide and heavy metals. Workers exposed to various hydrocarbons, alcohols, ketones, esters, or ethers typically exhibit altered autonomic function. Industrial exposure to acrylamide has caused peripheral sensory polyneuropathy, which often is preceded by blue skin color and excessive sweating of the extremities. **Arsenic** also produces abnormal extremity sweating. **Mercury** poisoning leads to acrodynia, which is characterized by hypertension, tachycardia, and pain and redness of the fingers, toes, and ears. Acrodynia is effectively treated with ganglionic blocking agents. Ingestion of **vacor** (N-3-pyridylmethyl-N9-p-nitrophenylurea), a rat poison that antagonizes nicotinamide metabolism, results in acute hyperglycemic ketoacidosis and a combined somatic and autonomic neuropathy.

Some commonly used chemotherapeutic agents also cause a dose-dependent and cumulative effect on autonomic function. **Vincristine,** a natural product of vinca alkaloids used to treat several cancers, has limited applications because of its neurotoxic effects revealed by prominent autonomic symptoms. **Cisplatin,** a nonspecific cytotoxic agent that inhibits the cell cycle, causes ototoxicity, retrobulbar neuritis, and peripheral neuropathy.

IMMUNE-MEDIATED AUTONOMIC SYNDROMES

The ANS can be a target of immunologic attack in several disorders. A rare but dramatic example is autoimmune autonomic neuropathy (AAN, described in 9–1).

Guillain-Barré Syndrome

This acute-onset, predominantly motor neuropathy commonly involves autonomic hypoactivity or hyperactivity. Approximately 65% of patients with Guillain-Barré syndrome have some dysautonomia, which is attributed to demyelination of preganglionic fibers of the sympathetic nervous system. Afferent baroreflex abnormalities in individuals with this syndrome can cause intermittent episodes of orthostatic hypotension, and abrupt fluctuations in blood pressure may precede fatal arrhythmias. Many cases of Guillain-Barré syndrome occur in the context of a viral infection or occasionally after immunizations, and are thought to be mediated by an autoimmune mechanism. In most patients, the syndrome is self-limited and resolves spontaneously over time.

Paraneoplastic Neurologic Syndromes

Patients with cancer may develop an autoimmune syndrome, where immune responses against the cancer cells cross-react with and damage normal tissues. The paraneoplastic disorders can affect any part of the nervous system including the ANS. The symptoms of autonomic dysfunction usually reflect impairment of both limbs of

---

9–1   Autoimmune Autonomic Neuropathy

The clinical features of AAN (also known as acute panautonomic neuropathy, idiopathic autonomic neuropathy, or acute pandysautonomia) reflect widespread involvement of sympathetic and parasympathetic components of the ANS but limited damage to somatic nerve fibers. Diverse autonomic symptoms (orthostatic hypotension and gastrointestinal abnormalities are most common) evolve over a few days to a few months in previously healthy individuals of all ages and both sexes. An antecedent viral infection is reported in about 60% of cases. Pure cholinergic neuropathy, which affects only postganglionic cholinergic neurons, most likely is a restricted expression of acute panautonomic neuropathy; it produces a markedly similar clinical picture, except that there is no orthostatic hypotension.

Over 50% of patients with the typical clinical features of AAN have high titers of autoantibodies directed against the ganglionic nicotinic ACh receptor (AChR). Serum levels of the antibody correlate with the severity of autonomic neuropathy. These antibodies directly bind to the ganglionic ACh receptors and thereby impair ganglionic transmission. Experimental autoimmune autonomic neuropathy (EAAN) can be induced in animals by introducing ganglionic ACh receptor antibodies. AAN is one of the few proven antibody-mediated neurologic disorders.

Most patients with AAN show spontaneous stabilization or recovery, and recurrences are uncommon. However, recovery is typically incomplete. The mainstay of treatment is symptomatic management of autonomic failure, including blood pressure support, bowel management, and supplemental moisture for dry eyes and mouth. **Acetylcholinesterase inhibitors** have been used to alleviate neurogenic orthostatic hypotension. Immunomodulatory therapies including plasma exchange, intravenous **immunoglobulin, steroids,** or **immunosuppressant** drugs, are beneficial in some cases.

the ANS. Paraneoplastic gastroparesis is an especially characteristic manifestation in patients with occult small-cell lung cancer and results from inflammation and destruction of myenteric ganglia that control gut motility.

The **Lambert-Eaton myasthenic syndrome** is another disorder that may present in patients with small cell carcinomas. Most patients have antibodies against neuronal voltage-gated calcium channels. These antibodies reduce presynaptic quantal release of acetylcholine at the neuromuscular junction and at other peripheral cholinergic synapses, including the autonomic ganglia. In addition to weakness, patients have characteristic autonomic symptoms: dry mouth, constipation, impotence, and reduced sweating.

SELECTED READING

Bannister R, Mathias CJ, eds. *Autonomic Failure.* New York: Oxford University Press; 1992.

Benarroch EE. The central autonomic network: functional organization, dysfunction, and perspective. *Mayo Clin Proc.* 1993;68:989–1001.

Carpenter MB. *Core Text of Neuroanatomy.* Baltimore: Williams & Wilkins; 1972.

Freeman R, Miyawaki E. The treatment of autonomic dysfunction. *J Clin Neurophysiol.* 1993;10:61–82.

Hoffman BB, Taylor P. Neurotransmission: the autonomic and somatic motor nervous systems. In: Hardman JG, Limbird LE, eds. *Goodman and Gilman's The Pharmacological Basis of Therapeutics,* 10th ed, New York: McGraw-Hill; 2001:115–153.

Hugdahl K. Cognitive influences on human autonomic nervous system function. *Curr Opin Neurobiol.* 1996;6: 252–258.

Klein CM, Vernino S, Lennon VA, et al. The spectrum of autoimmune autonomic neuropathies. *Ann Neurol.* 2003;53:752–758.

Low PA. *Clinical Autonomic Disorders: Evaluation and Management.* Rochester, MN: Mayo Foundation;1993.

Low PA, Gilden JL, Freeman R, et al. Efficacy of midodrine vs placebo in neurogenic orthostatic hypotension. A randomized, double-blind multicenter study. Midodrine Study Group. *J Am Med Assoc.* 1997;277: 1046–1051.

McLeod JG, Tuck RR. Disorders of the autonomic nervous system: Part 2. Investigation and treatment. *Ann Neurol.* 1987;21:519–529.

Pascuzzi RM, Kim YI. Lambert-Eaton syndrome. *Semin Neurol.* 1990;10:35–41.

Polinsky RJ. Biochemical and pharmacologic assessment of autonomic function. *Adv Neurol.* 1996;69:373–376.

Pourmand R. Diabetic neuropathy. *Neurol Clin.* 1997;15:569–76.

Rostami AM. Pathogenesis of immune-mediated neuropathies. *Pediatr Res.* 1993;33(suppl):S90–S94.

Schatz IJ, Low PA, Polinsky RJ. Disorders of the autonomic nervous system. *N Engl J Med.* 1997;337:278–280.

Singer W, Sandroni P, Opfer-Gehrking TL, et al. Pyridostigmine treatment trial in neurogenic orthostatic hypotension. *Arch Neurol.* 2006;63:513–518.

Vernino S, Low PA, Fealey RD, et al. Autoantibodies to ganglionic acetylcholine receptors in autoimmune autonomic neuropathies. *N Engl J Med.* 2000;343:847–855.

Neural and Neuroendocrine Control of the Internal Milieu

- Hormones are signaling molecules that reach their target cells via the bloodstream.

- The hypothalamus is the key regulator of the endocrine system by releasing hormones directly into the blood and by regulating the anterior pituitary.

- The hypothalamic–neurohypophyseal system secretes two peptide hormones directly into the blood, vasopressin and oxytocin.

- To regulate the anterior pituitary, hypothalamic neurons synthesize peptide releasing and inhibitory factors.

- The hypothalamic–pituitary–adrenal (HPA) axis. It comprises corticotropin-releasing factor (CRF), released by the hypothalamus; adreno-corticotropic hormone (ACTH), released by the anterior pituitary; and glucocorticoids, released by the adrenal cortex.

- The hypothalamic–pituitary–thyroid axis consists of hypothalamic thyrotropin-releasing hormone (TRH); the anterior pituitary hormone thyroid–stimulating hormone (TSH); and the thyroid hormones T_3 and T_4.

- The hypothalamic–pituitary–gonadal axis comprises hypothalamic gonadotropin–releasing hormone (GnRH), the anterior pituitary luteinizing hormone (LH) and follicle-stimulating hormone (FSH), and the gonadal steroids.

- Prolactin is synthesized and released by the anterior pituitary and triggers lactation in females; its release is inhibited by D_2 dopamine receptors.

- Growth hormone, also released by the anterior pituitary is under the stimulatory control of growth hormone–releasing hormone (GHRH) and inhibitory control of somatostatin.

- The hypothalamus contains a complex network of peptide-releasing neurons that regulate feeding and energy expenditure.

- Leptin released by adipocytes, regulates the long-term state of the body's energy reserves largely via its actions on the hypothalamus.

- The arcuate nucleus of the hypothalamus plays a key role in feeding and energy expenditure. It contains one set of neurons that express proopiomelanocortin (POMC) that suppress feeding and another set that express neuropeptide Y (NPY) that stimulate feeding.

- The POMC product, melanocortin (also called α-melanocyte-stimulating hormone) and NPY, in turn, regulate several other feeding peptides (eg, melanin concentrating hormone) to produce their ultimate effects on food intake and energy metabolism.

- The hypothalamus responds to inflammatory cytokines by causing fever and sickness behavior.

The brain controls bodily function and behavior through the motor system, the autonomic nervous system (Chapter 9), and hormones released by neuroendocrine neurons. Hormones are signaling molecules that reach their target cells by means of the bloodstream. They comprise three major classes: peptides, neurotransmitter-like small molecules such as epinephrine (adrenalin), and steroid-like molecules. Through its neuroendocrine system, the brain maintains homeostasis, regulates growth and maturation, and facilitates the body's response to environmental stressors, illness, and injury.

NEUROENDOCRINE HYPOTHALAMUS

Afferent Signals

The hypothalamus, located at the base of the diencephalon, is in a good position to integrate information about the state of the organism from diverse sources. It receives information about the external environment and the emotional response of the organism from the forebrain, information about the internal milieu from brainstem nuclei, and directly from the blood in regions where the blood-brain barrier gives way to fenestrated capillaries, eg, the median eminence at the base of the hypothalamus and near the circumventricular organs (Chapter 2). The hypothalamus also has reciprocal relationships with monoamine and cholinergic nuclei in the brainstem and basal forebrain that regulate states of arousal and attention (Chapter 6). Because they are lipophilic, circulating steroid hormones from the periphery can cross directly into the brain and bind receptors in the hypothalamus or in other brain areas, which send projections to the hypothalamus.

The hippocampus, amygdala, and septum, all of which are involved in processing the salience of environmental events (Chapters 14 and 15), project to the hypothalamus. Such connections enable adaptive responses; for example, they allow the hypothalamus to direct the release of stress hormones and activate the sympathetic nervous system in response to a threat. Communication between these regions and the hypothalamus is largely reciprocal; thus, the hippocampus, amygdala, and septum also receive input from the hypothalamus, which permits information about the internal milieu to affect cognition and other aspects of behavior. Accordingly, altered glucose metabolism and a trip to the refrigerator often go hand in hand. In addition to the many types of afferent signals directed toward the hypothalamus, there are extensive intrahypothalamic connections, which are involved in coordinating the many hormonal and autonomic outputs of this brain region.

Efferent Signals

The output of the neuroendocrine hypothalamus consists of peptide hormones released into the circulation. Hypothalamic neurons can affect bodily functions directly by releasing vasopressin or oxytocin into the systemic circulation via the posterior pituitary or indirectly via releasing hormones **10-1** into the portal hypophyseal circulation and thence to the anterior pituitary. Neuroendocrine neurons are specialized for the purpose of transducing neural signals into hormonal signals; in response to depolarization, they

10-1 **Hypothalamic Releasing Factors**

Releasing Factor	Cellular Origin	Function (Hormones Regulated in Anterior Pituitary)
Corticotropin-releasing factor (CRF; also called corticotropin releasing hormone, or CRH)	Parvocellular neurons of paraventricular nucleus	Stimulates ACTH release (in concert with vasopressin)
Gonadotropin-releasing hormone (GnRH)	Medial preoptic and arcuate nuclei	Stimulates LH and FSH release
Growth hormone–releasing hormone (GHRH)	Arcuate nucleus	Stimulates GH release
Somatostatin	Periventricular nucleus	Inhibits GH release
Thyrotropin-releasing hormone (TRH)	Parvocellular neurons of paraventricular and anterior hypothalamic nuclei	Stimulates TSH release
Dopamine	Arcuate nucleus	Inhibits prolactin release

release peptides into the bloodstream by means of axons that terminate on capillaries rather than at synapses **10-1**. These peptides are considered hormones because they travel through the bloodstream to reach their receptors. Many of these same peptides also act as neurotransmitters when they are released from other neurons in the brain and act at synapses.

Organization of the Hypothalamic–Pituitary Unit

The hypothalamus and pituitary gland may be seen as an interacting unit **10-2**. In humans, the pituitary

Neurotransmitter

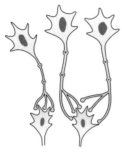

Neuroendocrine

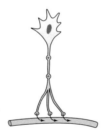

Endocrine

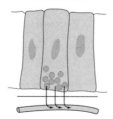

10-1 **Types of secretion.** Neurons secrete neurotransmitter into the synaptic space. Neuroendocrine neurons secrete hormones into the bloodstream through axon terminals embedded in capillaries. Endocrine cells secrete hormones into the bloodstream without the use of specialized terminals.

has two divisions: the neurohypophysis or posterior pituitary, which contains the axon terminals projecting from the hypothalamus, and the adenohypophysis or anterior pituitary, which is composed primarily of endocrine cells specialized to synthesize and release particular hormones. Rodents, but not humans, also possess a pituitary intermediate lobe.

In the neurohypophyseal system, the peptide hormones vasopressin and oxytocin are synthesized in magnocellular (large) neurons of the supraoptic and paraventricular nuclei (PVN) and transported to capillary-associated nerve terminals in the posterior pituitary, where they are released directly into the systemic circulation. In the adenohypophyseal system, peptide-releasing factors **10-1**, which are synthesized in hypothalamic neurons, are transported to nerve terminals in the median eminence; when the hypothalamic neurons are stimulated, peptide hormones are released into the hypophyseal–portal circulation, which drains into the blood vessels of the anterior pituitary. Such peptides act to stimulate or inhibit the release of anterior pituitary hormones into the systemic circulation. After reaching their targets, pituitary hormones cause the release of additional hormones, which subsequently act on diverse tissues of the body. Hypothalamic releasing factors that cause pituitary hormone release also have trophic influences on anterior pituitary cells; likewise, hormones of the anterior pituitary gland have trophic influences on their targets. Thus, hypersecretion of a hormone can lead to hypertrophy or hyperplasia of target endocrine cells, whereas the absence of a hormone can lead to the atrophy of such cells.

HYPOTHALAMIC–NEUROHYPOPHYSEAL SYSTEM

The hypothalamic–neurohypophyseal system secretes two major peptide hormones: vasopressin, also known as antidiuretic hormone (ADH), and oxytocin. Vasopressin and oxytocin are synthesized in distinct magnocellular neurons of the PVN and supraoptic nucleus (SON) of the hypothalamus, and are carried by axoplasmic flow to nerve endings in the posterior pituitary. Vasopressin also is synthesized in a distinct subset of parvocellular (small) PVN neurons that project to the median eminence. Vasopressin released from these neurons acts together with corticotropin-release factor (CRF; also known as corticotropin-releasing hormone, or CRH) to stimulate release of adrenocorticotropic hormone (ACTH; also known as corticotropin). Like most peptide transmitters, vasopressin and oxytocin are derived from large precursor proteins,

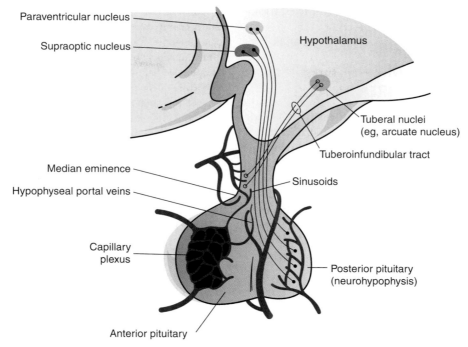

10-2 **Relationship of the hypothalamus and the pituitary gland.** The anterior pituitary, or adenohypophysis, receives rich blood flow from the capillaries of the portal hypophyseal system. This system delivers factors **10-1** released by hypothalamic neurons into portal capillaries at the median eminence. The figure shows one such projection, from the tuberal (arcuate) nuclei via the tuberoinfundibular tract to the median eminence. The posterior pituitary, or neurohypophysis, contains axon terminals of neurons projecting from the paraventricular and supraoptic nuclei of the hypothalamus.

which are cleaved to form active peptides. Associated cleavage events also produce carrier proteins, or neurophysins, which are coreleased with the peptides. Actions of vasopressin and oxytocin within the brain, where they act as neuropeptide neurotransmitters, are discussed in Chapter 7.

Vasopressin

Release of neurohypophyseal vasopressin occurs in response to central and peripheral monitoring of blood osmolality and blood pressure. Stimuli such as hemorrhage, pain, stress, and strenuous exercise can lead to vasopressin release. The primary systemic action of vasopressin occurs at the distal nephron within the kidney, where it increases reabsorption of water across the collecting duct epithelium. Many drugs can interfere with vasopressin action. **Lithium** inhibits vasopressin action by inhibiting the renal V_2 vasopressin receptor–linked adenylyl cyclase. Lithium thereby causes increased urine flow and, in some

individuals, nephrogenic **diabetes insipidus,** which is defined as the production of more than three liters of urine per day. Other drugs, including **nicotine** when taken in high doses, may cause a syndrome of inappropriate vasopressin (ADH) secretion (**SIADH**), which results in water retention and can lead to **dilutional hyponatremia** severe enough to produce seizures. Vasopressin and oxytocin have additional actions in the nervous system, most significantly, they regulate social behaviors including affiliation (Chapter 7).

Oxytocin

Oxytocin acts during parturition to cause uterine contractions. Synthetic forms of this hormone (**pitocin**) are used to induce labor. Oxytocin also mediates milk letdown in lactating mothers. Nipple stimulation causes oxytocin release, which in turn causes the myoepithelial cells of the nipple to contract, resulting in the ejection of milk. The release of oxytocin is subject to classical conditioning; thus, a lactating mother may experience milk letdown in response to the cry of a baby.

HYPOTHALAMIC–PITUITARY–ADRENAL AXIS

The hypothalamic–pituitary–adrenal (HPA) axis **10-3** produces a cascade of hormones that are central to the stress response **10-1**. This cascade begins with CRF produced by the parvocellular neurons of the PVN of the hypothalamus that project to the median eminence. CRF acts on the corticotroph cells of the anterior pituitary to synthesize and release ACTH. In turn, ACTH acts on the adrenal cortex to release **glucocorticoids**, **cortisol** in humans, and **corticosterone** in rodents. Glucocorticoids function as stress hormones

by causing cells to become catabolic, ie, to break down energy stores in order to release glucose. They also increase arousal and inhibit inflammation. (Inflammation both has a metabolic cost and might also impede fight or flight behaviors; it is appropriate as a component of healing processes after an emergency has passed.)

Basal CRF release is controlled partly by the circadian pacemaker, located in the suprachiasmatic nucleus (SCN) of the hypothalamus in mammals (Chapter 12). Maximum secretion of CRF occurs in the morning in humans near the time of waking; maximum secretion in rodents, which are nocturnal, typically occurs in the early evening. Superimposed on normal circadian variation in CRF release is release precipitated by stress. (Stressors also stimulate release of vasopressin by PVN neurons. Like CRF, vasopressin is a secretagogue for

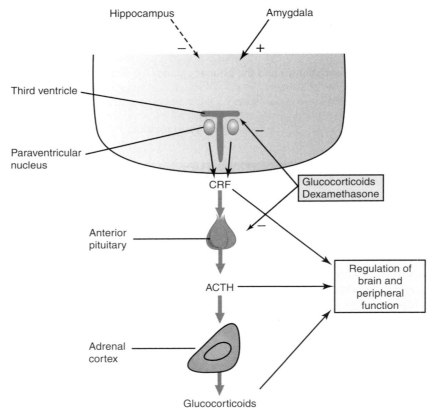

10-3 **The hypothalamic–pituitary–adrenal axis.** Corticotropin-releasing factor (CRF) and vasopressin are released from parvocellular neurons of the paraventricular nucleus of the hypothalamus into the hypophyseal portal system and act on the corticotrophs of the anterior pituitary to cause release of adrenocorticotropic hormone (ACTH). ACTH reaches the adrenal cortex by means of the bloodstream, where it stimulates the release of glucocorticoids. In addition to their diverse functions, glucocorticoids, including synthetic forms such as dexamethasone, repress CRF and ACTH synthesis and release. In this manner, glucocorticoids inhibit their own synthesis.

10–1　Stress

Cells, organs, and whole organisms must respond adaptively to changes in their environments if they are to function and ultimately survive. Adaptive responses to environmental challenges are described as *homeostasis*. Environmental challenges that are extreme, harsh, or aversive are described as *stressors*. Stressors can be both physical (eg, a wound, extreme cold, or lack of water) or psychological (eg, separation from or death of a parent, a consequential competition). There are large numbers of homeostatic mechanisms that act at the level of individual cells, organs, and organ systems. By controlling neuroendocrine hormone release and the autonomic nervous system, the hypothalamus plays a central coordinating role in the stress response of the whole organism. The result is a combination of physiologic and behavioral responses aimed at maintaining or restoring the internal milieu.

The typical response to a significant acute (phasic) stressor is traditionally called the *"fight or flight"* response. This response involves activation of the sympathetic nervous system, leading to release of epinephrine systemically from the adrenal medulla and norepinephrine at synapses with effector organs such as the heart and vascular smooth muscle, leading, for example, to more rapid and stronger cardiac contractions and elevated blood pressure (Chapter 9). In addition, the fight or flight response leads to the release of CRF and vasopressin into the portal hypophyseal circulation, resulting ultimately in release of systemic glucocorticoids from the adrenal cortex, with elevated levels observable within a few minutes, peaking at approximately 30 minutes and declining to basal levels after approximately an hour.

Glucocorticoids act together with the sympathetic nervous system to mobilize energy stores for the fight or flight response. Stressors also activate widely projecting monoamine systems (Chapter 6) to increase arousal and vigilance. Glucocorticoids appear to work in concert with monoamines to increase arousal and to encode memories of the circumstances under which the stressor was encountered (eg, see Chapter 14 for a description of the role of norepinephrine in the consolidation of fear-related memories).

While transient stress responses mounted in reaction to phasic physical or psychological threats are adaptive, indeed often critical for survival, during chronic stress, or failure to dampen the stress response when the danger has passed, they may produce illness in their own right. **Depression** and chronic stress have significant similarities (Chapter 14), and many patients with serious depression have elevated levels of CRF and cortisol secretion. Nonetheless, the precise relationship between stress and depression remains to be worked out.

There has been correlative evidence linking hippocampal atrophy with a history of major depression or posttraumatic stress disorder (PTSD). Given the concentration of glucocorticoid receptors (GR) and mineralocorticoid receptors (MR) in the hippocampus, it is hypothesized that chronically elevated levels of cortisol might lead to hippocampal atrophy by facilitating cell death or suppressing neurogenesis. While chronic glucocorticoid treatment per se can decrease hippocampal volumes in unaffected individuals, it is unknown whether the reductions seen in depression or PTSD are a result of chronic stress or a pre-existing risk factor for the disorders.

ACTH, as mentioned earlier.) PVN neurons receive stimulatory inputs from the amygdala and inhibitory inputs from the hippocampus (see 10–3). They also receive noradrenergic and other monoamine projections from the brainstem that relay information about the salience of stimuli. The effects of CRF and related peptides are mediated by two distinct G protein–coupled receptors, called CRF_1 and CRF_2. CRF binds selectively to CRF_1; the CRH-like peptide, urocortin 1, binds both CRF_1 and CRF_2; and urocortins II and III bind CRF_2 (Chapter 7). CRF appears to play the critical role in activating stress responses and acts via CRF_1.

Urocortins II and III may dampen the stress response acting via CRF_2 receptors. CRF_1 antagonists have been proposed as **antidepressant** and **anxiolytic drugs**, although key receptors for this indication may be outside the hypothalamus (Chapter 14).

ACTH and Glucocorticoids

CRF and vasopressin promote the synthesis of proopiomelanocortin (POMC) and release of its peptide derivatives. Glucocorticoids can feed back to inhibit POMC transcription. POMC is a large precursor protein (7-4 in Chapter 7) that gives rise to ACTH as well as β-endorphin and α-melanocyte-stimulating hormone (α-MSH). ACTH stimulates the adrenal cortex via Gs-coupled ACTH receptors to synthesize and secrete adrenal glucocorticoids. A cAMP-regulated pathway supports adrenal steroidogenesis by controlling transcription of the major synthetic enzymes. ACTH also stimulates the secretion of other adrenocortical steroids, including aldosterone (a major mineralocorticoid) and adrenal androgens.

Glucocorticoid Synthesis

Dietary **cholesterol** is the primary starting material for the biosynthesis of glucocorticoids and other adrenal steroids 10-4. Cholesterol enters one of three biosynthetic pathways in the adrenal cortex, which lead to the production of glucocorticoids (cortisol), mineralocorticoids (aldosterone), and adrenal androgens (eg, dehydroepiandrosterone). Cells within different zones of the adrenal cortex express distinct synthetic enzymes that catalyze the production of these specific hormones 10-2.

Glucocorticoid Receptors

The primary mode of action of all steroid hormones is to bind cytoplasmic receptors which, upon activation, translocate to the nucleus to regulate gene expression (Chapter 4). Certain metabolites of glucocorticoids and of the steroid hormone progesterone (including the so-called **neurosteroids**) appear to have an additional mechanism of action, however, interacting directly with distinct receptors on the plasma membrane to produce more rapid effects 10-2.

Glucocorticoids bind to two different cytosolic receptors: the glucocorticoid receptor (GR) and mineralocorticoid receptor (MR), both of which are members of the large superfamily of steroid hormone (nuclear) receptors (Chapter 4). Despite their names, the MR has a 10-fold higher affinity for glucocorticoids than the GR. Consequently, MR binding sites may be saturated, even with relatively low levels of circulating glucocorticoids, whereas significant GR binding requires high circulating glucocorticoid levels as might occur with a significant stressor or with peak levels of secretion under circadian control. In neurons that express both receptors, such as the hippocampus and amygdala, heterodimers may form with intermediate affinity.

The GR is expressed in essentially every tissue in the body including the brain, but with different levels of expression. Indeed, the lower affinity GR is anatomically well positioned to exert feedback control when levels of glucocorticoids are very high because it is concentrated in the PVN itself, in the hippocampus, which feeds back negatively on the PVN indirectly by activating GABAergic inputs, and on brainstem monoamine neurons (Chapter 6) that also project to the PVN.

MR expression is more restricted than GR expression; in addition to the brain, it is expressed in the kidney, gut, and heart. Some actions of GR and MR are DNA binding dependent and others occur independently of DNA binding. After they bind hormone, these receptors are freed from chaperone proteins including heat shock proteins, and are subsequently translocated to the nucleus 10-5. In the nucleus, MR and GR may bind as homodimers or heterodimers to their specific glucocorticoid response elements (GRE) in the regulatory regions of genes; alternatively they may inhibit or enhance the functions of other transcription factors by means of protein–protein interactions. Thus, glucocorticoid receptors may inhibit the actions of AP-1, CREB, NF-κB, and other transcription factors.

As their name suggests, glucocorticoids increase plasma glucose levels during periods of stress, including starvation; they do so by exerting catabolic effects on target tissues. Glucocorticoids also suppress the immune system by decreasing the synthesis and release of cytokines. In addition, they appear to affect the brain by rapidly increasing alertness and enhancing cognition. Chronic excessive glucocorticoid release or deficiency produces significant illness 10-3. Abnormally elevated CRF secretion and glucocorticoid levels may contribute to symptoms of **depression** in some patients (Chapter 14).

HYPOTHALAMIC–PITUITARY–THYROID AXIS

The synthesis and release of thyroid hormones are controlled by the hypothalamic–pituitary–thyroid (HPT) axis 10-6. Hypothalamic neurons synthesize and release

---

10-2 **Organization of Adrenal Hormone Synthesis**

Location	Layer	Significant Hormones
Deepest	Medulla	Epinephrine
Deepest cortical layer	Zona reticularis	Adrenal androgens, eg, androstenedione
Middle cortical layer	Zona fasciculata	Glucocorticoids, eg, cortisol
Superficial cortical layer	Zona glomerulosa	Mineralocorticoids, eg, aldosterone

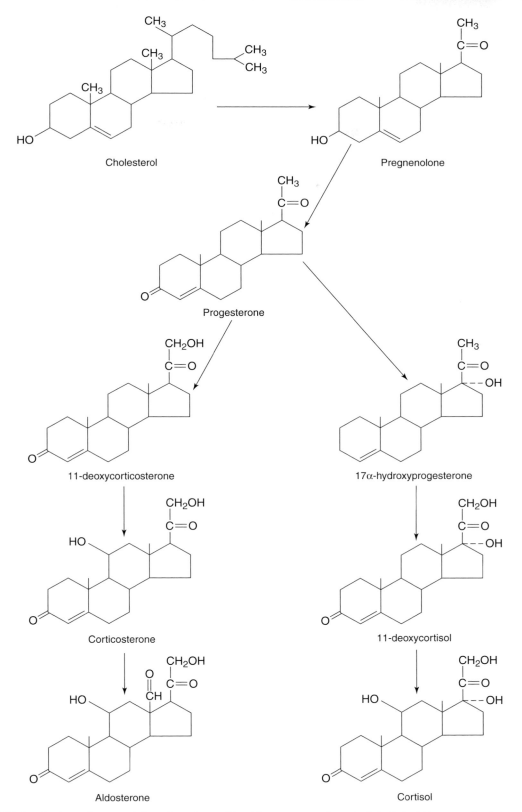

10-4 Synthetic pathways of the adrenal steroids aldosterone and cortisol. Synthesis of aldosterone and cortisol occur in different layers of the adrenal cortex (see **10-2**).

thyrotropin-releasing hormone (TRH), a 3-amino-acid peptide that is stored in axon terminals in the median eminence of the hypothalamus until it is released into the pituitary portal circulation. Normal TRH release is pulsatile and occurs in a circadian pattern; in humans, the highest levels of this hormone are released during the night. In the anterior pituitary gland, TRH binds to its receptors on thyrotroph cells and stimulates the release of the peptide hormone thyrotropin, also called thyroid-stimulating hormone (TSH). Neurons of the neuroendocrine hypothalamus synthesize and release somatostatin, a peptide that inhibits release of TSH and of growth hormone from the anterior pituitary (see **10–1**). Somatostatin also functions as a neuropeptide neurotransmitter in other brain regions including the hippocampus (see **7–4**, Chapter 7).

Because biologically active TSH requires glycosylation, it is described as a glycoprotein hormone. It is composed of two subunits; the α subunit is identical to that of two other pituitary hormones, luteinizing hormone (LH) and follicle-stimulating hormone (FSH). The β subunit is unique to each of these dimeric

hormones and provides specificity for receptor binding. TRH stimulates the synthesis of both α and β chains of TSH in thyrotroph cells.

Once released in response to TRH, TSH exerts trophic effects on cells of the thyroid gland, via activation of G_s-coupled TSH receptors. This action in turn stimulates the synthesis and release of two thyroid hormones: triiodothyronine (T_3) and tetraiodothyronine, or **thyroxine** (T_4) **10–6B**. T_4 is the predominant form of thyroid hormone secreted by the thyroid gland; it is subsequently converted to T_3 in target cells. All of the steps in the synthesis of these thyroid hormones are stimulated by TSH. Thyroid hormones are released into the general circulation to act on all tissues in the body. They also provide feedback control of transcription of the prepro-TRH gene by hypothalamic neurons and of the two subunits of TSH within pituitary thyrotrophs. Low levels of thyroid hormone stimulate transcription, and high levels lead to inhibition. Of the two thyroid hormones, T_3 exerts the more potent effects; consequently, altered rates of conversion of T_4 to T_3 can regulate the activity of the HPT axis.

10–2 **Neuroactive Steroids**

In addition to their slow-onset effects mediated via cytoplasmic receptors, a subset of steroids produces rapid effects on neuronal excitability by interacting with the GABA$_A$ receptor, the major inhibitory neurotransmitter receptor in the brain (Chapter 5). These **neuroactive steroids** (or **neurosteroids**) include the reduced metabolites of progesterone and deoxycorticosterone, such as **5α-pregnan-3α-ol-20-one** (3α, 5α-THPROG), **5β-pregnan-3α-ol-20-one** (3α, 5β-THPROG), and **5α-pregnan-3α,21-diol-20-one** (3α, 5α-THDOC). These compounds may be produced locally in the brain by metabolism of adrenal steroids that cross the blood–brain barrier because they are lipophilic. Certain neurons and glia express the enzymes both to synthesize pregnane steroids de novo or to produce them from peripheral starting materials (see figure).

3α, 5α-THPROG, 3α, 5β-THPROG, and 3α, 5α-THDOC are positive allosteric regulators of GABA$_A$ receptors and act by promoting the open state of the Cl$^-$ channel in response to GABA. This action is similar to that exerted by **benzodiazepines**, used in the treatment of anxiety (Chapter 14). The steroid binding sites on GABA$_A$ receptors are not certain, but recent evidence suggests two distinct binding sites that act in concert. At pharmacologic (ie, high) doses,

there is no question that these steroids elicit potent effects mediated by GABA$_A$ receptors. For example, steroids such as **alphaxolone** can be anesthetic. Less certain is the effect of endogenous neurosteroids on behavior. It is not yet clear how neurosteroids could exert selective effects in the brain and spinal cord, rather than acting as general depressants by facilitating GABAergic inhibition. Mechanisms by which neurosteroids might influence only subpopulations of GABA$_A$ receptors remain active areas of investigation; candidate mechanisms include region-specific variations in the subunit composition of GABA$_A$ receptors (Chapter 5), in posttranslational modification of the receptors (eg, phosphorylation), and in receptor location (synaptic vs. extrasynaptic). It is also possible that local synthesis of neurosteroids could permit them to act in an autocrine or paracrine fashion. Possible pharmacologic uses of neuroactive steroid-related drugs include not only **anesthetics**, but also **hypnotics, anticonvulsants**, and perhaps **analgesics**.

In addition to pregnane steroids, there is some evidence that estrogens (gonadal steroids) such as 17β-estradiol may have rapid effects at neuronal membranes.

Biosynthesis of GABA-modulatory neurosteroids. The pathway for the synthesis of 3α, 5α THDOC from cholesterol is shown. Also indicated is the proposed site of action of drugs that have been used to evaluate the influence of endogenous 3α, 5α THDOC on inhibitory neurotransmission. Steroidogenic acute-regulatory protein (StAR) might interact with the mitochondrial benzodiazepine receptor (MBR) to facilitate the transport of cholesterol across the mitochondrial membrane. 3α HSD, 3α hydroxysteroid dehydrogenase; 3β HSD, 3β hydroxysteroid dehydrogenase; 5α DHPROG, 5α dihydroprogesterone; P450scc, P450 side-chain cleavage. (From Belelli D, Lambert JJ. Neurosteroids: endogenous regulators of the GABA_A receptor. *Nature Rev Neurosci.* 2005;6:565–575.)

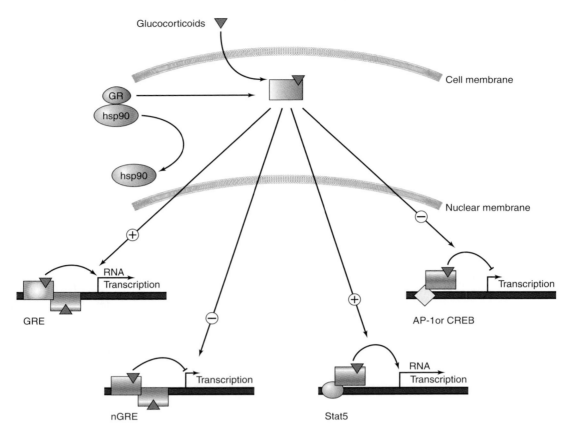

10-5 **Glucocorticoid receptor (GR) function.** After entering a cell, glucocorticoids bind to their receptors, which subsequently are released from their associations with chaperones such as heat shock proteins (hsp90). Ligand-bound GRs translocate to the nucleus, where they bind as dimers to positive glucocorticoid response elements (GREs) to activate gene expression or bind to negative GREs (nGREs) to repress gene expression. Alternatively, a ligand-bound GR can interact with other transcription factors to repress AP-1- or CREB-mediated transcription. Interaction with STAT5 can enhance the activation of target gene expression (Chapter 4).

The most common forms of **hypothyroidism** are caused by failure of the thyroid gland and are best detected through the measurement of serum TSH levels. These may become elevated in order to drive a failing thyroid gland even before levels of T_4 and T_3 become abnormal. Hypothyroidism caused by hypothalamic or pituitary failure is characterized by low levels of TSH. **Hyperthyroidism** is indicated by elevated levels of T_4 and T_3, which must be corrected to measure free thyroid hormone, because a considerable fraction of T_4 and T_3 in plasma is bound to thyroid-binding globulin or thyroglobulin (TBG) and is physiologically inactive.

Thyroid hormones exert genomic effects by regulating the transcription of target genes, and nongenomic effects by regulating intracellular ion concentrations and glucose transport. Genomic effects are mediated by two major thyroid hormone receptors: TRα-1 and TRβ-1. Like GR and MR, these receptors are members of the steroid hormone receptor superfamily. Like other ligand-regulated transcription factors, TRα-1 and TRβ-1 bind to a specific DNA element, known as the thyroid hormone–response element (TRE), which is found in the promoter region of many genes. The receptors bind as homodimers or, with other nuclear proteins such as thyroid hormone receptor auxiliary proteins (TRAPs), as heterodimers to stimulate or repress the transcription of target genes.

The action of thyroid hormones in the body is unusual in that these hormones are constitutively active. During stress or illness, however, thyroid axis function is suppressed, resulting in less secretion of

10-3   Cushing and Addison Syndromes

Cushing syndrome is the constellation of symptoms that results from sustained **hypercortisolemia**. Hypercortisolemia may be caused by adrenal tumors or by cancers associated with the ectopic production of ACTH; it also may occur in response to the administration of synthetic glucocorticoids, such as **prednisone** or **dexamethasone**, which are used to treat inflammatory conditions, autoimmune disease, and some types of cancer. When it is caused by microadenomas (small ACTH-secreting tumors) of the corticotroph cells of the anterior pituitary gland, it is called **Cushing disease**. Cushing syndrome is characterized by trunkal obesity, thinning skin, osteoporosis, and proximal muscle weakness. A substantial proportion of patients have insomnia or abnormalities of mood. Individuals with endogenous sources of cortisol are more often depressed; those receiving exogenous glucocorticoids may have manic-like symptoms.

Secondary adrenocortical insufficiency, or hypocortisolemia, caused by a lack of ACTH secretion results in **Addison syndrome**. This disorder most commonly occurs after discontinuation of long-term steroid treatment; such treatment leads to atrophy of corticotrophs and of the adrenal gland caused by glucocorticoid-mediated feedback inhibition. Classic symptoms include anorexia, nausea, and hypotension; in addition, hyperpigmentation often occurs in response to unrestrained POMC expression, which results in high levels of α-MSH. Apathy, fatigue, and irritability also are common among affected individuals. Moreover, sleep, appetite, and cognitive performance may be affected. **Addison disease** results from primary adrenocortical insufficiency, which is most often caused by an idiopathic autoimmune process that leads to destruction of the adrenal gland. This leads to loss not only of cortisol, but also of other adrenal hormones 10-2.

TSH and reduced conversion of T_4 to T_3 in peripheral tissues. During illness, binding of T_4 to TBG also increases, in turn further decreasing levels of free hormone. These are believed to be adaptations aimed at conserving energy. Some similar adaptations may occur during starvation.

HYPOTHALAMIC–PITUITARY–GONADAL AXIS

Reproductive function is controlled by the hypothalamic–pituitary–gonadal (HPG) axis 10-7 through the release of gonadotropin-releasing hormone (GnRH), previously known as luteinizing hormone–releasing hormone (LHRH). GnRH-expressing neurons are located in the medial basal hypothalamus and arcuate nucleus, and project to the median eminence. GnRH acts on gonadotrophs of the anterior pituitary gland to stimulate the synthesis and release of the gonadotropins, LH and FSH. GnRH release must be pulsatile to activate pituitary gondaotrophs. Accordingly, long-acting GnRH agonists such as **leuprolide**, which produce continuous stimulation of GnRH receptors, cause their desensitization and thereby inhibit release of LH and FSH. Leuprolide is used clinically to treat testosterone-sensitive **prostate cancers** and also to delay puberty in children who have precocious onset of puberty. A third gonadotropic hormone, *chorionic gonadotropin*, is secreted by the syncytiotrophoblast cells of the placenta during pregnancy; its presence in urine forms the basis of most **pregnancy tests**.

All gonadotropins are dimeric glycoprotein hormones that consist of a common α subunit (identical to the α subunit of TSH) and unique β subunits. GnRH stimulates the synthesis of both types of subunit and the glycosylation step required for their biologic activity. The targets of LH and FSH are the gonads. In the ovary, LH induces ovulation of the mature follicle and acts on theca cells to promote the synthesis of androgen precursors necessary for estrogen production 10-8A. Such precursors diffuse into nearby granulosa cells, where FSH stimulates the production of the steroid hormone estrogen. LH also sustains the ruptured follicle that forms the corpus luteum by stimulating progesterone synthesis; FSH stimulates development of the mature follicle. In the testes, LH stimulates testosterone biosynthesis in Leydig cells 10-8B.

Feedback control of gonadotropin secretion is complex, particularly in females, in whom such control

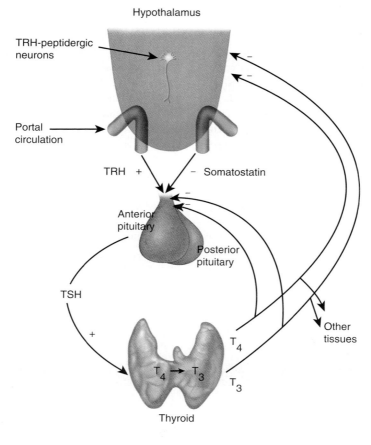

10–6 **Hypothalamic–pituitary–thyroid axis. A.** Thyrotropin-releasing hormone (TRH) stimulates and somato-statin inhibits release of TSH from anterior pituitary thyrotrophs. By means of the general circulation, TSH reaches the thyroid, where it stimulates the synthesis and release of triiodothyronine (T_3) and tetraiodothyronine or thyroxine (T_4) from the thyroid gland. **B.** The chemical structures of thyroid hormones T_3 and T_4.

varies during the different stages of the menstrual cycle. It comprises a complex integration of influences exerted by the gonadal steroids (estradiol, progesterone, and testosterone) and by the peptide hormones (inhibin and activin), which also are produced by the gonads. Moreover, GnRH release is influenced by several neuro-transmitter and neuromodulatory agents, including

catecholamines, endogenous opioids, γ-aminobutyric acid (GABA), neuropeptide Y, and possibly dopamine.

Among the actions that can be traced to gonadal steroids, their participation in gene transcription is best understood. Like glucocorticoids, gonadal steroids can regulate transcription either directly or indirectly. In some cases, they bind to estrogen or androgen response

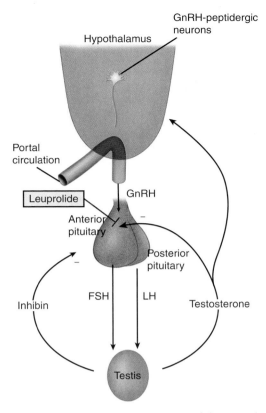

Gonadal steroids regulate neural function and behavior in adults. For example, changing levels of estrogen can have significant effects on mood 10–4. In addition, estrogens may exert rapid onset membrane effects of the sort better documented for the neuroactive steroids described in 10–2. They may also affect neural morphology; in female rats, for example, estradiol increases the density of dendritic spines on CA1 hippocampal pyramidal neurons. The physiologic and behavioral impacts of these changes are not yet clear.

A long-acting form of progesterone, **hydroxyprogesterone (Depo-Provera)**, and the selective estrogen receptor modulator (SERM) **tamoxifen** are used for reversible chemical castration of male sex offenders. The main use of Depo-Provera is for long-acting birth control in females, and of tamoxifen is for the treatment of estrogen receptor–positive breast cancer.

Diverse androgen derivatives (**anabolic steroids**) are used to increase muscle mass and athletic performance; such steroids often are used illegally and can produce deleterious effects on the brain. Anabolic steroids appear to be reinforcing, and hence potentially addicting, in some individuals; moreover, they may induce irritability and anger. A fraction of users, including females, have reported **hypomanic** symptoms during use and **depression** during withdrawal.

PROLACTIN

Prolactin, like growth hormone and placental lactogen, is a member of the somatotropic hormone family. It is synthesized and released by lactotrophs of the anterior pituitary gland. In males, serum prolactin levels normally are low throughout life. In females, such levels typically are only slightly higher but increase markedly during pregnancy. Pregnancy-related increases decline at term unless the mother breast feeds; suckling causes marked increases in prolactin levels, which serve to initiate lactation. Hypothalamic control of prolactin is primarily inhibitory. It is mediated by dopamine released into the portal circulation at the median eminence by neurons of the tuberoinfundibular dopaminergic system, which originates in the arcuate nucleus (10–9 ; see also Chapter 6). In the pituitary, dopamine binds to D_2 dopamine receptors to inhibit prolactin synthesis and release. TRH from the hypothalamus and vasoactive intestinal peptide (VIP), which is produced locally in the pituitary, act to increase the release of prolactin.

Although prolactin is released in response to stress, both the mechanism and function of such release in humans remain unclear. **Hyperprolactinemia** is most commonly caused by tumors, or microadenomas, of pituitary lactotrophs or by D_2 dopamine receptor

10–7 **Hypothalamic–pituitary–gonadal axis.** The male version of this axis is shown. Neurons that express gonadotropin-releasing hormone (GnRH) cause the pituitary to release luteinizing hormone (LH) and follicle-stimulating hormone (FSH), which in turn act on the testis (shown) or ovary. Gonadal steroids, such as testosterone or estrogen, inhibit both GnRH and LH release as part of a regulatory feedback process. The gonads also produce a peptide hormone known as inhibin, which inhibits FSH secretion. Leuprolide, a potent GnRH agonist, desensitizes the GnRH receptor and thereby inhibits this axis. It is used in the treatment of precocious puberty and to suppress testosterone secretion in prostate cancer. It also is used experimentally in the investigation and treatment of perimenstrual mood disorders (see 10–4).

elements in the regulatory regions of specific target genes and thereby influence the expression of those genes. In other cases, gonadal steroids affect transcription by interacting with AP-1, CREB, or other transcription factor families and in turn altering the expression of genes controlled by those transcription factors. Gonadal steroids also produce some of their physiologic effects by acting on cell surface proteins, as discussed in 10–2.

10–8A **Gonadal steroid synthesis.** Synthetic pathways in the female. Like all steroid hormones, gonadal steroids are derived from cholesterol.

antagonists, most commonly **antipsychotic drugs**. It can result in galactorrhea and dysmenorrhea in females. In males, it may produce galactorrhea and impotence. Because prolactin is under inhibitory control of dopamine, hyperprolactinemia can be treated with dopamine D_2 receptor agonists, such as **bromocriptine**.

The prolactin receptor belongs to the family of glycophosphatidylinositol (GPI)-linked receptors, which modulate the actions of many cytokines, including ciliary neurotrophic factor, leukemia inhibitory factor, and leptin (Chapter 8). Activation of GPI-linked receptors leads to the activation of the protein tyrosine kinase Janus kinase (JAK), which phosphorylates and activates the transcription factors called signal transducers and activators of transcription (STATs). This JAK-STAT signaling pathway is described in greater detail in Chapter 4.

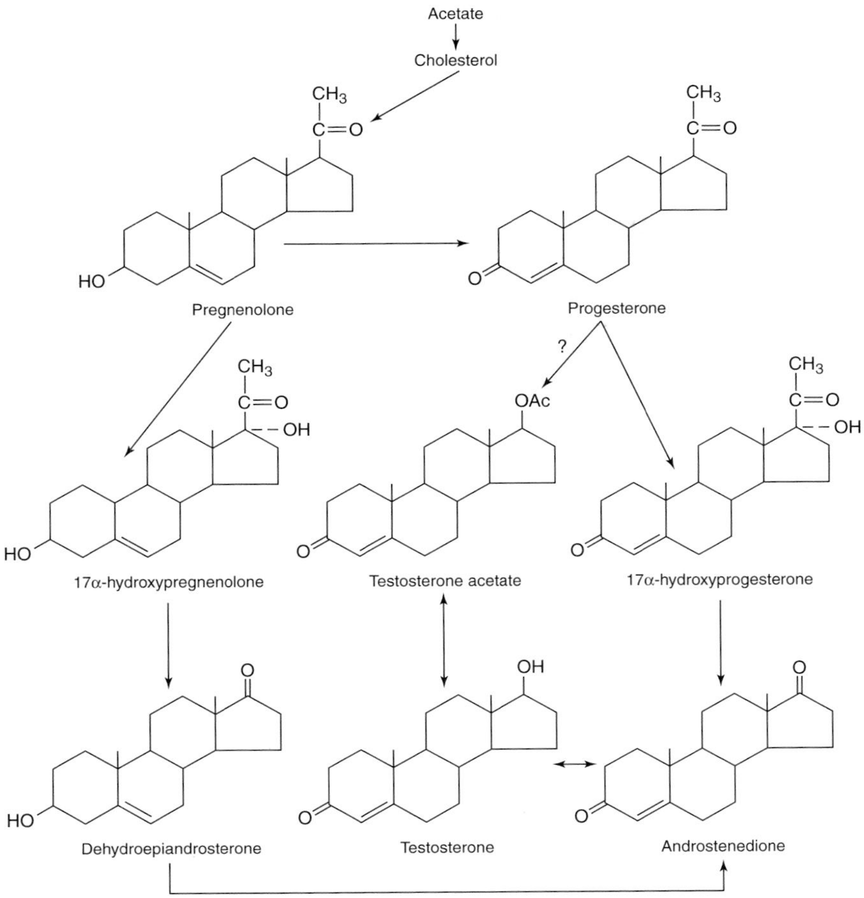

10-8B **Gonadal steroid synthesis.** Synthetic pathways in the male.

10-4 **Disorders of Mood Related to Reproductive Function**

Postpartum Mood Disorders

Many women develop transient blues after childbirth; however, a significant minority (up to 10%) go on to develop serious **postpartum depression** or **postpartum mania.** Such disorders are believed to be triggered by the rapid and dramatic changes in hormonal levels that occur perinatally. Both estrogen and progesterone levels rise during pregnancy and fall rapidly after delivery. Moreover, estrogen stimulates the production of thyroid-binding globulin, which leads to reduced levels of free thyroid hormone. Prolactin and cortisol levels also rise during pregnancy and subsequently return to a normal range within weeks of delivery. Although the pathophysiology is not fully understood, these postpartum alterations in mood are, fortunately, highly responsive to standard **antidepressant** or **antimanic** medications.

Premenstrual Mood Disorders

Some women with depression experience a premenstrual worsening of symptoms. Likewise, some women experience depressive or anxiety symptoms that recur during the luteal phase of the menstrual cycle and generally resolve shortly after the onset of menstruation. The GnRH receptor agonist **leuprolide,** which suppresses menstrual cycling (see **10-7**), causes remission of premenstrual dysphoria. Experimentally, symptoms were shown to recur when exogenous ovarian steroids were administered even with natural cycling being suppressed. In contrast, when **perimenopausal depression** does not respond to conventional antidepressants it may respond to administration of estradiol.

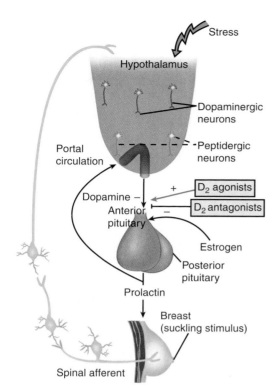

10-9 **Prolactin secretion.** Prolactin secretion is induced in lactotrophs of the anterior pituitary by thyrotropin-releasing hormone and perhaps other peptidergic signals, and is inhibited by dopamine acting at D_2 receptors. Antipsychotic drugs that are potent D_2 antagonists (Chapter 16) increase prolactin secretion. In lactating females, prolactin is strongly induced by suckling.

GROWTH HORMONE

The production of growth hormone by the somatotrophs of the anterior pituitary is under the stimulatory control of GHRH and the inhibitory control of somatostatin **10-10**. GH release must be pulsatile to stimulate skeletal growth.

GHRH is produced by cells of the infundibular and arcuate nuclei of the hypothalamus and is released at the median eminence. It binds to its G protein–linked receptor on the somatotroph membrane and stimulates transcription of growth hormone mRNA and release of mature growth hormone. Somatostatin, produced by neurons of the anterior periventricular region of the hypothalamus, is also released into the portal circulation at the median eminence; it acts via G protein–linked receptors coupled to $G_{i/o}$ on somatotrophs to inhibit the

release of growth hormone. Growth hormone provides negative feedback by stimulating somatostatin release. Growth hormone effects on target tissues are partly mediated by insulin-like growth factor 1 (IGF-1)/ somatomedin C, which among other actions suppresses the release of growth hormone from the pituitary.

Growth hormone is necessary for longitudinal growth; accordingly, levels of this hormone are high in children, reach maximal levels during adolescence, and decline during adulthood. In addition to the growth of long bones, the metabolic effects of this hormone, which generally are anabolic in nature, lead to increased muscle mass and decreased body fat. Growth hormone exhibits normal circadian patterns of release, but is also released in response to stressors, such as exertion, or emotional stress.

The growth hormone receptor, like the prolactin receptor, is GPI linked. It contains a single transmembrane domain, has a large extracellular N terminus involved in hormone binding and a large intracellular C terminus. Hormone binding causes the receptor to dimerize and results in the activation of the JAK-STAT pathway. Growth hormone has direct effects on some target tissues, and its induction of IGF-1 in peripheral tissues mediates some of its growth-promoting and anabolic actions. Certain forms of **dwarfism** are caused by loss of function mutations of the growth hormone receptor.

CONTROL OF FEEDING AND ENERGY BALANCE

The regulation of energy balance involves the exquisite coordination of food intake and energy expenditure. Experiments in the 1940s and 1950s showed that lesions of the *lateral hypothalamus (LH)* reduced food intake; hence, the normal role of this brain area is to stimulate feeding and decrease energy utilization. In contrast, lesions of the medial hypothalamus, especially the *ventromedial nucleus (VMH)* but also the *PVN* and *dorsomedial* hypothalamic nucleus (*DMH*), increased food intake; hence, the normal role of these regions is to suppress feeding and increase energy utilization. Yet discovery of the complex networks of neuropeptides **10-3** and other neurotransmitters acting within the hypothalamus and other brain regions to regulate food intake and energy expenditure began in earnest in 1994 with the cloning of the leptin (*ob*, for obesity) gene. Indeed, there is now explosive interest in basic feeding mechanisms given the epidemic proportions of **obesity** in our society, and the increased toll of the eating disorders, **anorexia nervosa** and **bulimia**. Unfortunately, despite dramatic advances in the basic

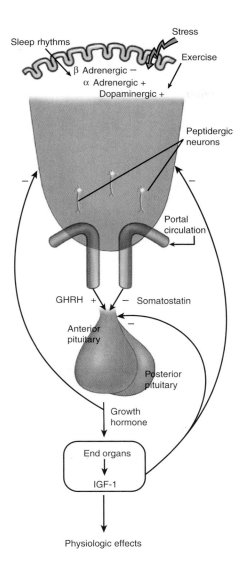

10–10 Growth hormone secretion. Growth hormone secretion is induced in somatotrophs of the anterior pituitary by growth hormone–releasing hormone (GHRH) and is inhibited by somatostatin. Release of these hypothalamic peptides is modulated by adrenergic and dopaminergic systems. Growth hormone acts on peripheral tissues largely through production of insulin-like growth factor-1 (IGF-1).

10–3 Examples of Peptides That Regulate Feeding

Peptides That Increase Feeding	Peptides That Decrease Feeding
Ghrelin	Leptin
NPY	α-MSH, β-MSH
Agouti-related peptide (ARP)	Cocaine- and amphetamine-regulated transcript (CART)
Orexin	CRH
Melanin-concentrating hormone (MCH)	Cholecystokinin (CCK)
Galanin	Insulin
	Glucagon-like peptide 1 (GLP-1)

neurobiology of feeding, our understanding of the etiology of these conditions and our ability to intervene clinically remain limited.

Leptin

Parabiosis studies, in which the circulation of two animals is joined, suggested that humoral factors are involved in energy balance. Rats with a medial hypothalamic lesion become obese; when a rat with a VMH lesion had its circulation joined with an unlesioned rat, the normal surgically joined circulatory partner ate less and lost weight. It was hypothesized that fat mass, which represents energy stores, releases a humoral "lipostatic" factor that inhibits feeding.

Obese (*ob/ob*) and diabetic (*db/db*) mice are two strains homozygous for different recessive mutations. Both strains are diabetic and typically weigh more than three times those of wild type mice even when fed an identical diet. When their circulations were joined, it could be concluded that the *ob/ob* mice lacked a circulating "lipostatic" factor and that the *db/db* mice were insensitive to it. The missing factor in the *ob/ob* mouse proved to be leptin, while the *db/db* mouse lacks the leptin receptor.

Leptin is produced primarily by adipocytes. Plasma levels of leptin correlate with adipose tissue mass; in both humans and rodents, such levels increase with increased adipose tissue and decrease with weight loss **10–11**.

Administration of leptin over time results in a dose-dependent decrease in body weight. Leptin levels do not change abruptly with meals; this finding

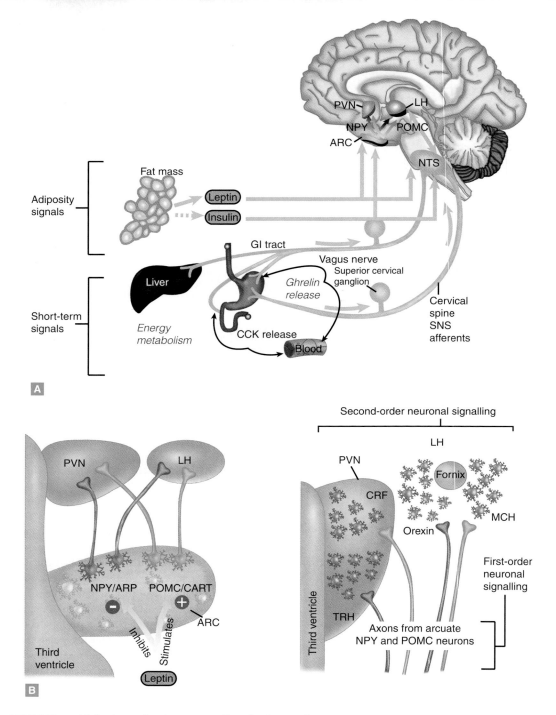

10-11 **Neurobiologic mechanisms controlling feeding and energy expenditure. A.** Shows the complex inter-play between peripheral and central factors in controlling feeding and energy metabolism. Peripheral factors include short-term or satiety factors, such as CCK, as well as signals that act over longer time periods, such as leptin. **B.** Shows how leptin influences the arcuate nucleus to stimulate POMC/CART neurons and inhibit NPY/ARP neurons (*left*). These arcuate neurons innervate the medial and lateral hypothalamus to regulate secondary orexigenic factors (MCH, orexin) and anorexigenic factors (CRF, TRH). Abbreviations: PVN, paraventricular nucleus; LH, lateral hypothalamus; ARC, arcuate nucleus; POMC, proopiomelanocortin; NPY, neuropeptide Y; NTS, nucleus of the solitary tract; CCK, chole-cystokinin; ARP, agouti-related peptide; CART, cocaine- and amphetamine-regulated transcript; CRF, corticotropin-releasing factor; TRH, thyrotropin release hormone. (Adapted from Schwartz MW, Woods SC, Porte D, Seeley RJ, Baskin DG. Central nervous system control of food intake. *Nature.* 2000;404:661–671.)

distinguishes alterations in leptin from short-term satiety signals such as levels of glucose, amino acids, or cholecystokinin (CCK) **10-5**. Mutations in leptin or in the leptin receptor in humans, which are very rare, produce morbid obesity and failure to undergo puberty.

The leptin receptor is most densely concentrated in the medial hypothalamus, the region known from lesion studies to be involved in suppression of feeding. Moreover, these nuclei are near the median eminence, a region of the brain with fenestrated capillaries that allows the entry of circulating leptin and other circulating peptides. The receptor is also highly expressed in the arcuate nucleus and more sparsely in other brain regions, including ventral tegmental area (VTA) dopamine neurons, which are important mediators of reward (Chapter 15). As will be seen later, activation of leptin receptors stimulates anorexigenic factors (antifeeding) and suppresses orexigenic factors (profeeding) to produce its powerful effects on feeding and energy utilization. The leptin receptor is a member of the GPI-linked receptor family, and leptin binding causes the activation of the JAK-STAT pathway.

Leptin influences other neuroendocrine functions. For example, *ob* mice exhibit many abnormalities characteristic of the starvation state, despite the animals' obesity and hyperphagia. Such mice exhibit decreased body temperature, decreased energy expenditure, infertility, and decreased immune function. Because leptin replacement corrects all of these abnormalities in the *ob* mouse, it is believed that leptin may play a role in multiple neuroendocrine cascades.

The discovery of leptin raised a great deal of excitement regarding its usefulness in the treatment of obesity. It turned out, however, that the vast majority of obese individuals already have appropriately high levels of leptin, which has turned the field's attention to other feeding factors, many of which are leptin targets.

Ghrelin

Ghrelin, also a peptide, is produced by the cells that line the stomach. Ghrelin secretion increases hours after the end of a meal and stimulates appetite for the next meal. Ghrelin receptors are G protein linked. The best described site of action of ghrelin is the VMH and arcuate nucleus, but ghrelin receptors are also expressed in the brain's reward pathways (eg, VTA dopamine neurons) and may stimulate feeding through this action as well. In addition to its role in stimulating feeding, ghrelin increases growth hormone release. Among many possible mechanisms, **bariatric surgery**, in which portions of the stomach are excised or constricted in the treatment of severe **obesity**, may reduce appetite in part by reducing ghrelin secretion. There is interest in the possible use of **ghrelin receptor antagonists**, still in early stages of development, in the treatment of obesity.

POMC, NPY, and the Arcuate Nucleus

The arcuate nucleus of the hypothalamus plays a central role in energy balance. It contains two groups of GABAergic neurons that produce opposite effects **10-11B**.

10-5 **Cholecystokinin**

Satiety signals act more rapidly than the leptin signal and are released in response to meals. Glucose and amino acids absorbed from meals can serve as satiety signals. Another satiety signal is the peptide, cholecystokinin (CCK). It is synthesized in the gut wall and released into the circulation in response to the presence of certain nutrients in the gut. It stimulates G protein–coupled receptors located on the vagus nerve, which in turn transmit information to the nucleus of the solitary tract in the brainstem and subsequently to the hypothalamus. Blockade of

peripheral CCK receptors leads to increased food intake. Cholecystokinin is also synthesized and released by certain neuronal cell types in the brain, where it functions as a peptide neurotransmitter. CCK is reported to exert diverse behavioral effects via actions on CCK_1 and CCK_2 receptors (see **7-4**, Chapter 7). While there remains interest in the development of CCK receptor antagonists for the treatment of obesity and neuropsychiatric conditions, no clinical validation is yet available.

One group expresses POMC and cocaine- and amphetamine-regulated transcript (CART) and exerts anorexigenic effects and increases energy utilization; these cells are potently stimulated by leptin. The other group expresses neuropeptide Y (NPY) and agouti-related peptide (ARP) and exerts orexigenic effects and reduces energy expenditure; these cells are inhibited by leptin.

As described above in the discussion of the HPA axis, POMC is a large precursor that is cleaved to produce ACTH, α-, β-, and γ-MSH (also called melanocortins), and β-endorphin (see also 7–4 in Chapter 7). α- and β-MSH reduce feeding and increase energy expenditure acting via melanocortin receptors 3 and 4 (MC_3 and MC_4, which are G_s linked) in the arcuate nucleus itself and also in the lateral hypothalamus, PVN, and DMH, those regions of the hypothalamus known to suppress feeding (and which, when lesioned, release excessive feeding behavior). Recent evidence indicates that POMC neurons express the serotonin $5HT_{2C}$ receptor, which, when activated, stimulates melanocortin release. This likely explains the mechanism by which serotonin-promoting drugs (eg, **fenfluramine** or **fenfluramine-phentermine** combinations; Chapter 6) cause weight loss. MC_4 receptors are also rich in the nucleus accumbens, a major brain reward region (Chapter 15), which may provide a mechanism by which α-MSH suppresses motivation for feeding in addition to suppressing food consumption and increasing energy utilization per se.

In contrast to melanocortins, NPY is a potent activator of feeding and suppressor of energy expenditure acting at its Y_1 and Y_5 receptors, which are linked to $G_{i/o}$. The NPY neurons of the arcuate nucleus also express ARP that acts as an inverse agonist at the MC_3 and MC_4 receptors. ARP not only blocks α- and β-MSH binding, but serves as an inverse agonist: it independently inhibits MC_3 and MC_4 function and thereby stimulates feeding and inhibits energy expenditure. In addition to being inhibited by leptin, NPY/ARP cells are stimulated by ghrelin.

Based on this evolving model of feeding regulation, one would predict that **melanocortin agonists** or **NPY antagonists** would be useful in the treatment of **obesity**. Numerous agents are in development but have not yet been tested extensively in the clinic.

Lateral Hypothalamus

Both the POMC and the NPY neurons of the arcuate nucleus project to the lateral hypothalamus. As mentioned earlier, this brain area is the site of potent orexigenic factors. One of the most important is melanin-concentrating hormone (MCH), which stimulates appetite and suppresses energy utilization. MCH receptors, which are $G_{i/o}$ linked, are enriched in the hypothalamus as well as in the nucleus accumbens. **MCH antagonists**, beyond serving as potential antiobesity treatments, are being evaluated for their possible **antidepressant** use, based on a growing number of studies in animal models.

More recently, the lateral hypothalamus was also found to play a central role in arousal. Neurons in this region contain cell bodies that produce the orexin (also called hypocretin) peptides (see also Chapter 6, 6–25). These neurons project widely throughout the brain and are involved in sleep, arousal, feeding, reward, aspects of emotion, and learning. In fact, orexin is thought to promote feeding primarily by promoting arousal. Mutations in orexin receptors are responsible for **narcolepsy** in a canine model, knockout of the orexin gene produces narcolepsy in mice, and humans with narcolepsy have low or absent levels of orexin peptides in cerebrospinal fluid (Chapter 12).

LH neurons have reciprocal connections with neurons that produce monoamine neurotransmitters (Chapter 6). It should not be surprising that arousal and feeding are jointly regulated since feeding is absolutely central to survival, and the wake period for free-living organisms must be associated with the ability to find and consume food.

Dopaminergic Reward Circuits

Reward circuits, which are described in detail in Chapter 15, play a key role in feeding behavior. New, palatable foods cause dopamine release from VTA neurons of the midbrain that project to the nucleus accumbens, prefrontal cortex, and other limbic structures that regulate emotion. Dopamine acts in the nucleus accumbens to attach motivational significance to stimuli associated with rewards (such as food). It acts in the orbital prefrontal cortex to set a value on rewards, and dopamine released from the substantia nigra acts in the dorsal striatum to consolidate efficient motor programs to obtain rewards. It is very interesting then, as mentioned above, that orexin, leptin, and ghrelin receptors are expressed in the VTA, and MC_4 and MCH receptors are enriched in the nucleus accumbens. There is increasing evidence that some of the actions of these feeding peptides are mediated at the level of the VTA-NAc circuit: recent studies, for example, have shown that injection of leptin into the VTA suppresses feeding behavior, while RNAi (RNA interference; Chapter 4)-mediated knockdown of leptin receptors in the VTA increases food intake, sensitivity to highly palatable foods, and locomotor activity.

HYPOTHALAMIC RESPONSE TO INFECTION AND INFLAMMATION

Inflammation plays a critical role in fighting infection, in wound healing, and in responses to many forms of tissue damage. At the same time, infections and tissue damage represent substantial challenges to homeostasis. Immune mediators such as cytokines help defend the organism against infection, for example, but can have their own toxic effects if released in excess or as a result of autoimmunity.

Multiple microbial antigens and toxins activate cells of the immune system to secrete cytokines, including interleukin-1β (IL-1β), tumor necrosis factor-α (TNF-α), and interleukin-6 (IL-6) (Chapter 8). Such inflammatory mediators not only act locally at the site of an infection, but also act systemically. As has been described in this chapter, the hypothalamus plays the central role in regulating homeostasis; moreover, some regions of the hypothalamus lie outside the blood–brain barrier and are thus able to detect circulating cytokines. It also has been hypothesized that cytokines interact with capillary endothelial cells on the blood side of the blood–brain barrier to produce lipid messengers, such as prostaglandins, that diffuse directly into the brain. As such, the hypothalamus is central in mediating systemic effects of cytokines, including the generation of **fever** and of "sickness behaviors" such as decreased appetite, reduced activity, fatigue, and altered hormonal output (eg, increased CRF secretion and decreased GnRH and TRH release).

Fever results from the action of prostaglandin PGE_2 acting on EP_3 prostaglandin receptors. Prostaglandins are synthesized by endothelial cells within small venules near the surface of the brain. Anatomically selective genetic deletion of EP_3 receptors within the median pre-optic nucleus (MnPO) of the hypothalamus demonstrates that this site is required for the generation of fever. GABAergic MnPO neurons project to and tonically inhibit neurons within the PVN and DMH and to a region of the medulla that regulates sympathetic nervous system activity. Activation of EP_3 receptors disinhibits these neurons, and thereby facilitates thermogenic responses such as constriction of blood vessels in the skin.

Pharmacologic blockade of the enzymes that generate PGE_2 are antipyretic. Such drugs include **aspirin** and other salicylates and **nonsteroidal anti-inflammatory drugs** (**NSAIDs**) such as **ibuprofen** and **naproxen.** These drugs block production of PGE_2 by inhibiting type 2 cyclooxygenase (COX2), which converts arachadonic acid to prostaglandins. Selective inhibitors of COX2 such as **celecoxib** and **rofecoxib** were developed to avoid blocking COX1, expressed in the gut, thus avoiding risk of peptic ulcers. However, by failing to block COX1, these drugs also permit relative increases in the production of thromboxane and therefore increase the risk of thrombosis. This has led to the recent removal of several COX2 inhibitors from the market.

SELECTED READING

Bale TL, Vale WW. CRF and CRF receptors: role in stress responsivity and other behaviors. *Annu Rev Pharmacol Toxicol.* 2004;44:525–575.

Belelli D, Lambert JJ. Neurosteroids: endogenous regulators of the GABA_A receptor. *Nature Rev Neurosci.* 2005;6:565–575.

Brown ES, J Woolston D, Frol A, et al. Hippocampal volume, spectroscopy, cognition, and mood in patients receiving corticosteroid therapy. *Biol Psychiatry.* 2004;55:538–545.

Castro MG, Morrison E. Posttranslational processing of proopiomelanocortin in the pituitary and in the brain. *Crit Rev Neurobiol.* 1997;11:35–57.

De Kloet ER, Joels M, Holsboer F. Stress and the brain: from adaptation to disease. *Nature Rev Neurosci.* 2005;6:463–475.

Elmquist JK, Coppari R, Balthasar N, et al. Identifying hypothalamic pathways controlling food intake, body weight, and glucose homeostasis. *J Comp Neurol.* 2005;493:63-71.

Gao Q, Horvath TL. Neurobiology of feeding and energy expenditure. *Annu Rev Neurosci.* 2007;30: 367–398.

Friedman JM. Modern science versus the stigma of obesity. *Nature Med.* 2004;10:563–569.

Fulton S, Pissios P, Manchon RP, et al. Leptin regulation of the mesoaccumbens dopamine pathway. *Neuron.* 2006;51:811–822.

Hosie AM, Wilkins ME, da Silva, et al. Endogenous neurosteroids regulate GABA_A receptors through two discrete transmembrane sites. *Nature.* 2006;444:486–489

Halford JC, Blundell JE. Pharmacology of appetite suppression. *Prog Drug Res.* 2000;54:25–58.

Hommel JD, Trinko R, Georgescu D, et al. Leptin receptor signaling in midbrain dopamine neurons regulates feeding. *Neuron.* 2006;51:801–810.

Itoi K, Jiang YQ, Iwasaki Y, et al. Regulatory mechanisms of corticotropin-releasing hormone and vasopressin gene expression in the hypothalamus. *J Neuroendocrinol.* 2004;16:348–355.

Lazarus M, Yoshida K, Coppri R, et al. EP3 prostaglandin receptors in the median preoptic nucleus are critical for fever responses. *Nature Neurosci.* 2007;10:1131–1133.

McEwen BS. Stress and hippocampal plasticity. *Annu Rev Neurosci.* 1999;22:105–122.

McEwen BS, Alves SE. Estrogen actions in the central nervous system. *Endocr Rev.* 1999;20:279–307.

Richards M, Rubinow DR, Daly RC, et al. Premenstrual symptoms and perimenopausal depression. *Am J Psychiatry.* 2006;163:133–137.

Schwartz MW, Woods SC, Porte D, et al. Central nervous system control of food intake. *Nature.* 2000;404:661–671.

Sheline YI. Neuroimaging studies of mood disorder effects on the brain. *Biol Psychiatry.* 2003;54:338–352.

Smith GW, Aubry J-M, Dellu F, et al. Corticotropin-releasing factor receptor 1-deficient mice display decreased anxiety, impaired stress response, and aberrant neuroendocrine development. *Neuron.* 1998;20:1093–1102.

Spiegelman BM, Flier JS. Obesity and the regulation of energy balance. *Cell.* 2001;104:531–543.

Pain and Inflammation

KEY CONCEPTS

- Nociception is the form of somatic sensation that detects noxious, potentially tissue-damaging stimuli. Pain has both a localizing somatic sensory component and an aversive emotional and motivational component.

- Pain begins with peripheral nociceptors, which have their cell bodies in dorsal root ganglia (DRG) and in the trigeminal ganglia in the head; these neurons synapse, respectively, in the dorsal horn of the spinal cord or the trigeminal nucleus, the medullary extension of the dorsal horn.

- Peripheral nociceptors express a set of channels, most notably transient receptor potential (TRP) channels, that are sensitive to noxious mechanical, thermal, and chemical stimuli. These neurons also express receptors for inflammatory mediators and substances released by damaged cells.

- Sensitization is a clinically significant process in which nociceptors in an area extending beyond a tissue injury exhibit decreased thresholds for activation. Sensitization can be initiated by inflammatory mediators such as prostaglandins and leukotrienes.

- Nonsteroidal anti-inflammatory drugs (NSAIDs) act by blocking prostaglandin-mediated sensitization, specifically by inhibiting the enzyme cyclooxygenase that is required for the synthesis of prostaglandins from arachidonic acid.

- Primary nociceptors release a large number of neuropeptide and nonpeptide neurotransmitters in the dorsal horn of the spinal cord. The dorsal horn is an important site of integration for both ascending nociceptive information and descending antinociceptive influences.

- Opiate drugs selectively suppress nociception, but not other sensory modalities, by binding to endogenous opioid receptors in descending analgesic pathways.

- Damage to neurons in nociceptive pathways can lead to severe chronic pain syndromes, termed neuropathic pain.

- Plasticity within the dorsal horn, mediated by NMDA glutamate receptors, may be key in the initiation of chronic pain syndromes by increasing the excitability of neurons in nociceptive pathways.

Chronic pain is a significant public health problem associated with severe patient suffering and disability and, in some cases, drug abuse. Pain begins, however, as an adaptive response to actual or potential harm to the body with the stimulation of *peripheral nociceptors*, neurons specialized to detect noxious stimuli. Pain is not simply a modality of somatic sensation like touch or vibration sense, however. Pain also has physiologic, behavioral, and aversive emotional components. Without its alerting and aversive components, its activation of withdrawal reflexes and avoidance behaviors, or its capacity to inscribe powerful emotional memories, pain would not reliably trigger escape from danger and avoidance of future harm **11-1**. When it becomes chronic, however, pain loses its adaptive role as a defender of the body's tissues and instead becomes a pressing medical problem. The aversive emotions associated with pain no longer serve a protective function, but rather produce suffering and, all too often, maladaptive behaviors. Chronic pain may result from continuing tissue damage, as can occur with cancer, but much chronic pain results from chronic inflammatory processes or damage to the pain pathways themselves (eg, by trauma, nerve compression, diabetes, or Herpes varicella-zoster infection), in which case it is termed **neuropathic pain**. Neuropathic pain continues long after tissues have healed, and thus becomes a persistent false alarm.

In sum, pain has both a discriminative sensory aspect and an emotional and motivational aspect. Because of its discriminative sensory component a person can describe where the pain seems to arise (although, as will be discussed, pain from viscera can seem to come from the body surface) and can delineate its characteristics (eg, sharp, pricking, aching, burning). Because of its emotional and motivational component, pain interrupts ongoing behaviors and demands attention; it also powerfully motivates learning and thereby suppresses behaviors that put an organism in harm's way. The emotional and motivational component gives pain its survival value, but also can produce suffering and disability when pain is chronic.

11-1 **Congenital Inability to Perceive Pain**

Three consanguineous families from northern Pakistan were found to contain individuals who had never experienced pain. These individuals possess morphologically normal nociceptive neurons, intact somatic sensation aside from nociception, and exhibit normal intelligence. They understood something about pain (and the dangers it portends) by observing others, but were simply incapable of experiencing it themselves. What they were lacking, as a result of homozygosity for a loss of function mutation in the SCN9A gene, was a functional protein to form the α-subunit of a particular voltage-gated Na$^+$ channel, known as Na$_v$1.7, which is highly expressed in nociceptive neurons (Chapter 2). This is a remarkable finding because it demonstrates that in humans—the same is not true in the mouse—a single protein plays an absolutely essential role in the function of otherwise normal-looking peripheral nociceptors. Because the affected individuals are otherwise healthy, the finding also suggests that Na$_v$1.7 could be a very significant target for the development of new **analgesic** (or antipain) medications.

These families also illustrate the protective role of pain. All affected members had significant injuries to their lips and tongues from biting themselves. All had frequent bruises and cuts and most had limb fractures, often diagnosed as a result of a limp or inability to use a limb. The index case for the study, a 10-year-old child, worked as a street performer. He placed knives through his arms and walked on hot coals—and died before his 14th birthday from jumping off a roof.

Other families with hereditary sensory and autonomic neuropathy type 4 lack nociceptive neurons because of a mutation in the TrkA receptor (the receptor for nerve growth factor or NGF; Chapter 8). TrkA is expressed in all normally developing peripheral nociceptors, and is required for their survival. Similar to individuals with mutations in SCN9A, people lacking TrkA have injuries to lips and tongue and to limbs. The latter are reported to include joint damage and loss of finger tips. Even though individuals who do not feel pain learn second hand to be aware of injury risks, they cannot overcome the loss of pain, which while troublesome is ultimately a protective form of experience.

PRIMARY NOCICEPTORS

Pain begins with primary afferent nociceptors that have cell bodies in *dorsal root ganglia* (*DRG*) and that make synapses in the *dorsal horn* of the spinal cord **11-1**. Primary nociceptors in the face and head have their cell bodies in *trigeminal ganglia* and synapse in the brainstem continuation of the dorsal horn, called the trigeminal nucleus. Throughout this discussion we will use the terms DRG and dorsal horn with the understanding that the same principles apply to their rostral extensions in the head.

The peripheral terminals of primary afferent nociceptors are morphologically undifferentiated free nerve endings. However, these nerve endings express a large panoply of receptors and channels **11-2**. They express a large number of G protein-coupled receptors, including bradykinin B_2, eicosanoid, purine nucleoside P2Y, histamine, serotonin $5HT_1$ and $5HT_{2A}$, $GABA_B$, α_2-adrenergic, somatostatin, neuropeptide Y, and μ, δ, and κ opioid receptors. They also express ligand-gated channels, such as the ATP-gated $P2X_3$ receptor, and a subset of mature nociceptors express TrkA, the protein tyrosine kinase that binds nerve growth factor (NGF). (All developing nociceptors express TrkA and are dependent on NGF; see **11-1**.) In addition, nociceptive terminals express diverse channels involved in transducing noxious signals, including transient receptor potential (TRP) channels **11-2**; **11-1**, heat-sensitive K^+ channels, and acid-sensing ion channels (ASICs). These ion channels may be gated directly by noxious heat, cold, mechanical stimulation, acid, or irritant chemicals. Alternatively, TRP channels may be coupled to activation of G protein-coupled receptors, as appears to be the case for the bradykinin B_2 receptor **11-3**.

Many of the TRP channels transduce environmental stimuli such as temperature and exogenous chemicals. Many of the G protein-coupled receptors and ligand-gated channels detect tissue damage that causes, for example, release of ATP and of K^+ and H^+ ions from damaged cells. In the vicinity of an injury, serotonin is released from platelets, and histamine from tissue mast cells. Bradykinin, one of the most potent activators of nociception, is produced from plasma kininogen by the actions of kallikreins, enzymes that are activated rapidly at the site of an injury **11-3**. However, the interactions of G protein-coupled receptors and of TRP and other channels is complex and an important avenue for research on pain and analgesia.

Because nociceptors are specialized to respond only to noxious stimuli, the channels that transduce environmental signals have high thresholds for activations—in marked contrast to the transducers for light touch. When activated, noxious stimulus-detecting channels produce inward (depolarizing) currents within the peripheral terminals of primary nociceptors that can initiate trains of action potentials that are then transmitted to the dorsal horn of the spinal cord. Nociceptive neurons of dorsal root ganglia represent "first order" neurons that synapse on "second order" neurons within the dorsal horn of the spinal cord. These second order neurons may be local interneurons or projection neurons that carry nociceptive information to the brainstem and thalamus.

Finally, not all receptors and channels expressed on primary nociceptors transmit pain signals. Cannabinoid CB_1 and μ, δ, and κ opioid receptors expressed on nociceptors have been demonstrated to mediate analgesia. Indeed, evidence from genetically engineered mice, with CB_1 receptors deleted only in primary nociceptors, suggests that peripheral CB_1 receptors play a major role in cannabinoid-mediated analgesia. This might permit development of cannabinoid analgesics that do not cross the blood-brain barrier and are thus free of cognitive and psychotropic effects.

Peripheral nerves contain several different types of axons that carry sensory information; the greater the diameter and thickness of myelination of the axons, the greater their conduction velocity. The axons of cutaneous afferent nerves belong to one of three main classes. The largest and most heavily myelinated axons that originate from the skin are called A_β fibers. A_α axons, which are thicker, innervate muscles and joints; these axons are involved in proprioception, the transmission of sensory information related to posture, motion, and position. A_β fibers include cutaneous mechanoreceptors, which are free nerve endings that respond to light touch and the bending of hairs. Primary nociceptive neurons have small-caliber axons, some of which are thinly myelinated A_δ and most of which are unmyelinated C fibers. Given their lack of myelination, C fibers conduct impulses very slowly (<2 m/s) compared with that of A_δ fibers (approximately 20 m/s) **11-2**; **11-4**.

Primary nociceptive neurons must convey signals that distinguish between innocuous and noxious stimuli. Nociceptors accomplish this in one of two ways. They either possess high thresholds for stimulation or possess the capability of coding the intensity of a stimulus in the frequency of impulses relayed centrally, so that noxious stimuli produce the highest firing rates **11-3**. A_δ nociceptors, or high-threshold mechanoreceptors, respond to noxious mechanical stimuli, especially sharp objects; approximately half of the mechanothermal nociceptors

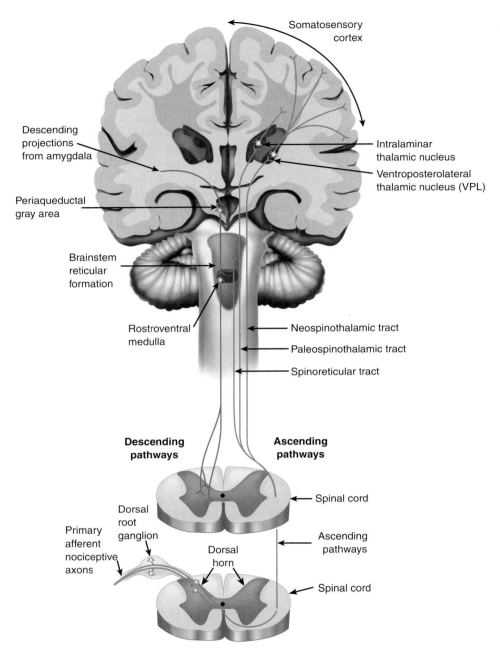

11-1 **Nociceptive pathways.** A primary afferent (or first order) nociceptive neuron synapses in the superficial layers of the dorsal horn. Morphologically, these are bipolar neurons with cell bodies in the dorsal root ganglion (or in the head, the trigeminal ganglion) and bifurcated axons that project both to the periphery and to the spinal cord (or in the head to the trigeminal nucleus of the brainstem). Axons of dorsal horn (or second-order) nociceptive neurons cross the midline and ascend in the spinoreticular or spinothalamic tracts (*right*). The spinothalamic tract comprises the neospinothalamic and paleospinothalamic tracts. In the neospinothalamic tract, second-order neurons synapse in the ventroposterolateral nucleus of the thalamus (VPL), and third-order neurons project to somatosensory regions of the cerebral cortex. In the paleospinothalamic tract, second-order neurons synapse in the intralaminar thalamic nuclei and project to association cortex and limbic structures. Descending analgesic systems believed to originate with cortical neurons and neurons of the amygdala (*left*) activate descending analgesic systems by activating neurons in periaqueductal gray area (PAG) of the brainstem. A projection from the PAG to the rostral ventral medulla that descends to the dorsal horn mediates opiate-dependent descending analgesia.

Primary nociceptor peripheral terminal

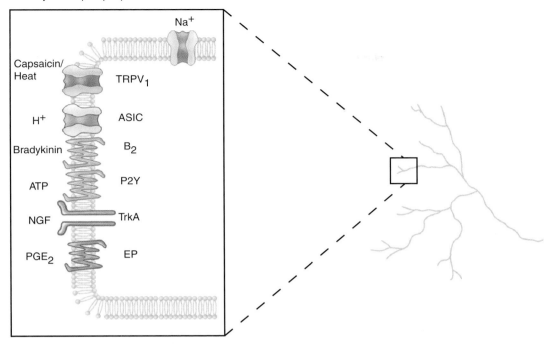

11-2 **Receptors and channels on the peripheral terminals of primary nociceptors.** The detail is from a section of a hypothetical cutaneous free nerve ending. It shows a transient receptor potential (TRP) channel, the TRPV$_1$ channel, that is gated by capsaicin and heat, an acid-sensing ion channel (ASIC), and a voltage-gated Na$^+$ channel that might be activated by the generator potentials caused by stimulating the TRP and ASIC channels. Voltage-gated K$^+$ and Ca^{2+} channels (not shown) would also be expressed. Many G protein-coupled receptors might be expressed as described in the text. Shown are the bradykinin B$_2$ and P2Y ATP receptors, which signal primarily via G$_q$, and the prostaglandin PGE$_2$ EP receptors different subtypes of which signal via G$_{i/o}$ or other G proteins. Another receptor family, the tyrosine receptor kinases, is represented by TrkA, the nerve growth factor (NGF) receptor.

also respond to noxious thermal stimuli. The majority of C fibers in cutaneous nerves have higher thresholds than those of myelinated axons, and respond nonselectively to noxious mechanical, thermal, and chemical stimuli. They are therefore known as polymodal nociceptors. Activation of C fibers is mediated by a wide range of endogenous chemicals that are released in response to damaged tissue or inflammation.

SENSITIZATION

At sites of tissue damage, diffusable mediators, including arachidonic acid metabolites such as *prostaglandins* and *leukotrienes*, cytokines such as *interleukin-1 (IL-1)*, chemokines, and growth factors such as NGF, induce a form of neural plasticity within nociceptors called *sensitization*. The area of sensitized nociceptors usually extends beyond the borders of

tissue damage **11-4**. While some mediators such as bradykinin **11-3** can both activate and sensitize nociceptors, sensitization per se does not cause pain. Instead, sensitization decreases the thresholds for activation of nociceptors. Thus, previously innocuous stimuli, such as light touch, now activate nociceptors and are experienced as painful; this is termed *allodynia*. Moreover, the response to noxious stimuli is exaggerated, referred to as *hyperalgesia*. At its most extreme, sensitization might produce pain in the absence of a stimulus (ie, spontaneous pain). Possible mechanisms of sensitization include second messenger–dependent phosphorylation of TRP channels and Na$^+$ channels in pain pathway neurons in a manner that alters their thresholds for opening.

Heightened sensitivity to previously innocuous stimuli presumably serves the adaptive purpose of leading an organism to protect an injured area in the

11-2 The Capsaicin Receptor and TRP Channels

Capsaicin, the compound that gives chili peppers (capsicums) their heat, has turned out to be a powerful experimental tool for the study of pain. Many individuals who have touched their eyes after cutting chili peppers can attest to the intense burning pain that capsaicin can produce. The discovery of the capsaicin receptor, first described as the *vanilloid receptor* (*VR_1*) for the family of pungent chemicals that includes capsaicin, opened an important door in the study of nociception. VR_1 was the first of a family of channels that are the key detectors of noxious stimuli on peripheral nociceptors.

VR_1 turned out to be structurally homologous to *transient receptor potential* (*TRP*) channels, already known from *Drosophila* photoreceptors; thus VR_1 is now denoted as *TRPV1*. Across phylogeny TRP channels serve as major sensory transducers, with diverse ligands and gating mechanisms. In humans, they are gated not only by noxious thermal, chemical, and mechanical stimuli, but also by nonnoxious heat and cold. As well, TRP receptors transduce sweet, bitter, and umami tastes in humans and other animals, and detect pheromones in the mouse.

TRP channels are formed in different cell types by a large number of different but related proteins of which there are six mammalian subfamilies based on amino acid homology. TRP channels are composed of six transmembrane subunits that assemble into tetramers with a central pore that forms a nonselective cation channel. In general, channel opening will admit Na^+ and Ca^{2+}, thus depolarizing cells. Gating of TRP channels is complex **11-1**; different channels can be activated by changes in ambient temperature (eg, TRPV1, 2, 3, and 8), by mechanical stimuli, by exogenous small molecules (eg, capsaicin), endogenous lipids (eg, arachidonic acid metabolites, anandamide, diacylglycerol), and perhaps by ions such as Ca^{2+} and Mg^{2+}. Knockout experiments demonstrate quite clearly that response to a single stimulus, eg, a particular temperature, does not map to a single channel. Moreover, there is growing evidence that TRP channel subunits may form heteromultimers.

In addition to direct gating by exogenous stimuli, TRP channels can be gated or modulated by G protein-coupled receptor-activated second messengers, such as phosphatidylinositol (4,5)-bisphosphate (PIP_2) and diacylglycerol (DAG), by protein phosphorylation, and by lipid signals such as anandamide (an endocannabinoid; Chapter 8). The precise TRP channels expressed in a cell determine, to a great extent, the ability of that cell to sense important features of the environment.

short term, but it is a major cause of clinically significant pain if it persists. Sensitization of primary nociceptors may lead to sensitization of second-order neurons within the dorsal horn. The combination of peripheral and central sensitization underlies neuropathic pain, resulting in chronic allodynia, hyperalgesia, and spontaneous pain.

ASPIRIN AND NONSTEROIDAL ANTI-INFLAMMATORY DRUGS (NSAIDs)

Aspirin, acetaminophen (**paracetamol**), and the **NSAIDs** **11-5**, including **indomethacin, ibuprofen,** and **naproxen,** among others, produce analgesia primarily by diminishing sensitization. They accomplish this by inhibiting the enzyme *cyclooxygenase-2 (COX2)*, which is induced at sites of inflammation and which catalyzes a necessary step in the generation of the sensitizing mediator, prostaglandin E_2 (PGE_2) from arachidonic acid **11-6**. Given the multiple signaling pathways that produce sensitization, which do not all involve arachidonic acid metabolism, the analgesic efficacy of aspirin, acetaminophen, and NSAIDs is ultimately limited; nonetheless they remain the most widely used nonopiate analgesics. All three drugs are also antipyretic (Chapter 10), but only aspirin and the NSAIDs are anti-inflammatory. Acetaminophen's lack of significant anti-inflammatory effects presumably reflects at least a partially different interaction with cyclooxygenase than aspirin and NSAIDs.

There are two forms of cyclooxygenase, encoded by different genes. Cyclooxygenase-1 (COX1) is constitutively expressed in most cells and is the only isoform in mature platelets. As mentioned above, COX2 is induced by inflammation. In the stomach, COX1-derived prostaglandins protect the gastric mucosa

11-1 Selected TRP Channels Involved in Pain

Channel	Family	Exemplary Stimuli[1]	Location
TRPV1	TRPV	$T > 43°C$[2] Capsaicin Resiniferatoxin H^+, anandamide, 2APB[4]	PN[3]
TRPV2	TRPV	$T > 52°C$, 2APB	PN
TRPV3	TRPV	$T > 30–39°C$, camphor, 2APB	PN, tongue
TRPV4	TRPV	$T > 25°C$ Noxious mechanical stimuli H^+, hypotonicity, arachidonic acid metabolites	PN
TRPM8	TRPM[5]	Cold sensing. $T < 23–28°C$ Menthol, icilin	PN
TRPA1	TRPA	Cold sensing. $T < 18°C$ Mechanical stimuli Bradykinin Mustard, wasabi, garlic	PN

[1] TRP channels typically respond to multiple stimuli. Most studies have utilized cellular expression systems and investigated single stimuli, but TRP channels can integrate multiple stimuli through allosteric mechanisms.
[2] The heat-sensing TRP channels, TRPV1-4, share a C-terminal domain that is responsible for this property.
[3] PN = peripheral nociceptor (with cell bodies in dorsal root ganglia).
[4] 2APB = 2-aminoethoxydiphenyl borate.
[5] Another member of the TRPM family, TRPM5, is expressed on the tongue where it is involved in transducing sweet, bitter, and umami taste.

11-3 **Bradykinin**

Bradykinin, a 9-amino-acid peptide, is one of the most potent pronociceptive, or *algesic*, substances known. It is capable of eliciting intense pain and burning sensations when administered to humans. The term *bradykinin* (*brady*, slow; *kinin*, movement) refers to the substance's ability to produce a slow-onset contraction of smooth muscle in the gut in vitro.

Bradykinin and kallidin are products of the kininogen propeptides (resulting from two splice variants) released by the enzymatic action of kallikreins, which are primarily concentrated in plasma but also can be found in smaller quantities in tissues. Kallikreins are inactive in their basal state; they become activated when they are cleaved by factor VII, a protease that also plays a role in blood clotting cascades. Factor VII is activated in response to contact with collagen and other negatively charged substances exposed during tissue injury. After they are formed, bradykinin and kallidin promote pain and inflammation; thus factor VII is primarily responsible for the coordinated response of blood clotting, pain, and inflammation that occurs after tissue is damaged.

Bradykinin acts via two G protein-coupled receptors, termed B_1 and B_2. B_2 receptors are highly expressed by primary nociceptors, and are important in acute pain and inflammation; B_1 receptors may contribute more to chronic pain and inflammation. Surprisingly, mice lacking TRPA1 or TRPV1 channels have a markedly diminished nociceptive response to bradykinin. It appears that the B_2 receptor is coupled to these channels via activation of phospholipase $C\beta$ (PLCβ), which is activated by G_q-linked receptors (Chapter 4). This observation raises the interesting possibility that other neurotransmitter receptors expressed in nociceptors, such as $5HT_{2A}$ and P2Y receptors, that are also G_q linked and activate PLCβ, may stimulate TRPA1 and TRPV1. Additionally, it suggests that TRP channels may serve as effectors of G protein-coupled receptor activation.

11-2   **Characteristics of Primary Nociceptive Fibers**

	A$_\delta$ Fibers	C Fibers
Diameter	2–5 μm	0.2–1.5 μm
Conduction velocity	6–30 m/s	0.5–2 m/s
Myelination	Thinly myelinated	Unmyelinated
Time to conduct 1 meter	Approximately 0.05 sec	Approximately 2.0 sec
Responsiveness to stimuli	High-threshold mechanoreceptors, mechanothermal receptors	Polymodal
Blocked by	Pressure	Low doses of local anesthetics

from the acid environment; accordingly, aspirin and nonselective NSAIDs such as ibuprofen, which inhibit COX1 can produce gastric ulceration. This side effect of NSAIDs motivated the development of **selective COX2 inhibitors (coxibs)**, such as **rofecoxib** and the less selective **celecoxib.** Unfortunately, selective COX2 inhibitors alter the balance between the eicosanoids thromboxane and prostacyclin leading to cardiovascular

risks. Thromboxane A$_2$ (TXA$_2$) is produced in platelets from prostaglandin H$_2$. TXA$_2$ induces platelet aggregation and is a potent vasoconstrictor. Given its platelet source, it is largely COX1 derived. Prostacyclin is synthesized in endothelial cells from prostaglandin H$_2$. Prostacyclin has a homeostatic role in limiting platelet aggregation; it also acts as a vasodilator. An unintended consequence of selective COX2 inhibitors is to

---

11-4   **First and Second Pain**

When a person forcefully stubs a toe or otherwise hurts a distal extremity, he or she experiences two distinct sensations. The first sensation arrives swiftly and is sharp and brief; the second sensation, which arrives after a brief delay, typically burns, is more unpleasant, and tends to be more prolonged. The first sensation, or *first pain,* is caused by more rapidly conducting A$_\delta$ fibers, whereas the more aversive *second pain* is caused by slowly conducting C fibers.

Differences in the timing of first and second pain are directly related to the conduction velocities of A$_\delta$ and C fibers. Imagine accidentally placing a finger tip into a cup of scalding coffee. If the distance from finger tip to spinal cord were one meter, an A$_\delta$ fiber conducting at 20 m/s would deliver the message to the CNS in 0.05 seconds. A C fiber conducting at 0.5 m/s would require two seconds to deliver the same message. Under such circumstances, the response of A$_\delta$ fibers leads to a rapid spinal reflex that causes the finger to be withdrawn and thus rescued from further harm. In contrast, the response of

C fibers is slow enough that, by itself, it would have permitted serious tissue damage to occur.

These two types of fibers can be separated in other ways summarized in **11-2** with a view to better understanding pain. A$_\delta$ fibers are relatively sensitive to pressure but are relatively insensitive to low doses of local anesthetics. Conversely, C fibers are more sensitive to **local anesthetics.** Because of such differences it is possible to selectively suppress the firing of A$_\delta$ fibers, for example, by inflating a blood pressure cuff around a limb, and the firing of C fibers, for example, by an appropriate injection of local anesthetic. The blocking of A$_\delta$ fibers by such means suppresses the sharp first pain that occurs in response to an acute noxious stimulus, but, interestingly, that may cause the delayed second pain to be stronger and more aversive. These findings suggest that A$_\delta$ fiber stimulation may reduce C fiber–mediated nociception. This may be the reason why slapping or rubbing a patch of skin prior to receiving an injection may decrease the overall aversiveness of the experience.

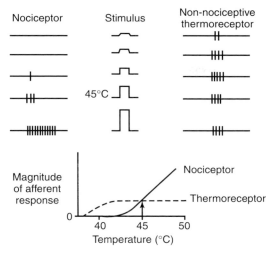

11-3 **Physiologic recordings from two cutaneous primary sensory neurons.** Action potentials from both are compared as the intensity of a stimulus increases (*top to bottom*); 45°C is the threshold for tissue damage. The nociceptor (*left*) has a higher threshold, but exhibits an increasing firing rate once within the noxious range. The thermoreceptor, which detects nonnoxious heat, has a low threshold and exhibits no change in firing rate as the stimulus intensity increases.

tip the balance between TXA_2 and prostacyclin toward TXA_2 and thus a prothrombotic state. As is now well known, selective COX2 inhibitors initially became very popular as analgesic and anti-inflammatory drugs, but an increased incidence of cardiovascular side effects has sharply limited their use.

NEUROGENIC INFLAMMATION

Neurogenic inflammation results from the release of peptides from the peripheral terminals of nociceptive neurons into surrounding tissues. Such "retrograde" release occurs in response to tissue damage, to endogenous inflammatory mediators, or perhaps to exogenous chemicals. Neurogenic inflammation is a normal homeostatic response to inflammation or tissue damage in diverse organs, including skin, joints, gut, bladder, and the respiratory system. When inappropriate or excessive, however, it may contribute to several diseases, possibly including **arthritis** and **asthma**.

Peptides released by nerve terminals in neurogenic inflammation are the tachykinins, substance P and neurokinin A, and calcitonin gene-related peptide (CGRP) **11-7** and **11-9**. Recall from Chapter 7 that CGRP is

generated from the calcitonin gene via alternative splicing. Substance P causes vasodilation and extravasation of plasma proteins from capillaries, which contributes to the generation of bradykinin from kininogen (see **11-3**) and release of other proinflammatory mediators such as prostaglandins. In addition, it causes mast cell degranulation with release of histamine. Neurogenic inflammation is attenuated by antagonists of the NK_1 (substance P) receptor and in genetically engineered mice lacking NK_1 receptors. CGRP causes vasodilation and has pronociceptive effects, but its role in extravasation of plasma proteins from blood vessels is unclear. Recently, neurogenic inflammation and, in particular, CGRP released from primary nociceptors with cell bodies in the trigeminal ganglion have been hypothesized to be major contributors to **migraine**, which is covered in Chapter 19.

PROCESSING OF PAIN-RELATED INFORMATION BY THE CNS

Dorsal Horn of the Spinal Cord

The gray matter of the spinal cord is organized as a laminar structure; generally 10 layers are identified

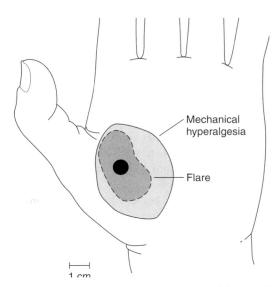

11-4 **Sensitization of tissue.** A burn (*solid dark circle*) produces an area of reddening, or a flare (*dashed line*), that extends beyond the injury and is caused by increased blood flow. An even larger area (*solid line*) is characterized by enhanced sensitivity to subsequent stimulation, which reflects the sensitization of nociceptive neurons.

11-5. **Chemical structures** of aspirin, acetaminophen, representative nonselective NSAIDs (indomethacin, ibuprofen, and naproxen), and the COX2 selective celecoxib.

11-8. Laminae I–VI make up the dorsal horn, with lamina VI discernible only in the cervical and lumbar enlargements of the cord. Based on the appearance of freshly cut sections, lamina II often is referred to as the substantia gelatinosa. Primary nociceptive neurons synapse in the dorsal horn of the spinal cord on neurons in laminae I, II, IV, and V. (Axons from the face and head synapse in the trigeminal nucleus in the brainstem as noted earlier.) Within these laminae, the primary nociceptive neurons synapse on both projection neurons, which relay information to the brainstem, hypothalamus, and thalamus, and to local circuit neurons, including both excitatory and inhibitory interneurons. Local circuit neurons not only process afferent information but also convey nociceptive information to the autonomic nervous system and to motor neurons involved in local withdrawal reflexes. Diverse inputs may converge on a single dorsal horn cell. Such inputs include those from descending

analgesic pathways, discussed below. Consequently, the dorsal horn is not a simple relay station but an important site of integration for both nociceptive and analgesic information.

The existence of multiple inputs on individual dorsal horn neurons may help to explain the phenomenon of *referred pain*. Such pain arises in viscera but is experienced as emanating from the body surface. Pain that originates in particular deep structures tends to correspond to the same sites of referred pain in all individuals. The pain of cardiac ischemia, for example, is commonly experienced as running from the chest down the left arm. Likewise, pain that originates in the diaphragm is often referred to the shoulder. These and other types of referred pain are most likely caused by the convergence of axons of visceral and cutaneous nociceptive neurons on the same neurons in the dorsal horn of the spinal cord. When a single neuron in the dorsal horn receives both visceral and cutaneous

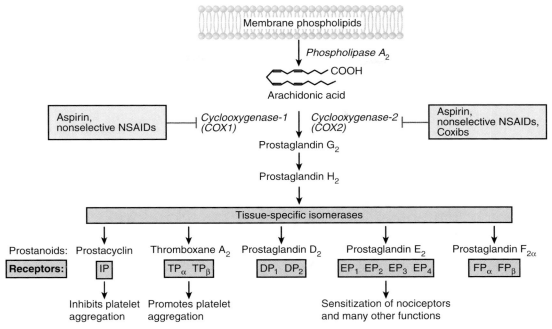

11–6 **Metabolism of arachidonic acid.** A variety of stimuli, including inflammatory, mechanical, and chemical stimuli, activate phospholipase A_2 (PLA_2), which releases arachidonic acid from membrane phospholipids. Arachidonic acid is converted by prostaglandin G/H synthases, which include cyclooxygenases-1 (COX1) or -2 (COX2) and hydroperoxidase. Tissue-specific isomerase enzymes then produce various prostanoids of which prostaglandin E_2, produced in a variety of tissues, is important in sensitization of nociceptors. Aspirin and nonselective NSAIDs inhibit both COX1 and COX2. Coxibs inhibit only COX2.

inputs, higher processing centers of the brain cannot distinguish the source of pain and refer it to the body surface.

Neurotransmitters and Receptors in the Dorsal Horn

Stimulation of afferent A_δ and C fibers evokes fast excitatory postsynaptic potentials in dorsal horn neurons, which appear to be mediated by glutamate, the major neurotransmitter used by dorsal root ganglion neurons. These fast responses to glutamate are mediated by both AMPA and NMDA receptors. Certain projection neurons with cell bodies in the dorsal horn, which are described as nociceptive specific, exhibit high electrophysiologic thresholds. Others, which are referred to as wide dynamic range (WDR) neurons, receive inputs from both nonnociceptive and nociceptive neurons and respond to stimuli of increasing intensity with a corresponding increase in their rate of firing.

High-intensity stimulation of primary nociceptive neurons produces additional slow excitatory postsynaptic potentials in dorsal horn neurons, which most likely are caused by the release of various neuropeptides or other substances. Indeed, primary nociceptive neurons contain a complex array of neuropeptides, among which the most abundant are CGRP and the tachykinins, substance P and neurokinin A (Chapter 7). Substance P is synthesized in some C fiber neurons and is coreleased with glutamate; CGRP is found in subsets of both A_δ and C fiber neurons. It was long believed that substance P played a central role in pain. However, mice with disruption of the gene encoding substance P exhibit only subtle differences in pain behavior compared with wild-type mice. Moreover, **NK1 receptor antagonists** failed in clinical trials for pain.

The plasticity of dorsal horn neurons is believed to be an important factor in persistent pain. As previously mentioned, the sensitization of cutaneous nociceptors can cause the sensitization of dorsal horn neurons. Evidence suggests, for example, that nerve injury leads to neuropathic pain because it triggers an

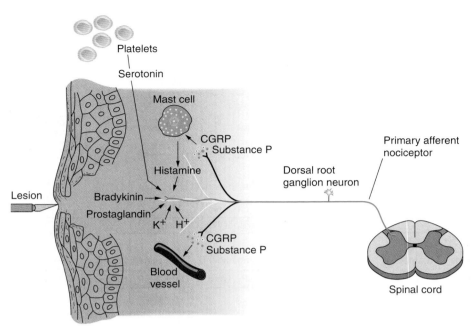

11-7 **Neurogenic inflammation.** Tissue injury causes the release of bradykinin and the activation of cyclooxygenases, which in turn leads to the generation of prostaglandins and other mediators, such as K^+ and H^+. Bradykinins and prostaglandins activate and sensitize neurons. Substance P and CGRP, released in retrograde fashion from free nerve endings, dilate local blood vessels. Substance P has also been shown to cause fluid and protein to extravasate from vessels and to trigger the release of histamine from mast cells. (Adapted with permission from Kandel ER, Schwartz JH, Jessell TM. *Principles of Neural Science*. 4th ed. New York: McGraw-Hill; 2000.)

NMDA receptor–mediated, long-lasting increase in the excitability of dorsal horn neurons **11-5**.

Multiple Pathways to the Brain

Axons of projection neurons from the dorsal horn cross the midline and ascend into the anterolateral quadrant of the spinal cord (see **11-1**). However, a small but significant number of axons remain ipsilateral. These uncrossed axons may contribute to the return of pain after unilateral neurosurgical lesions of the anterolateral spinal cord have been made to alleviate intractable pain. Most of the nociceptive neurons that ascend into the anterolateral quadrant terminate in the reticular formation of the brainstem (spinoreticular tract) and in the thalamus (spinothalamic tract). The spinoreticular tract, which originates largely in laminae VII and VIII of the dorsal horn of the spinal cord, lacks precise topographical information in that the reticular neurons receive dorsal horn inputs that represent wide receptive fields. The reticular neurons send projections to many brain regions, among which

is a prominent input to the thalamus (the reticulothalamic tract). Consistent with this wiring pattern is the theory that the spinoreticular tract contributes to general aspects of pain perception; for example, it may alert an individual to the onset of pain.

Neurons in the spinothalamic tract originate in laminae I and V–VII. A related projection extends from laminae I and V of the dorsal horn to the midbrain (spinomesencephalic tract). A major target of this spinomesencephalic tract is the periaqueductal gray matter (PAG) of the midbrain. Neurons of the PAG represent an important site of convergence between ascending axons that carry sensory information from the spinal cord and descending axons that arise from neurons in brain structures involved in the processing of emotion, such as the amygdala (Chapter 14). Although the PAG receives nociceptive input from the spinal cord, it is not a pain relay nucleus because destruction of the PAG does not alter pain threshold. Rather, the PAG appears to be involved in the brain's endogenous system of analgesia. Other nociceptive neurons project to the

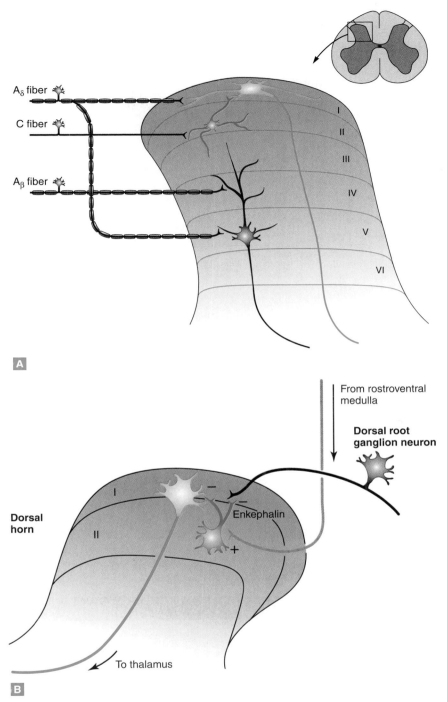

11-8 **Laminae of the dorsal horn of the spinal cord. A.** One of several possible synaptic arrangements of A_δ and C fibers. A_δ fibers synapse on projection neurons in lamina I. These neurons receive indirect input from C fibers that synapse on interneurons in lamina II. Lamina V neurons are projection neurons that receive direct inputs from both A_δ fibers and C fibers that carry information about innocuous stimuli (not shown). (Adapted with permission from Kandel ER, Schwartz JH, Jessell TM. *Principles of Neural Science*, 4th ed. New York: McGraw-Hill; 2000.) **B.** Descending analgesia in the dorsal horn. Projections from the rostral ventral medulla synapse on enkephalinergic interneurons in lamina II. These interneurons in turn synapse on dorsal horn neurons in lamina I, inhibiting their firing and thereby interrupting the flow of nociceptive information.

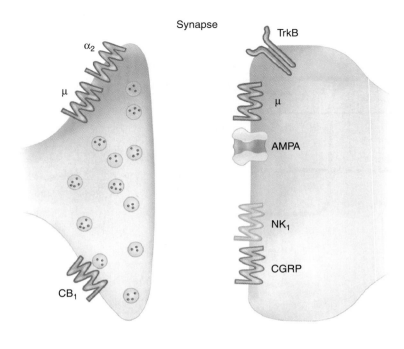

11-9 **Neurotransmitters and receptors on synapses in the dorsal horn.** The nerve terminal on the left is the central terminal of a primary nociceptive neurons (with its cell body in the dorsal root ganglion, or DRG). The process on the right is from the dendrite of a dorsal horn nociceptive neuron. Shown in the extrasynaptic regions of the primary nociceptive terminal are three G protein-coupled receptors (μ opiate, CB_1 cannabinoid, and α_2-adrenergic) that can inhibit neurotransmitter release in response to analgesic signals described in the text. This presynaptic terminal releases glutamate and multiple peptides, perhaps substance P and CGRP. The dorsal horn neuron is shown expressing the AMPA glutamate receptor, which mediates fast synaptic transmission, the substance P (NK_1) receptor, and the CGRP receptor, all of which mediate pronociceptive signals. It is also shown expressing the μ opioid receptor, which could mediate antinociceptive signals. Finally, it expresses TrkB, the receptor for brain-derived neurotrophic factor (BDNF), which may be released from activated microglia, to contribute to central sensitization, a process that can contribute to chronic neuropathic and inflammatory pain.

hypothalamus and amygdala, where they most likely mediate some of the autonomic, emotional, and neuroendocrine responses to pain.

Neurons that project from the dorsal horn (or from the trigeminal nucleus) to the thalamus segregate into two divisions. In the *lateral division* of the spinothalamic tract, axons that relay information from the trunk and extremities terminate in the ventroposterolateral (VPL) nucleus of the thalamus, and axons that relay information from the trigeminal system terminate in the ventroposteromedial (VPM) nucleus of the thalamus. In the *medial division,* axons terminate mostly in the intralaminar nuclei of the thalamus.

Because the lateral division is phylogenetically recent, it is often called the *neospinothalamic tract* (see **11-1**). It is somatotopically organized and is responsible for the localizing and discriminative aspects of pain. Consistent with this function, the dorsal horn neurons of laminae I and V, from which the neospinothalamic tract originates, have small receptive fields that permit accurate localization of nociceptive stimuli. The VPL and VPM nuclei of the thalamus receive inputs from all modalities of somatic sensation. Less than 10% of the neurons in these thalamic nuclei respond to nociceptive stimuli; the majority respond to touch and proprioceptive inputs from

11-5 Neuropathic Pain

Damage to neurons in nociceptive pathways generally causes some loss of normal pain sensation. However, after a delay, such damage can, rather unpredictably, result in neuropathic pain. Neuropathic pain can be produced by several disease processes that injure nociceptive neurons or lead to cell death either in the periphery or the central nervous system. Common causes include **postherpetic neuralgia**, **diabetic neuropathy, nerve compression** (including spinal disc disease)**, or **cutting of nerves** (as may occur in accidents, amputations, or even in routine surgical procedures). Postherpetic neuralgia, or **shingles,** is caused by the reactivation of a latent Herpes varicella-zoster virus, or **chicken pox** virus. This type of virus can remain dormant in primary sensory neurons for decades and become reactivated by unknown mechanisms. Shingles generally affects a single spinal nerve or cranial nerve branch and thus affects a single dermatome. Because of damage to the nerve, persistent and sometimes severe neuropathic pain may result. One well-known and dramatic example of neuropathic pain is **trigeminal neuralgia** (also called **tic douloureux**) which produces severe lancinating pain in a trigeminal nerve distribution. The cause appears to be compression damage to the trigeminal nerve where it exits the skull. Patients with neuropathic pain may experience allodynia, hyperalgesia, and spontaneous pain, which may include persistent burning, paresthesias such as pins and needles, or unprovoked paroxysms of sharp pain.

Neuropathic pain is initiated by damage to peripheral or central nociceptive neurons. Persistent pain syndromes can therefore result not only from damage to cutaneous nociceptors, as in postherpetic neuralgia, but also from damage to spinal or thalamic neurons involved in nociception. Sensitization of damaged peripheral (or central) nociceptors is thought to produce high-intensity action potentials that cause plasticity in the higher order neurons to which they project. One implication is that surgical interruption of damaged peripheral nerves (eg, resection of a neuroma that may form after injury) or lesioning of central structures in an effort to relieve pain may not only prove ineffective, but also may produce new neuropathic pain on its own account.

Even severed nerves may contribute to central plasticity, not only by releasing K^+, H^+, and ATP onto surrounding neurons, but also as a result of the significant molecular changes that they undergo; a large number of genes are activated or suppressed within the cell body of a deafferented neuron. If these neurons retain their central connections, they may also contribute to the process of sensitization. Indeed, it is still unclear whether central sensitization is due more to the damaged nociceptors or the surrounding nociceptors they influence.

In a rodent model, central sensitization that produces tactile allodynia has been attributed to *brain-derived neurotrophic factor (BDNF)* released by a highly circuitous route. Damage to peripheral nociceptors may lead, by unknown mechanisms, to activation of microglia in the spinal cord, which then express $P2X_4$ receptors. These respond to ATP stimulation with release of BDNF, which, in turn, sensitizes dorsal horn nociceptive neurons. Whether or not this scenario turns out to be correct, it serves as a reminder that microglia, other glia, growth factors, and perhaps additional mediators may play an important role in sensitization and persistent pain.

Treatment of neuropathic pain has proved challenging. **NSAIDs** are not adequately effective for most people. **Opiates** only partially alleviate neuropathic pain and, as discussed later in this Chapter and in Chapter 15, their long-term use poses the risk of dependence and the far more consequential risk of addiction. Much treatment relies, therefore, on a variety of **antidepressants** and **anticonvulsants**, which are useful in some patients but not others. The mechanisms underlying the antipain action of these treatments remain poorly understood. It is generally believed that the utility of certain antidepressants in the treatment of pain syndromes is related to blockade of norepinephrine reuptake (Chapters 14). Safer and more effective treatments are very much in need.

dorsal column neurons that reach the thalamus by way of the medial lemniscus. VPL and VPM neurons, including those that receive nociceptive inputs, project somatotopically to the primary somatic sensory cortex of the parietal lobe.

Because the medial division of the spinothalamic tract is phylogenetically old it is often called the *pale-ospinothalamic tract*. Unlike VPL and VPM neurons, whose projections are restricted to somatosensory cortex, intralaminar thalamic neurons have widespread cortical projections, in particular, to association cortex and prefrontal cortex. The paleospinothalamic tract, like the spinoreticular tract, lacks precise soma-totopic organization. The dorsal horn neurons from which it originates, which are typically found in lam-inae that lie deeper in the spinal cord than those that give rise to the neospinothalamic tract, have large and complex receptive fields; indeed, the receptive fields of some of these cells comprise the entire body. Such large receptive fields are consistent not with the pre-cise localization of pain but with more generalized responses. Thus, it is believed that the pale-ospinothalamic tract, like spinoreticular, reticu-lothalamic, and spinohypothalamic projections, is involved in the alerting, emotional, and motivational aspects of pain.

Itch Pathways

While just an annoyance for many people, itch can be a persistent and debilitating symptom for individuals with **atopic dermatitis**, **liver disease**, **renal disease**, or **HIV infection**. One of the most potent stimulators of itch is histamine acting on H_1 receptors. A class of histamine-responsive unmyelinated C fibers and second-order lamina I dorsal horn neurons 11-8 have been found; these respond poorly, if at all, to nociceptive stimuli. Experiments in mice have found *gastrin-releasing peptide (GRP)* containing neurons that project to laminae I and II of the dorsal horn, but the GRP receptor is expressed only in lam-ina I. Mice lacking the GRP receptor have normal pain responses to thermal, mechanical, and inflam-matory stimuli, but have a marked reduction in the itch response to chemicals that cause histamine release from mast cells. Because multiple animal models have been used, it is not clear how the story adds up, but it would be useful to have additional antipruritic compounds because the current **hista-mine H_1 receptor antagonists** (that do not cross the blood–brain barrier and thus do not produce drowsi-ness) have only limited efficacy. Examples of such agents are given in Chapter 6.

ENDOGENOUS MECHANISMS OF ANALGESIA

Endogenous Opioids and Related Peptides

The endogenous opioid peptides (Chapter 7) are derived from three distinct genes that encode large precursor proteins—proopiomelanocortin (POMC), proenkephalin, and prodynorphin. A fourth precursor, proorphanin FQ–nociceptin, encodes the ligand for the orphanin FQ–nociceptin receptor 11-10 . Despite significant homologies with opioid peptides, orphanin FQ–nociceptin may exert antiopioid effects and may promote nociception. Two additional putative opioid peptides, endomorphin 1 and 2, also have been described. In vitro, these peptides bind to the μ opioid receptor with greater affinity and selectivity than that of any other endogenous peptide. However, their sta-tus as endogenous signaling peptides will remain uncertain until their mode of synthesis is clarified.

Molecular cloning studies have identified three types of opioid receptors: μ, δ, and κ. Pharmacologic studies have suggested that subtypes of opioid receptors may exist, perhaps as a result of alternative splicing or post-translational modifications of μ, κ, and δ receptors, and perhaps as a result of their ability to form het-erodimers, which exhibit unique ligand binding and functional properties. The relative affinities of differ-ent opioid peptides for these receptors are described in Chapter 7. Despite its homology to the δ opioid recep-tor, ORL_1, the orphanin FQ–nociceptin receptor lacks significant affinity for opioid ligands, including the nonselective opioid antagonist **naloxone**.

All of the opioid receptors, as well as ORL_1, are seven-transmembrane domain receptors linked to het-erotrimeric $G_{i/o}$ proteins. $G_{i/o}$-coupled receptors inhibit the electrical firing of many types of neurons through activation of inwardly rectifying K^+ channels

Met-enkephalin	Y G G F M
Leu-enkephalin	Y G G F L
Dynorphin A	Y G G F L R R I R P K L K W D N Q
α-endorphin	Y G G F M T S E K S Q T P L V T
Orphanin FQ	F G G F T G A R K S A R K L A N Q

 11-10 **Amino acid sequences of endogenous opioid peptides and the related orphanin FQ-nociceptin peptide.**

(GIRKs) and the closing of voltage-gated Ca^{2+} channels (Chapter 2). Opioid receptors also inhibit adenylyl cyclase and the cAMP-protein kinase A pathway (Chapter 4), which may partly mediate their longer-term effects such as tolerance, dependence, withdrawal, and **addiction** (Chapter 15).

Descending Analgesic Pathways

Because severe pain can disorganize behavior and thereby interfere with the ability to fight or escape danger, mechanisms that suppress pain at times of extreme emergency have significant survival value. Some of the most striking examples of such phenomena have been observed during combat situations in which severely wounded soldiers may deny that they are feeling pain. The threshold level of stress for activating descending analgesic systems must be high, or pain would lose its survival value.

Rodent models of *stress-induced analgesia*, which can be produced, for example, by foot shock, reveal that this phenomenon is partly opioid dependent (blocked by **naloxone**) and partly opioid independent. A key neural substrate for stress-induced analgesia is the PAG of the brainstem, which receives projections from pain pathways (as discussed earlier) and from the amygdala (Chapter 14). Microinjection of **morphine** directly into the PAG produces analgesia independently of stress. Microinjections of naloxone into this region partially block stress-induced analgesia. The nonopioid component appears to be dependent on endogenous cannabinoids. Foot shock in rats causes release of two endocannabinoids, *2-arachidonylglycerol (2-AG)* and *anandamide* (Chapter 8), and the resulting analgesia is blocked by **CB₁ receptor antagonists** (eg, **rimonabant**).

The rostral ventral medulla (RVM), a region of the brainstem that includes the nucleus raphe magnus, the nucleus gigantocellularis, and the adjacent reticular formation, is another important site for analgesia. Microinjections of morphine in the RVM produce analgesia; local electrical stimulation of either the PAG or RVM also produces analgesia, presumably causing release of opioids and other analgesic endogenous neurotransmitters.

The PAG projects to the RVM, which in turn projects to the dorsal horn by means of the dorsolateral funiculus of the spinal cord **11–1**. Cutting fibers that descend in the dorsolateral funiculus blocks analgesia produced by electrical stimulation of the PAG. High levels of endogenous opioid peptides and opioid receptors are found within the PAG, RVM, and dorsal horn, and neurons of both the PAG and RVM can be activated by opioids. Because opioid receptors generally produce inhibitory effects on neuronal firing, the ability of endogenous opioid peptides or opiate drugs to activate neurons within the PAG, RVM, and other brain regions is dependent on an anatomic arrangement whereby opioid receptors inhibit inhibitory GABAergic interneurons in these brain regions. Neurons of the RVM that project to the dorsal horn activate enkephalinergic interneurons that are located in the dorsal horn. The neurotransmitter involved in opioid-mediated descending analgesia was long believed to be serotonin from the nucleus raphe magnus (Chapter 6). Indeed, serotonergic neurons do project to the dorsal horn but do not appear to be directly involved in opioid analgesia. Rather, they are thought to play a more complex modulatory role. This theory is consistent with the clinical observation that selective serotonin reuptake inhibitor (**SSRI**) antidepressants, such as **fluoxetine** (Chapter 14), lack analgesic properties.

Within the RVM, three physiologic classes of cells project to the dorsal horn. "On" cells are excited by noxious stimuli and inhibited by opioids; "off" cells are inhibited by noxious stimuli and excited by opioids; and neutral cells do not respond to noxious stimuli or opioids. The "off" cells are involved in the classic descending analgesic circuit, and glutamate may be the critical neurotransmitter that conveys descending analgesic information to the dorsal horn. Serotonin is found in neutral cells. Orphanin FQ–nociceptin appears to inhibit opiate-activated descending analgesic outflow from the RVM, and may be responsible for similar activity in the PAG.

Within the dorsal horn, enkephalin-containing interneurons inhibit dorsal horn neurons at the origin of the spinothalamic tract by making direct postsynaptic contact with them. Indirect evidence suggests that presynaptic inhibition of primary nociceptive neurons by opioid-containing interneurons also occurs, but anatomic evidence for this arrangement is lacking.

ANALGESIC MEDICATIONS

Opiates

In contrast to local anesthetics, which produce numbness, analgesia produced by stimulation of the PAG or RVM and analgesia produced by morphine are modality specific with regard to somatic sensation: they suppress only nociception, and do not affect touch, proprioception, or sensation of nonnoxious temperatures. This specificity can be confirmed electrophysiologically:

nociceptive neurons in lamina V of the dorsal horn are inhibited by analgesia produced by PAG stimulation or by opiates, but nonnociceptive neurons in lamina III are unaffected by either type of analgesia.

The combination of efficacy in treating pain and, while oft forgotten, the lack of degradation of other sensory modalities has made opiates **11-11** the most important class of drugs for treating severe pain in the history of medicine. The dark side of opiates is well known. They have a significant risk for producing addiction (Chapter 15).

Opiates often are called narcotics because of their potent sedative effects. However, the term *narcotic* also has a legal definition in the United States and many other countries, which is used for regulatory purposes by the Food and Drug Administration and the Drug Enforcement Agency. For legal purposes, the term narcotic is applied to both opiate and nonopiate drugs with substantial abuse liability. The production, distribution, and prescription of these drugs is closely monitored and regulated. Some of these drugs, such as **heroin**, have no legally acceptable use outside of research in the United States.

Morphine-like opiates comprise the most important class of compounds used in the treatment of severe acute pain and severe cancer pain. These drugs bind preferentially to the μ opioid receptor, which appears to be the most significant opioid receptor involved in both supraspinal and spinal sites of analgesia. μ Receptors are located in areas known to be involved in descending analgesia, including the PAG, RVM, and dorsal horn of the spinal cord. They also are found in regions such as the ventral tegmental area (VTA) of the midbrain and the nucleus accumbens (ventral striatum), where they are responsible for the reinforcing effects of opiates, and in the locus ceruleus (LC) and other regions that mediate aspects of physical dependence on opiates (Chapter 15).

The usefulness of morphine-like drugs is limited by their side effects, such as constipation and respiratory depression, and the risks associated with their use, including dependence and addiction. Repeated use of these drugs also results in tolerance to their analgesic effects. Considerable progress has been made in understanding the molecular adaptations that contribute to tolerance at the cellular level, as will be discussed in Chapter 15.

A large number of morphine-like opiates are available clinically **19-2**. These drugs differ in their pharmacokinetic properties, particularly with regard to their suitability for oral administration, time of onset, and half-life, and their relative affinity for the μ receptor.

11-11 Chemical structures of representative opiate analgesics.

Codeine and **oxycodone** are examples of lower-potency μ agonists; both are effective when administered orally and are commonly combined with **aspirin** or **acetaminophen** (eg, **Percocet**). **Dilaudid** and **fentanyl** are examples of very high-potency μ agonists; the former is suitable for oral administration, whereas the latter is suitable for parenteral or transdermal administration. As previously discussed, the use of each of these μ agonists is associated with tolerance and physical dependence and the risk for addiction. Indeed, abuse of these various prescription opiates, of low and high potency, is a growing problem in the United States today.

The use of partial agonists at the μ receptor, such as **buprenorphine,** may be associated with fewer liabilities; it is believed that such agents sufficiently activate the receptor to induce some analgesia but not so much as to induce the molecular adaptations that underlie tolerance and dependence. Partial agonists also may carry a lower risk for abuse because higher doses of the drug do not lead to greater behavioral effects.

Benzomorphan opiate drugs, such as **pentazocine,** exhibit a high affinity for κ opioid receptors **11-3** . Like many opiates, κ receptor agonists produce sedation and miosis. Although in contrast to μ agonists they are often aversive, resulting in negative emotional effects, they can be abused and can produce addictive behaviors. κ Receptors are found in the dorsal horn of the spinal cord, in deep cortical layers, and in many other brain regions. Many κ agonist drugs possess properties of μ receptor antagonists and may precipitate withdrawal symptoms in individuals who are dependent on morphine-like drugs. Despite their aversive properties, κ agonists frequently are used instead

of μ agonists for obstetric analgesia to reduce the risk of respiratory depression in the newborn.

Considerable effort has been aimed at the development of small-molecule δ agonists during the past two decades; however, only peptides, which lack substantial clinical utility, remain the available ligands with a high affinity for the δ receptor. δ Receptors are concentrated not only in the limbic system and in the dorsal horn of the spinal cord, but also in regions of the brain that have no clear association with pain. Like κ opioid receptors, δ receptors appear to mediate analgesia at the level of the dorsal horn. These receptors also mediate hypotension and miosis.

Opiate antagonists have clinical utility as well. **Naloxone,** a nonselective antagonist with a relative affinity of μ > δ > κ, is used to treat heroin and other opiate overdoses. Such treatment often is life saving, because opiate overdose can be fatal when it results in severe respiratory depression. A longer-acting nonselective antagonist, **naltrexone,** is used to prevent relapse to opiate use after detoxification and to limit relapse in alcoholism (Chapter 15).

Nonopioid, Non-NSAID Analgesics

The limitations of opiates and NSAIDs (discussed in an earlier section of this chapter) have spurred intense interest in the development of analgesics with novel mechanisms of action. Many of the chemical mediators outlined earlier in this chapter represent potential targets for new drugs, although some, including bradykinin and substance P antagonists, have proven disappointing to date. Currently there is interest in **CGRP receptor antagonists**, especially for the treatment of **migraine** (Chapter 19).

Descending noradrenergic projections from the LC or from related noradrenergic nuclei in the pons inhibit dorsal horn neurons, and thereby contribute to descending analgesia. The involvement of norepinephrine in descending analgesia may explain the analgesic effects of **tricyclic antidepressants,** including those selective for norepinephrine reuptake such as **desipramine** (Chapters 6 and 14), or combined serotonin-norepinephrine reuptake inhibitors (**SNRIs**) such as **duloxetine,** which often are effective in the treatment of **neuropathic pain**. Although many individuals with chronic neuropathic pain experience depression, the analgesic effects of these agents are clearly independent of their antidepressant effects, because the analgesic effects occur at lower doses and after shorter periods of treatment. In contrast to tricyclic antidepressants, SSRIs appear to lack analgesic properties. Norepinephrine is believed to exert its

---

11-3 **Classification of Representative Opiate Drugs**

μ Receptor Agonists

Codeine	Diacylmorphine (heroin)
Fentanyl	Hydrocodone
Hydromorphone	Levorphanol
Meperidine	Methadone
Morphine	Oxycodone

Partial μ Receptor Agonist

Buprenorphine

κ Receptor Agonists and μ Receptor Antagonists

Butorphanol	Dezocine
Nalbuphine	Pentazocine

antinociceptive effects by means of α_2-adrenergic receptors on dorsal horn neurons.

SELECTED READING

Agarwal N, Pacher P, Tegeder I, et al. Cannabinoids mediate analgesia largely via peripheral type 1 cannabinoid receptors in nociceptors. *Nature Neurosci.* 2007;10:870–879.

Akil H, Mayer DJ, Liebeskind JC. Antagonism of stimulation-produced analgesia by naloxone, a narcotic antagonist. *Science.* 1976;191:961–962.

Bautista DM, Jordt SE, Nikai T et al. TRPA1 mediates the inflammatory actions of environmental irritants and proalgesic agents. *Cell.* 2006;124:1269–1282.

Beecher HK. Pain in men wounded in battle. *Ann Surg.* 1946;123:96–105.

Calixto JB, Cabrini DA, Ferreira J, et al. Kinins in pain and inflammation. *Pain.* 2000;87:1–5.

Caterina MJ, Schumacher MA, Tominaga M, et al. The capsaicin receptor: A heat-activated ion channel in the pain pathway. *Nature.* 1997;389:816–824.

Cox JJ, Reimann F, Nicholas AK, et al. An SCN9A channelopathy causes congenital inability to experience pain. *Nature.* 2006;444:894–898.

Coull JA, Beggs S, Boudreau D, et al. BDNF from microglia causes the shift in neuronal anion gradient underlying neuropathic pain. *Nature.* 2005;438:1017–1021.

Craig AD. Pain mechanisms: labeled lines versus convergence in central processing. *Annu Rev Neurosci.* 2003;26:1–30.

Dhaka J, Viswanath V, Patapoutian A. TRP ion channels and temperature sensation. *Annu Rev Neurosci.* 2006;29:135–161.

FitzGerald GA, Patrono C. The coxibs, selective inhibitors of cyclooxygenase-2. *N Engl J Med.* 2001;345:433–442.

Gao K, Chen DO, Genzen JR, et al. Activation of serotonergic neurons in the raphe magnus is not necessary for morphine analgesia. *J Neurosci.* 1999;18:1860–1868.

Hohlmann AG, Suplita RL, Bolton NM, et al. An endocannabinoid mechanism for stress-induced analgesia. *Nature.* 2005;435:1108–1112.

Jordt SE, McKemy DD, et al. Lessons from peppers and peppermint: the molecular logic of thermosensation. *Curr Opin Neurobiol.* 2003;13:487–492.

Marchand F, Perretti M, McMahon SB. Role of the immune system in chronic pain. *Nature Rev Neurosci.* 2005;6:521–532.

Ramsey IS, Delling M, Clapham DE. An introduction to TRP channels. *Annu Rev Physiol.* 2006;68:619–647.

Sun Y-G, Chen Z-F. A gastrin-releasing peptide receptor mediates the itch sensation in the spinal cord. *Nature.* 2007;448:700–703.

Woolf CG, Ma Q. Nociceptors-noxious stimulus detectors. *Neuron.* 2007;55:353–364.

Zimmer A, Zimmer AM, Baffi J, et al. Hypoalgesia in mice with a targeted deletion of the tachykinin 1 gene. *Proc Natl Acad Sci.* 1998;95:2630–2635.

Sleep and Arousal

- Sleep and arousal are both active processes mediated by specific brain regions.

- Sleep can be divided into two phases, non-REM and REM sleep, the latter being characterized by brain activity resembling that observed during the waking state.

- The different physiologic functions of sleep are unknown; a role in memory consolidation is likely.

- The initiation of non-REM sleep is controlled in part by neurons in the preoptic/anterior hypothalamic area; the initiation of REM sleep is controlled by cells in the pontine tegmentum.

- Sleep is controlled both by circadian rhythms and by the homeostatic drive produced by periods of wakefulness.

- The suprachiasmatic nucleus is the primary pacemaker for the circadian regulation of sleep and other physiologic processes.

- Circadian rhythms are produced, in part, by the complex transcriptional regulation of "clock" genes that have been conserved throughout evolution.

- Sleep disorders are a primary cause of morbidity. A major advance is the finding that decreases in the hypothalamic neuropeptide orexin (also called hypocretin) contributes to narcolepsy.

- Benzodiazepines and related drugs are the most common pharmacologic treatments for insomnia.

- General anesthetics, comprising diverse classes of compounds, induce a non-REM sleep-like state characterized by amnesia, analgesia, immobility, and hypnosis. Most general anesthetics act by facilitating inhibitory ion channels (including ligand-gated channels) or inhibiting excitatory ion channels.

Defining sleep and arousal is not a simple matter. Sleep is clearly different from hibernation, coma, or states produced by general anesthesia. The first part of this chapter presents a broad overview of the neurobiology of sleep and arousal states. The second part covers some of the major sleep disorders, the mechanisms of which are slowly being elucidated. The third part discusses the pharmacologic treatment of these disorders.

As with other behavioral states such as fear and reward (Chapters 14 and 15), sleep states, such as rapid eye movement (REM) and nonrapid eye movement (NREM) sleep depend on specific neural circuits. However, certain phenomena that occur during sleep may also employ some of the circuitry that contributes to behavioral states during waking hours. **Night terrors**, for example, involve a partial arousal out of deep NREM sleep; patients exhibit powerful sympathetic activation including tachycardia, mydriasis, and diaphoresis, despite the fact that they remain asleep. In contrast, patients with **REM behavior disorder** may have bouts of violent behavior during REM sleep that are not accompanied by elevations in heart rate or blood pressure. Hence, states of sleep and arousal are complex and heterogeneous and cannot be explained by a simple rheostat model.

HISTORICAL OVERVIEW

Before the beginning of the 20th century, sleep was conceptualized as a passive process; sleep and arousal were believed to reflect a continuous gradient of levels of consciousness. It was believed that the level of arousal corresponded to the number of neurons that were actively engaged in processing information, in much the same way that the illumination from a light bulb varies depending on the amount of electric current it receives. During the second half of the 20th century, however, it was discovered that distinct cell groups in the brainstem and basal forebrain are active during periods of wakefulness versus sleep, demonstrating that the existing model was too simplistic.

An early clue that sleep is not merely a passive state but an active process emerged with the finding that particular brain regions must be intact for sleep to occur. It was discovered, for instance, that lesions of the anterior hypothalamus create a state of chronic insomnia, which suggested that activity in this region is necessary for sleep. In contrast, lesions involving the posterior hypothalamus create a state of hypersomnolence.

The advent of the electroencephalogram (EEG) in the 1930s permitted noninvasive assessment of brain function in humans. EEG is a technology that uses scalp electrodes to detect electrical signals produced by surface areas of the brain. The EEG has excellent temporal resolution, but because it integrates information coming from a very large number of neurons, it has very limited spatial resolution. For many years, EEG has been the central tool in studies of sleep and wakefulness. Accordingly, sleep states have been defined by EEG patterns.

In 1948 it was discovered that stimulation of the reticular formation of the brainstem elicits EEG arousal that is independent of sensory afferent pathways. Thus, arousal began to be viewed as an intrinsic property of the brain mediated by specific areas rather than a simple correlate of increased sensory input. This change in perspective roughly coincided with the discovery that alertness and arousal have a circadian rhythmicity that is independent of the number of hours an individual sleeps. Studies of sleep-deprived individuals indicated that alertness increases in the midmorning from a nadir that occurs late at night despite a longer period of continuous wakefulness. Such findings demonstrated that arousal is not a simple function of previous rest.

An important finding occurred during the late 1950s; cats with pontine lesions were reported to have undergone REM sleep without normal loss of muscle tone (atonia). In these studies the lesioned cats walked and exhibited attack and defense behaviors while they were unresponsive to external stimuli and their EEGs were in a REM state. Subsequent histochemical studies of the brainstem suggested that REM is a complex state that is controlled by several neurotransmitter systems; these studies laid the groundwork for electrophysiologic experiments in the 1970s that showed that the onset of REM is generated by cholinergic cells in the pontine tegmentum (PT) and that inputs from the noradrenergic locus ceruleus (LC) and serotonergic raphe nuclei (RN) inhibit REM (Chapter 6). These findings in turn led to the development of an influential reciprocal interaction model of REM regulation, which is described later in this chapter.

NORMAL STRUCTURE OF HUMAN SLEEP

Normal sleep exhibits fairly stereotypic patterns as measured by the EEG **12-1**. In adults, in the first hour of sleep, brain activity descends through a series of NREM stages into deep sleep. NREM stage 1 occurs during the transition between wakefulness and sleep and is defined by the presence of background theta

Awake – low voltage – random, fast

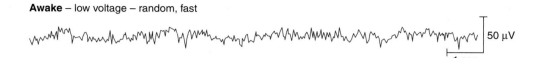

50 μV

1 sec

Drowsy – 8 to 12 cycles/s (cps) – alpha waves

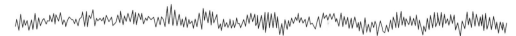

Stage 1 – 3 to 7 cps – theta waves

Theta waves

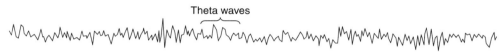

Stage 2 – 12 to 14 cps – sleep spindles and K complexes

Sleep spindles

K complex

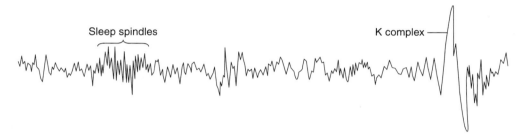

Delta sleep – $\frac{1}{2}$ to 2 cps – delta waves > 75 μV

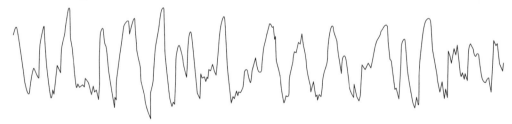

REM sleep – low voltage – random, fast with sawtooth waves

Sawtooth waves

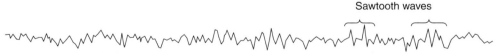

12-1 **EEG recordings of brain activity during various stages of sleep.** (Adapted with permission from Hauri P, Orr W. *Current Concepts: The Sleep Disorders*. Kalamazoo, MI: Upjohn; 1982.)

activity (4 to 7 Hz) that comprises more than 50% of each 30-second epoch. NREM stage 2 is composed of a background rhythm of theta activity with superimposed burst–pause waveforms such as K-complexes (high-amplitude, slow-frequency electronegative waves followed by electropositive waves) and spindles (brief bursts of 7 to 14 Hz activity). NREM stages 3 and 4, together referred to as slow-wave sleep, are defined by the presence of slow-wave (0.1 to 4 Hz), or delta, sleep activity that comprises 20% and 50% of each epoch of sleep, respectively. The predominance of low-frequency activity in slow-wave sleep indicates greater synchrony in neuronal firing and leads to a summed polarization and depolarization large enough to be recorded by the EEG.

After approximately 90 minutes of NREM sleep, the brain's electrical activity reascends through the same stages toward the first cycle of REM sleep. REM sleep is characterized by low-amplitude, mixed-frequency and desynchronized EEG activity that appears similar to the EEG of the normal waking state **12-1**. The desynchronization of the EEG results from individual neurons being in many different states of activity. This EEG pattern is accompanied by rapid eye movements—hence the name REM sleep—and profound relaxation of limb muscles. The NREM-REM sleep cycle repeats itself four or five times in the course of the night, with decreasing amounts of slow-wave sleep and increasing amounts of REM sleep in successive cycles **12-2**.

Intermittent awakenings are part of normal sleep and may serve an adaptive function; for example, they may enable changes in posture to minimize circulatory pooling or nerve compression, or appraisals of the environment to guard against possible threats. Humans are unaware of most of these brief awakenings because they experience retrograde amnesia for several minutes after resuming sleep. A common misperception is that dreams occur only during REM. In fact, dreams occur during all stages of sleep but tend to be more dramatic, varied, and vivid in the latter part of the night during REM.

DEVELOPMENTAL CHANGES IN SLEEP PATTERNS

Newborns spend 20 hours a day in sleep. These hours are characterized by an incomplete segregation between REM-like, or *active* sleep, and NREM-like, or *quiet* sleep. By 6 months of age, REM and NREM sleep can be reliably distinguished. During the first 3 years of life, humans begin to segregate sleep and waking until they become 2 distinct, consolidated periods. During adolescence a precipitous drop in slow-wave sleep activity occurs. With advancing age a gradual decline in total hours of sleep occurs together with an increase in the number of awakenings. The sixth and seventh decades of life are characterized by a decline in total slow-wave sleep

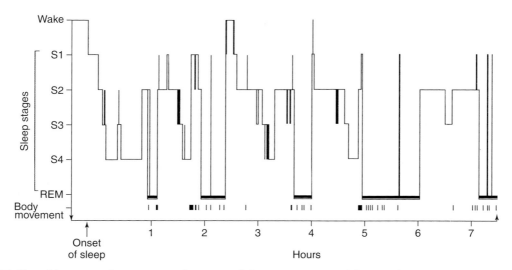

12-2 **Sleep histogram shows a normal pattern of sleep in a young adult**. Note that the time spent in REM increases as the night progresses. (Adapted with permission from Kryger MH, Roth T, Dement WC, eds. *Principles and Practice of Sleep Medicine,* 2nd ed. Philadelphia: WB Saunders; 1994.)

activity, which correlates with a decline in EEG amplitude. Elderly people experience more awakenings, complain more often of insomnia, and shift more of their sleep time to the day in the form of naps. Older people have a propensity to fall asleep at earlier hours and to have more early morning awakenings (phase advance of circadian rhythms). The decline in total sleep time in healthy older subjects is relatively modest, however, with more severe declines often related to medical conditions, pain, or untreated depression.

NORMAL PHYSIOLOGIC CHANGES DURING HUMAN SLEEP

Each sleep stage is accompanied by specific physiologic changes. Slow-wave sleep is associated with a reduced metabolic rate and a decline in brain and body temperature. Electrophysiologic features of all four NREM stages of sleep include increased firing of sleep-active centers in the anterior hypothalamus, hyperpolarization of thalamocortical neurons, and burst–pause activity driven by the reticular thalamic nucleus. Broad systemic features of stages 1 to 4 include behavioral quiescence, low muscle activity, reduced blood pressure, reduced heart and respiration rates, reduced cortisol and thyroid hormone levels, and increased growth hormone, testosterone, prolactin, insulin, and glucose levels (Chapter 10).

REM sleep, in contrast, is a unique state of arousal characterized by brain electrical activity, cerebral blood flow, and brain glucose metabolism similar to that of wakefulness. REM sleep is accompanied by a generalized muscular atonia except for the extraocular muscles (thus the rapid eye movements) and the diaphragm. Clitoral or penile tumescence, phasic bursts of eye movements, and alternating acceleration and deceleration of heart and respiratory rates also characterize REM.

Electrophysiologic recordings during REM sleep have documented tonic cerebral activity, synchronized firing of hippocampal neurons in the theta frequency range, and phasic ponto-geniculo-occipital (PGO) spikes originating in the pons. Several limbic structures and regions of the hypothalamus and brainstem reach their highest firing rate during REM. Positron emission tomography (PET) studies in humans have shown that limbic structures such as the amygdala become metabolically active during REM sleep. Interestingly, despite the pattern of cerebral activation, the threshold for arousal from REM sleep is higher than that from NREM sleep.

FUNCTIONS OF SLEEP

The need to sleep is universal among mammals, birds, and reptiles and has been conserved in evolution. It has even been reported in *Drosophila*. Despite the obvious disadvantages of sleep, such as reduced vigilance against predators, it is necessary to sustain life. It is claimed that total sleep deprivation in rodents can result in death. Another striking observation that supports the importance of sleep has come from marine mammals, which must remain awake constantly in order to surface every few minutes for air. These mammals sleep unihemispherically; that is, one cerebral hemisphere exhibits sleep patterns detectable by EEG, while the other hemisphere remains awake. The persistence of sleep states in animals that must remain awake to breathe is a powerful indication that sleep serves an essential function.

Despite intense scientific research, no theory has convincingly explained the function of sleep. Questions regarding the amount of sleep that is needed, the stage of sleep that is most restorative, and the interventions that best promote healthy sleep remain unanswered. The popular belief that sleep is needed to restore the integrity of body functions makes some intuitive sense. Yet, this theory is accompanied by a false assumption that sleep is an inactive state. Because quiet wakefulness and sleep differ very little in terms of energy expenditure, it is unlikely that sleep and its attendant reduction in vigilance were conserved in evolution simply to save energy. Furthermore, no compelling evidence suggests that tissue rebuilding or an increase in protein synthesis is associated with sleep. Many types of external and internal stimuli, including ambient temperature, darkness, food intake, exercise, and endogenous immune factors affect sleep, but none of these variables has provided clues to the core function of sleep.

Many hypotheses have been used to explain the functions of REM sleep, but these frequently focus on a particular feature of REM, such as PGO spikes, and ignore other features. One prominent and intriguing hypothesis is that REM is needed to enhance learning or to discard irrelevant memory traces. While sleep may be important for enhancing the consolidation of memories (see below), the evidence in support of a specific role for REM in this process is limited. Another interesting hypothesis, which arises from observed relationships between the proportion of sleep spent in REM by species based on their degree of maturity at birth, is that REM is needed for early neurodevelopment in species, such as our own, characterized by marked immaturity at birth. However, this hypothesis does not adequately explain the persistence of REM in adulthood and the increased amount of REM sleep that occurs after sleep deprivation. Current hypotheses also fail to explain the functional significance of alternations between REM and NREM sleep cycles, although it appears that the length of these cycles in mammals correlates closely with brain size. Consequently, the function of sleep may relate to crucial molecular and cellular processes not yet adequately understood.

Sleep in general seems to be important for memory processing: long-term memory consolidation and reconsolidation seem to occur during sleep. For example, during early nocturnal sleep when slow-wave sleep is predominant, hippocampus-dependent declarative memories are replayed, stabilized, and likely enhanced. On the other hand, late sleep, when REM sleep predominates, has been associated with amygdala-dependent emotional memory. There is also evidence suggesting a role for sleep in motor learning, specifically in post-training consolidation.

NEURAL SUBSTRATES OF SLEEP

Several neural systems mediate the switching between wakefulness and sleep and between the different stages of sleep **12-3**. These systems include the ascending

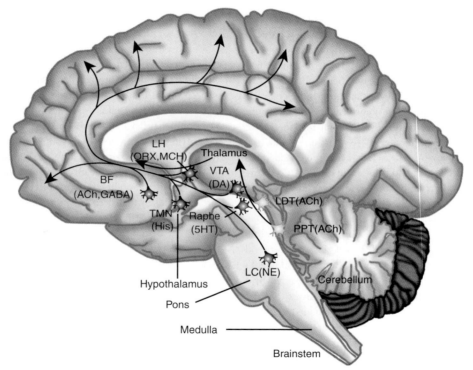

12-3 **A schematic drawing showing key components of the ARAS.** A major input to the relay and reticular nuclei of the thalamus (blue pathway) originates from cholinergic (ACh) cell groups in the upper pons, the pedunculopontine (PPT) and laterodorsal tegmental nuclei (LDT). These inputs facilitate thalamocortical transmission. A second pathway (red) activates the cerebral cortex to facilitate the processing of inputs from the thalamus. This arises from neurons in the monoaminergic cell groups, including the tuberomammillary nucleus (TMN) containing histamine (His), the ventral tegmental area (VTA) containing dopamine (DA), the dorsal and median raphe nuclei containing serotonin (5HT), and the locus coeruleus (LC) containing norepinephrine (NE). This pathway also receives contributions from peptidergic neurons in the lateral hypothalamus (LH) containing orexin (ORX) or melanin- concentrating hormone (MCH), and from basal forebrain (BF) neurons that contain γ-aminobutyric acid (GABA) or ACh. Note that all of these ascending pathways traverse the region at the junction of the brainstem and forebrain where lesions cause profound sleepiness. (From Saper CB, Scammell TE, Lu J. Hypothalamic regulation of sleep and circadian rhythms. *Nature*. 2005;437:1257–1263.)

reticular activating system (ARAS), the ventrolateral pre-optic (VLPO) area, and the orexin/hypocretin system (Chapters 6 and 7).

The ARAS is a complex structure consisting of several different circuits including the four monoaminergic pathways discussed in Chapter 6. The norepinephrine pathway originates from the locus ceruleus (LC) and related brainstem nuclei; the serotonergic neurons originate from the raphe nuclei within the brainstem as well; the dopaminergic neurons originate in ventral tegmental area (VTA); and the histaminergic pathway originates from neurons in the tuberomammillary nucleus (TMN) of the posterior hypothalamus. As discussed in Chapter 6, these neurons project widely throughout the brain from restricted collections of cell bodies. Norepinephrine, serotonin, dopamine, and histamine have complex modulatory functions and, in general, promote wakefulness. The PT in the brain stem is also an important component of the ARAS. Activity of PT cholinergic neurons (REM-on cells) promotes REM sleep. During waking, REM-on cells are inhibited by a subset of ARAS norepinephrine and serotonin neurons called REM-off cells.

The VLPO area of the anterior hypothalamus consists mainly of inhibitory neurons that release γ-aminobutyric acid (GABA) and the neuropeptide galanin. The VLPO neurons are likely to have reciprocal interactions with the ARAS and orexin neurons. The VLPO neurons inhibit and are inhibited by the TMN histamine neurons and REM-off monoamine neurons. Orexin neurons are located in the lateral hypothalamus. They are organized in a widely projecting manner, much like the monoamines (Chapter 6), and innervate all of the components of the ARAS. They excite the REM-off monoaminergic neurons during wakefulness and the PT cholinergic neurons during REM sleep. They are inhibited by the VLPO neurons during NREM sleep.

NREM Sleep

According to a simplified model, the onset of NREM sleep is driven by VLPO area neurons that exert an inhibitory effect on TMN histamine neurons 12–3 . Consistent with this hypothesis is the finding that VLPO and TMN neurons exhibit opposite patterns of activity during the sleep–wake cycle. In contrast to the VLPO neurons, which are active during sleep, the TMN neurons are persistently active during wakefulness, reduce their firing during NREM sleep, and become inactive during REM sleep. The role of the TMN histamine neurons in sleep–wake activity explains how the

older **antihistamines** such as **diphenhydramine** and **chlorpheniramine**, which are H_1 **receptor antagonists** (or inverse agonists), promote drowsiness and sleep. Newer antihistamines, such as **loratadine**, do not cross the blood-brain barrier and are without sedative effects. The older antihistamines are still marketed as over-the-counter sleep aids.

In the absence of tonic activity from the ARAS and TMN, which promotes wakefulness, higher-frequency oscillations in the cortex disappear, giving rise to the synchronous firing of a large thalamocortical neuronal ensemble. Thus, the delta wave and spindling rhythms observed during NREM sleep most likely reflect intrinsic properties of thalamic neurons, which synchronize the large thalamocortical network. Because a large number of neurons fire in synchrony at this stage, EEG recordings detect high-amplitude waves.

The brain structures involved in the control of NREM sleep are also crucial to thermoregulation. Some neurons in the preoptic area of the hypothalamus (POAH) are thermosensitive; they respond to changes in temperature by activating broad thermoregulatory mechanisms. In fact, as indicated previously, NREM sleep is associated with a lowering of the set point for body temperature, a loss of body heat, and a decline in energy metabolism. Warm-sensitive cells in the POAH area appear to be sleep active, whereas cold-sensitive cells are active during wakefulness. Consistent with these observations, warm-sensitive POAH neurons increase their firing rates during the transition from wakefulness to NREM sleep, whereas cold-sensitive neurons reduce their firing rates during the onset of sleep. Furthermore, warming of the POAH induces NREM sleep, increases the length of NREM periods, and increases delta activity during slow-wave sleep. In contrast, POAH lesions result in chronic disruption of both NREM sleep and thermoregulation. It therefore appears that warm-sensitive neurons in the POAH regulate the onset and maintenance of slow-wave sleep. Interestingly, passive heating of the body improves sleep continuity in patients with **insomnia.**

REM Sleep

In contrast to the diffuse brain structures involved in NREM sleep, the neuroanatomy of REM-active structures is relatively circumscribed. As previously mentioned, the primary oscillator that drives REM sleep appears to be located in the PT 12–3 . REM-on cholinergic neurons in the pedunculopontine tegmental (PPT) and laterodorsal tegmental (LDT) nuclei have high discharge rates during wakefulness and REM sleep and low discharge rates during NREM sleep. During NREM sleep, the VLPO area neurons start inhibiting the orexin neurons of the lateral hypothalamus. Consequently, the norepinephrine and serotonin REM-off cells, which are excited by orexin neurons during wakefulness, start to wane in activity, which gradually releases the cholinergic REM-on cells from their inhibitory effect. At the end of NREM sleep, the VLPO area neurons directly inhibit the REM-off cells, which completely disinhibits the REM-on cholinergic neurons and initiates REM sleep. Consistent with the inhibition of REM-on cells by serotonergic and noradrenergic inputs, **antidepressant** drugs, which increase the availability of synaptic serotonin or norepinephrine (Chapter 14), reduce REM sleep. Older tricyclic antidepressants, which are also anticholinergic, likely reduce REM sleep by this latter mechanism as well.

Via their heavy projections to thalamic nuclei and the reticular formation, the REM-on cells result in EEG desynchronization. Not surprisingly, application of **cholinergic agonists** or **acetylcholinesterase inhibitors** to the target cells in the thalamic nuclei or the reticular formation activates REM sleep, whereas **muscarinic cholinergic antagonists** suppress REM sleep.

Activity in the PT is responsible not only for initiating REM sleep but also for the physical manifestations of REM sleep. For example, cholinergic projections from the pons to the medulla and spinal cord regulate muscle atonia, most likely by hyperpolarizing motor neurons and associated interneurons. REM-associated cortical asynchrony, phasic eye movements, and cardiopulmonary accelerations and decelerations involve projections from the pons to the hypothalamus and thalamus. Although discrete pontine structures initiate most tonic and phasic elements of REM sleep, other structures are involved in REM regulation. For example, the orexin neurons in the lateral hypothalamus appear to be critical for the regulation of REM sleep, as discussed in the section on **narcolepsy** below. In addition, inputs from the amygdala and other limbic structures can influence phasic REM activity. This finding may explain why stress and **depression** are associated with increased phasic REM activity. Furthermore, lesions caudal and rostral to pontine REM-on cells profoundly alter the characteristics of REM sleep; for instance, such lesions can cause REM sleep without atonia, which can lead to the motoric expression of dreams. Such motor activity in humans during sleep has been associated with nocturnal violence against sleeping partners and injury from falls.

HOMEOSTATIC AND CIRCADIAN CONTROL OF THE SLEEP–WAKE CYCLE

Sleep is partly controlled by a homeostatic drive that increases the propensity to fall asleep in response to the amount of prior wakefulness. A student who has "pulled an all-nighter" may take an afternoon nap in response to a strong homeostatic drive resulting from an unmet need for sleep. This homeostatic drive is reflected by the amount of EEG slow-wave activity. However, the propensity to sleep is also affected by a circadian process **12-4**. The student who stays awake to study may feel increasingly tired throughout the night, and yet may feel more alert at 8:00 am than at 4:00 am, despite the fact that by 8:00 am four additional hours of sleep debt have accumulated.

Homeostatic Control of Sleep

The homeostatic control of sleep is still poorly understood. A number of sleep-modulating substances have been identified, including *adenosine*, muramyl dipeptide, interleukin-1, delta sleep-inducing peptide, prostaglandin D_2, and tumor necrosis factor (TNF). Extracellular adenosine decreases during slow-wave sleep and increases after prolonged wakefulness. During sleep deprivation, adenosine accumulates in the basal forebrain, especially in the substantia innominata extracellular spaces, and promotes sleep by inhibiting cholinergic neurons. Recovery sleep leads to a decline in adenosine levels. Adenosine may, therefore, serve to mark the duration of wakefulness as well as indicate an increased need for sleep. However, the evidence from

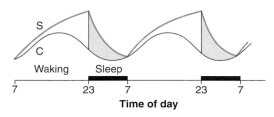

12-4 **A two-process model of sleep regulation.** The graph indicates the time course of the homeostatic process that promotes sleep (S) and the circadian process (C) that influences wakefulness. Awakening occurs at the intersection of S and C. (Adapted with permission from Kryger MH, Roth T, Dement WC, eds. *Principles and Practice of Sleep Medicine*, 2nd ed. Philadelphia: WB Saunders; 1994.)

adenosine receptor knockout mice suggests that adenosine has a modulatory rather than a direct sleep-generating effect. The alertness associated with the use of **caffeine** and related **methylxanthines** (**theophylline**, **theobromine**) is mediated primarily by their ability to block adenosine A_1 receptors, and to thereby block inhibition of the cholinergic arousal centers by adenosine (Chapter 8). The drugs also antagonize adenosine A_{2A} receptors, which are enriched in striatum; antagonism of the receptors is locomotor-activating, particularly in rodents, which contributes indirectly to arousal. Prostaglandin D_2, acting on prostaglandin D (PGD) receptors has been shown to indirectly activate adenosine-dependent pathways in the basal forebrain, and thereby promote sleep indirectly. Interleukin-1 and TNF appear to modulate sleep in the context of acute inflammation or infection.

Circadian Control of Sleep

Circadian variations have been observed in virtually all organisms and physiologic processes. Such circadian cycles prepare an organism to feed, avoid predators, and cope with environmental fluctuations, such as changes in light and temperature. To be useful, circadian cycles must correspond to environmental events. Environmental variables that entrain the circadian pacemaker are called *zeitgebers* (time givers). Light is the primary zeitgeber that helps an organism adapt to the light–dark cycle as it varies across the seasons. Other zeitgebers that entrain the circadian clock are temperature, food availability, and social cues.

Most mammalian circadian rhythms are controlled by the *suprachiasmatic nucleus (SCN)* `12-5`, which is the primary pacemaker for neuroendocrine rhythms, the temperature cycle, and REM sleep periods. The SCN is located in the midline anterior hypothalamus immediately above the optic chiasm. Its importance is indicated by the loss of most circadian rhythms and the disorganization of sleep–wake patterns that occur when the SCN is lesioned.

In mammals, a connection between retinal ganglion cells and the SCN (the retinohypothalamic pathway) allows the latter to receive direct input about ambient light that helps entrain circadian rhythms. Light-derived input to the SCN is conveyed also indirectly via the intergeniculate leaflet of the thalamus and the geniculohypothalamic tract. On exposure to light, retinal ganglion cells release melanopsin into the SCN, which in turn activates the sympathetic intermediolateral cell column in the thoracic spinal cord, which has a negative feedback loop with the pineal gland, resulting in inhibition of melatonin release

`12-1`. See Chapter 6 for synthesis and structure of melatonin.

The SCN also receives serotonergic input from the raphe nuclei and cholinergic inputs from the forebrain and brainstem. Moreover, it exerts control over circadian neuroendocrine and thermal rhythms through its projections to the paraventricular nucleus and to lateral and posterior areas of the hypothalamus. The SCN neurons influence the release of orexin, corticotrophin-releasing factor, thyrotropin-releasing hormone, and gonadotrophin-releasing hormone, and the activity of autonomic neurons (Chapters 9 and 10). Although SCN cells are predominantly GABAergic, the peptide neurotransmitters somatostatin, vasopressin, and vasoactive intestinal peptide (VIP) also may be released by SCN neurons to modulate the activities of certain sleep- and wake-promoting cells.

Molecular Control of Circadian Rhythms

In the last decade of the 20th century, several discoveries helped to elucidate the molecular basis of circadian timekeeping. The identification of the *Clock* gene in mammals, the *Period* and *Timeless* genes in *Drosophila*, and the *Frequency* gene in the fungus *Neurospora* illuminated conserved mechanisms for circadian regulation.

Each of the ~20 000 cells of SCN neurons expresses a molecular circadian clock. Intracellular circadian rhythms are maintained by the transcription of three period genes (*Per1–3*), two cryptochrome genes (*Cry1,2*), the *Clock* gene, and the *Bmal 1* gene `12-6`. Clock and Bmal 1 proteins form a heterodimer that is an active transcription factor (Clock:Bmal 1). At the beginning of an organism's wake-time, the transcription and translation of *Per* and *Cry* genes are accelerated by Clock:Bmal 1 heterodimers that have accumulated during the preceding sleep-time. Cry and Per proteins start accumulating during the wake-time and their levels peak at the beginning of the organism's subjective night. Complexes of Cry and Per proteins exert a negative feedback by inhibiting the Clock:Bmal 1 heterodimers, hence, Per and Cry protein levels start to decline. Meanwhile, Per2 protein had activated the transcription of Bmal 1. Bmal 1 protein starts accumulating and its level peaks during the night. New Clock:Bmal 1 heterodimers are formed and start the cycle again the next day after they are released from the feedback inhibition of the Cry complexes, the levels of which have been declining throughout the preceding night. In addition to exerting interlocking negative and positive feedback effects on each other, some of these gene products regulate the expression of many other

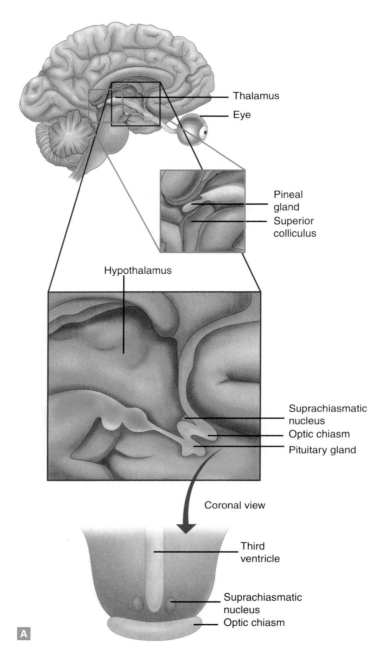

12–5 **The suprachiasmatic nucleus (SCN). A.** The SCN is situated in the hypothalamus immediately above the optic chiasm on either side of the third ventricle. It consists of about 16 000 neurons distributed bilaterally and connected with the retina. (From http://thebrain.mcgill.ca/flash/a/a_02/a_02_cr/a_02_cr_vis/a_02_cr_vis.html [accessed on March 1, 2007].)

genes (eg, growth hormone) which in turn mediate circadian regulation of many physiologic functions.

Molecular circadian mechanisms are sensitive to changes in light–dark cycles via the photoactivation of

neuroreceptors in SCN neurons. As most airplane travelers have experienced, circadian rhythms can shift to conform to new light–dark cycles, although they do not always shift as efficiently as one might wish. How do

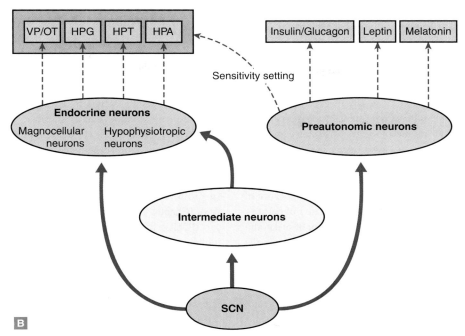

12-5 **B.** Three main types of SCN outputs have been identified: connections with endocrine, preautonomic, and intermediate neurons. In addition to this diversity of connections, the SCN uses different neurotransmitters to fine-tune its control of each specific endocrine function. Also note how the SCN uses its autonomic outputs to prepare the target tissue for the upcoming change in hormone release mediated via its endocrine outputs. VP, vasopressin; OT, oxytocin; HPG, hypothalamo-pituitary-gonad; HPT, hypothalamo-pituitary-thyroid; HPA, hypothalamo-pituitary-adrenal. (From Kalsbeek A, Palm IF, La Fleur SE, Scheer FAJL, Perreau-Lenz S, Ruiter M, Kreier F, Cailotto C, Buijs RM. SCN outputs and the hypothalamic balance of life. *J Biol Rhythms*. 2006;21:458.)

circadian gene products, oscillating in their own time zone, adjust to a shift in the light–dark cycle? The exact mechanisms that underlie such adjustments are unknown. However, the administration of bright light at times other than those predicted by the regular light–dark cycle can result in altered patterns of gene expression in SCN cells. This finding indicates that external stimuli can affect the expression of specific genes, which in turn may influence the production or activity of circadian gene products.

While the SCN is the master circadian control region, and certainly the most important region for entraining circadian rhythms to environmental light, it is crucial to note that *Clock* and most other circadian genes are expressed ubiquitously in brain and peripheral tissues where they also exhibit circadian cycles. Indeed, circadian rhythms in certain forebrain structures, independent of the SCN, may contribute to circadian regulation of **mood**, **reward**, and other complex functions. Moreover, several genes homologous to *Clock*, such as

NPAS (neuronal pas domain–containing transcription factor), can mediate molecular circadian rhythms in the absence of Clock protein itself. This information underscores the complexity of the molecular and neural circuit basis of circadian rhythms in physiology and behavior.

SLEEP DISORDERS

Difficulties related to sleep affect virtually all individuals at some point during their lives. Up to 10% of the general population has recurrent sleep difficulties. Sleep disturbances can be categorized as primary or secondary sleep disorders, the latter resulting from primary neuropsychiatric or general medical conditions. Examples of primary sleep disorders are given in **12-1**.

Dyssomnias

Dyssomnias include primary insomnia, primary hypersomnia, narcolepsy, breathing-related sleep disorders, circadian rhythm sleep disorder, and other conditions.

12-1 Circadian Regulation of Melatonin

Although a great deal is known about the regulation of endogenous melatonin, its physiologic function in humans has yet to be determined. In lower vertebrates, melatonin dramatically affects skin pigmentation: it lightens the skin by inducing pigment granule aggregation in melanocytes. This skin-lightening effect also occurs to a lesser degree in mammals. The reproductive systems and diurnal rhythms of some vertebrates, including some mammals, also are affected by melatonin. However, the significance of these effects in humans remains a matter of debate.

The nocturnal synthesis and release of melatonin is indirectly driven by the circadian oscillator in the suprachiasmatic nucleus (SCN). Interestingly, melatonin is released in the dark phase of all mammalian species, regardless of whether the animal is diurnal or nocturnal. In this respect, melatonin is very different from many factors that exhibit circadian cycles; for example, cortisol exhibits daytime peaks in diurnal species and nighttime peaks in nocturnal species. Among its many actions, the SCN induces nocturnal release of norepinephrine from sympathetic nerve endings that innervate the pineal gland. Released

norepinephrine acts by means of β-adrenergic receptors to induce high levels of cAMP in the pineal gland. High levels of cAMP activate protein kinase A, which in turn induces transcription of the rate-limiting enzyme in melatonin synthesis known as arylalkylamine-N-acetyltransferase (NAT). This norepinephrine-dependent diurnal variation in NAT transcription and melatonin synthesis is mediated by a switch between levels of phosphorylated CREB (p-CREB), the cAMP-dependent transcriptional activator (Chapter 4), and inducible cAMP early repressor (ICER), the cAMP-dependent transcriptional inhibitor. p-CREB accumulates when darkness begins and declines as the amount of ICER rises. p-CREB mediates the induction of NAT transcription during the first half of the night, and ICER mediates the repression of transcription during the second half. This knowledge of melatonin regulation has aided our understanding of the molecular mechanisms that generate circadian oscillations, and should assist investigations aimed at better appreciating the physiologic function of melatonin in humans.

12-1 Categorization of Primary Sleep Disorders

Dyssomnias

Primary insomnia
Primary hypersomnia
Narcolepsy
Breathing-related sleep disorder
Circadian rhythm sleep disorder
  Delayed sleep phase type
  Jet lag type
  Shift work type
  Unspecified
Other dyssomnias

Parasomnias

Nightmare disorder
Sleep terror disorder
Sleepwalking disorder
Other parasomnias

Most of these disorders are syndromes that are defined only by clinical signs and symptoms. Many are heterogeneous and the molecular and cellular underpinnings remain poorly understood.

Primary insomnia   This disorder, which is characterized by difficulty in initiating and maintaining sleep, causes significant psychological distress and impairment at school or work. Primary insomnia can be characterized objectively with polysomnography, which demonstrates an increased number of awakenings 12-7. Although the biology of insomnia is not well understood, it is increasingly viewed as a disorder of hyperarousal. Subjects with primary insomnia have an elevated 24-hour metabolic rate and a decreased propensity to sleep when given the opportunity to nap during sleep latency tests. Nonpharmacologic interventions that reduce arousal, including biofeedback, meditation, and relaxation therapy, are effective in the treatment of primary insomnia. Sleep hygiene also promotes healthy sleep through nonpharmacologic,

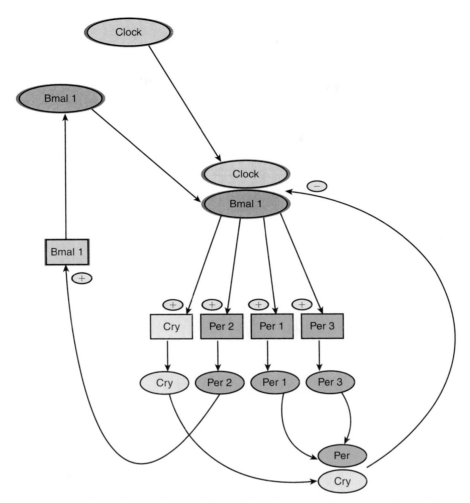

12-6 **Molecular basis of circadian oscillators.** Clock and Bmal 1 proteins form a heterodimer that promotes the transcription of cryptochrome (*Cry*) and period (*Per1-3*) genes. Cry and Per1 and 3 proteins form complexes and exert a negative inhibitory feedback on the Clock:Bmal 1 heterodimer, slowing the transcription of Cry and Per genes. Meanwhile, Per2 protein complexes promote the transcription of the Bmal 1 gene. Bmal 1 proteins accumulate and form complexes with available Clock proteins to resume the cycle.

common-sense measures; these include adherence to a stable sleep–wake schedule, a reduction in the use of **caffeine** and other stimulants, a reduction in the use of **alcohol**, regular exercise, and reduction of alerting stimuli in the sleep environment. Behavior modification therapy helps reduce the conditioned association between the sleep environment and wakeful arousal. Sleep restriction therapy and stimulus control behavior modification reduce the amount of awake time spent in bed. Patients who undergo sleep restriction therapy are instructed to get out of bed after a given period of wakefulness (approximately 15 minutes), and are advised not to return to bed until they feel tired enough to sleep. In this way, the association between being in bed and going to sleep is strengthened, and the association between being in bed and "tossing and turning" is weakened.

Primary hypersomnia Patients who experience excessive somnolence are diagnosed with primary hypersomnia when other disorders of somnolence, such as narcolepsy and sleep apnea, have been ruled out. Subjects with this disorder appear to sleep longer during the day and have a greater propensity to fall asleep compared with normal controls. Primary hypersomnia

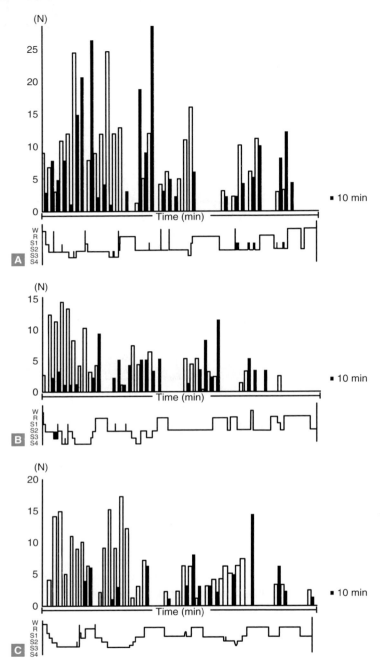

12-7 **Polysomnogram findings.** Polysomnogram (PSG) findings from a representative patient with unmedicated primary insomnia (**A**) or following hypnotic medication (**B**); and from a different subject without sleep complaints (**C**). Per 10 minutes of NREM sleep, a white bar counts the number of interruptions of a predominantly synchronized EEG activity (SWS), while a black bar counts the number of interruptions of mixed or predominantly desynchronized EEG activity (non-SWS NREM). The bars are matched with the sleep histogram. Untreated insomnia (**A**) is associated with a reduction of slow-wave sleep (stages 3 and 4), increased intrusions of wakefulness, and an impressively increased number of interruptions compared to control (**C**). Active medication (**B**) elicits a recovery of slow-wave sleep and reduction of nocturnal wakefulness, and drastically curtails the number of switches. Note that because each bar indicates the number of interruptions in the previous 10 minutes, there may be the false impression of interruptions occurring in REM sleep. W, wakefulness; R, REM sleep; S1, S2, S3, S4, stages 1, 2, 3, 4, respectively. (From Terzano MG, Parrino L, Spaggiari MC, Palomba V, Rossi M, Smerieri A. CAP variables and arousals as sleep electroencephalogram markers for primary insomnia. *Clin Neurophysiol.* 2003;:1715–1723.)

is not well understood biologically but is believed to involve a disturbance of pathways that mediate wakeful arousal. Treatment primarily involves the use of **psychostimulants**, as discussed later in this chapter.

Narcolepsy Narcolepsy was first described during the late 1800s. It is characterized by abnormal transitions between REM and NREM sleep during the night and across the sleep–wake cycle. Narcoleptic patients do not sleep more than normal individuals; however, they have intrusive episodes of REM sleep during the day and fragmented sleep at night. The characteristic symptoms of narcolepsy, which include pathologic sleepiness, sleep paralysis, hypnagogic hallucinations (hallucinations that occur with the onset or termination of sleep), and cataplexy, are caused by the sudden intrusion of REM sleep into wakefulness. *Cataplexy* is pathognomonic for narcolepsy and is characterized by the sudden loss of muscle tone during wakefulness. During a cataplectic attack, a narcoleptic may suddenly fall to the floor from a standing position and be unable to move even though fully conscious. Interestingly, cataplectic attacks often are elicited by positive emotional stimuli. The primary treatment for narcolepsy consists of **psychostimulants** or **modafinil** to counter the hypersomnolence, and REM-suppressing drugs, such as **tricyclic antidepressants**, which reduce cataplexy. Nonpharmacologic treatment, such as scheduled naps, also is effective for treating daytime hypersomnolence.

Narcolepsy can be a heritable disorder, but in humans most cases appear sporadic. In some families, narcolepsy has been linked to a gene that is near the human leukocyte antigen (HLA) alleles DQB1 and DQA1 on chromosome 6, suggesting an autoimmune basis. In a dog model of narcolepsy, transmission is autosomal recessive, which is clearly different from human transmission, and is due to loss-of-function mutations in the orexin OX_2 receptor gene. Disruption of the gene encoding orexin peptides in mice also causes a narcolepsy-like disorder. Orexin neurons, located in the lateral and posterior hypothalamus **6–25** and **12–3** excite monoaminergic neurons during wakefulness and cholinergic neurons during REM sleep. They are inhibited by VLPO during NREM sleep.

Orexin neurons are significantly decreased in number in narcoleptic patients. Hence, one hypothesis is that because of the small number of these neurons in narcolepsy there is less excitation of the monoaminergic neurons during wakefulness and consequently a tendency for the cholinergic neurons to escape from the monoaminergic inhibition resulting in sudden attacks of atonia and REM periods. This hypothesis is supported by the observation that administration of cholinomimetic agents exacerbates cataplexy in narcoleptic dogs, while administration of anticholinergic agents decreases cataplexy; drugs that block the reuptake of norepinephrine (ie, certain antidepressants)—and therefore enhance noradrenergic transmission at REM-off terminals—are powerful anticataleptic agents.

Most cases of narcolepsy in humans are not linked to mutations in the genes encoding orexin peptides or receptors, but are associated with significantly reduced, often undetectable, levels of orexin in cerebrospinal fluid and brain tissues **12–8**. Together, the linkage of narcolepsy with HLA alleles, its peak and trough incidence among those born in March and September, respectively (suggesting an environmental influence during the fetal or perinatal period), and the loss of orexin neurons raise the interesting possibility that narcolepsy may be caused by an autoimmune-mediated destruction of these neurons in analogy with the autoimmune destruction of insulin-secreting β-islet cells in type I diabetes. A search for small-molecule agonists at orexin receptors is underway and could lead to a treatment for narcolepsy.

Sleep apnea Sleep apnea, a breathing-related sleep disorder, is a common, age-related condition characterized by oropharyngeal collapse during sleep. Such collapse causes sleep fragmentation, hypoxia, pulmonary and systemic hypertension, and cardiac arrhythmias. Obstructive sleep apnea can be caused by obesity or anatomic factors, such as micrognathia, that predispose patients to airway occlusion during sleep. Central sleep apnea is secondary to impaired central respiratory drive; it is associated with congestive heart failure and advanced age, and occurs in 30% of men older than 60 years of age. Treatment may involve behavior modification, including weight loss and sleep position therapy; the use of mechanical devices to eliminate airway collapse, such as continuous positive airway pressure (CPAP); the use of dental appliances that adjust the position of the jaw and tongue; or surgery to enhance the size of the oropharynx.

Circadian rhythm sleep disorders Some of these disorders, which are caused by a misalignment between behavioral waking activity and the endogenous circadian cycle, are perhaps not properly classified as primary sleep disorders. They are chronobiologic disorders caused artificially by jet travel across multiple time zones, or by shift work that results in a rapidly changing sleep–wake cycle. Clinical manifestations of these disorders, which include sleepiness, insomnia, diminished attention, gastrointestinal discomfort, and fatigue, vary depending on the juxtaposition of the underlying circadian cycle and sleep–wake behavior.

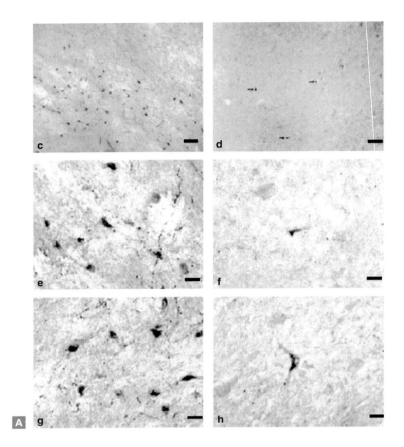

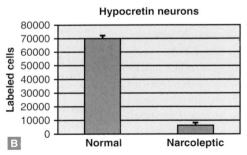

12–8 **Neurons expressing orexin are decreased in narcolepsy. A.** Distribution of cells expressing orexin in perifornical and dorsomedial hypothalamic regions of normal (left panels) and narcoleptic (right panels) humans. Many orexin somas and axons can be seen in the brain sections of normal controls but few in the narcoleptic patients. **B.** Number of orexin-containing neurons is dramatically decreased in hypothalamic brain tissues of narcoleptic patients compared to healthy controls. (From Thannickal TC, Moore RY, Nienhuis R, et al. Reduced number of hypocretin clinical study neurons in human narcolepsy. *Neuron.* 2000;27:469–474.)

Advanced sleep phase syndrome (ASPS) is a rare autosomal dominant disorder that results in abnormal circadian behavior. Individuals sleep and wake earlier than desired (from about 1900 hours in the evening to 0400 hours in the morning). The first described gene mutation for familial ASPS was a missense mutation in the *Per2* gene (serine-to-glycine). Recently, another single missense mutation in the casein kinase I delta (CKIdelta) gene (threonine-to-alanine) was found to be associated with familial ASPS I humans. CKIdelta binds and phosphorylates mammalian Per proteins, thereby regulating their stability, subcellular localization, and the timing of the molecular clock. However, most cases of familial ASPS are not caused by this mutation.

Delayed sleep phase syndrome (DSPS) is the most frequent sleep disorder among young adults. It is characterized by persistently delayed sleep-wake timing (sleep from 0400 hours in the morning to noon). A number of gene polymorphisms have been associated with DSPS. A higher percentage of patients with DPSP have been found to carry the short allele of the *Per3* gene compared to controls. DSPS has also been associated with a single nucleotide polymorphism in the arylalkylamine *N*-acetyltransferase gene, the rate-limiting enzyme in the synthesis of **melatonin**, resulting in an amino acid substitution from alanine to threonine at position 129. DSPS has been associated with the HLA-DR1 antigen as well. How exactly these genetic variations alter the sleep-wake cycle remains poorly understood.

Parasomnias

Parasomnias are represented by nightmares, sleep or night terrors, sleepwalking, and other conditions that arise during stage 4 sleep. They are considered disorders only when their frequency, severity, or persistence disrupts the normal functioning of an individual. Excessive and severe nightmares are strongly associated with psychological trauma and often are seen in the context of posttraumatic stress disorder (Chapter 14). Night terrors and sleepwalking occur predominantly in children and involve a partial awakening out of slow-wave sleep. Children affected by night terrors experience extreme fear and sympathetic activation without fully awakening; consequently they are difficult to console, much to the consternation of alarmed parents. In most cases, night terrors represent a benign condition that a child is likely to outgrow. Sleepwalking similarly involves partial arousal from deep slow-wave sleep. Although this disorder typically is innocuous, the persistence of sleepwalking in adults can be associated with psychopathology, including **schizophrenia** and **mood disorders**. Medications that are effective in the treatment of these parasomnias have yet to be developed.

PHARMACOLOGY OF SLEEP–WAKE DISORDERS

Benzodiazepines

Benzodiazepines became available in the late 1950s and rapidly replaced the **barbiturates** as preferred sedative–hypnotics. Their wide acceptance resulted from their greater safety, including lower risks associated with overdose and abuse compared with those of the barbiturates and related sedative–hypnotics such as **methaqualone**, **ethchlorvynol**, **meprobamate**, and **chloral hydrate**; benzodiazepines also are less likely to induce hepatic metabolism of other drugs. Yet, like barbiturates and related sedative–hypnotics, benzodiazepines and related drugs bind to and facilitate the functioning of GABA$_A$ receptors. Their mechanisms of action and general pharmacology are discussed in greater detail in Chapters 5 and 14. The chemical structures of representative benzodiazepines used as sedative–hypnotics are shown in `12–9`.

Benzodiazepines promote the onset of sleep and sleep continuity in the treatment of insomnia. They also are commonly used as **anxiolytics** (Chapter 14). Much of the clinical art of benzodiazepines and other treatments for insomnia involves an understanding of the importance of drug half-life in determining appropriate drug therapy and minimizing adverse effects `12-2`. Long-acting benzodiazepines, such as **flurazepam** and **chlordiazepoxide**, have active metabolites with half-lives in excess of 200 hours; their use often interferes with daytime alertness and is associated with more errors while driving an automobile compared with the use of shorter-acting agents. In contrast, benzodiazepines with extremely short half-lives (2–4 hours), such as **triazolam**, are useful for promoting the onset of sleep, but may be of less benefit to those who have difficulty maintaining sleep. Such short half-life agents can cause rebound insomnia during the latter half of the night, which can be viewed as a mild withdrawal syndrome that occurs in response to a single dose of the benzodiazepine. Repeated use of these agents can lead to more significant rebound insomnia and anxiety; however, the slow tapering of these agents can minimize the occurrence of a discontinuation syndrome. For these reasons, compounds with intermediate half-lives are optimal for most individuals. Benzodiazepines are also associated with anterograde amnesia, especially if used in high doses or taken with **alcohol**. The drugs suppress the total amount of REM sleep and alter the time spent in stages 1 through 4; consequently, sleep produced by a sedative-hypnotic may not be as physiologically useful as normal sleep.

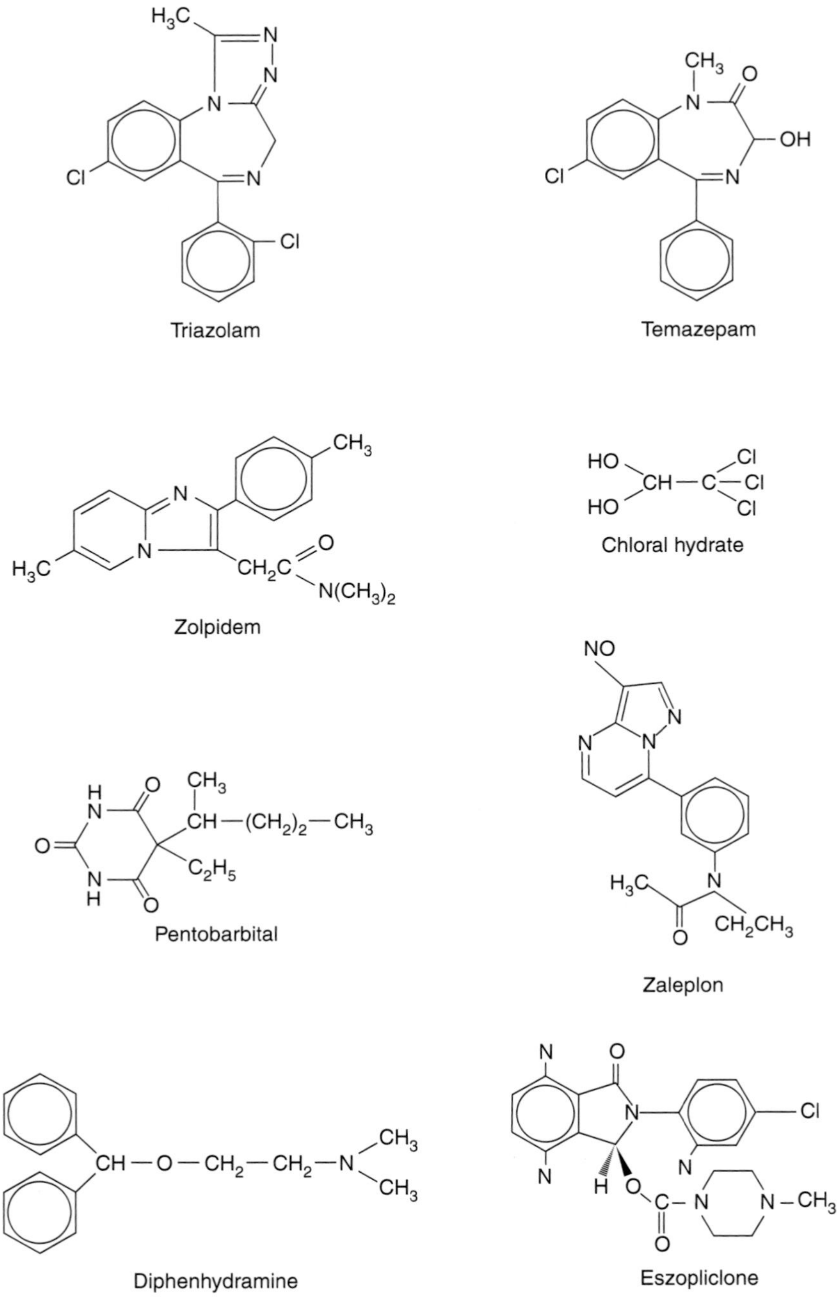

Triazolam

Temazepam

Zolpidem

Chloral hydrate

Pentobarbital

Zaleplon

Diphenhydramine

Eszopiclone

12-9 **Chemical structures of representative benzodiazepines and other drugs used to treat insomnia.**

Although **zaleplon**, **zolpidem**, and **eszopiclone** are not chemically classified as benzodiazepines **12-9**, they act on the benzodiazepine site of the $GABA_A$ receptor with similar results. They have many of the same benefits and liabilities of short-to-intermediate half-life benzodiazepines.

Attempts to improve the long-term treatment of insomnia have addressed the various liabilities of drugs that act at the benzodiazepine site of the $GABA_A$ receptor. One strategy, which remains speculative, might involve the use of partial agonists at this site; such drugs might be designed to cause sedation

12-2 Comparison of Representative Benzodiazepines for Insomnia Therapy

Drug	Half-Life	Advantages	Disadvantages
Estazolam	Intermediate		Some daytime sedation and performance decrements
Flurazepam	Long	Delayed rebound insomnia	Daytime sedation; high risk of falls and driving errors
Temazepam	Intermediate		Some daytime sedation and performance decrements
Triazolam	Short	No daytime sedation	Rebound insomnia
Zolpidem[1]	Short	No daytime sedation	Rebound insomnia

[1]Zolpidem does not have a benzodiazepine structure, but acts at the same site on the GABA$_A$ receptor as do the benzodiazepines (see **12-9**). A new sustained release preparation has extended its half-life to avoid rebound insomnia.

without producing tolerance. Another strategy might be to take advantage of the molecular diversity of GABA$_A$ receptor subunits. Because the sedative effects of benzodiazepines appear to be mediated predominantly by one particular GABA$_A$ receptor α subunit, the α_1 subunit (Chapters 5 and 14), drugs might be developed that are selective for this subunit and therefore unlikely to cause the deleterious cognitive effects of previously mentioned agents. Certain currently available drugs (eg, zolpidem and eszopiclone) show some preference for this subunit, but true subunit-selective benzodiazepine-like drugs are not yet available. Such drugs are in preclinical and clinical stages of development.

Nonbenzodiazepine Sedative–Hypnotic Agents

Several nonbenzodiazepine classes of drugs are currently used to promote sleep. Antihistamines, specifically the first generation H$_1$ receptor inverse agonists—commonly referred to as antagonists—are frequently used and in fact are the active ingredients in most over-the-counter sleep remedies. They are able to penetrate the blood-brain barrier because of their lipophilicity, relatively low molecular weight, and lack of recognition by the P-glycoprotein efflux pump (Chapter 2). Examples of these medications include **diphenhydramine** **12-9**, **dimenhydrinate**, **chlorpheniramine**, **hydroxyzine**, and **promethazine**. However, these drugs are less effective than benzodiazepines and are associated with more adverse daytime effects. Antihistamines also can adversely affect memory and psychomotor performance, even after the

drugs are no longer detectable in the general circulation. Many people report the sensation of being "in a fog" for as many as 24 hours after taking an antihistamine.

As H$_1$ inverse agonists, antihistamines combine with and stabilize the inactive form of the H$_1$ receptor, shifting the equilibrium toward the inactive state. However, because the histaminergic neurons of the TMN of the hypothalamus are quiescent during sleep, antihistamines may cause more sedation during waking hours than promotion of sleep during the sleep cycle. Several **tricyclic antidepressants** and **antipsychotic drugs** block H$_1$ receptors, which contributes to the sedative effects of these agents. Another strategy for promoting sleep may involve the use of an **H$_3$ receptor agonist**. As described in Chapter 6, H$_3$ receptors are inhibitory autoreceptors on histaminergic neurons of the TMN. An agonist at these receptors, for example, **R-α-methylhistamine**, would be expected to reduce the activity of the neurons and thereby promote sleep. This approach has not yet been tested in humans.

Sodium oxybate (γ-hydroxybutyrate, GHB) is a naturally occurring CNS metabolite. It is found in highest concentration in the hypothalamus and basal ganglia. GHB is given to consolidate sleep, increase total nocturnal sleep time, and decrease sleep paralysis, hypnagogic hallucinations, and nightmares. Patients report progressive restfulness upon awakening. Patients with narcolepsy report a decrease in cataplexy frequency. GHB is often referred to as a **date rape drug**, used to induce sleep in unsuspecting victims. The mechanism of action of GHB is poorly understood. It may be an agonist at GABA$_B$ receptors; it also may be metabolized into GABA and thereby activate other GABA receptors. Another date rape drug, **fluni-trazepam**, is a benzodiazepine agonist.

γ-aminobutyric acid (GABA)

γ-hydroxybutyrate (GHB)

Trazodone is marketed as an antidepressant but is less effective in the treatment of depression than many other available agents. However, trazodone is sedating and is sometimes used to promote sleep. It improves sleep continuity and also subjective sleep quality. Although it is frequently recommended because of a putative lack of associated tolerance, data regarding its long-term efficacy have not been obtained. Although trazodone appears to be an agonist at several 5HT receptors, its mechanism of action in promoting sleep remains undetermined. **Mirtazapine** is another antidepressant known clinically for its sedative effect. This effect is thought to be related to the blockade of serotonin $5HT_2$ receptors.

There has been great interest in the **melatonin** system as a potential target for new sedative–hypnotic agents. Endogenous melatonin is synthesized exclusively in the pineal gland from tryptophan and serotonin (Chapter 6). Its physiologic role in the control of circadian rhythms and sleep remains uncertain. Exogenous melatonin has been shown to help reset the circadian clock in some experimental situations `12–1`. It is commonly used to treat jet lag in individuals who travel across multiple time zones. Moreover, it has been used to help shift workers better adjust to new work hours, although its efficacy when used for these purposes has not been established in well-designed clinical trials. Its efficacy in the treatment of noncircadian insomnia also has not been supported by convincing evidence. Moreover, the safety of over-the-counter melatonin preparations in the United States has yet to be determined; indeed, even the composition of most of these preparations remains unknown because of the lack of regulatory oversight by the Food and Drug Administration (FDA). The dose commonly available

in health food stores has been determined to produce a level of melatonin that is 10 times greater than peak physiologic levels. Elevated concentrations of melatonin have been associated with endocrine disturbances such as amenorrhea in females and hypogonadism in males. Melatonin also can lead to the asynchrony of circadian physiology if used frequently at different times of the day. Melatonin produces its effects in mammals via activation of two $G_{i/o}$-linked receptors, termed MT_1 (Mel_{1a}) and MT_2 (Mel_{1b}), and knockout mice are now being used to determine their selective physiologic functions. The pharmaceutical industry currently is attempting to develop agonists that are selective for these melatonin receptors, such as the recently marketed **ramelteon**; whether these drugs will prove to be safer and more effective than melatonin remains to be seen.

Because of the prevalence of insomnia, and the imperfect treatment offered by available medications, many individuals have turned to so-called **natural products** that are marketed to promote and improve sleep. These products include not only melatonin but also herbal products and hormones. The public often believes that a natural product is unquestionably safe and likely to be efficacious. Yet the dangers of **digitalis**, originally derived as an herbal preparation from foxglove, and natural hormonal products such as **insulin** demonstrate that any drug powerful enough to have a desired effect may also have serious side effects. Moreover, reliance on natural products can prevent individuals from seeking medical attention, which in turn can cause serious disorders to remain undiagnosed. Insomnia, for example, can be a symptom of illnesses as diverse as depression and congestive heart failure. As with any pharmacologic treatment, treatment with natural products requires that manufacturers: (1) establish standardized preparations; (2) establish the safety and mechanism of action of these preparations in animals; and (3) establish safety and efficacy in humans. Just as identification and examination of the active ingredients in digitalis leaf led to the development of digoxin, it is hoped that the active ingredients in certain natural products can be identified so that their mechanisms of action can be studied and improved preparations can be formulated.

Drugs That Increase Alertness

The drugs used most commonly to promote wakefulness are **caffeine**—for example, in coffee, soda, and over-the-counter stimulants—and related substances such as **theophylline** in tea and **theobromine** in chocolate. Although these drugs have several mechanisms of action, their stimulant properties are most closely associated with antagonism of adenosine receptors, particularly that of A_1 and possibly A_{2A} receptors as stated earlier (Chapter 8). The medicinal use of these drugs is limited by side effects such as nausea, headache, and tremulousness, which are common at clinically relevant doses. More selective antagonists of adenosine receptors, which have yet to be developed, may offer the clinical benefits of these agents without such unpleasant side effects.

The most potent agents that promote wakefulness are amphetamine-like psychostimulants, including D-**amphetamine**, **methamphetamine**, **methylphenidate**, **mazindol**, and **pemoline**. These drugs increase the synaptic levels of dopamine, serotonin, and norepinephrine primarily by blocking their reuptake or promoting their release (Chapters 6, 14, and 15). Actions on the dopamine system are believed to be most important for the stimulant effects of these drugs. Amphetamines remain the treatment of choice for **narcolepsy**. Although these drugs offer important symptomatic improvement in many patients, their use is associated with complications such as nighttime insomnia, tolerance, dependence, and in some cases addiction.

Modafinil, a (diphenyl-methyl)-sulfinyl-2-acetamide derivative, is another wakefulness-promoting drug approved by the FDA. It increases alertness and vigilance in normal individuals and in patients with narcolepsy, although it is clearly less efficacious than amphetamines. However, modafinil shows fewer cardiovascular side effects and less abuse potential compared with amphetamines. The mechanism of action of modafinil is unknown. The drug may partially inhibit the dopamine transporter, to which it binds with micromolar affinity, although some investigators have suggested that it acts by means of nondopaminergic mechanisms, eg, affecting the histaminergic system, inhibiting the release of GABA in the hypothalamus, or influencing serotonin release. Of note, modafinil reduces subjective sleepiness and improves wakefulness; however, it does not reduce cataplexy.

Several **antidepressants** alter the sleep–wake cycle. Some of these drugs exhibit strong antagonism of H_1 histamine and muscarinic cholinergic receptors, which mediates the ability of these drugs to promote sleep independently of their antidepressant actions. However, several antidepressants such as **fluoxetine** and **bupropion**, which have an amphetamine-like structure (Chapter 14), exert the opposite effect in some patients and can lead to insomnia. Why some serotonin-acting antidepressants, such as **trazodone**, promote sleep while others, for example, **fluoxetine**, disrupt sleep in a subset of patients remains unknown but may be related to the different groups of 5HT receptors that are activated by these medications.

Many distinct but interdependent neural pathways regulate the sleep–wake cycle. Because each of these pathways is subserved by distinct neurotransmitters, many pharmacologic agents can influence sleep patterns. The cellular and molecular mechanisms involved in the regulation of sleep and circadian rhythms require more investigation, but it is anticipated that the elucidation of these mechanisms will lead to new targets for the effective pharmacologic treatment of sleep disorders.

General Anesthetics

Despite 160 years of widespread use, the mechanisms through which drugs produce a state of anesthesia remain poorly understood. Initial hypotheses revolved around the discovery that an anesthetic drug's potency correlated with its solubility in olive oil. This finding, coupled with the low potency of most general anesthetics (micromolar to millimolar), slowed identification of specific molecular targets and led to the lipid theory of anesthetic action, in which anesthetic effects were thought to be mediated by nonspecific interactions within lipid membranes. This lipid theory of anesthetic action dominated thinking for more than 80 years until the 1980s when anesthetics were shown to interact directly with the firefly luciferase protein in a lipid free preparation. Rapidly thereafter, researchers focused on ion channels as anesthetic targets.

At clinically relevant concentrations, general anesthetics (including all volatile **ether**-based anesthetics—**isoflurane**, **sevoflurane**, **desflurane**, and **enflurane**—as well as the halogenated volatile alkane anesthetic, **halothane**) act as positive or negative allosteric modulators of many ligand-gated ion channels, eg, $GABA_A$, NMDA and AMPA glutamate, nicotinic acetylcholine, and glycine receptors (Chapters 5 and 6). The anesthetics also regulate several types of ion channels, such as two-pore K^+ channels, voltage-gated

Modafinil

Na⁺ channels, and the hyperpolarization-activated, cyclic nucleotide-modulated (HCN) channels (Chapter 2). The net effect of anesthetics is to hyperpolarize resting membrane potentials (mainly by activating 2-pore K⁺ channels) and to enhance synaptic inhibition and inhibit excitation. For example, at $GABA_A$ receptors, most volatile and intravenous anesthetics (eg, **propofol** and **etomidate**) prolong the channel open time by enhancing the gating of the receptor by GABA. At glutamatergic synapses, volatile anesthetics act presynaptically to decrease glutamate release. Other nonhalogenated inhaled anesthetics (**xenon, nitrous oxide**, and **cyclopropane**) and the intravenous dissociative anesthetic **ketamine** depress glutamatergic transmission postsynaptically by blocking NMDA glutamate receptors; some also activate two-pore K⁺ channels.

While the molecular targets of anesthetic action have been the focus of intense investigation over the past 2 decades, the critical neuroanatomic substrates on which anesthetic drugs act have received relatively little attention. *General anesthesia* is a state defined by a collection of specific behavioral endpoints including amnesia, analgesia, immobility, and hypnosis. We focus here on anesthetic-induced unconsciousness as an example of how the behavioral features of general anesthesia are being understood neurobiologically, although parallel efforts are underway to understand other features of anesthesia.

The *hypnotic* component of general anesthesia (defined experimentally as a lack of perceptive awareness of nonnoxious stimuli) shares many similarities to that of NREM sleep **12-3**. However, one crucial difference is that even the deepest sleeper can be awakened by external stimuli, while the anesthetized individual will not reawaken until the anesthetic drugs are discontinued. Nonetheless, similarities led to the hypothesis that anesthetic drugs may exert their hypnotic effects via specific interactions on NREM sleep promoting circuits. Anesthetic drugs appear to close the thalamic gates, functionally depriving the cortex of peripheral sensory inputs. **Propofol** and the barbiturate anesthetics (eg, **pentobarbital**) have been shown to activate the VLPO while simultaneously inhibiting the TMN. Meanwhile, **dexmedetomidine**, an α_2-adrenergic agonist, appears to induce a hypnotic state by inhibiting the LC, which in turn disinhibits the VLPO, and culminates in inhibition of the TMN. Finally, volatile anesthetics such as **isoflurane** and **sevoflurane** inhibit the wake-promoting orexin neurons while undoubtedly affecting other sleep- and wake-active centers as well.

Like general anesthesia, sleep was once considered to be a passive state caused by deprivation of peripheral inputs to the cortex. The preponderance of evidence now demonstrates that sleep is an actively generated state dependent on the integrated contribution of multiple neuronal loci. Whether future studies

12-3 **Comparison Between Non-REM Sleep and General Anesthesia**

	NREM Sleep	General Anesthesia
Arousal state	Transient unconsciousness	Transient unconsciousness
Cerebral metabolic rate	Decreased globally	Decreased globally
Cerebral blood flow	Decreased globally with more specific reductions in thalamic and midbrain reticular formation activity	Decreased globally with more specific reductions in thalamic and midbrain reticular formation activity
EEG pattern	Increased delta power	Increased delta power
EEG entropy (measure of disorder)	Decreased	Decreased
EMG activity	Decreased	Decreased to totally absent
Thalamic sensory relay	Impaired	Impaired
Effect of agents that promote sleep (such as adenosine)	Promote sleep	Potentiate general anesthesia
Cardiac output	Decreased	Decreased
Minute ventilation	Decreased	Decreased
Core body temperature	Decreased	Decreased

will similarly overturn the concept of passive inactivation of the brain leading to general anesthesia remains to be discovered.

SELECTED READING

Blanco-Centurion C, Xu M, Murillo-Rodriguez E, et al. Adenosine and sleep homeostasis in the basal forebrain. *J Neurosci*. 2006;26:8092–8100.

Boivin DB, Duffy JF, Kronauer RE, et al. Dose-response relationships for resetting of human circadian clock by light. *Nature*. 1996;379:540–542.

Campagna JA, Miller KW, Forman SA. Mechanisms of actions of inhaled anesthetics. *N Engl J Med*. 2003;348:2110–2124.

Chemelli RM, Willie JT, Sinton CM, et al. Narcolepsy in orexin knockout mice: molecular genetics of sleep regulation. *Cell*. 1999;98:437–452.

Czeisler CA. The effect of light on the human circadian pacemaker. *Ciba Found Symp*. 1995;183:254–290.

Dauvilliers Y, Arnulf I, Mignot E. Narcolepsy with cataplexy. *Lancet*. 2007;369:499–511.

Dauvilliers Y, Carlander B, Molinari N. Month of birth as a risk factor for narcolepsy. *Sleep*. 2003;26:663–665.

Deboer T, Vansteensel MJ, Détári L, et al. Sleep states alter activity of suprachiasmatic nucleus neurons. *Nature Neurosci*. 2003;6:1086–1090.

Dement WC. The study of human sleep: a historical perspective. *Thorax*. 1998;53(suppl):S2–S7.

Dijk DJ, Duffy JF. Circadian regulation of human sleep and age-related changes in its timing, consolidation, and EEG characteristics. *Ann Med*. 1999;31: 130–140.

Fredholm BB, Chen JF, Masino SA, et al. Actions of adenosine at its receptors in the CNS: insights from knockouts and drugs. *Annu Rev Pharmacol Toxicol*. 2005;45:385–412.

Gvilia I, Xu F, McGinty D, et al. Homeostatic regulation of asleep: a role for preoptic area neurons. *J Neurosci*. 2006;26:9426–9433.

Hemmings HC Jr, Akabas MH, Goldstein PA, et al. Emerging molecular mechanisms of general anesthetic action. *Trends Pharmacol Sci*. 2005;26:503–510.

Hirayama J, Sassone-Corsi P. Structural and functional features of transcription factors controlling the circadian clock. *Curr Opin Genet Dev*. 2005;15:548–556.

Hobson JA, Pace-Schott EF. The cognitive neuroscience of sleep: neuronal systems, consciousness and learning. *Nature Rev Neurosci*. 2002;3:679–693.

Hosie AM, Wilkins ME, da Silva HMA, et al. Endogenous neurosteroids regulate $GABA_A$ receptors through two discrete transmembrane sites. *Nature*. 2006;444:486–489.

Jin X, von Gall C, Pieschl RL, et al. Targeted disruption of the mouse Mel(1b) melatonin receptor. *Mol Cell Biol*. 2003;23:1054–1060.

Jones BE. Arousal systems. *Front Biosci*. 2003;8: s438–s451.

Kelz MB, Sun Y, Chen J, et al. An essential role for orexins in emergence from general anesthesia. *Proc Natl Acad Sci USA*. 2008;105:1309–1314.

King D, Takahashi JS. Molecular genetics of circadian rhythms in mammals. *Annu Rev Neurosci*. 2000;23:713–742.

Lin L, Faraco JU, Li R, et al. The sleep disorder canine narcolepsy is caused by a mutation in the hypocretin (orexin) receptor 2 gene. *Cell*. 1999;98:365–376.

Lowrey PL, Shimomura K, Antoch MP, et al. Positional syntenic cloning and functional characterization of the mammalian circadian mutation tau. *Science*. 2000;288:483–492.

Maronde E, Pfeffer M, Olcese J, et al. Transcription factors in neuroendocrine regulation: rhythmic changes in pCREB and ICER frame melatonin synthesis. *J Neurosci*. 1999;19:3326–3336.

McCarley RW, Strecker RE, Porkka-Heiskanen T, et al. Modulation of cholinergic neurons by serotonin and adenosine in the control of REM and non-REM sleep. In: *Sleep and Sleep Disorders: From Molecule to Behavior*. Tokyo, Academic Press; 1997; 63–79.

McGinty D, Szymusiak R. Brain structures and mechanisms involved in the generation of NREM sleep: focus on the preoptic hypothalamus. *Sleep Med Rev*. 2001;5:323–342.

Nakahata Y, Grimaldi B, Sahar S, et al. Signaling to the circadian clock: plasticity by chromatin remodeling. *Curr Opin Cell Biol*. 2007;19:230–237.

Nelson LE, Guo TZ, Lu J, et al. The sedative component of anesthesia is mediated by GABA(A) receptors in an endogenous sleep pathway. *Nat Neurosci*. 2002;5:979–984.

Nishino S, Ripley B, Overeem S, et al. Hypocretin (orexin) deficiency in human narcolepsy. *Lancet*. 2000;355:39–40.

Pace-Schott EF, Hobson JA. The neurobiology of sleep: genetics, cellular physiology and subcortical networks. *Nature Rev Neurosci*. 2002;3:591–605.

Peyron C, Faraco J, Rogers W, et al. A mutation in a case of early onset narcolepsy and a generalized absence of hypocretin peptides in human narcoleptic brains. *Nature Med*. 2000;6:991–997.

Porkka-Heiskanen T, Strecker RE, Thakkar M, et al. Adenosine: a mediator of the sleep-inducing effects of prolonged wakefulness. *Science*. 1997;276:1265–1268.

Rechtschaffen A. Current perspectives on the function of sleep. *Perspect Biol Med*. 1998;41:359–390.

Reppert SM, Weaver DR. Molecular analysis of mammalian circadian rhythms. *Annu Rev Physiol.* 2001;63:647–676.

Saper CB, Scammell TE, Lu J. Hypothalamic regulation of sleep and circadian rhythms. *Nature.* 2005;437:1257–1264.

Siegel JM. Brainstem mechanisms generating REM sleep. In: Kryger MH, Roth T, Dement WC (eds). *Principles and Practice of Sleep Medicine,* 2nd ed. Philadelphia: WB Saunders; 1994;125–144.

Simons FE. Advances in H1-antihistamines. *N Engl J Med.* 2004;351:2203–2217.

Steriade M. Arousal: revisiting the reticular activating system. *Science.* 1996;272:225–226.

Steriade M, McCarley RW. *Brainstem Control of Wakefulness and Sleep.* New York: Plenum Press; 1990.

Toh KL, Jones CR, He Y, et al. An h*Per2* phosphorylation site mutation in familial advanced sleep phase syndrome. *Science.* 2001;291:1040–1043.

Weitz CJ. Circadian timekeeping: loops and layers of transcriptional control. *Proc Natl Acad Sci USA.* 1996;93:14308–14309.

Xu Y, Padiath QS, Shapiro RE, et al. Functional consequences of a CKIdelta mutation causing familial advanced sleep phase syndrome. *Nature.* 2005;434:640–644.

Zeitzer JM, Nishino S, Mignot E. The neurobiology of hypocretins (orexins), narcolepsy and related therapeutic interventions. *Trends Pharmacol Sci.* 2006;27:368–374.

Zeman A, Britton T, Douglas N, et al. Narcolepsy and excessive daytime sleepiness. *Br Med J.* 2004;329:724–728.

CHAPTER 13

Higher Cognitive Function and Behavioral Control

- Executive function, the cognitive control of behavior, depends on the prefrontal cortex, which is highly developed in higher primates and especially humans.

- Working memory is a short-term, capacity-limited cognitive buffer that stores information and permits its manipulation to guide decision-making and behavior.

- Attention permits the selection of relevant information from the enormous welter of sensory inputs. Attention may be effortful or may result "bottom-up" from the appearance of a salient stimulus.

- Attention depends on working memory and on mechanisms that filter sensory inputs for access to working memory.

- Attention and working memory are modulated by drugs that directly or indirectly stimulate dopamine D_1 receptors and noradrenergic receptors. Such drugs, most notably the psychostimulants methylphenidate and amphetamine, are used to treat attention deficit hyperactivity disorder (ADHD).

- Obsessive-compulsive disorder (OCD) and Tourette syndrome may represent related abnormalities in the circuitry connecting the prefrontal cortex, striatum, and thalamus.

- Declarative or explicit memory, which is the memory of facts and events, and nondeclarative or implicit memory, which includes all other forms such as procedural memory and habits, are the two broad categories of memory.

- Structures in the medial temporal lobe, such as the hippocampus, are particularly important for the temporary storage of declarative memories.

- The striatum plays a central role in procedural and habit memory.

- Long-lasting changes in synaptic efficacy (synaptic plasticity) are thought to be important mechanisms for storing memories.

- Strong emotions enhance memory formation, likely because of the associated activation of diffusely projecting neurotransmitter systems (eg, monoamines, acetylcholine).

- Despite intense interest in finding drugs that enhance memory under pathologic conditions (eg, Alzheimer disease) or normal conditions (eg, aging), no robustly effective agents have yet been developed.

The simplest nervous systems sense survival-relevant stimuli in the environment and respond reflexively for self defense, to obtain nourishment, and to reproduce. As organisms became more complex, an increasing number of neurons were interposed between sensory inputs and motor outputs, creating what has been called "the great intermediate net." In the human nervous system, this net has reached remarkable levels of complexity, making possible diverse and subtle forms of cognition and behavioral control including many kinds of learning and memory, abstract thought, the creation of fiction, music, and visual art, and the ability to navigate flexibly in uncertain and changing social situations. For the sake of survival, humans retain simple reflexive responses (eg, to noxious stimuli), simple unconscious homeostatic behaviors such as swallowing and control of respiration, and more complex but automatized behavioral responses to salient stimuli (eg, to certain types of threats or to rewards such as attractive foods).

Most human behavior, however, whether automatic or requiring effortful conscious control, whether learned or improvised, results from interactions among sensory stimuli, innate drives (eg, hunger, thirst, sexual arousal), memories, emotions, and diverse types of cognitive processing. This complexity, which brings with it the possibility of flexible and creative responses to sensory stimuli, also creates the potential for conflict among goals and confusion among possible responses. Without coordination among inputs and outputs, and some mechanism to supervise the selection of goals and behavioral outputs, the result could be self-defeating confusion rather than evolutionary advantage.

The first part of this chapter focuses on prefrontal regions of cerebral cortex and their connections with sensory and emotional centers in the brain that exert control over an individual's behavior under normal and pathological conditions. The second section covers different types of memory, including explicit memories, which are dependent on hippocampal function, and implicit procedural memories, which are dependent on the striatum.

COGNITION, EMOTION, AND THE CONTROL OF BEHAVIOR

Anatomy and Function of the Prefrontal Cortex

The prefrontal cortex is the region that subserves *executive function*, the ability to exert *cognitive control* over decision-making and behavior. It is also important for

anticipating reward and punishment and for empathy and complex emotions. This brain area has grown disproportionately large in our near primate relatives and especially in humans compared with other mammals **13–1**. Different subregions **13–2** participate in a large number of distinct circuits that permit the integration and processing of diverse types of information. The prefrontal cortex receives inputs not only from other cortical regions, including association cortex, but also, via the thalamus, inputs from subcortical structures subserving emotion and motivation, such as the amygdala (Chapter 14) and ventral striatum (or nucleus accumbens; Chapter 15). The prefrontal cortex is also innervated by widely projecting neurotransmitter systems, such as norepinephrine, serotonin, acetylcholine, and orexin/hypocretin, and is the only

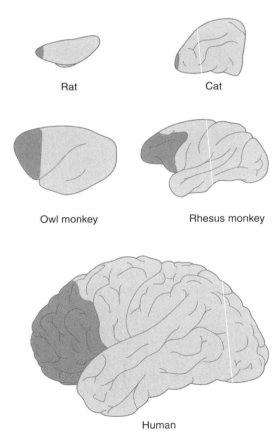

Rat

Cat

Owl monkey

Rhesus monkey

Human

13–1 **Phylogenetic comparison of the proportion of the brain taken up by prefrontal cortex in five different mammalian species.** (Adapted with permission from Kandel ER, Schwartz JH, Jessel TM. *Principles of Neural Science,* 3rd ed. New York: Elsevier; 1991:837.)

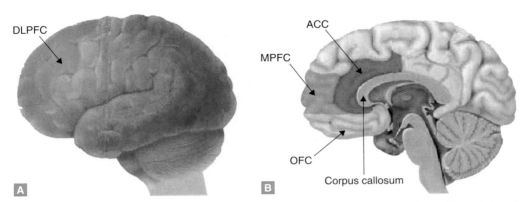

13-2 **Regions of the prefrontal cortex involved in complex cognitive function.** *Left panel,* lateral view showing the dorsolateral prefrontal cortex (DLPFC). *Right panel,* sagittal section showing the medial prefrontal cortex (MPFC), orbital frontal cortex (OFC), and anterior cingulate cortex (ACC).

region of cerebral cortex to receive substantial dopaminergic innervation (Chapter 6). These diverse inputs and back projections to both cortical and subcortical structures put the prefrontal cortex in a position to exert what is often called "top-down" control or cognitive control of behavior. Because behavioral responses in humans are not rigidly dictated by sensory inputs and drives, behavioral responses can instead be guided in accordance with short- or long-term goals, prior experience, and the environmental context. The response to a delicious-looking dessert is different depending on whether a person is alone staring into his refrigerator, at a formal dinner party attended by his punctilious boss, or has just formulated the goal of losing 10 pounds. The response to a rattlesnake will differ depending on whether a person is a novice hiker or a herpetologist looking for specimens. Adaptive responses depend on the ability to inhibit automatic or prepotent responses (eg, to ravenously eat the dessert or run from the snake) given certain social or environmental contexts or chosen goals and, in those circumstances, to select more appropriate responses. In conditions in which prepotent responses tend to dominate behavior, such as in **drug addiction**, where drug cues can elicit drug seeking (Chapter 15), or in **attention deficit hyperactivity disorder** (ADHD; described below), significant negative consequences can result.

Because the prefrontal cortex does not subserve primary sensory or motor functions, language production, or basic intelligence (eg, arithmetic calculation), it was once thought to be silent or nearly so. As late as the 1950s, prefrontal lobotomy was used to treat **schizophrenia** and other severe mental disorders and was rationalized, in part, because basic intelligence survived the surgery. However, damage to the prefrontal cortex has a significant deleterious effect on social behavior, decision making, and adaptive responding to the changing circumstances of life. An important role for regions of the prefrontal cortex was demonstrated as early as the 19th century by the case of Phineas Gage **13-1**.

Several subregions of the prefrontal cortex **13-2** have been implicated in partly distinct aspects of cognitive control, although these distinctions remain somewhat vaguely defined. The *anterior cingulate cortex* is involved in processes that require correct decision-making, as seen in conflict resolution (eg, the Stroop test, see **16-3** in Chapter 16), or cortical inhibition (eg, stopping one task and switching to another). The *medial prefrontal cortex* is involved in supervisory attentional functions (eg, action-outcome rules) and behavioral flexibility (the ability to switch strategies). The *dorsolateral prefrontal cortex*, the last brain area to undergo myelination during development in late adolescence, is implicated in matching sensory inputs with planned motor responses. The *ventromedial prefrontal cortex* seems to regulate social cognition, including empathy. The *orbitofrontal cortex* is involved in social decision making and in representing the valuations assigned to different experiences. It is also implicated in impulsive and compulsive behaviors.

13-1 Phineas Gage

Phineas Gage was a 25-year-old construction foreman, whose team was laying new track for the Rutland and Burlington Railroad when, on a September day in 1848, he became the victim of a dramatic accident. While using a tamping iron to pack blasting powder into a hole drilled in rock, he accidentally set off an explosion that sent the fine-pointed iron through his face, skull, and brain (see figure). The force of the explosion was such that the iron landed yards away. Remarkably, Gage rapidly regained consciousness and was able to talk and, with the help of his men, to walk. As remarkably, during the preantibiotic era, he returned to physical health and showed no signs of paralysis, impaired speech, or loss of memory or general intelligence.

Despite his recovery, Gage was a transformed man, and not for the better. Prior to the accident, he had been polite, responsible, capable, and well socialized; indeed, he had earned the role of foreman at an early age. After the accident he became an unreliable man who would not be trusted to keep his commitments and thus lost his job. He no longer observed social convention; it is documented, for example, that his language became quite profane. He wandered over the next several years and died in the custody of his family, never having held a responsible position again.

Gage's physician, John Harlow, who had related Gage's altered behavior to his brain injury, learned of Gage's death from his family some five years after its occurrence and convinced them to exhume the body. As a result, Gage's skull and the tamping iron, with which he had been buried, are available for study, thus permitting the reconstruction shown in the figure: left, reconstruction of path of tamping bar through the skull; right, midlevel transverse section of the brain showing damaged area of medial prefrontal cortex and preserved Broca area (yellow), motor cortex (red), Wernicke area (blue), and sensory cortex (green).

Gage's lesion involved portions of the left orbital prefrontal cortex and portions of both left and right anterior medial prefrontal cortices. Based on Harlow's reports of Gage's behavior, and on what we now know of the functioning of these brain regions (see text), Gage's lesions explain the degradation of his social behavior and his inability to guide his behavior in accordance with long-term goals. It appears that Gage's dorsolateral prefrontal cortex was spared, thus preserving other domains of cognitive control.

Since the time of Phineas Gage, there have been many studies of human brain damage affecting the prefrontal cortex and more recently functional imaging studies. The case of Phineas Gage illustrates the central importance of the prefrontal cortex in integrating emotion and cognition in the service of executive function.

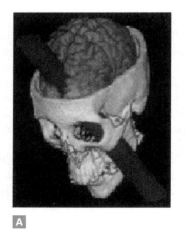
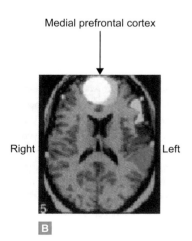

Medial prefrontal cortex

Right   Left

A   B

(From Damasio H, Grabowski T, Frank R, Galaburda AM, Damasio AR. The return of Phineas Gage: clues about the brain from the skull of a famous patient. *Science.* 1994;264:1102–1105.)

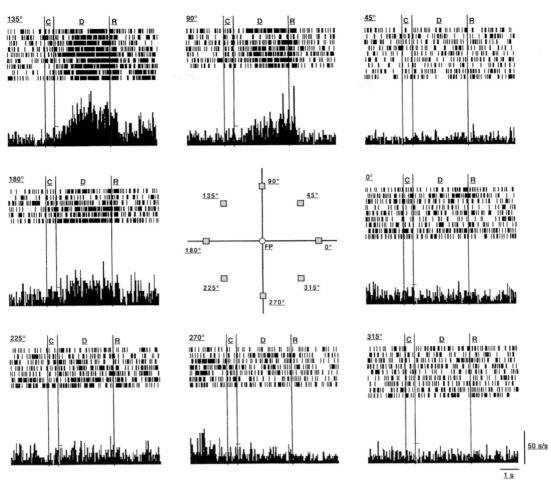

13-3 Repeated recordings from a single neuron during many trials over which a rhesus monkey performed an oculomotor delayed-response working memory task. During a test session, the monkey's ability to make correct memory-guided responses is evaluated 10 to 12 times per target location. The neuron's response is collated over all the trials for a given target location (eg, 135°, 45°) as a histogram of the average response per unit time for that location. The activity is also shown in relation to task events (C, cue; D, delay; R, response) on a trial-by-trial basis for each target location. The particular neuron being recorded fires maximally during the delay period when the target at the 135° location disappears and the monkey is maintaining fixation. This neural activity is maintained throughout the delay period until a response is made. Activity is also seen in the 90° and 180° targets during the delay period but less than that observed for this neuron's best direction. Different neurons code different spatial locations providing a spatial map in working memory. (From Funahashi S, Bruce CJ, Goldman-Rakic, PS. Mnemonic coding of visual space in the primate dorsolateral prefrontal cortex. *J Neurophysiol.* 1989;61,331–349.)

Working Memory

Executive function depends on *working memory*, a short-term, capacity-limited cognitive buffer that maintains a representation of sensory information. Working memory permits the integration and manipulation of this information to guide thought, emotion, and behavior. Working memory can be demonstrated in a range of mammals and has been studied extensively in nonhuman primates as well as humans. Findings drawn from primate research have been used to examine the mechanisms of working memory and its role in executive function. A classic experiment involved the placement of bilateral lesions in the prefrontal cortex of a chimpanzee and subsequent testing of the animal for delayed spatial responses. The chimpanzee watched as a piece of food was placed under one of several opaque containers. After a brief delay, the animal was allowed to choose a container. Unlesioned control animals uniformly chose the container with food, whereas lesioned animals made random selections. After several additional experiments were performed to determine the types of cognitive deficits involved, it became apparent that basic sensory and cognitive functions were intact in the lesioned chimps. What the chimpanzees lacked was the ability to maintain an internal representation of the food and its significance. These chimps needed ongoing sensory stimulation to track the food.

· Our understanding of working memory has expanded considerably since these initial experiments. Subsequent studies, for example, have examined the electrical activity of particular neurons in prefrontal cortex in experimental paradigms that require working memory. In one such study, a monkey was conditioned to fix its eyes on a central point on a video screen 13-3. Subsequently a box was displayed briefly in one of eight areas on the screen. After a 3- to 6-second delay, the central fixation point was removed from the screen, and the monkey was trained to shift its gaze to the area where the box previously had been displayed. This study enabled the identification of neurons in prefrontal cortex that are specific for the region of the screen where the box was displayed. Such neurons become more active during the delay phase of the task and return to baseline levels of activity when the gaze returns to the area in which the box appeared. The increased activity of neurons in the prefrontal cortex during the delay phase of a task is the signature of working memory. This activity appears to provide an internal representation of the box even when it is not visible.

The pharmacologic manipulation of working memory has been the focus of considerable investigation, in part because of the working memory deficits that characterize **schizophrenia** (Chapter 16) and in part because working memory may be impaired in **ADHD**, the most common childhood psychiatric disorder seen in clinical settings, and in several other conditions, including severe stress.

Mild dopaminergic stimulation of the prefrontal cortex enhances working memory; in contrast, higher levels of stimulation profoundly disrupt this function. Because stress is known to increase dopaminergic transmission from the ventral tegmental area to the prefrontal cortex, the actions of dopamine in this brain region may explain why low levels of stress can enhance performance in working memory tasks, whereas higher levels of stress can disrupt performance. These findings are consistent with evidence that

working memory depends on an optimal level of stimulation of D_1 dopamine receptors (see also Chapter 16). D_1 **agonists** have, therefore, been studied as enhancers of working memory, although it has not yet been possible to generate such agonists devoid of troubling side effects such as nausea and vomiting.

Manipulation of the norepinephrine system also affects working memory. For example, α_2-**adrenergic agonists** such as **clonidine** and **guanfacine** (13-4 ; see Chapter 6) appear to enhance working memory, a finding that may explain the utility of these agents in the treatment of **ADHD**. The **selective norepinephrine reuptake inhibitor** (**NRI**), **atomoxetine** 13-4 , is approved for the treatment of ADHD, although its effects on working memory per se have not been established. Atomoxetine does not appear to be distinct in its therapeutic properties from older **tricyclic** NRIs (eg, **desipramine**) that are approved for the treatment of depression (Chapter 14), although it does have milder side effects.

Therapeutic (relatively low) doses of **psychostimulants,** such as **methylphenidate** and **amphetamine** 13-4 , improve performance on working memory tasks both in individuals with **ADHD** and in normal subjects. Positron emission tomography (PET) demonstrates that methylphenidate decreases regional cerebral blood flow in the dorsolateral prefrontal cortex and posterior parietal cortex while improving performance of a spatial working memory task. This suggests that cortical networks that normally process spatial working memory become more efficient in response to the drug. Both methylphenidate and amphetamines act by triggering the release of dopamine, norepinephrine, and serotonin, actions mediated via the plasma membrane transporters of these neurotransmitters and via the shared vesicular monoamine transporter (Chapter 6). Based on animal studies with micro-iontophoretic application of selective D_1 dopamine receptor agonists (such as the partial agonist **SKF38393** or the full agonist **SKF81297**) and antagonists (such as **SCH23390**), and clinical evidence in humans with **ADHD**, it is now believed that dopamine and norepinephrine, but not serotonin, produce the beneficial effects of stimulants on working memory. At abused (relatively high) doses, stimulants can interfere with working memory and cognitive control, as will be discussed below. It is important to recognize, however, that stimulants act not only on working memory function, but also on general levels of arousal and, within the nucleus accumbens, improve the saliency of tasks. Thus, stimulants improve performance on effortful, but tedious tasks, probably acting at different sites in the brain through indirect stimulation of dopamine and norepinephrine receptors.

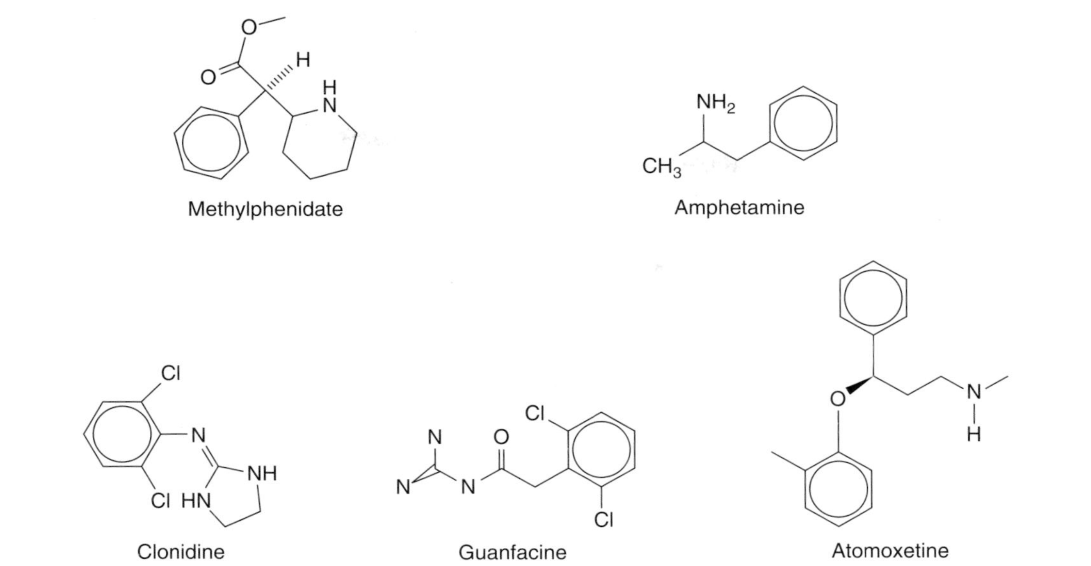

13-4 **Medications used in the treatment of ADHD.**

Methylphenidate

Amphetamine

Clonidine

Guanfacine

Atomoxetine

Although the animal studies described above involve very simple mental representations, working memory is at the heart of many complex mental tasks in higher mammals. When viewed as a rudimentary form of abstraction, working memory can be seen as crossing from the realm of the brain into that of the mind, where internal representations of the external world are consistent and reliable. The ability to think in abstract terms presumably allows humans to create a sense of identity, to establish goals, and to plan for the future.

Attention

In the mass of sensory stimulation by which an animal is bombarded at all times, it must have mechanisms to select the information that is most relevant for its particular situation and ultimately its survival. Selection of relevant information is the role of attention. Once attended to, information gains access to working memory, and can thereby be used to plan appropriate responses. In humans, responses may be simple, but may also involve complex trains of cognition, the activation of emotional circuits, and production of elaborate behaviors. It must be emphasized that much important sensory information is processed by the brain unconsciously, and need not be made conscious to elicit significant responses. For example, subliminal processing of fearful faces can activate physiological aspects of the fear response in humans without ever reaching consciousness (Chapter 14). However,

information that is processed consciously is, at some point, attended to and entered into working memory.

Attention is not a simple unitary function. Attention may be commanded by "bottom-up" sensory information such as a stabbing pain or the sudden appearance of a loud noise or bright flashing light. The concept of attention also includes effortful "top-down" processing involving the prefrontal cortical circuits that connect with other specialized brain regions. For instance, we can purposefully allocate attention, eg, to a particular spatial location (which involves parietal cortex), we can pay selective attention to specific features of the world, eg, the color of an object (which involves the inferior temporal cortex), and we divide our attention, suppress distractions, and concentrate (ie, sustain attention over time).

In one model, four basic cognitive processes are considered to be the building blocks of attention **13-5**: (1) Working memory, as mentioned earlier, is required to exert top down control over those sensory representations that will be attended to and for effortful direction of "the searchlight" of attention. Working memory acts by guiding orientation, such as the direction of the body, the head, or the eyes, and also produces signals that influence the sensitivity of neural circuits that represent information. (2) The allocation of attention, eg, to a point in space, can be shown by functional neuroimaging in humans and by physiological recordings in monkeys to alter activity in relevant brain regions or

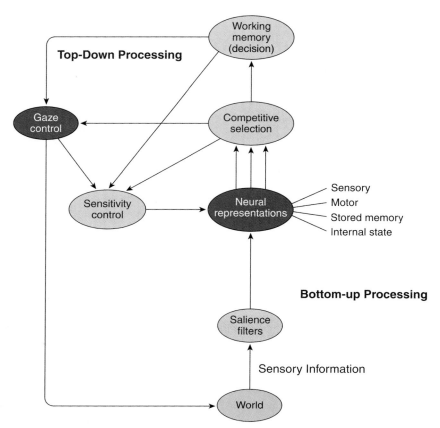

13-5 **Cognitive building blocks of attention.** These cognitive modules can have distributed implementation in the brain. The processes that contribute to attention are in red type. Bottom-up processing occurs when sensory information is permitted to pass by salience filters tuned to innate or learned survival-relevant stimuli and to novel or highly salient stimuli. The neural representations of these stimuli are processed in circuits relevant to the type of information they contain (eg, different sensory modalities, interoceptive information). These neural representations then enter a competitive process that selects the one with the highest signal strength for access to working memory. Working memory directs gaze and other orienting behaviors as well as signals that modulate sensitivity to representations for access to working memory. (Adapted from Knudsen EI. Fundamental components of attention. *Annu Rev Neurosci.* 2007;30:57–78.)

relevant neurons. Thus working memory can exert *sensitivity control* over neural representations and thereby influence the selection of representations that are attended to. Patients with **ADHD** have difficulty sustaining attention or ignoring distractions, suggesting problems with sensitivity control. (3) Diverse sensory information is subjected to *salience filters* so that irrelevant information does not gain access to working memory. Patients with psychotic disorders including **schizophrenia** attend to irrelevant and to hallucinatory stimuli, suggesting a failure of filtering processes. Salience is determined, for example, by innate or learned predictors of threat or reward or by the appearance of rare or

high intensity stimuli. (4) Sensory representations that pass salience filters are subjected to competitive processes that select the strongest signals for access to working memory.

The monoamine neurotransmitters and orexin have a critical permissive role in attention by regulating arousal (Chapters 6 and 12). Performance on cognitive tasks has different optimal levels of arousal depending on the degree of effort required. This is captured in simplistic form by the Yerkes-Dodson principle **13-6** which expresses the relationship of arousal to performance for specific tasks as an inverted U-shaped curve. Such a curve also captures the effects of pharmacologic

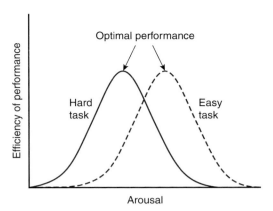

13-6 **Yerkes-Dodson Principle.** This principle (dating from 1908) captures the inverted U-shaped relationship between arousal and performance. Performance on diverse cognitive tasks improves with arousal, but only up to a point; when arousal becomes too great, performance declines. Shown here are two Yerkes-Dodson curves illustrating that lower levels of arousal are optimal for hard tasks (eg, tasks that demand greater cognitive resources) and higher levels for easy tasks or tasks that require greater persistence.

agents that influence arousal, ranging from **psychostimulants** and **caffeine** (Chapter 12) among those drugs that increase arousal to β-**adrenergic antagonists** and **benzodiazepines** that might decrease maladaptive arousal in an extremely anxious person. Beyond these general permissive effects, dopamine (acting via D_1 receptors) and norepinephrine (acting at several receptors) can, at optimal levels, enhance working memory and aspects of attention. Drugs used for this purpose include, as stated above, **methylphenidate, amphetamines, atomoxetine,** and **desipramine. Modafinil** is effective in improving both arousal and attention, yet its mechanism of action remains unknown (Chapter 12).

Attention deficit hyperactivity disorder ADHD is characterized by symptoms in three dimensions of behavior: inattention, impulsiveness, and hyperactivity. Hyperactivity may be absent, in which case the term **attention deficit disorder** (**ADD**) may be used. These dimensions are continuous with normality, but, when severe, ADHD produces significant impairment. ADHD can be a profound obstacle to success in school or work, despite normal intelligence. ADHD also increases the risk for substance abuse and accidents, as well as for comorbid depression, anxiety disorders, and conduct disorders.

ADHD begins in childhood, often very early, but is typically diagnosed when children enter school. While symptoms often remit during teen years, a substantial fraction of individuals with ADHD remain symptomatic in adulthood. Based on current diagnostic criteria, worldwide prevalence ranges between 3% and 5%, but widely divergent diagnostic practices in different regions of the world produce varying local estimates. Indeed, the diagnosis and treatment of ADHD varies widely in the United States, with far higher rates in affluent, suburban communities compared with poorer, inner city areas.

Risk of ADHD is highly influenced by genes; however, like all major psychiatric disorders, including **depression, bipolar disorder,** and **schizophrenia,** ADHD is genetically complex, making the identification of risk alleles very challenging. Multiple studies have reported an association of ADHD with an allele of the D_4 dopamine receptor, which contains seven repeats of a 48 base-pair variable number tandem repeat (VNTR) in exon 3. However, this finding has not been universally replicated. Discovery of other candidate alleles and clear delineation of the contribution of the D_4 receptor and other gene candidates to ADHD risk awaits large-scale genetic studies using advanced methods.

ADHD can be conceptualized as a disorder of executive function; specifically, ADHD is characterized by reduced ability to exert and maintain cognitive control of behavior. Compared with healthy individuals, those with ADHD have diminished ability to suppress inappropriate prepotent responses to stimuli (impaired response inhibition) and diminished ability to inhibit responses to irrelevant stimuli (impaired interference suppression).

The ability to suppress prepotent responses is thought to require the action of *frontal-striatal-thalamic circuits* **13-7**. A series of parallel loops connect the prefrontal cortex with specific regions of the basal ganglia and, via the thalamus, project back to prefrontal cortex. These loops are thought to be involved in the initiation and control of motor behavior, attention, cognition, and reward responses. Functional neuroimaging in humans demonstrates activation of the prefrontal cortex and caudate nucleus (part of the striatum) in tasks that demand inhibitory control of behavior. Subjects with ADHD exhibit less activation of the medial prefrontal cortex than healthy controls even when they succeed in such tasks and utilize different circuits.

Early results with structural MRI show thinning of the cerebral cortex in ADHD subjects compared with age-matched controls in prefrontal cortex and posterior parietal cortex, areas involved in working memory

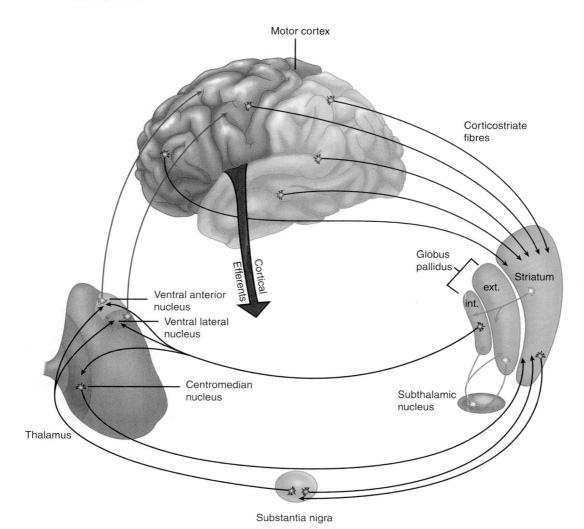

13-7 **Cortical-striatal-thalamic loops.** The basal ganglia are a set of related subcortical nuclei comprised of the striatum (composed of the caudate nucleus, the putamen, and the ventral striatum), the globus pallidus, the substantia nigra (composed of the dopaminergic pars compacta and the pars reticulata) and the subthalamic nucleus. The striatum receives major inputs from the cerebral cortex, thalamus, and brainstem (including dopamine from the substantia nigra) and projects via the globus pallidus and substantia nigra pars reticulata to the thalamus and thence to the prefrontal cortex. As shown, this arrangement gives rise to a series of parallel loops. Different sets of cortico-striatal-thalamic loops have specialized functions depending on the cortical areas that give rise to them and that receive their input. A motor loop that passes through the putamen may be involved in Tourette syndrome, while a cognitive loop through the caudate nucleus may be involved in the obsessions that characterize obsessive-compulsive disorder. See **17-9** for more detail on striatal circuits.

and attention. More recent longitudinal studies comparing ADHD and control populations find that cortical thickness tends to normalize during adolescence. These results, while still preliminary, suggest that ADHD represents an abnormal rate of cortical maturation rather than a unique pattern of cortical development. It is hypothesized that residual symptoms in adulthood might result from incomplete normalization, but at this point the data are not available.

As suggested by the previous discussions of the pharmacology of working memory and attention, ADHD can be treated with **psychostimulants,** such as methylphenidate and amphetamine, which remain by far the most effective treatments available. The most widely used treatments are sustained release preparations of methylphenidate that compensate for its short half-life, or mixtures of amphetamine derivatives with different half-lives to provide both early and extended treatment during the day. The main side effects of stimulants are appetite suppression, growth delay, and insomnia. Atomoxetine or other NRI antidepressants such as desipramine represent an alternative for patients who do not tolerate stimulants, although these drugs are not as effective as stimulants in most cases. The α_2-adrenergic agonists, clonidine and guanfacine, show beneficial effects in a subset of patients, but their use is not well supported by clinical trials data. Children and adults with ADHD can also benefit from behavioral treatments aimed at enhancing top-down control of behavior.

Stimulant prescriptions have engendered controversy because these drugs are potentially abusable (when the drugs are used at higher than therapeutic doses), because they are used even in young children (as early as age three), and because they may be used with benefit by individuals with only mild or even absent symptoms, in which case they are being used for cognitive enhancement rather than treatment. Controversy notwithstanding, there are extensive clinical trials data that demonstrate that stimulants effectively reduce ADHD symptoms, albeit with little data bearing on long-term academic and employment outcomes. Several longitudinal studies suggest that untreated ADHD is associated with elevated risk of substance abuse and conduct disorders, as stated earlier, and that stimulant treatment decreases that risk. Two factors may be at play. First, supervised use of stimulants at therapeutic doses may decrease risk of experimentation with drugs to self-medicate symptoms. Second, untreated ADHD may lead to school failure, peer rejection, and subsequent association with deviant peer groups that encourage drug misuse.

Obsessive-Compulsive Disorder Spectrum Disorders

Obsessive-compulsive disorder (OCD) is characterized by *obsessions* (intrusive, unwanted thoughts) and *compulsions* (highly ritualized behaviors intended to neutralize the anxiety and negative thoughts resulting from the obsessions). Individuals with OCD experience the obsessions as unwanted and even nonsensical, but powerfully insistent. Attempts to resist the performance of compulsions result in high levels of anxiety. Typical symptom patterns are remarkably similar

across cultures, such as repetitive hand washing, sometimes hours a day to the point of skin damage, to neutralize fears of contamination, or repeatedly checking the front door because affected individuals cannot be sure the door is locked. OCD often begins in childhood or teen years, although later onset can occur.

OCD is often accompanied by depression. A smaller fraction of individuals with OCD have other disorders that are thought to be related etiologically or pathophysiologically to OCD, specifically Tourette syndrome and body dysmorphic disorder (relentless obsessions about one's supposed bodily deformities). These are sometimes described as part of an OCD spectrum.

Tourette syndrome is characterized by motor and phonic *tics* that wax and wane in severity over time. Tics are habitual movements or vocalizations that appear suddenly and that mimic fragments of normal behaviors. Tics usually begin during childhood, and may start as early as age three. Patients with Tourette syndrome may also have OCD, ADHD, and other behavioral disorders characterized by poor impulse control. While stress can exacerbate the symptoms of Tourette syndrome, as seen for most neurologic and psychiatric disorders, there is no evidence that stress per se contributes to the pathogenesis of the illness.

Frontal-striatal-thalamic circuits are thought to be involved in implicit learning that consolidates fragments of motor behavior, speech, or thought into smooth, but flexible routines, eg, the ability to drive one's car home without effortful attention, or the ability of an actor to deliver her lines without thinking. These well-learned assembled routines are often described as *habits*. The striatum and other nuclei of the basal ganglia are thought to recode both cortical (eg, cognitive and motor) and subcortical (eg, emotional and motivational) inputs into sequences, sometimes called "chunks" that permit appropriate cues to release automatic responses, as will be described in greater detail in later sections of this chapter.

Structural MRI studies of OCD patients show reduced gray matter volume in the medial frontal gyrus, medial orbitofrontal cortex, and other regions. Functional imaging studies of OCD have reported increased activity in components of cortical-striatal-thalamic circuitry including the orbitofrontal cortex and the caudate nucleus. Similarly, in Tourette syndrome, increased activity has been observed in other regions of the prefrontal cortex as well as in the caudate. These and similar observations, combined with increasing basic knowledge of the functioning of basal ganglia circuits (see below), have led to the hypothesis that OCD and Tourette syndrome result from abnormal activity in different cortical-striatal-thalamic loops inappropriately releasing unwanted intrusive thoughts (OCD) or fragments of motor behavior (Tourette).

Despite the hypothesized similarities in pathophysiology and the frequent co-occurrence of OCD in Tourette patients, the pharmacologic treatments differ. OCD is treated with **selective serotonin reuptake inhibitors** (**SSRIs**) such as **fluoxetine** or **sertraline**, or with **tricyclic antidepressants** that have relative selectivity for the serotonin transporter such as **clomipramine** (Chapter 14). OCD is also responsive to cognitive behavioral therapies focused on stopping unwanted thoughts and rituals, presumably acting to facilitate top-down cognitive control. The doses of SSRIs required for OCD are usually higher than those for depression, and the onset of therapeutic benefit is often even slower (up to 10 weeks). SSRIs are also effective in the treatment of **body dysmorphic disorder**.

In contrast to OCD, Tourette syndrome is most often treated with both first- and second-generation D_2 dopamine receptor antagonist **antipsychotic drugs** at lower doses than those used to treat schizophrenia. α_2-Adrenergic agonists (eg, **clonidine** and **guanfacine**) are also effective in many patients. These drugs are not efficacious in treating OCD. Such differences in treatment response suggest that ascending serotonin and dopamine projections may modulate parallel but separate cortical-striatal-thalamic loops quite differently.

MEMORY

Our ability to learn and remember is such an integral part of our lives that it is difficult to function with any significant memory impairment. Memory permeates existence, from the mundane (Where did I put my keys?) to the profound (Who am I? What are my beliefs?). It is only a slight exaggeration to say that our memories are *who we are*. Memory depends on the precise functioning of healthy neurons. Age, trauma, malnutrition, and genetic factors can diminish our ability to store and recall information, and severe forms of memory impairment, as seen in common dementias such as **Alzheimer disease**, can have tragic consequences. This section considers the neural mechanisms that underlie learning and memory.

Declarative and Nondeclarative Memory

Learning and memory are closely related to one another, but the terms are not interchangeable. Learning refers to the process by which behavior can be changed as a result of experience or practice. Memory refers to the ability to recall what has been learned. There are several different types of memory that can be divided into two major classes termed *declarative* and *nondeclarative* **13-8**. Declarative memory, which also is

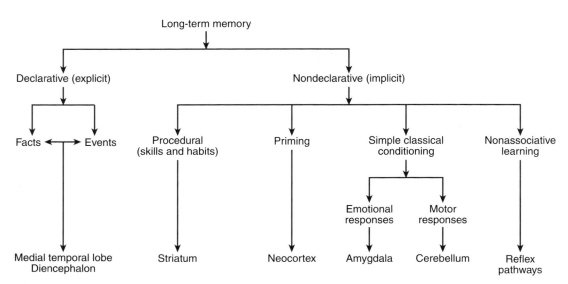

13-8 **Taxonomy of mammalian memory systems.** This categorization of the different types of memory recognized by psychologists and neuroscientists indicates the brain structures and neural connections believed to be especially important for each kind of memory. (Adapted with permission from Milner B, Squire LR, Kandel ER. Cognitive neuroscience and the study of memory. *Neuron.* 1998;20:445.)

known as *explicit memory,* refers to the process that enables us to recall facts or events. Memorizing the Gettysburg Address and remembering where you parked your car this morning involve declarative memory. This type of memory also may be thought of as *conscious memory* or as memory that is capable of being verbalized. In contrast, nondeclarative memory, also known as *implicit memory,* can be thought of as subconscious or unable to be verbalized. The term nondeclarative memory is used broadly and may refer to several learning processes, including those that involve procedural skills and the formation of habits.

Procedural memory is a type of nondeclarative memory involved in learning skilled behaviors; it is used, for example, when an individual learns to type or to play tennis. Procedural memory is distinct from a declarative memory of the actual training episode; for instance, typing is distinct from remembering when you learned how to type. The formation of *habits,* or the gradual acquisition of behavioral tendencies that are specific to a set of stimuli, also involves nondeclarative memory. Habit learning is exhibited during *operant conditioning,* as when an animal learns to perform a task to obtain some reward, such as food or a drug of abuse. Significantly, declarative and nondeclarative memory processes can be experimentally distinguished, are mediated by distinct neural substrates, and are affected by different types of diseases **13–8**.

The Medial Temporal Lobe System

In 1953, a patient referred to as H.M. underwent a bilateral resection of the medial structures of the temporal lobe—including the anterior two-thirds of the hippocampus—as a desperate measure to treat intractable epilepsy. This surgery had tragic consequences that caused H.M. to become one of the best known neurologic patients. After his operation, H.M. had severe *anterograde amnesia:* he lost his ability to store new memories. Although he could recall the names of people he had known for many years before his operation, he could not remember the names of individuals he met postoperatively, including those of nurses and doctors whom he would meet repeatedly over a period of several months. In addition to his inability to form new memories, H.M. lost memories of events that had occurred up to a decade before his surgery. Yet his ability to recall more remote events remained intact and his I.Q. test scores rose (from 104 to 118), an improvement that can be attributed to postsurgical control of his seizures. Moreover, H.M. retained some memory capacity; with great exertion he was able to remember facts, such as short strings of digits, for approximately 15 minutes. However, as soon as he was distracted, such facts would vanish from his memory. Thus H.M. did have the ability to store facts for brief periods of time, ie, he had normal working memory. However, he appeared unable to transfer a fact from working memory to *long-term memory,* which enables facts to remain accessible for long periods of time.

Despite his difficulty in storing facts, H.M. was capable of procedural learning as evidenced by his ability to learn how to trace an object while viewing his hand in a mirror. Although such a task is quite tricky, H.M. learned to perform this task as quickly and as well as control subjects. However, after repeating the task many times he was completely unable to recall whether he had ever previously performed the task. This demonstrated that procedural learning can occur independently of declarative learning and that declarative memory, but not procedural or other types of nondeclarative memory or working memory, is critically dependent on at least one of the brain structures that had been removed during H.M.'s surgery.

Patients such as H.M., who have well defined brain lesions with otherwise good health, are relatively rare. Thus, our knowledge of the brain structures that are crucial for declarative learning has been drawn primarily from animal experiments. It may seem problematic to attribute declarative learning to animals that cannot talk to human experimenters. However, it is possible to distinguish "learning what" (declarative memory) from "learning how" (nondeclarative memory) in primates and rodents. One method of testing declarative memory in animals involves the use of the "delayed nonmatching to sample task." During this task, a test subject is shown an object that is subsequently taken away. Next, two objects—a new object and the original object—are presented. To receive a reward, the subject must choose the object that has *not* been seen before. Consequently, to choose correctly, the subject must be able to retain a declarative memory of the original object between the two presentations. Normal monkeys perform this task well. Monkeys with bilateral medial temporal lobe lesions perform at chance levels, except when the intervals between presentations are short. Extensive lesion studies have revealed that the specific crucial structures underlying the ability to store declarative memories are the hippocampus, the subicular complex, and the entorhinal cortex **13–9**. Importantly, these findings are consistent with what has been learned from the small number of human patients with lesions restricted to medial temporal lobe structures.

Does the medial temporal lobe store our declarative memories? The answer is that it probably does not,

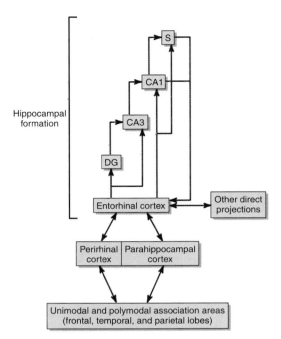

Hippocampal formation

13-9 **The medial temporal lobe memory system.** Some of the interconnections among the structures of this system and connections between the medial temporal lobe and the neocortex are shown. S, subiculum; DG, dentate gyrus. (Adapted with permission from Milner B, Squire LR, Kandel ER. Cognitive neuroscience and the study of memory. *Neuron.* 1998;20:445.)

at least not permanently. As previously mentioned, H.M. did not lose all of his declarative memories. He was able to recall his name and his date of birth, and he appeared to have accurate and normal memories of events that had occurred 10 or more years before his operation. Results of animal experiments are consistent with H.M.'s experience. In one type of experiment, animals are trained in a task, and at varying times thereafter undergo bilateral damage to the hippocampus. Retention of the task is then assessed shortly after the surgery. These studies reveal that such damage causes a retrograde amnesia of days to months depending on the time interval between the training and the surgery. Experiments such as these and observations of human amnesiacs have led investigators to postulate that structures in the medial temporal lobe coordinate a process by which memories or associations are gradually imprinted on the cerebral cortex. How this occurs has not been determined, but it is believed that inputs from the medial temporal lobe to specific cortical regions gradually reorganize synaptic

connections in the cortex until memories are somehow stored and available for recall. Recent work suggests that some of this *consolidation* of declarative memories in the cortex occurs during sleep.

The Striatum and Habit Memory

In contrast to declarative memory, nondeclarative memory does not appear to be supported by a single brain region, but by diverse neural circuits that underlie the behavior that comes to be modified by learning. For example, the basal ganglia play a central role in the acquisition of stimulus-response associations that, as described above, can ultimately be reorganized into automatic behavioral repertoires or habits. Stimulus-response associations result from the gradual modification of neural circuits that comprise the basal ganglia. Evidence that the caudate nucleus and putamen influence stimulus-response learning comes from lesion studies in rodents and primates and from neuroimaging studies in humans and from studies of human disease.

In **Parkinson disease**, the dopaminergic innervation of the caudate and putamen is severely compromised by the death of dopamine neurons in the substantia nigra pars compacta (Chapter 17). Patients with Parkinson disease have normal declarative memory (unless they have a co-occurring dementia as may occur in **Lewy body disease**.) However, they have marked impairments of stimulus-response learning. Patients with Parkinson disease or other basal ganglia disorders such as **Huntington disease** (in which caudate neurons themselves are damaged) have deficits in other procedural learning tasks, such as the acquisition of new motor programs.

Synaptic Plasticity: How Do Neurons Remember?

Whether we consider declarative or nondeclarative memory, a key question is how do the properties of neurons change in a manner that allows new memories to form. A major mechanism by which this occurs is synaptic plasticity, which refers to the ability of neural activity itself to modulate the strength of synaptic communication. Indeed, as discussed in Chapter 5, it is now well established that in virtually all brain regions different patterns of activity can bidirectionally influence synaptic strength by eliciting either long-term potentiation (LTP), a long-lasting increase in synaptic strength, or long-term depression (LTD), a long-lasting decrease. In the context of learning and memory, NMDA receptor-dependent LTP has received the most attention and we will briefly review its properties and the evidence of its functional importance. Molecular mechanisms underlying LTP and LTD are covered in Chapter 5.

LTP and memory formation LTP was first described in the hippocampus where it was shown that repetitive, brief (one sec) high-frequency stimulation of axons sufficient to strongly depolarize postsynaptic cells caused a long-lasting increase in the size of the postsynaptic response lasting for hours and in some cases even weeks 13–10. Not only can LTP be elicited in the hippocampus, a structure known to be important for learning and memory, but it also has properties that seem ideal for a synaptic mechanism that underlies the storage of new information: it can be elicited rapidly by a short stimulus (high-frequency stimulation) and exhibits both *input-specificity* and *associativity*. Input specificity indicates that LTP occurs only at synapses that are stimulated by a given pattern of afferent activity, and not at adjacent, unstimulated synapses

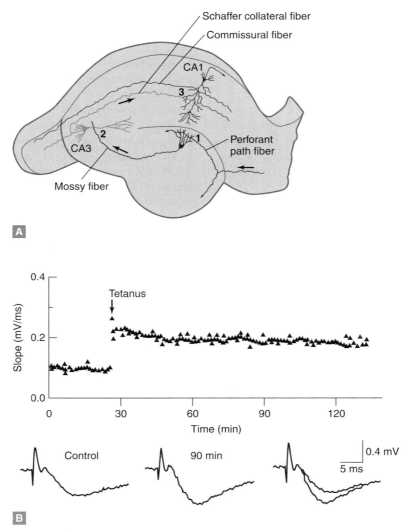

13–10 A. Diagram of the major excitatory pathways (1, 2, 3) in the hippocampus. B. Long-term potentiation (LTP) obtained from a hippocampal slice preparation. Schaffer collateral and commissural fibers were stimulated to generate a synaptic response in CA1 pyramidal cells; after baseline recordings were obtained for 30 minutes, a high-frequency train of stimuli (tetanus) was given. This tetanus elicited a stable, long-lasting increase in the size of the postsynaptic response. Sample extracellular synaptic responses are shown below the graph. (Adapted with permission from Nicoll RA, Kauer JA, Malenka RC. The current excitement in LTP. *Neuron.* 1988;1:97.)

on the same postsynaptic cell. Limiting the number of synapses on a given cell that are modified by afferent activity greatly increases the storage capacity of the neural circuit in which that cell participates. The property of associativity refers to the fact that the generation of LTP requires coincident presynaptic and postsynaptic activity. Importantly, a weak input that is incapable of significantly depolarizing the cell is potentiated only if it is active at the same time that the postsynaptic cell is depolarized by a strong input.

These properties of LTP derive from the fact that it is triggered by a large Ca^{2+} influx through postsynaptic NMDA receptors and that activation of these receptors requires coincident presynaptic release of glutamate to depolarize the postsynaptic neurons, which relieves the Mg^{2+} block of the NMDA receptor channel (Chapter 5). Thus, LTP does not occur at synapses unless they are active when the postsynaptic cell is strongly depolarized. Because a neuron generally has thousands of inputs and several of these must be active simultaneously to cause significant depolarization of the neuron, the firing of a single or small numbers of inputs does not generate LTP.

A great deal of experimental evidence supports the requirement of NMDA receptor activation and Ca^{2+} influx for the induction of LTP. As discussed in Chapter 5, this NMDA receptor–mediated rise in Ca^{2+} activates intracellular signaling pathways (in particular, Ca^{2+}-activated protein kinases), which increase synaptic strength by inserting AMPA receptors into the postsynaptic membrane. The enzymatic alteration of preexisting synaptic proteins by means of phosphorylation is sufficient to change synaptic efficacy for relatively short periods of time. Therefore, the maintenance of LTP for days or weeks involves additional mechanisms. LTP is associated with the structural enlargement of synapses and possibly the growth of new dendritic spines. Such changes in synapse structure can explain how the initial increase in synaptic strength becomes permanent since larger synapses in general are stronger synapses and would allow the new "information" encoded by LTP to become more permanent.

The prolonged enhancement of synaptic strength also likely requires the activation of particular genes and new protein synthesis. Although the critical gene products are unknown, the cAMP pathway and its regulation of the transcription factor CREB (see Chapter 4) have been strongly implicated in the long-term maintenance of LTP and also in the maintenance of long-term memory. In diverse invertebrate and vertebrate species, for example, manipulations that decrease functioning of the cAMP pathway or CREB have been shown to impair certain memory tasks,

whereas manipulations that enhance CREB function often have the opposite effect.

An important question is how altered gene expression, which occurs in the nucleus of the cell body, leads to the maintenance of potentiation only in previously stimulated synapses, and not in the neuron's thousands of other synapses. One possibility is that the modification of preexisting synaptic proteins that occurs immediately after the induction of LTP might somehow tag these synapses so that the newly synthesized proteins generated through the stimulation of gene transcription are targeted to these synapses and not to adjacent synapses on the same cell.

Although LTP displays characteristics that might be expected of a memory mechanism, attempts to perform experiments that directly link LTP per se to real memory processes are difficult. Based on the hypothesis that LTP underlies learning and memory, two major predictions can be made. First, the prevention of LTP should be able to prevent or at least disrupt the establishment of memories. Consistent with this prediction, genetic manipulations in mice that lead to the absence of the NMDA receptor in various regions of the hippocampus cause profound deficits in spatial learning. Conversely, mutant mice with enhanced NMDA receptor function in this brain region, achieved through the overexpression of $NMDAR_{2B}$ receptor subunits, which increases receptor-mediated currents (Chapter 5), perform better than wildtype mice in memory tasks. Furthermore, when injected into the hippocampus of rats one day after they had been trained in a spatial memory task, agents that reverse LTP caused the loss of the memory. These findings strongly suggest that LTP in the hippocampus is required for at least some forms of learning and memory known to be dependent on this brain region.

A second prediction is that if LTP underlies learning and memory, it also should occur during the formation of memories. However, its presence during memory formation is not easy to demonstrate since it is very difficult to isolate the small proportion of neural connections that are responsible for a given learning event. Nonetheless, LTP-like phenomena have been observed to occur in parallel with learning in the hippocampus and in the amygdala during a form of learning termed *fear conditioning*. As described in Chapter 14, one form of conditioned fear is produced in experimental animals when a neutral tone is paired with an electric shock. This fear conditioning involves the amygdala, which receives glutamatergic inputs that undergo NMDA receptor–dependent LTP. Consistent with a role for LTP, blocking NMDA receptors in the amygdala prevents the development of the conditioned fear response. A subsequent critical experiment, in which auditory-evoked responses in the amygdala were recorded while an animal underwent a conditioning procedure, demonstrated that fear conditioning induces LTP in the auditory pathway to the amygdala **13-11**. Taken together, these findings make an impressive case for a connection between memory processes and LTP.

Other forms of neural plasticity Although LTP remains the synaptic mechanism most commonly thought to mediate learning and memory, other forms of synaptic plasticity are also likely to play important roles. These include several different forms of LTD, a generic term used to describe a long-lasting, activity-dependent decrease in synaptic strength (Chapter 5). Evidence suggests, for example, that a form of LTD observed in the cerebellum is critically important for mediating certain types of motor learning. As well, LTD may be important for reversing LTP because, without such a mechanism, LTP might completely saturate synaptic strength at large numbers of synapses and thereby limit the storage capacity of any given neural circuit. Indeed, computational models of neural networks have demonstrated that the ability to bidirectionally modify synaptic strength, that is, utilizing both LTP and LTD, greatly increases the power of these circuits to store and retrieve information.

Although synaptic plasticity (LTP and LTD) is the best understood mechanism by which neuronal responsiveness can be regulated, there is evidence that *nonsynaptic plasticity* may also be important, particularly for more generalized forms of learning and memory such as emotional memory versus memory of a specific event. Nonsynaptic plasticity comprises changes in the electrical excitability of neurons that are generalized to many synapses or perhaps the entire cell and not localized to a particular dendritic spine. For example, altered levels of expression of ion channels in a neuron or even changes in the subtypes of ion channels expressed in response to some stimulus would be expected to either increase or decrease that neuron's excitability by a host of inputs. Similarly, general growth or retraction of dendritic arborizations would have significant effects on neuronal responsiveness that would not be limited to specific synapses. It is easy to imagine how such nonsynaptic plasticity might mediate changes in the responsiveness of neurons to certain types of environmental exposures, for example, tolerance or sensitization to a **drug of abuse**, which can be viewed as a type of memory (Chapter 15). Further work is needed to determine whether nonsynaptic plasticity also contributes to memory of

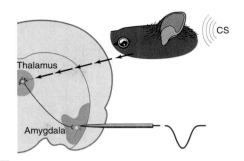

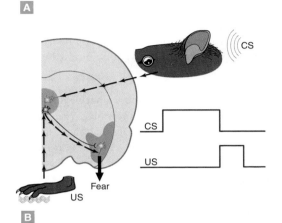

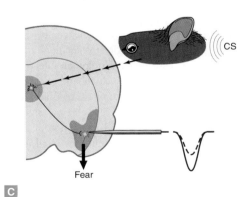

13-11 **The occurrence of long-term potentiation (LTP) during fear conditioning. A.** An auditory conditioned stimulus (CS) evokes a synaptic response (generated by way of the thalamus) in the amygdala. **B.** The CS is paired with a foot shock, which is referred to as the unconditioned stimulus (US). **C.** After repeated training (pairing of the CS and US), the CS causes a larger synaptic response in the amygdala and is capable of eliciting fear. (Adapted with permission from Malenka RC, Nicoll RA. Learning and memory: Never fear, LTP is hear. *Nature.* 1997;390:552.)

nonpharmacologic, that is, behavioral–environmental stimuli.

A detailed understanding of the physical changes in the nervous system that are responsible for learning and memory will require a great deal of additional research. However, the elucidation of some of the basic mechanisms underlying LTP and LTD and other mechanisms of plasticity has focused attention on what for many decades was believed to be an intractable problem. Thus, it seems likely that major discoveries are on the horizon and that during the next decade new pharmacologic agents will be developed to facilitate learning and memory by targeting proteins that have been shown to be involved in neural plasticity.

Beyond LTP: why we remember what we remember
It is impossible to remember everything. Therefore, an important goal for research on learning and memory is to understand the factors that allow us to remember certain events or associations and forget others. One factor that can enhance memory is extreme emotion. Almost everybody will remember a car accident or where they were during a public tragedy such as 9/11. This type of declarative memory, which is enhanced by strong emotion, is often called *flashbulb memory*. In general, the stronger the associated emotion when a memory is encoded, the more vivid the memory is. This cognitive enhancement of declarative memory, which is hippocampal dependent, also requires an intact amygdala. Evidence suggests that such enhancement can be inhibited, without associated amnesia, by β-**adrenergic antagonists** (eg, **propranolol**). This observation is consistent with the well-established promotion of certain forms of LTP in the hippocampus by β-adrenergic receptor activation, which involves stimulation of the cAMP-CREB pathway.

Strong emotion also produces amygdala-dependent *emotional memories* (see Chapter 14). This form of nondeclarative memory can be observed even in individuals with hippocampal lesions that have no conscious recall of the circumstances under which the memory was acquired. Emotional memories are usually activated by cues that are reminiscent of the original stimulus and that produce physiologic and behavioral responses appropriate to the emotion. In the case of fear, such responses include activation of the sympathetic nervous system and may result in a freezing response in prey species. Conversely, in strongly rewarding situations, responses elicited by emotional memory lead to approach behavior and physiologic preparation for activities such as eating, drinking, or sex. Both the declarative and nondeclarative

components of memories when encoded in the context of strong emotional stimuli have survival value: a vivid memory of a dangerous situation helps an organism avoid similar situations in the future, and memory of a rewarding situation helps an organism obtain future rewards.

However, emotional memory can be maladaptive in some situations; for example, when it is activated under the pathologic circumstances that characterize **posttraumatic stress disorder** (**PTSD;** Chapter 14) or **drug addiction** (Chapter 15). Most research on the neural substrates of emotional memory has focused on the amygdala in studies of aversive stimuli and on the ventral striatum in studies of reinforcing stimuli. Currently, a major challenge is to understand how these subcortical structures interact with more traditional memory structures, such as the hippocampus and prefrontal cortex, to produce fully integrated emotional memories, and how such circuits malfunction in pathologic conditions. The view that pathological emotional memories may contribute to disorders such as PTSD and drug addiction has led to the novel idea of enhancing *extinction* of these memories during treatment. Rather than simply undoing the earlier memory, extinction is now thought to represent a second learning event on top of the underlying memory. Current clinical trials are testing whether stimulation of pathological memories in patients with PTSD or drug addiction (eg, by use of virtual reality of combat or drug-taking situations) coupled with drugs that promote new memory might enhance extinction and lead to clinical improvement. One such drug used for this purpose is D-**cycloserine,** a partial agonist at NMDA glutamate receptors. There is also evidence in animal studies that **glucocorticoids** may exert similar actions.

Pharmacological Regulation of Memory

There has been intense interest in developing medications that correct the cognitive impairments commonly seen in many neurologic and psychiatric illnesses, in particular, **schizophrenia** and **Alzheimer disease**, not to mention medications that promote cognitive function in normal individuals, so-called **cognitive enhancers**. Numerous strategies are currently under investigation and several show promise in preclinical studies; however, no drug mechanism has yet been definitively validated in humans.

Among the neurotransmitters with the greatest influence on memory is acetylcholine. In both humans and animals, muscarinic cholinergic antagonists, such as **atropine** and **scopolamine,** produce memory deficiencies at low doses and a more profound disruption of memory and consciousness known as **delirium**. Delirium may be caused by any of several common psychiatric medications which have muscarinic cholinergic antagonist properties, such as **tricyclic antidepressants** (Chapter 14) and first-generation **antipsychotic drugs** (Chapter 16). Delirium is particularly common among the elderly, where it can be confused with dementia **13–1**.

In the mammalian brain, cholinergic nuclei—most notably the nucleus basalis, or Meynert's nucleus, in the basal forebrain—project heavily to the neocortex and hippocampus (Chapter 6). The release of acetylcholine by these nuclei generally promotes depolarization or rhythmic firing of postsynaptic neurons through the activation of muscarinic and nicotinic cholinergic receptors. **Carbachol,** for example, a muscarinic cholinergic agonist, produces rhythmic, synchronized firing of hippocampal CA1 pyramidal neurons. This synchronized firing occurs at a frequency of approximately 5 to 7 Hz and is described as a *theta rhythm*. The precise role of theta rhythm in memory storage is not completely understood; however, when it is induced in a hippocampal slice preparation, weak stimuli that ordinarily do not produce potentiation can evoke LTP. One current view is that cholinergic activity decreases the threshold of neural activity necessary for learning. Nicotinic receptors are similarly implicated in hippocampal function and in the formation of memory.

This body of knowledge led to the introduction of acetylcholinesterase inhibitors (eg, **donepezil** and **tacrine**) for the treatment of memory deficits in Alzheimer disease. However, the efficacy of these agents is weak at best (Chapter 17). Current efforts are focused on agonists at specific muscarinic or nicotinic receptors. For example, animal studies suggest that **agonists at nicotinic α_7 homomeric receptors,** which predominate in hippocampus, can improve learning and memory (Chapter 6). Clinical studies are now needed to validate this mechanism in humans.

Several other mechanisms are being considered to improve cognitive function under pathological and normal conditions. Drugs that promote glutamate function might be expected to enhance learning and memory, based on the essential role of glutamate in synaptic plasticity as discussed earlier. D-**Cycloserine,** a partial agonist at the glycine site of the NMDA glutamate receptor, is under clinical evaluation as discussed above. So-called **AMPA-kines,** drugs that are positive allosteric regulators of AMPA glutamate receptors (Chapter 5), show promise in animal studies and are also in clinical trials. **Agonists or antagonists at particular metabotropic glutamate receptors** might also be expected to promote glutamate-mediated synaptic plasticity and thereby enhance learning and memory.

The ability of **dopamine D_1 receptor agonists,** in prefrontal cortical circuits, to promote working memory was discussed earlier in this chapter. Similarly effective in these brain regions in some animal models are protein kinase A (PKA) activators or phosphodiesterase (PDE) inhibitors; these agents would be expected to mimic the activation of D_1 receptors, which signal via the G_s-cAMP-PKA pathway (Chapters 4 and 6). Such agents might also be expected to promote memory formation in hippocampal and other circuits, where they would mimic the pro-memory effects of β-adrenergic receptors, which couple to this same signaling pathway. The precognitive effects of stimulating the cAMP pathway is consistent with this pathway's activation of CREB, a mediator of long-term memory as discussed earlier. **Rolipram,** an inhibitor of PDE4, shows moderate cognitive-enhancing activity in preclinical studies, although it has unacceptable side effects (eg, nausea and vomiting). Accordingly, there has been great effort to develop more selective inhibitors of PDE4 subtypes, which might be devoid of these side effects, as well as inhibitors of several other PDE subtypes highly expressed in memory-related circuits in the brain.

13–1   **Comparison Between Delirium and Dementia**

	Delirium	Dementia
Course	Acute	Chronic
Symptoms	Fluctuating	Persistent
Level of consciousness	Reduced	Alert
Orientation	Impaired	Variable
Attentional deficit	Prominent	Variable
Thought processes	Disorganized	Variable
Perceptual abnormalities	Present	Variable
Sleep–wake cycle	Disrupted	Variable
Memory	Impaired (particularly recent memory)	Impaired (short- and long-term memory)

Based on the ability of high potency, short-acting **benzodiazepines** (eg, **midazolam** and **triazolam**) to disrupt learning and memory, there has been interest in developing inverse-agonists at the benzodiazepine site of the $GABA_A$ receptor as cognitive enhancers. While full inverse agonists would cause seizures, it is possible that weak partial inverse agonists might be sufficiently safe and effective. This strategy has not yet been tested in humans. Finally, there is interest in the potential of **adenosine receptor antagonists** in promoting learning and memory (Chapters 8 and 12).

While most efforts are being devoted toward developing drugs that enhance memory, there are a small number of clinical situations where disruption of memory is advantageous. The high-potency, short-acting **benzodiazepines** mentioned in the previous paragraph are useful in the context of medical procedures (eg, colonoscopy, dental surgery) in part because they disrupt memory. Moreover, as previously indicated, it appears that β-adrenergic antagonists such as **propranolol** may be useful in preventing memories of traumatic events.

SOCIAL COGNITION

Social cognition refers to cognitive and emotional processes that explicitly underpin social processes, such as social judgments or social affiliation. Other cognitive processes, such as language, that enable social interaction are considered outside the purview of social cognition or of social neuroscience more broadly. Humans are a social species and, as such, are constantly emitting social signals, both consciously (effortfully and automatically) and, more commonly, unconsciously. Similarly, we receive and automatically process a large number of social signals throughout the day. Along with our biases and nonsocial sensory inputs the social signals we receive influence diverse social judgments. These include: (1) judging the likely mental states and motives of others (eg, by observing the direction of their gaze and their other actions); (2) forming empathy, ie, not only judging the other's feelings from the outside, but feeling the emotion the other seems to feel; (3) forming moral and esthetic judgments about the actions and motives of others; and (4) becoming aware of how one's own internal thoughts and emotions are influenced by others.

Signals that communicate emotional states have potent effects on social behaviors, although at present the best experimentally characterized example of the effect of emotional signals comes from outside the social domain. Faces, and most especially eyes, that express emotion can influence not only social emotions

such as pride, shame, guilt, trust, or jealousy, but also basic "survival emotions" such as fear, anger, happiness, and disgust. Fearful faces, which might signal a threat, activate the amygdala in functional imaging experiments (Chapter 14). Interestingly, a fearful face can still elicit amygdala activation and a change in the autonomic nervous system even if it is presented for a very short period and then followed by a "mask," a neutral face. Subjects who participate in such experiments have no conscious recall of having seen the fearful face, despite their brains having clearly processed the information.

Much of our information on human social cognition is based on human brain injuries and on functional imaging with social tasks. As one example, the ventromedial prefrontal cortex appears to be activated when thinking about the mental states of both self and others, and patients with lesions of the ventromedial prefrontal cortex have deficits in social emotions such as shame, guilt, and empathy. Emerging evidence suggests that social cognition is highly dependent on prefrontal cortex, and on the integration of more purely cognitive processing with emotional information coming from the amygdala, hypothalamus, and ventral striatum. Much remains to be learned in this young field and there is little specific pharmacology as yet with the exception of experiments using the peptides oxytocin and vasopressin (Chapter 7).

Oxytocin and *vasopressin* are evolutionarily closely related nonapeptides that cross the blood–brain barrier when given intranasally. In different species both have physiologic functions based on their release from the posterior pituitary (neurohypophysis; Chapter 10) and central functions based on their action within the hypothalamus, amygdala, and other structures. Within the brain, these peptides regulate anxiety and social behavior. In humans, vasopressin increases anxiety, acting on circuits within the amygdala (thus **vasopressin V_{1a} receptor antagonists** are being studied as possible antianxiety agents), and oxytocin decreases anxiety acting on different cells in the amygdala. In rodent species, oxytocin is well known to increase social recognition, pair bonding, and affiliation. In humans, oxytocin nasal spray has been shown to increase trust in a laboratory-based economic trust game. We are just embarking on the beginning of the exploration of the neural substrates and pharmacologic manipulation of social emotions, with all of the complex therapeutic and ethical implications waiting to be addressed.

Autism   Autism is a disorder in which social cognition is powerfully disturbed. Autism is characterized by abnormal social function, by language delay (or in severe cases absence of language function), and restricted interests and repetitive behaviors. Autism is highly genetically influenced, but given the complexity of genetic risk, significant information about risk genes is only just starting to emerge. The diagnosis is made in early childhood; the disorder can best be thought of as a spectrum, ranging in severity from very high functioning individuals (**Asperger syndrome**) with normal language function to children who also suffer from **mental retardation** and **seizures**. In addition to deficits, individuals with autism often have remarkable islands of cognitive strength.

The restriction of behaviors and interests in autism has been hypothesized to reflect abnormal functioning of the cortical-striatal-thalamic loops discussed above. Far more investigation is needed to confirm this theory. Whatever the pathogenesis, however, this aspect of autism can lead to significant impairment and can warrant both behavioral and pharmacologic interventions. Autistic people forced to break routine can be angry, anxious, and extremely stubborn. Severely affected individuals may have repetitive behaviors that are self-injurious, which are nonetheless extremely difficult to terminate. In these cases, when behavioral interventions fail, pharmacologic agents are used empirically, eg, **SSRIs** to control anxiety or low-dose second-generation **antipsychotic drugs** to control highly problematic behavioral outbursts.

The core deficit in the social cognitive abilities of individuals with autism is thought to be an inability to form empathy. This deficit makes it difficult or impossible for the autistic person to attribute mental states to others and thus to make sense of their motives and actions, resulting in severe impairments of social interaction. Unfortunately, there are currently no pharmacologic treatments for this disabling aspect of autism spectrum disorders.

Recent work is beginning to identify genes that cause or predispose individuals to autism spectrum disorders. Mutations in *MeCP2* (a methylated DNA binding protein) cause Rett syndrome (Chapter 4), while mutations in *FMRP* (Fragile X mental retardation protein) cause Fragile X syndrome, which often presents with autism-like symptoms (Chapter 5). Mutations in several synaptic proteins (eg, *neuroligins* and *neurexins*) are associated with a small number of cases of autism. Interestingly, neuroligins are postsynaptic proteins that bind to the presynaptic neurexins, interactions which are thereby believed to specify neuronal connections in the developing brain. These advances are enabling better animal models of autism spectrum disorders; thus, mice with mutations in the aforementioned proteins show abnormalities in social behavior. It is hoped that such models will lead eventually to a better understanding of the neurobiologic basis of the disorders and to more rational and effective pharmacotherapies.

SELECTED READING

Adolphs R. Cognitive neuroscience of human social behaviour. *Nat Rev Neurosci.* 2003;4:165–178.

Aston-Jones G, Cohen JD. An integrative theory of locus coeruleus-norepinephrine function: adaptive gain and optimal performance. *Annu Rev Neurosci.* 2005;28:403–450.

Baddeley A. Working memory: looking back and looking forward. *Nat Rev Neurosci.* 2003;4:829–839.

Baron-Cohen S, Belmonte MK. Autism: a window onto the development of the social and analytic brain. *Annu Rev Neurosci.* 2005;28:109–126.

Cai WH, Blundell J, Han J, et al. Postreactivation glucocorticoids impair recall of established fear memory. *J Neurosci.* 2006;26:9560–9566.

Damasio H, Grabowski T, Frank R, et al. The return of Phineas Gage: clues about the brain from the skull of a famous patient. *Science.* 1994;264:1102–1105.

Davis M, Ressler K, Rothbaum BO, et al. Effects of D-cycloserine on extinction: translation from preclinical to clinical work. *Biol Psychiatry.* 2006;60:369–375.

Desimone R, Duncan J. Neural mechanisms of selective visual attention. *Annu Rev Neurosci.* 1995;18:193–222.

Frith CD, Frith U. Social cognition in humans. *Curr Biol.* 2007;17:R724–R732.

Goldman-Rakic PS. Cellular basis of working memory. *Neuron.* 1995;14:477–485.

Graybiel AM. The basal ganglia: learning new tricks and loving it. *Curr Opin Neurobiol.* 2005;15:638–644.

Kirsch P, Esslinger C, Chen Q, et al. Oxytocin modulates neural circuitry for social cognition and fear in humans. *J Neurosci.* 2005;25:11489–11493.

Knudsen EI. Fundamental components of attention. *Annu Rev Neurosci.* 2007;30:57–78.

Kosfeld M, Heinrichs M, Zak PJ, et al. Oxytocin increases trust in humans. *Nature.* 2005;435:673–676.

Malenka RC, Bear MF. LTP and LTD: an embarrassment of riches. *Neuron.* 2004;44:5–21.

McGaugh JL. The amygdala modulates the consolidation of memories of emotionally arousing experiences. *Annu Rev Neurosci.* 2004;27:1–28.

Mehta MA, Owen AM, Sahakian BJ, et al. Methylphenidate enhances working memory by modulating discrete frontal and parietal lobe regions in the human brain. *J Neurosci.* 2000;20:RC65.

Miller EK, Cohen JD. An integrative theory of prefrontal cortex function. *Annu Rev Neurosci.* 2001;24: 167–202.

Milner B, Corkin S, Teuber HL. Further analysis of the hippocampal amnesic syndrome: 14-year follow-up study of HM. *Neuropsychologia.* 1968;6: 215–234.

MTA Cooperative Group. A 14-month randomized clinical trial of treatment strategies for attention-deficit/hyperactivity disorder. *Arch Gen Psychiatry.* 1999;56:1073–1086.

Packard MG, Knowlton BJ. Learning and memory functions of the basal ganglia. *Annu Rev Neurosci.* 2002;25:563–593.

Pastalkova E, Serrano P, Pinkhasova D, et al. Storage of spatial information by the maintenance mechanism of LTP. *Science.* 2006;313:1141–1144.

Robbins TW. Chemistry of the mind: neurochemical modulation of prefrontal cortical function. *J Comp Neurol.* 2005;493:140–146.

Shaw P, Eckstrand K, Sharp W, et al. Attention-deficit/hyperactivity disorder is characterized by a delay in cortical maturation. *Proc Natl Acad Sci U S A.* 2007;104:19649–19654.

Squire LR, Kandel ER. *Memory: From Mind to Molecules.* New York: WH Freeman; 1999.

Tabuchi K, Blundell J, Etherton MR, et al. A neuroligin-3 mutation implicated in autism increases inhibitory synaptic transmission in mice. *Science.* 2007;318: 71–76.

Tonegawa S, Nakazawa K, Wilson MA. Genetic neuroscience of mammalian learning and memory. *Phil Trans R Soc Lond B Biol Sci.* 2003;358:787–795.

Turner DC, Robbins TW, Clark L, et al. Cognitive enhancing effects of modafinil in healthy volunteers. *Psychopharmacol.* 2003;165: 260–269.

Vaidya CJ, Bunge SA, Dudukovic NM, et al. Altered neural substrates of cognitive control in childhood ADHD: evidence from functional magnetic resonance imaging. *Am J Psychiatry.* 2005;162: 1605–1613.

Volkow ND, Wang G-J, Fowler JS, et al. Evidence that methylphenidate enhances the saliency of a mathematical task by increasing dopamine in the human brain. *Am J Psychiatry.* 2004;161:173–180.

Whitlock JR, Heynen AJ, Shuler MG, et al. Learning induces long-term potentiation in the hippocampus. *Science.* 2006;313:1093–1097.

CHAPTER 14

Mood and Emotion

- Emotions activate physiologic, cognitive, and behavioral outputs that facilitate adaptive responses to salient external and internal stimuli.

- A crucial emotion, important in several mental disorders, is fear. The neural circuitry of fear is well understood because fear can be reliably elicited in animal models, and because its effects can readily be measured.

- Information about threatening stimuli is transmitted from the thalamus and cerebral cortex to the amygdala where it is processed; neurons carrying fear-related information then project to diverse downstream sites in the brain responsible for adaptive responses.

- Anxiety, a state characterized by arousal, vigilance, physiologic preparedness, and in humans, negative subjective states, may share some critical circuits with fear.

- Because of the evolutionary conservation of key neural circuits, animal research on fear has relevance to humans. Several anxiety disorders may involve abnormal regulation of amygdala-based fear circuitry.

- Mood disorders are divided into unipolar disorders, which are characterized by depression only, and bipolar disorder, which is diagnosed if the person has ever had an episode of mania.

- Mood disorders are influenced by both genes and environment, with genes playing a greater role in bipolar than in unipolar disorders.

- Animal models to study mood regulation and mood disorders are far from perfect. However, in concert with human experiments involving functional neuroimaging and clinical trials of deep brain stimulation, a picture of mood-regulating circuits is beginning to emerge.

- Individuals with major depression often exhibit excessive activation of the hypothalamic–pituitary–adrenal axis; thus, depression shares some physiologic mechanisms with chronic stress.

- Most of the effective pharmacologic treatments for depression act on protein targets within monoamine synapses, generally enhancing neurotransmission by norepinephrine, serotonin, or both. A similar role for dopamine is postulated but unproven.

- Although the initial molecular targets of antidepressants are well characterized, the actual mechanism of action is not understood. The several-week latency of onset of therapeutic effects suggests that slowly developing adaptive responses to initial enhancement of monoamine neurotransmission are required for efficacy.

- Therapies for bipolar disorder include lithium and several drugs, including valproic acid, that were originally developed as anticonvulsants.

- The mechanism of action of lithium is not well understood. Two leading candidate mechanisms are inhibition of the inositol phosphate and Wnt signaling glycogen synthase kinase 3β pathways.

Emotions are critical to survival and represent transient physiologic, cognitive, and behavioral outputs that constitute adaptive responses to survival-relevant or otherwise salient stimuli. *Mood* is a term used to characterize the predominant emotional state over time. Moods (eg, happy, sad, irritable) interact bidirectionally with emotional responses to particular stimuli.

Although there are many subtle forms of emotion, they may be divided into two broad categories by their valence. Negative emotions, such as fear, are elicited under normal circumstances by stimuli that connote danger, pain, or other noxious conditions and generally lead to avoidance, escape, or protective responses. Positive emotions are elicited by stimuli that connote food, safety, comfort, or reproductive opportunities and lead to approach behaviors.

Many common human diseases produce pathologic emotional states that may be transient or enduring. Although most individuals with these disorders can be treated, at least in part, with available pharmacologic agents, their mechanisms of action are generally not deeply understood. For example, the initial molecular targets of **anxiolytic** (antianxiety) and **antidepressant** drugs have been determined, but the mechanisms by which these drugs ultimately produce their therapeutic effects have yet to be adequately characterized.

REPRESENTATION OF EMOTION IN THE BRAIN

Emotion processing circuits in the brain appraise the valence and potency of stimuli and activate appropriate responses. The neural substrates of emotion involve, in part, evolutionarily old brain regions lying deep to the neocortex **14-1**, including the amygdala, hippocampus, parahippocampal gyrus, and cingulate gyrus. These structures have strong interconnections with the hypothalamus, ventral striatum (nucleus accumbens), and the orbital and medial prefrontal cortex. Although the older term *"limbic system"* (comprising an inexact collection of forebrain structures) is still in use, suggesting some central processor for emotion, it is clear based on lesion studies in animals, strokes and other brain injuries in humans, and functional neuroimaging that different emotions (eg, fear, disgust, trust) utilize distinct circuits involving limbic structures, frontal regions of cortex, and the hypothalamus.

Appraisal of a stimulus (eg, as dangerous, novel, or desirable) requires that highly processed sensory and cognitive information from the association cortex gain access to emotion processing circuits, which then activate adaptive responses. These downstream responses include stimulation of arousal and attention, mediated via activation of monoamine, cholinergic, and other

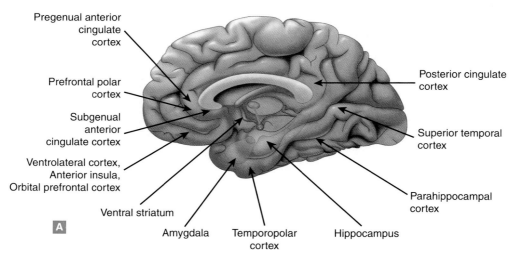

14-1A **Limbic regions involved in emotion and mood. A.** A ring of tissue (limbus) comprised of the hippocampus and amygdala as well as the cingulate and parahippocampal gyri encircles the upper brainstem. It consists of evolutionarily older forms of cortex than the six layered neocortex. This ring has been called the limbic lobe or limbic system, but is no longer thought to represent a single purpose system involved in emotion. Rather "limbic" structures play important roles in diverse circuits that interact with the prefrontal cortex and the hypothalamus.

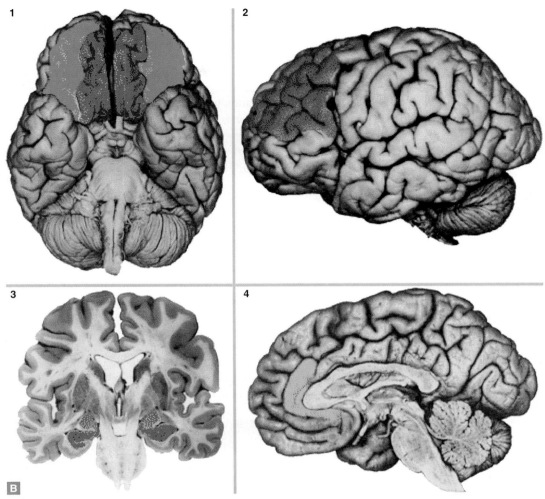

14-1B **Limbic regions involved in emotion and mood.** **B.** Multiple views of the prefrontal cortex and related areas. *Panel 1:* View from the bottom of the brain showing the orbital (pink) and medial (green) prefrontal cortex. *Panel 2:* Dorsolateral prefrontal cortex (purple). *Panel 3:* Hippocampus (bottom, pink) and amygdala (top, stippled pink). *Panel 4:* Anterior cingulate gyrus (yellow). (From Davidson RJ, Pizzigalli D, Nitschke JB, Putnam K. Depression: perspectives from affective neuroscience. *Annu Rev Psychol.* 2002;53:545–574.)

widely distributed neurotransmitter systems in the brain (Chapter 6) as well as by activation of the autonomic nervous system (Chapter 9) and certain neuroendocrine systems (Chapter 10). Strong emotion suppresses ongoing behaviors in favor of automatic defensive or approach behaviors. Experiences encoded under the influence of strong emotion also lead to the enhancement of diverse types of memory processes to make subsequent responses to similar stimuli maximally efficient (Chapter 13). Whether in avoidance of a predator or in

hunting food, a few hundred milliseconds can have enormous implications for success and even survival.

Fear

Research on fear in animal models has relevance to humans in both health and disease because of the evolutionary conservation of significant aspects of fear circuitry across mammalian species. Fear can be roughly divided into innate fear and learned (or conditioned) fear. Innate fear is exemplified by the inborn avoidance of brightly lit, open spaces by rodents. Conditioned fear results when an animal learns to associate predictive stimuli with danger, harm, or pain. Fear conditioning has been exploited in the laboratory to delineate fear circuitry in the brain **14–1**.

Experiments in rat and mouse models have indicated that information about threatening stimuli is transmitted from the sensory thalamus and sensory and association areas of the cerebral cortex to the lateral nuclear complex of the amygdala (there are some species-specific differences in the organization of the amygdala), the amygdala's major input nuclei. Information is processed and sent by both direct and indirect routes to the central nucleus, the major output nucleus of the amygdala, although some information may bypass the central nucleus and be transmitted directly to effector sites of the fear response. Efferent projections from the central nucleus activate numerous effector sites for cognitive, physiologic, and behavioral aspects of the fear response **14–2**.

14–1 **Studying Fear Circuitry**

Classical conditioning experiments have been used to analyze fear circuitry. In such experiments, a neutral stimulus such as a tone or light is consistently presented prior to a strongly aversive stimulus—the unconditioned stimulus (US)—such as foot shock. After a period of learning, known as conditioning, the animal regards the previously neutral stimulus, now the conditioned stimulus (CS), as a predictor of the aversive event. The resulting associative learning causes a tone previously paired with foot shock to produce fear-related behaviors, the conditioned response (CR), such as freezing or enhanced startle. (With a strongly aversive stimulus, conditioning can be apparent after a single episode.) With the use of precise lesions and anatomic methods, investigators have been able to trace the pathways between areas in the brain that receive auditory input (the tone) and the areas responsible for various physiologic and behavioral outputs (see **14–2**). Such mapping studies have identified the amygdala, a complex nucleus in the temporal lobes, as a critical node in fear-processing circuits.

Corroboration of the importance of the amygdala in fear comes from observation of humans with lesions due to disease or injury and by functional neuroimaging studies following presentation of fearful stimuli. For example, the figure shows a coronal section of a functional MRI (fMRI) image. The right amygdala is significantly activated by a masked fearful face compared with a masked happy face. The rapid masking of the fearful face interferes with conscious recollection of seeing the fearful face; hence the amygdala activation represents a rapid unconscious response. The bar graph shows the percent change in blood oxygen level dependent (BOLD) fMRI signal for successive epochs in which individuals were exposed to masked fearful versus masked happy faces. Note that the fear response (signal elevation in amygdala) desensitizes over time.

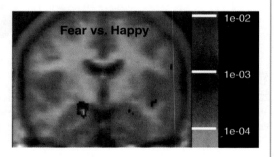

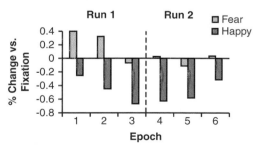

Whalen PJ, Rauch SL, Etcoff NL, et al. Masked presentations of emotional facial expressions modulate amygdala activity without explicit knowledge. *J Neurosci.* 18:411–418.

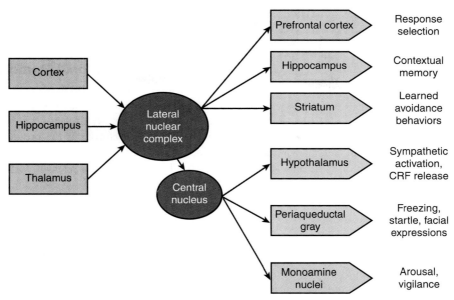

14–2 **Flow of information into and out of the amygdala.** Fear-related information enters the amygdala by means of its lateral nuclear complex. These nuclei project to the central nucleus, which projects to structures that produce the diverse physiologic and behavioral responses characteristic of fear, including the central or periaqueductal gray area, lateral hypothalamus, paraventricular nucleus of the hypothalamus (PVN), monoaminergic nuclei such as locus ceruleus, raphe nuclei, ventral tegmental area, and many regions not shown. Some outputs bypass the central nucleus.

Projections to the lateral hypothalamus mediate activation of the sympathetic nervous system, and projections to the paraventricular nucleus (PVN) of the hypothalamus induce the synthesis and release of corticotropin-releasing factor (CRF) (Chapters 7 and 10). The release of CRF activates a cascade that ultimately leads to the release of glucocorticoids from the adrenal cortex. Glucocorticoids cause the body to enter a catabolic state; they suppress inflammatory responses and heighten arousal. The hypothalamic–pituitary–adrenal (HPA) axis often becomes chronically hyperactive in individuals with **depression,** as discussed in subsequent sections of this chapter. Because CRF also serves as a neurotransmitter for neurons in the central nucleus of the amygdala, through which it may contribute to fear and anxiety, **CRF antagonists** are being developed as potential antidepressants and anxiolytics.

Projections from the amygdala to the periaqueductal gray matter (PAG) in the core of the brainstem activate descending analgesic responses that involve endogenous opioid peptides, which can suppress pain in response to intense fear and stress (Chapter 11). Projections to a different region of the PAG activate

species-specific defensive responses, such as behavioral freezing in rats and mice. Projections to the noradrenergic locus ceruleus, the serotonergic raphe nuclei, and the dopaminergic ventral tegmental area increase arousal and vigilance and enhance the formation of explicit and implicit memories of circumstances under which danger has occurred (Chapter 6).

Under normal circumstances, fear responses enhance survival. It has been hypothesized, however, that abnormal fear processing gives rise to disabling anxiety disorders.

Anxiety

Anxiety is a state of preparation for danger, which is characterized by arousal, vigilance, physiologic preparedness, and, in humans, negative subjective states that are qualitatively similar to those associated with fear. Yet anxiety differs from fear in that it is triggered in the absence of an immediately threatening stimulus. Anxiety can be elicited by diverse cues ranging from the specific to the general. Moreover, in circumstances in which there are no "safety" signals, the state of anxiety may be prolonged.

The circuitry underlying anxiety may differ somewhat from that of fear responses in that the *bed nucleus of the stria terminalis (BNST)* may partly take the place of the central nucleus of the amygdala in giving rise to projections involved in physiologic and behavioral expressions of anxiety. The BNST is considered an extended region of the amygdala, and indeed resembles the central nucleus of the amygdala with regard to its cellular organization; yet it is hypothesized that this area may respond to less specific stimuli than the central nucleus and thus may mediate the more generalized symptoms of anxiety. CRF may act in this region to induce anxiety-like behaviors. An example of an animal test of anxiety is shown in **14–2**.

Anxiety and Emotional Memory

The memories produced by fearful situations have both a cognitive and an emotional component. The cognitive component, which depends at least in part on the hippocampus, records the precise setting in which danger was experienced and details of the experience. The emotional component of fear-related memories, which depends in part on the lateral

---

14–2 **Elevated Plus Maze**

A long-established device for observing anxiety-like behavior in rodents is the elevated plus maze (see figure). This apparatus is elevated above a table and consists of two arms that intersect to form the shape of a plus sign. The sides of one arm are closed, and the sides of the other arm are open. An animal is placed at the intersection of the arms, and the amount of time it chooses to spend in each arm is measured. Rodents normally prefer the closed arm; this preference has led investigators to hypothesize that rodents experience an aversive state akin to anxiety in the open arm. The elevated plus maze has become a screening tool to identify drugs with anxiolytic properties. **Benzodiazepines** such as **diazepam** dramatically increase the amount of time an animal spends in the open arm, as indicated on the hypothetical bar graph. In contrast, β-**carboline** (β-**CCE**), an inverse agonist at the benzodiazepine binding site of the GABA$_A$ receptor, which is anxiogenic in humans, reduces the amount of time an animal spends in the open arm. Drugs that do not produce anxiolytic or anxiogenic responses in humans are without effect when administered to animals placed in the elevated plus maze.

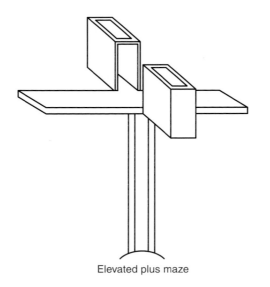
Elevated plus maze

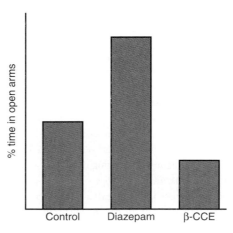
% time in open arms

Control   Diazepam   β-CCE

nuclear complex of the amygdala, activates physiologic and behavioral responses to danger when learned predictors of danger are encountered. Normally, we experience the cognitive and emotional components of fear-related memories as completely intertwined, but their dependence on different circuits can be revealed by lesions. Patients who have had lesions of the amygdala from stroke, viral infections, or head injury lack autonomic and other conditioned responses to previously learned fearful stimuli, even though their declarative memory (their ability to consciously recall a specific stimulus) is intact. Conversely, patients with hippocampal lesions may not consciously recall exposure to fear-associated stimuli, but retain their autonomic responses.

The cognitive component of memories encoded under strong emotion are markedly enhanced compared with ordinary memories. Contrast, for example, the memories of Americans for the details of where they were on the morning of September 11, 2001 versus September 10, 2001. Based on pharmacologic experiments in human subjects and invasive experiments in rodents, this enhancement has been shown to depend on β-adrenergic receptors in the amygdala, which then interacts strongly with the hippocampus. Moreover, this enhancement can be blocked by β-adrenergic receptor antagonists such as **propranolol** administered prior to certain stages of memory consolidation. A pilot clinical trial of propranolol given in

the emergency room after a trauma is suggestive that it might be efficacious under realistic circumstances in humans, although the results are not yet conclusive. It is important that propranolol does not cause amnesia; the hoped for goal in this trial is to cause traumatic memories to recede to the level of ordinary memories, perhaps decreasing the risk of **posttraumatic stress disorder** (**PTSD**; 14-3).

Positive emotional experiences also promote memory. Under normal circumstances these memories produce reinforcement in response to natural rewards such as food, safety, and mating opportunities. Just as abnormal function of fear circuitry can produce disabling symptoms, abnormal stimulation of reward circuitry by certain drugs may be a central cause of addiction. Interestingly, the amygdala, acting in concert with the brain's reward circuitry, has been implicated in mediating such reward-enhanced memory formation (Chapter 15).

Mood Regulation

Compared with the neural mechanisms that underlie emotions such as fear and anxiety, those that underlie mood regulation are less well understood. Experimental models of fear and anxiety in animals do not have obvious counterparts that might facilitate the investigation of moods such as sadness or happiness. Yet considerable overlap or interaction likely exists among the neural

---

14-3 Posttraumatic Stress Disorder

PTSD initially was identified in veterans exposed to life-threatening combat situations, and has more recently been demonstrated in response to severe civilian trauma. Symptoms include hyperarousal, sleep disturbance, cue-induced reexperiencing of the traumatic event accompanied by physiologic aspects of the fear response, and emotional numbing. Fear-related memories enable us to avoid putting ourselves in harm's way a second time after we have been burned, bitten, or chased. Such memories enable us to identify cues that predict danger so that when we encounter them we are physiologically and behaviorally ready to fight or flee. In PTSD, these memories are too strong and overly generalized and can lead to severe impairment in an individual's ability to function.

The strength and persistence of memories encoded in the presence of intense fear may underlie not only PTSD, but other anxiety disorders as well, such as **agoraphobia**. In PTSD, reminders of the original trauma elicit both explicit (conscious) memories of the experience and emotional memories, including physiologic and behavioral fear responses. Agoraphobia, or a fear of public places, often results from the association of extremely frightening symptoms known as a **panic attack** with previously neutral contexts in which panic attacks have occurred. PTSD and related syndromes have been hypothesized to involve powerful stimulation of amygdala-based fear pathways, resulting in powerful, maladaptive associative emotional memories.

systems that regulate emotions such as fear and anxiety, and moods such as sadness. Not only do moods and emotions influence each other, but anxiety and mood disorders often co-occur in the same individuals and appear to have shared genetic risk factors. Because of the lack of fully convincing animal models of mood, much of the investigation of mood regulation has required the use of noninvasive neuroimaging techniques such as positron emission tomography (PET) and functional magnetic resonance imaging (fMRI) in studies of human subjects. Accumulated data suggest that circuits involved in mood regulation and mood disorders include the orbital and medial prefrontal cortex, the cingulate gyrus, amygdala, ventral striatum, hippocampus, and hypothalamus.

PET studies from several laboratories have focused attention on the region of the anterior cingulate gyrus that bends under the genu of the corpus collosum (subgenual cingulate cortex) also known as Broadmann area 25 based on traditional mapping of the cerebral cortex **14-1** and **14-3**. One subregion of the anterior cingulate gyrus is activated by pain. Others are activated when task performance deviates from successful attainment of goals. Thus, the anterior cingulate cortex may monitor performance for signs of failure, just as the amygdala monitors sensory inputs for signs of threat. This cortical region exhibits, on average, increased levels of metabolic activity in major depression, which return to normal with successful pharmacologic treatment. It is also activated in normal subjects in response to scripts that induce sadness **14-3**. Based on these findings, patients with unremitting major depression, who have not achieved relief from multiple drugs, psychotherapy, or electroconvulsive therapy, have been treated by **deep brain stimulation (DBS)** with placement of the stimulating electrode within the subgenual cingulate cortex **14-4**. Such DBS would be expected to quiet an overactive region. To date, approximately two-thirds of the

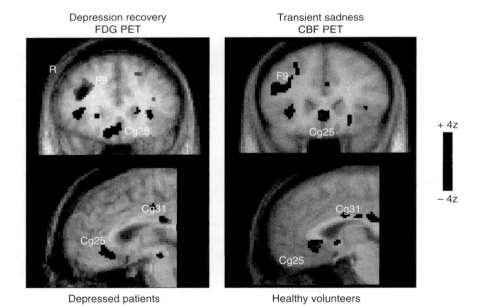

Depression recovery
FDG PET

Transient sadness
CBF PET

Depressed patients

Healthy volunteers

14-3 **Subgenual cingulate cortex responds to changes in mood state.** PET scanning following injection of fluorine 18-labeled deoxyglucose permits measurement of metabolic activity in the brain. The left panel shows patients after successful pharmacologic treatment of depression. The right panel shows normal subjects following transient induction of sadness. The top views are coronal sections, the bottom show midsagittal sections. In the pseudocolor scale (right) red shows increased activity and blue shows decreased activity compared with the comparison state (depressed for the patients; prior to inducing sadness for the normal subjects). Successful treatment of depression decreases activity in subgenual cingulate cortex (cingulate gyrus area 25–cg25), while induction of sadness increases activity in this area. F9 is an area in dorsolateral prefrontal cortex. Cg31 is an area in the posterior cingulate gyrus. (From Mayberg HS. Reciprocal limbic-cortical function and negative mood: converging PET findings in depression and normal sadness. *Am J Psychiatry*. 1999;156:675–682.)

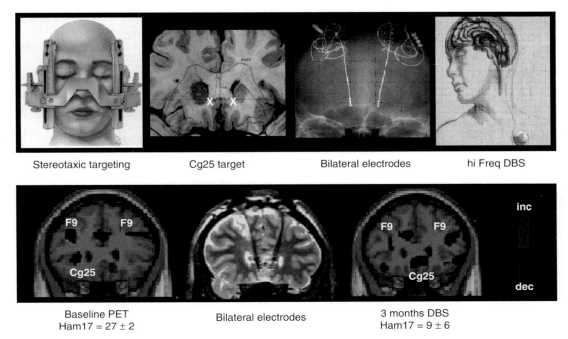

| Stereotaxic targeting | Cg25 target | Bilateral electrodes | hi Freq DBS |

| Baseline PET
Ham17 = 27 ± 2 | Bilateral electrodes | 3 months DBS
Ham17 = 9 ± 6 |

14–4 **Deep brain stimulation for major depression.** *Top panel* (from left to right): Stereotactic frame used in surgery; coronal section showing cg25 target; placement of bilateral electrodes, and placement of stimulator in the chest (similar to a pacemaker). *Bottom panel:* Activity in cg25 is elevated in depressed patient (with elevated 17-item Hamilton depression rating scale) as measured by PET scanning following administration of fluorine 18–labeled deoxyglucose; MRI scan showing electrode placement; activity in cg25 diminishes, correlating with improvement in the Hamilton depression rating scale, measured 3 months after beginning DBS. (From Mayberg HS, et al. Deep brain stimulation for treatment-resistant depression. *Neuron.* 2005;45;651–660.)

patients have had sustained improvement. Whether or not this proves to be a practical treatment for severe depression, these trials of DBS corroborate imaging findings in suggesting that the subgenual cingulate cortex is a critical node in mood-regulating circuits in the brain. Related studies have suggested that DBS of the nucleus accumbens, a major brain reward region, may also have mood-elevating effects.

PHARMACOLOGY OF ANXIETY AND ANXIETY DISORDERS

Anxiety disorders refer to a heterogeneous group of conditions, each of which features some type of anxiety as a prominent symptom **14-1**. The current categorization of these disorders is based exclusively on syndromal groupings of subjective and behavioral symptoms. Thus, the classification should be considered provisional and should not guide all scientific investigation. Family and twin studies suggest a

genetic component of risk for these disorders. Nonetheless, the lack of objective markers for phenotyping and the likely genetic complexity of all common behavioral disorders (involvement of multiple genetic and nongenetic factors of small effect) have, to date, impeded the discovery of risk genes. Neuroimaging studies using PET or fMRI have demonstrated hyperactive responses of the amygdala in humans with **PTSD**, both in response to scripts recalling their trauma and in response to more generalized stimuli such as fearful faces. Overall it appears that patients with certain anxiety disorders exhibit hyperresponsiveness of amygdala-based fear circuitry and decreased activity of medial and orbital prefrontal cortical regions that normally serve to suppress fear and anxiety. However, greater specificity in delineating the neural circuits as well as the cellular and molecular pathophysiology of anxiety disorders has not yet emerged from research.

Despite gaps in our understanding of the genetics and pathophysiology of anxiety disorders, several

14-1 Anxiety Disorders

Panic Disorder

Panic attacks are discrete episodes of intense anxiety accompanied by somatic symptoms such as tachycardia, tachypnea, and dizziness. Panic disorder is diagnosed when multiple panic attacks occur or when one or a few attacks are followed by persistent fear of having another attack.

Generalized Anxiety Disorder (GAD)

GAD is characterized by unrealistic and excessive worry for more than six months accompanied by specific anxiety-related symptoms, such as motor tension, sympathetic hyperactivity, and excessive vigilance.

Posttraumatic Stress Disorder (PTSD)

PTSD occurs after serious trauma and is characterized by numbing, cue-elicited reliving of the traumatic experience, increased startle, and nightmares.

Simple Phobias

Simple phobias are characterized by intense fear of and avoidance of specific stimuli, such as snakes, dogs, airplane travel, or exposure to heights.

Social Phobia (Social Anxiety Disorder)

Social phobia is a persistent fear of one or more social situations involving possible exposure to scrutiny by others, and associated fear of humiliation. An example of a specific social phobia is stage fright. A social phobia may generalize, in which case it may lead to avoidance of all social situations, resulting in substantial social and occupational disability. The boundary between shyness and this type of social phobia has not been well clarified.

The anxiety disorders listed here are described in the American Psychiatric Association's *Diagnostic and Statistical Manual of Mental Disorders*, 4th ed. (American Psychiatric Association, 1993). Obsessive–compulsive disorder also is listed in the manual as an anxiety disorder but appears to be pathophysiologically distinct. The disorders listed in this table have, as their primary symptom, dysregulation of fear, whereas the primary symptom of obsessive-compulsive disorder appears to be intrusive, unwanted thoughts, which most likely are the products of different neural circuits (Chapter 13).

highly effective treatments are available. **Acute anxiety,** for example, is successfully treated with **benzodiazepines, generalized anxiety disorder** with **antidepressant drugs** or benzodiazepines, **panic disorder** with long-term administration of antidepressants or with high-potency benzodiazepines (often in combination with cognitive-behavioral therapies), and obsessive–compulsive disorder (OCD) with long-term administration of **selective serotonin reuptake inhibitor (SSRI) antidepressants** or the serotonin reuptake inhibitor **tricyclic antidepressant clomipramine** together with behavioral therapies. Treatment of **PTSD** remains challenging, although various antidepressants provide modest relief. For some patients, **cognitive–behavioral therapies** are highly effective adjuncts or alternatives to medication therapy; the efficacy of these

therapies emphasizes the importance of learning and memory in the pathogenesis of many anxiety disorders. Although neurobiologic causes of anxiety are not well understood, much is known about the mechanisms by which pharmacologic agents act to reduce anxiety. Therefore the discussion that follows approaches the topic of anxiety disorders from a treatment perspective.

Molecular Pharmacology of the GABA$_A$ Receptor

As discussed in Chapter 5, the GABA$_A$ receptor, like many other ligand-gated channels, is a heteropentamer with its subunits arranged like staves around a barrel. Four major types of GABA$_A$ receptor subunits—α, β, γ, and ρ—are known, and multiple subtypes have been identified. GABA$_A$ receptors containing ρ subunits are expressed in the retina and sometimes referred to as GABA$_C$ receptors. They play no role in neuropsychopharmacology and will not be discussed further. Significant binding sites on the GABA$_A$ receptor complex are summarized in 14-2. **Benzodiazepines** bind to a site on the α subunit of the GABA$_A$ receptor complex and thereby increase the affinity of the β subunit for GABA; a γ subunit must be present in the heteropentamer for benzodiazepine binding and must therefore allosterically regulate the binding site on the α subunit. Benzodiazepines facilitate the ability of GABA to activate the GABA$_A$ receptor's intrinsic Cl$^-$ channel and in turn facilitate inhibitory neurotransmission. In the absence of GABA, benzodiazepines exert little effect on GABA$_A$ receptors.

Competitive antagonists of anxiolytic benzodiazepines have been discovered and include agents such as **flumazenil**. These antagonists do not exert independent effects on GABA$_A$ receptor function, but competitively block effects on the receptor produced by benzodiazepine agonists such as **diazepam**. Clinically, flumazenil is useful in the treatment of benzodiazepine overdoses; however, this drug can precipitate withdrawal in benzodiazepine-dependent patients in much the same way that opiate antagonists such as **naloxone** produce withdrawal symptoms in opiate-dependent patients (Chapter 15).

Inverse agonists, which decrease GABA-activated Cl$^-$ conductance, bind at or near the benzodiazepine binding site on the GABA$_A$ receptor α subunit but exert opposite effects on receptor function compared with those produced by benzodiazepines (see 14-2). The prototypical inverse agonist is β-carboline-3-carboxylic acid ethyl ester (**β-CCE** or β-**carboline**). β-CCE is proconvulsant. It is also proconflict when administered

14-2 Pharmacologically Significant Binding Sites on GABA$_A$ Receptors

Site	Agonists	Antagonists	Inverse Agonists
GABA	GABA Muscimol	Bicuculline	
Benzodiazepine	Diazepam	Flumazenil	β-Carbolines RO-15-4513
Barbiturate	Pentobarbital		
Convulsant[1]	Picrotoxin Pentylenetetrazole		
Neuroactive steroid[2] (site uncertain)	3α and 5α-THP	DHEA-S	

[1] The categorization of picrotoxin and pentylenetetrazole as agonists at this site may seem paradoxical because these agents antagonize GABA$_A$ receptor function. The term *agonist* is used to indicate that the drugs bind to an allosteric site in the receptor complex that exerts an effect (albeit an inhibitory one) on the receptor.

[2] See Chapter 10 for a more in-depth discussion of neuroactive steroids.

3α and 5α-THP, tetrahydroprogesterone; DHEA-S, dehydroepiandrosterone sulfate.

to animals undergoing the conflict test. During this test, which is used to screen for benzodiazepine effects in animals, a rat presses a lever for food or water and simultaneously receives a shock, which tends to inhibit further pressing of the lever. The pairing of these events is believed to create a state of conflict in the animal, which is faced with both the desire for food and the expectation of punishment. Benzodiazepines are anticonflict: they release behaviors inhibited by conflict. Thus, under the influence of a benzodiazepine, the rat continues to eat or drink despite the threat of punishment. β-CCE exerts the opposite effect in this assay. In nonhuman primates, β-CCE produces dose-related behavioral agitation and increases plasma cortisol, blood pressure, and heart rate. In human volunteers, inverse agonists produce sympathetic arousal and intense feelings of inner tension and impending doom.

Effects of GABAergic Drugs on Anxiety

Benzodiazepines Benzodiazepines are a class of drugs with anxiolytic, sedative, muscle relaxant, and anticonvulsant properties **14-3**. Benzodiazepines also produce anterograde amnesia, a property that is exploited when high potency, short-acting benzodiazepines are used as preoperative anxiolytics, but that otherwise represents an unwanted side effect. All

benzodiazepines exert their pharmacologic effects by facilitating GABA$_A$ receptor function, as previously mentioned. A series of chemically distinct (nonbenzodiazepine) compounds, such as **zolpidem, eszopiclone**, or **zaleplon**, bind to the same site on the GABA$_A$ receptor and exert similar pharmacologic effects. Many benzodiazepines and other drugs that bind to the benzodiazepine site are available for clinical use; the major distinguishing features of these agents are

14-3 Benzodiazepines and Related Drugs

Agonists

Alprazolam	Flurazepam	Prazepam
Chlordiazepoxide	Halazepam	Quazepam
Clonazepam	Lorazepam	Temazepam
Clorazepate	Midazolam	Triazolam
Diazepam	Nitrazepam	Zolpidem[1]
Estazolam	Oxazepam	Eszopiclone[1]
		Zaleplon[1]

Antagonist

Flumazenil

[1] These nonbenzodiazepines act on the same site of the GABA$_A$ receptor as do benzodiazepines.

their pharmacokinetic properties. Some of these drugs exhibit particularly short half-lives, and thus are desirable for use as hypnotics or sleeping pills; examples include zolpidem, eszopiclone, and the benzodiazepine lorazepam. Drugs with longer half-lives are preferable for generalized anxiety; examples include **diazepam** and **chlordiazepoxide**. **Alprazolam** and **clonazepam** are widely prescribed for the treatment of panic disorder because of their high-potency. The chemical structures of representative benzodiazepines used in the treatment of anxiety disorders appear in **14-5**; the structures of related agents that are more commonly used to treat insomnia are provided in Chapter 12.

The diverse clinical effects of benzodiazepines and chemically unrelated drugs that bind the benzodiazepine site are mediated by $GABA_A$ receptors of different subunit composition expressed in different regions of the brain. Anxiolytic properties of benzodiazepines at least partly reflect actions in the amygdala. GABAergic inhibition of serotonergic, noradrenergic, and many other types of neurons that project to brain structures involved in emotional processing also may contribute to anxiolysis. Sedative and amnestic actions are exerted in more widespread locations, including the cerebral cortex. Anticonvulsant actions of benzodiazepines are believed to occur in the cerebral cortex, hippocampus, or amygdala.

The binding site for benzodiazepines was first identified by means of radioreceptor binding assays. It is best conceptualized as an allosteric regulatory binding site on the $GABA_A$ receptor. Evidence that this site is related to the clinical efficacy of benzodiazepines was drawn from classic pharmacologic investigations that demonstrated that the affinities of various benzodiazepine drugs for this site neatly corresponded to their clinical potencies (eg, clonazepam > lorazepam > diazepam > oxazepam). However, these early studies were carried out before the molecular cloning of multiple subtypes of benzodiazepine binding sites (ie, multiple α subunits of the $GABA_A$ receptor). Based on in vitro binding studies and in vivo observations performed on mice with a gene knockout (α_1, α_5, α_6 subunits), or with knockin (α_1, α_2 α_3, α_5 subunits) mutations that destroy benzodiazepine binding sites with point mutations, it has been possible to investigate the pharmacology of benzodiazepines and related drugs and to link specific α subunits with clinical effects. Diazepam and other benzodiazepines in current use have high affinity for $GABA_A$ receptors containing α_1, α_2, α_3, or α_5 subunits. Zolpidem and eszopiclone, widely used hypnotics, have higher affinity for $GABA_A$ receptors containing an α_1 subunit. One

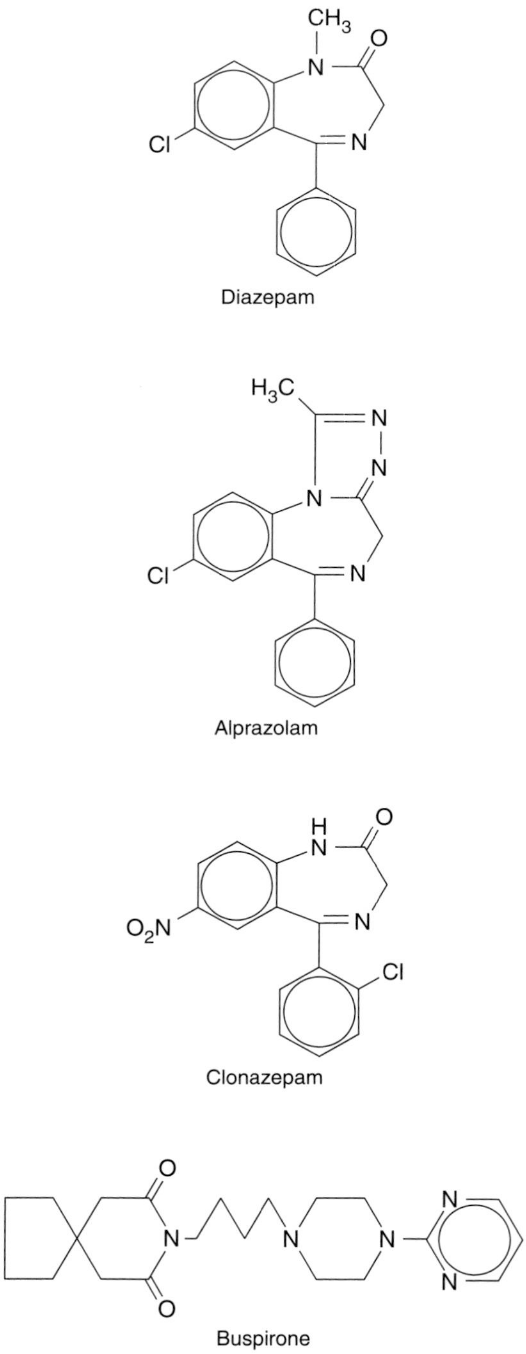

Diazepam

Alprazolam

Clonazepam

Buspirone

14-5 **Chemical structures of representative anxiolytics.** (See Chapter 12 for the structures of benzodiazepines and related compounds that are used primarily in the treatment of insomnia.)

goal of current research is to design drugs selective for particular α subunits thus limiting side effects. The α_1 subunit has been associated with hypnotic effects, the α_5 subunit with some of the cognitive effects, and the α_2 subunit with anxiolysis. A drug selective for α_2 subunit containing GABA$_A$ receptors might produce anxiolysis without sedation and anterograde amnesia. Indeed, alprazolam and clonazepam may exert greater anxiolysis versus sedation due to higher affinity for α_2-containing GABA$_A$ receptors.

Barbiturates Like benzodiazepines, barbiturates interact with the GABA$_A$ receptor; however, they bind to a physically different site on the receptor, which is believed to be in close proximity to the Cl$^-$ channel (see **14-2**; also see Chapter 5). Whereas benzodiazepines increase the likelihood that Cl$^-$ channels will open in a GABA-dependent manner, barbiturates increase not only the probability that they will open but also the duration of their opening. Moreover, at high doses barbiturates can act independently of GABA; consequently, they can lead to far greater inhibition of the nervous system than can benzodiazepines. Accordingly, a much greater risk of serious respiratory depression and death are associated with barbiturate overdose. Overdoses of benzodiazepines can result in coma but very rarely cause death unless combined with the use of a cross-reactive substance such as a barbiturate or **alcohol**. Many barbiturate-like drugs, including **methaqualone (quaalude)**, **ethchlorvynol**, **meprobamate**, and **chloral hydrate**, were introduced into clinical practice in the past with the hope that their use might result in fewer side effects and less abuse compared with barbiturates. None have stood the test of time; today barbiturates and related compounds are rarely used for sedation or anxiolysis. Short-acting barbiturates currently are used primarily for anesthesia. A prototypical agent used for this purpose is **pentobarbital**. A long-acting barbiturate, **phenobarbital**, is still used for certain seizure disorders (Chapter 18).

Neuroactive steroids represent yet another class of molecules that modulate the function of GABA$_A$ receptors; however, their precise mechanisms of action remain unknown. These molecules are discussed in greater detail in Chapter 10.

Alcohol Concentrations of ethanol produced in humans from the consumption of alcoholic beverages (millimolar range) facilitate the GABA-mediated opening of GABA$_A$ receptor Cl$^-$ channels. Thus, it should not be surprising that a reduction in anxiety is among the most prominent effects of ethanol, at least

at low doses and while blood levels continue to rise. This characteristic helps to explain why ethanol is widely self-administered to enhance social interaction. When ethanol is taken with benzodiazepines or barbiturates, its effects are greatly intensified because each of these agents alters GABA$_A$ receptor conformation to increase the efficacy of the others. Because of this cross-reactivity, which is synergistic, mixtures of these drugs can be lethal. Such cross-reactivity is exploited in ethanol detoxification regimens, which typically replace ethanol with a benzodiazepine which is then slowly tapered. Benzodiazepines, such as **chlordiazepoxide**, are used for detoxification because they have a longer half-life than ethanol; thus they permit a smoother detoxification process (ie, less risk of withdrawal symptoms), cause fewer side effects, and may reduce the likelihood of relapse.

Tolerance and Dependence Associated with Benzodiazepines and Ethanol

Benzodiazepines, barbiturates and related compounds, and ethanol can produce tolerance to many of their behavioral effects, although tolerance does not seem to occur to the anxiolytic effects of benzodiazepines. In addition, the drugs can cause dependence, which leads to potentially fatal withdrawal syndromes upon cessation of their use. Barbiturates and ethyl alcohol, and rarely benzodiazepines, can also produce compulsive use, ie, addiction (Chapter 15).

The molecular mechanisms that underlie tolerance and dependence caused by drugs that act at GABA$_A$ receptors are not fully understood. Covalent modification of the GABA$_A$ receptor, for example, by phosphorylation, may explain such phenomena as "acute tolerance," which can be observed even within dose. As a result of acute tolerance, individuals may recover from the sedative effects of a benzodiazepine or ethanol even when blood levels remain elevated above the level that produced sedation to begin with. Longer-term tolerance and dependence may be explained by altered expression of GABA$_A$ receptor subunits leading to altered receptor levels. Chronic administration of ethanol to laboratory animals, for example, causes region-specific alterations in the patterns of expression of several GABA$_A$ receptor subunits in the brain, and increasing evidence has linked these changes to tolerance, dependence, or specific withdrawal symptoms.

Nonbenzodiazepine Anxiolytics

Considerable effort has been devoted to the development of anxiolytic agents with novel mechanisms of action. One mechanism in clinical trials is **CRF$_1$ receptor**

antagonism. Another mechanism in clinical use, albeit with only modest efficacy, is partial agonism at $5HT_{1A}$ serotonin receptors. This mechanism is exemplified by **buspirone** `14-5`, an azaspirodecanedione marketed as an anxiolytic. $5HT_{1A}$ receptors serve as autoreceptors on serotonin neurons and also as postsynaptic receptors (Chapter 6). When administered to animals, buspirone has a taming effect on rhesus monkeys, inhibits conditioned avoidance responses in rats, and reduces shock-elicited fighting in mice. However, it is generally ineffective as an anticonflict agent in rats and monkeys. Buspirone is approved for use in the treatment of **generalized anxiety disorder**, although it is less effective than benzodiazepines or SSRI antidepressants when used for this or related purposes. The major advantage of buspirone and SSRIs compared with benzodiazepines is that they are less likely to give rise to dependence, and they are virtually without abuse liability.

Adenosine receptor agonists   Another target under consideration for anxiolytic drugs is the adenosine A_1 receptor (Chapter 8). Adenosine is a purine neurotransmitter that inhibits the release of other neurotransmitters, including acetylcholine, norepinephrine, glutamate, dopamine, 5HT, and GABA, in specific regions of the brain through actions at its A_1 receptor. This action is mediated through the opening of K^+ channels, the inhibition of Ca^{2+} channel opening, and the inhibition of adenylyl cyclase—all by means of the $G_{i/o}$ family of G proteins. Adenosine is sedative, anticonvulsant, analgesic, and anxiolytic. Adenosine receptor antagonists, including methylxanthines such as **caffeine** and **theophylline**, produce stimulant effects. Large doses of caffeine are anxiogenic, and high doses administered into the brain may produce seizures.

Although the role of adenosine in human anxiety is unclear, A_1 adenosine receptor agonists may prove to be useful in the treatment of various types of anxiety disorders.

Treatment of Anxiety Disorders

As previously suggested, both benzodiazepines and some antidepressants have efficacy in the treatment of anxiety (see `14-1`). Although beyond the scope of this text, it is important to point out that **cognitive** and **behavioral psychotherapies**, focused on the management of symptoms, are very useful in the treatment of anxiety disorders and obsessive compulsive disorder. The preferred pharmacologic treatment for **generalized anxiety disorder (GAD)**, **panic disorder, and posttraumatic stress disorder (PTSD)** is an antidepressant, generally an **SSRI** or newer serotonin-norepinephrine reuptake inhibitors (SNRIs) such as **venlafaxine** and **duloxetine**. Older antidepressants, such as **tricyclics** and **monoamine oxidase inhibitors** (**MAOIs**), are efficacious but have less tolerable side effects for many patients. The most common alternative for GAD is a low-potency benzodiazepine, such as diazepam; for panic disorder the most common alternatives are high-potency benzodiazepines such as **alprazolam** or **clonazepam**. The benzodiazepines have the advantage of rapid onset (hours versus weeks for antidepressants), but the disadvantages of sedation (at least initially, before tolerance occurs), cognitive impairment, and, especially for the high potency drugs, dependence.

Social anxiety disorder is characterized by a persistent fear of experiencing humiliation in one or more social situations in which an individual may be exposed to scrutiny by others. It can be treated by cognitive-behavioral therapies, antidepressants, or benzodiazepines. One interesting exception is a form of social anxiety called performance anxiety, such as stage fright. This is generally associated with sympathetic arousal giving rise to a pounding heart, dry mouth, and tremor. Because benzodiazepines can adversely affect mental acuity, preferred pharmacologic treatment is with a β-adrenergic receptor antagonist such as **propranolol** taken immediately prior to the performance.

Obsessive–Compulsive Disorder

Obsessive–compulsive disorder (OCD) is characterized by (1) recurrent intrusive thoughts that an individual recognizes as products of his or her own mind (obsessions); and (2) repetitive, seemingly purposeful behavior designed to prevent or neutralize a dreaded occurrence, often as a consequence of the obsession (compulsions). Although it traditionally has been classified as an anxiety disorder based on the anxiety that drives the compulsions, growing evidence suggests that OCD differs from other anxiety disorders with regard to its neurobiologic substrates. Current evidence, based largely on structural and functional imaging, and to a lesser degree on animal models, suggests that OCD results from abnormal functioning of striatal-thalamic-prefrontal cortical circuits (Chapter 13). **Tourette syndrome,** also believed to reflect abnormal striatal functioning, is characterized by multiple tics, but also may feature obsessive–compulsive symptoms. In contrast, the other anxiety disorders appear to represent abnormal function of amygdala-based fear circuitry, as discussed earlier.

14-4 Effects of Tricyclic and Related Tetracyclic Antidepressants on Receptors and Transporters

Drug	Transporters		Receptors		
	NE	5HT	Muscarinic Acetylcholine	H$_1$ Histamine	α$_1$ Adrenergic
Amitriptyline	+/−	++	++++	++++	+++
Amoxapine	++	0	0	+/−	++
Clomipramine	+	+++	++	+	++
Desipramine	+++	0	+	0	+
Doxepin	++	+	++	+++	++
Imipramine	+	+	++	+	++
Maprotiline	++	0	+	++	+
Nortriptyline	++	+/−	++	+	+
Protriptyline	++	0	+++	+	+
Trimipramine	+	0	++	+++	++

Number of plus (+) signs indicates binding affinity. 0, undetectable. All effects listed are antagonistic. Desipramine is the desmethyl metabolite of imipramine, and nortriptyline is the desmethyl metabolite of amitriptyline.

OCD currently is treated with **SSRIs** at high doses, or with the tricyclic drug **clomipramine**, which also preferentially inhibits the 5HT transporter **14-4**. Cognitive-behavior therapy has proven to be useful in the treatment of some patients, especially with regard to reducing or eliminating compulsive rituals. Treatment of Tourette syndrome focuses on the use of various **antipsychotic drugs** as well as α$_2$-adrenergic agonists, such as **clonidine** or **guanfacine** (Chapter 13). How these various drugs alleviate the symptoms of OCD or Tourette syndrome remains unknown.

PHARMACOLOGY OF MOOD DISORDERS

Mood disorders rank among the leading causes of disability worldwide and are the leading cause of suicide. Based on symptoms and patterns of familial transmission, these disorders can be assigned to one of two broad categories. Individuals with **unipolar depression** experience episodes of depression only; those with **bipolar disorder** experience at least one episode of mania, and most commonly experience multiple episodes of depression and mania **14-5**. Yet it must be emphasized that these clinical entities, much like anxiety disorders, likely represent a heterogeneous group of disparate pathophysiologic processes. Moreover, many individuals with mood disorders also experience significant symptoms of anxiety. Risk of bipolar

14-5 Mood Disorders

Major Depression

Characterized by sad mood or loss of interest in usual pursuits, accompanied by abnormalities of sleep, appetite, energy, sex drive, and motivation. Other features may include psychomotor retardation or agitation, and abnormal thoughts, such as guilt, hopelessness, and suicidal ideas.

Dysthymia

Represents chronic milder depression. Its course is often punctuated by episodes of major depression.

Bipolar Disorder (Manic-Depressive Illness)

Characterized by episodes of mania, with or without distinct episodes of depression. The symptoms and signs of depression are the same whether the disorder is unipolar or bipolar. Mania is characterized by euphoria or irritability, increased energy, and a decreased need for sleep. Patients often are intrusive, hypersexual, and impulsive; they have inflated self-esteem, which may be delusional. Cognitively, they are distractible; their speech is often rapid and pressured. Psychotic symptoms are common.

Based on the American Psychiatric Association's *Diagnostic and Statistical Manual of Mental Disorders,* 4th ed. (American Psychiatric Association, 1993).

disorder is highly influenced by genetics, risk of unipolar disorders more moderately so. Given the heterogeneity and genetic complexity of these disorders, it is not surprising that convincingly replicated risk genes have not yet been identified.

Mood disorders generally are characterized by an episodic course, although they can become chronic. A striking feature of mood disorders is that their symptoms appear to reflect abnormal functioning in many different regions of the brain. Sleep disturbances may be traced to alterations in brainstem monoamine or cholinergic nuclei or to disruptions of the circadian pacemaker in the suprachiasmatic nucleus (SCN) of the hypothalamus (Chapter 12). Changes in appetite and energy may reflect abnormalities in various hypothalamic nuclei. Depressed mood and anhedonia (lack of interest in pleasurable activities) in depressed individuals, and euphoria and increased involvement in goal-directed activities in patients, who experience mania, may reflect opposing abnormalities in the nucleus accumbens, medial prefrontal cortex, amygdala, or other structures. Anxiety, which is a common symptom of depression, may reflect abnormalities in the functioning of the amygdala and BNST, as previously mentioned. The excessive release of stress hormones, such as cortisol, which occurs in many individuals with mood disorders, may result from hyperfunctioning of the PVN of the hypothalamus, hyperfunctioning of the amygdala (which activates the PVN), or hypofunctioning of the hippocampus (which exerts a potent inhibitory influence on the PVN). Alterations in the content of thought, which are a cardinal feature of depression and mania, most likely reflect abnormal functioning of the cerebral cortex. A neurobiologic explanation of mood disorders must be able to demonstrate how diverse brain regions are affected, why associated abnormalities are episodic, and how both genes and environment can affect the pathogenesis of these disorders. Circuits that can directly or indirectly influence all of the structures affected by these disorders are currently a focus of research. Because of their widespread projections, and because of their role in antidepressant action, monoamine systems in the brain historically have been thought to play an important role in the pathophysiology of mood disorders. Even if they are not the primary cause of mood disorders, monoamine systems may serve to generalize an abnormality initiated elsewhere so that it affects much of the rest of the brain.

One obstacle to research in depression has been a lack of good animal models. Several tests (eg, forced swim or learned helplessness) are used to predict antidepressant responses in rodents, but are limited in terms of whether they model depression per se 14–4. Models in which rodents are subjected to various types of chronic stress more accurately reflect certain aspects of depression, although they are not yet validated clinically. Limitations associated with animal models have required the use of human subjects for much research on mood disorders.

A substantial focus of research has been the documentation of abnormalities in monoamine systems because of the efficacy of antidepressant drugs that target norepinephrine, serotonin, and, less commonly, dopamine systems. Although it is widely recognized that such pharmacologic treatments may act on synapses that are unrelated to the pathophysiology of depression or mania, a large number of studies have examined monoamine turnover, monoamine receptors on accessible peripheral blood cells, and the neuroendocrine and behavioral effects of various pharmacologic challenges such as the depletion of monoamine systems. Many of these active challenges can provoke symptoms or alter physiologic responses, but they have yielded little specific information about disease pathophysiology or even mechanisms of drug action. Certain antidepressant drugs have proved efficacious for a wide range of emotional and other disorders, including depression, panic disorder, OCD, PTSD, eating disorders, enuresis (bed wetting), and chronic pain syndromes. Thus serotonin and norepinephrine are not exclusively related to depression. Rather, it appears that modulation of the brain's serotonergic or noradrenergic systems can result in palliative effects on many pathophysiologic mechanisms.

Neuroendocrine Abnormalities Associated with Depression

Abnormal, excessive activation of the HPA axis (see Chapter 10, 10–3) occurs in approximately half of all individuals who experience an episode of major depression. These individuals may exhibit increased cortisol production, as measured by increases in free cortisol in urine, and a reduced ability to suppress plasma cortisol, adrenocorticotropic hormone (ACTH), and β-endorphin after administration of dexamethasone, a potent synthetic glucocorticoid. Direct and indirect evidence suggests that these individuals also exhibit hypersecretion of CRF. Moreover, ACTH responses to intravenously administered CRF are blunted, and concentrations of CRF in cerebrospinal fluid (CSF) tend to be increased. As previously indicated, increases in cortisol induce catabolism, suppress the immune system, and may have temporary elevating effects on mood, energy, and

---

14-4 The Search for Animal Models of Depression

A major obstacle to research on depression has been the lack of good animal models. Three tests that are commonly used to predict the efficacy of antidepressant drugs illustrate the weaknesses in current models. The Porsolt test, or *forced swim test*, involves placing a rodent in a bucket of water. Most rodents struggle for a time before adopting a floating position without further struggle. The administration of an antidepressant, regardless of the type, increases the amount of time the animal spends struggling. Consequently it has been hypothesized that such drugs cause these animals to avoid "despair" and to work harder and refuse to give up. This interpretation is not at all obvious. Moreover, the effects of the antidepressants administered during this test are observed immediately, even though their clinical effects in humans require long-term administration.

Two other tests, *tail suspension* and *learned helplessness*, are very similar. In the tail suspension test, mice hung upside down by their tails after a time stop struggling; an acute antidepressant dose increases the time they struggle. In learned helplessness, rodents are repeatedly given a mild foot shock but are not permitted to escape from the environment in which they receive the shock. After a suitable training period, these animals are permitted to escape after receiving a shock. Under these circumstances, a subpopulation of rodents fails to attempt escape, that is, they show signs of having "given up." Administration of an antidepressant facilitates escape behavior.

All clinically validated antidepressants are active in these tests. However, this should not be surprising because only compounds that are active in the tests are pursued as antidepressants for human use. This has created a "catch-22." Although these tests are good predictors of available antidepressants, it is not known whether they can detect the effectiveness of agents with truly novel mechanisms of action. A non-monoamine-based agent, for example, might be effective in humans despite its failure to produce expected results in these tests. On the other hand, these tests have detected antidepressant-like activity of numerous novel, non-monoamine-based manipulations, but these various manipulations have not yet been validated clinically. Hence, another catch-22.

The novelty suppressed feeding test measures the time it takes a mouse to approach food in a novel environment. An attractive feature of this test is that chronic, but not acute, administration of an antidepressant reduces this latency. However, acute administration of anxiolytic drugs causes the same effect, and this test, like the despair-based tests outlined above, are performed in normal animals.

Recent research has focused on developing models of depression that have greater validity and that can be reversed only with long-term antidepressant administration. Various types of chronic stress models have been proposed, some of which involve animals subjected to low levels of stress for relatively long periods of time (weeks to months), termed *chronic mild stress*. In some laboratories, stress is created by exposing animals to highly aggressive dominant males, a paradigm referred to as *social defeat*. Some of these models have yielded encouraging results, but it has, in general, been difficult to induce long-lasting behavioral abnormalities in response to stress in normal rodents. The hope is that the identification of human depression genes, once placed into mice, will facilitate efforts to develop bona fide animal models of this disorder.

---

cognition. Although short-term administration of glucocorticoids often produces euphoria and increased energy, the impact of long-lasting increases in endogenous glucocorticoids produced during depression can involve complex adaptations such as those that occur in **Cushing syndrome** (Chapter 10). For example, evidence indicates that prolonged increases in cortisol may be damaging to hippocampal neurons and can suppress hippocampal neurogenesis (the generation of new neurons postnatally). Because the hippocampus is required for feedback inhibition of CRF neurons 14-6 , episodes of depression could conceivably produce a vicious cycle of impairment in feedback regulation of the HPA axis and thus predispose to future recurrences.

Significant parallels exist among melancholic depression, the stress response, and behavioral and physiologic effects produced by CRF injected into

Hippocampus

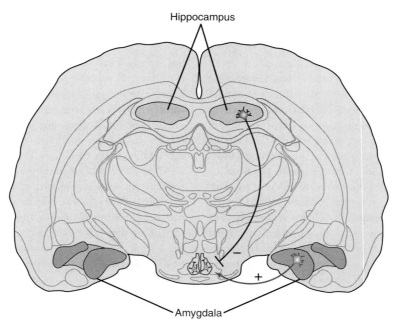

Amygdala

14–6 **Regulation of the hypothalamic–pituitary–adrenal (HPA) axis shown in rat brain.** Neurons of the paraventricular nucleus (PVN) of the hypothalamus containing corticotropin-releasing factor integrate information relevant to stress. Prominent neural inputs include excitatory afferent signals from the amygdala and inhibitory (though indirect) afferent signals from the hippocampus. Other important inputs are received from ascending monoamine pathways and from the periphery, the latter of which include inhibitory inputs from circulating endogenous glucocorticoids such as cortisol (Chapter 10).

cerebral ventricles. These include increased arousal and vigilance, decreased appetite, decreased sexual behavior, and increased heart rate and blood pressure. Thus, even if hypothalamic abnormalities are not a primary cause of depression, they very likely contribute to the generation of serious symptoms and have an impact on the course of depression and its somatic sequelae. Accordingly, new pharmacologic agents currently under investigation have been designed to correct some of these abnormalities. Although **mifepristone** (**RU486**) is marketed as an abortifacient based on its progesterone receptor antagonist properties, it is also a **glucocorticoid receptor antagonist** and has shown some promise in early trials in patients with severe, psychotic depression. As well, **CRF₁ receptor antagonists** are in development for depression as well as anxiety, as mentioned earlier. Interestingly the logic behind their development may not bear out, even if they eventually prove efficacious. It may be that their most important clinical effects occur by blocking CRF_1 receptors in amygdala circuits. It appears that CRF_1 antagonists do not

cause hypocortisolism, which would represent a dangerous side effect, because ACTH synthesis and release are controlled by vasopressin as well as by CRF (Chapter 10).

Antidepressant Drugs

Antidepressant drugs are a heterogeneous group of compounds that are effective in the treatment of major depression **14–6**. As previously mentioned, most are also effective in the treatment of anxiety disorders, and serotonin-selective agents (ie, **clomipramine** and **SSRIs**) are effective in the treatment of **OCD**. Based on structural and neurochemical properties, antidepressant drugs often are subdivided into groups that include **tricyclic** and related cyclic antidepressants; **SSRIs;** selective norepinephrine reuptake inhibitors (**NRIs**); serotonin and norepinephrine reuptake inhibitors (**SNRIs**); **MAOIs;** and miscellaneous antidepressants whose acute mechanisms of action are unknown. The chemical structures of representative antidepressants are shown in **14–7**.

14–6 Commonly Used Antidepressant Medications

Tricyclics[1]
5HT-selective reuptake blockers

Amitriptyline[2]
Imipramine[2]
Clomipramine

NE-selective reuptake blockers

Nortriptyline
Desipramine

SSRIs

Citalopram
Fluoxetine
Fluvoxamine
Paroxetine
Sertraline

NE-selective reuptake inhibitors (NRIs)

Reboxetine
Atomoxetine

Mixed 5HT/NE reuptake inhibitors (SNRIs)

Venlafaxine
Duloxetine

MAOIs

Tranylcypromine
Phenelzine

Antidepressants with other mechanisms

Bupropion
Mirtazapine
Nefazodone
Trazodone

[1]See 14–4 for additional examples of tricyclic and related cyclic antidepressants.
[2]Although these compounds predominantly inhibit 5HT reuptake, they are metabolized into nortriptyline and desipramine, antidepressants in their own right that are NE reuptake inhibitors.
5HT, serotonin; NE, norepinephrine; MAOIs, monoamine oxidase inhibitors.

Tricyclic antidepressants inhibit serotonin and norepinephrine reuptake to varying extents 14–4 and 14–6 . They also antagonize several neurotransmitter receptors, particularly muscarinic cholinergic, H_1 histaminergic, and α_1 adrenergic receptors; such antagonism explains their many side effects, including sedation, dry mouth, and constipation. SSRIs were developed to selectively inhibit the serotonin transporter, without activity at cholinergic, histaminergic, or adrenergic receptors; their use has represented a rational means of avoiding some of the side effects associated with tricyclic agents. Likewise, **reboxetine** and **atomoxetine** are NRIs that lack many side effects associated with tricyclic agents by avoiding activity at the same receptors. **Venlafaxine** and **duloxetine** inhibit both serotonin and norepinephrine reuptake and also lack many of the side effects of tricyclic antidepressants. The newer drugs have their own side effects, such as sexual dysfunction with SSRIs, but the side effects are generally better tolerated by most patients. The development of MAOIs resulted from the serendipitous discovery in the 1950s that the antitubercular drug iproniazid alleviated depression, and the subsequent discovery that such alleviation stems from MAO inhibition (Chapter 6).

The mechanisms of action of other antidepressant agents, which often are described as atypical, remain poorly understood. **Bupropion,** an aminoketone, is an effective antidepressant that does not produce appreciable effects on the serotonin or norepinephrine systems. Its effectiveness has been attributed to its inhibition of dopamine reuptake; however, this is unlikely, because cocaine also inhibits dopamine reuptake but does not serve as an effective antidepressant, and because brain imaging studies have shown minimal occupancy of the dopamine transporter at clinically effective doses. **Mirtazapine,** also an effective antidepressant, is reported to be an antagonist at α_2-adrenergic and $5HT_{2A}$ and $5HT_3$ serotonin receptors; however, the relationship between these actions and its antidepressant effects has not been ascertained. **Trazodone** and **nefazodone,** both triazoloperidine derivatives of modest efficacy, influence serotonin systems in several ways.

Electroconvulsive therapy (**ECT**), which typically involves a series of six to eight generalized seizures under light anesthesia over 2 to 3 weeks, remains one of the most effective treatments for depression, but its therapeutic effects often are short lived; for this reason, ECT is often combined with a chemical antidepressant. ECT no longer induces a motor seizure because of the concurrent use of muscle paralyzing agents such as **succinylcholine** (Chapter 9); to be effective, however, it must produce electroencephalographic evidence of a seizure. The mechanism by which ECT treats depression is unknown. As described, **deep brain stimulation (DBS)** is in early trials for treatment-refractory major depression. There is also interest in magnetic stimulation therapies, **transcranial magnetic stimulation (rTMS)** or **magnetic seizure therapy (MST),** but the efficacy of these treatments is not yet established. Antidepressant activity of **vagal nerve stimulation (VNS)** has been reported, but the effects seem to be modest at best in most patients.

14-7 **Chemical structures of representative antidepressants.**

Monoamine systems and antidepressant action
Altered synaptic levels of modulatory neurotransmitters, such as serotonin or the catecholamines, have a marked influence on behavior, which they regulate through their effects on information processing in multiple circuits that underlie sensation, cognition, emotion, and motor and neuroendocrine outputs. However, their actions must be understood in the proper context. Historically, hypotheses linking mood disorders to norepinephrine and serotonin systems in the brain were overly simplistic, based not on the anatomy and

physiology of these systems but on pharmacologic observations alone. It was observed, for example, that approximately 15% of patients who received long-term treatment with the antihypertensive drug **reserpine** developed a syndrome indistinguishable from naturally occurring depression; concomitantly it was discovered that reserpine depletes neurons of norepinephrine, serotonin, and dopamine (Chapter 6). Likewise, studies of the first antidepressants revealed that they influence monoamines; for example, it was discovered that MAOIs inhibit the enzyme that metabolizes monoamine neurotransmitters, as mentioned earlier. Furthermore, it was proposed that because this enzyme is located in certain presynaptic terminals, its inhibition prolongs the life of monoamine neurotransmitters in the presynaptic cytoplasm and in turn increases the amount of these transmitters available for packaging into vesicles and subsequent release. Similarly, it was discovered that imipramine and other tricyclic antidepressants inhibit the reuptake of norepinephrine and serotonin in varying ratios. Because reuptake was known to be the primary mechanism by which the synaptic actions of monoamines are terminated, it was posited that tricyclic antidepressants act by increasing the amount of these neurotransmitters in synapses.

Pharmacologic observations such as these led to a simple hypothesis: depression is the result of inadequate monoamine neurotransmission, and clinically effective antidepressants work by increasing the availability of monoamines. Yet this hypothesis has failed to explain the observation that weeks of treatment with antidepressants are required before clinical efficacy becomes apparent, despite the fact that the inhibitory actions of these agents—whether in relation to reuptake or monoamine oxidase—are immediate. This delay in therapeutic effect eventually led investigators to theorize that long-term adaptations in brain function, rather than increases in synaptic norepinephrine and serotonin per se, most likely underlie the therapeutic effects of antidepressant drugs. Consequently, the focus of research on antidepressants has shifted from the study of their immediate effects to the investigation of effects that develop more slowly.

The anatomic focus of research on antidepressants also has shifted. Although monoamine synapses are believed to be the immediate targets of antidepressant drugs, more attention is given to the target neurons of monoamines, where chronic alterations in monoaminergic inputs caused by antidepressant drugs presumably lead to long-lasting adaptations that underlie effective treatment of depression. The identification of molecular and cellular adaptations that occur in response to antidepressants, and the location of the cells and circuits in which they occur, are the chief goals that guide current research. The work described toward the beginning of the chapter on mood-regulating circuits that involve the subgenual cingulate gyrus, for instance, represent a significant advance over a narrow focus on monoamine neuron function.

Although the remainder of this section is devoted to a discussion of antidepressant-induced neuroadaptations, a series of clinical studies conducted during the past 10 years, which supports a role for serotonergic and noradrenergic systems in antidepressant action, deserves comment. According to these studies, patients with depression who respond to treatment with an **SSRI** exhibit a brief relapse when their body stores of tryptophan, the precursor of serotonin, are depleted (Chapter 6). In contrast, such tryptophan depletion does not cause relapse in patients treated with **NRIs**. Moreover, patients treated with NRIs experience relapse in response to inhibition of catecholamine synthesis with α-**methylparatyrosine** (**AMPT**), an inhibitor of tyrosine hydroxylase (Chapter 6), whereas patients treated with SSRIs do not. Overall, these findings indicate that monoamine systems are important substrates for the clinical efficacy of antidepressants. In addition, the brief relapses described here may represent withdrawal phenomena akin to those associated with benzodiazepine antagonists. However, the studies that produced these findings do not reveal the specific changes in the brain that mediate such clinical responses and do not offer information about the pathophysiology of depression.

Long-term adaptations in antidepressant action
The several weeks latency in onset of the therapeutic actions of antidepressants contributes to distress and clinical risk for those with severe depression. In the search for treatments of more rapid onset, great effort has gone into trying to understand the delay in efficacy of current antidepressants. All current ideas posit that antidepressant-induced increases in synaptic monoamine concentrations cause slowly accumulating adaptive changes in target neurons. Two broad classes of theories have emerged: (1) Changes in protein phosphorylation, gene expression, and protein translation occur in target neurons that ultimately alter synaptic structure or function in a way that relieves symptoms; and (2) antidepressant-induced neurogenesis in the hippocampus and the incorporation of those new neurons into functional circuits is a required step in the therapeutic response. Before considering specific hypotheses, however, it is important to discuss obstacles in relating research in animal models to human depression.

Obstacles to research Whether experimental findings in laboratory animals can be generalized to humans is often difficult to determine, and this issue represents a major difficulty associated with antidepressant research. Changes in the levels of most neurotransmitters and neurotransmitter receptors currently cannot be measured in specific brain regions of living human patients. Changes in postreceptor messenger systems are even more difficult to trace. Although advances in PET, single-photon emission computed tomography (SPECT), and magnetic resonance spectroscopy (MRS) technology may eventually enable us to assess some of these changes, human studies have thus far relied on indirect methods of assessment. One such method involves the measurement of monoamine metabolite levels in CSF, blood, or urine—an approach that is compromised by many confounding variables, including peripheral sources of monoamines. The amount of a monoamine metabolite detected in one of these fluids, for example, is not a dependable indicator of the functioning of monoaminergic neurons in the brain. Even metabolite levels measured in CSF reflect a complicated integration of monoaminergic function throughout the brain; they reveal very little about the functioning of specific monoaminergic pathways and nothing about their target neurons. Studies of the function of neural circuits that regulate mood and emotion using PET and fMRI, as mentioned above, have added a great deal to narrower studies of neurotransmitter levels and receptor binding.

The pharmacologic challenge paradigm, which is analogous to methods used in endocrinology, was enlisted in an attempt to understand the pathophysiology of mood disorders. This approach allowed the sensitivity of a receptor system to be measured based on altered responses to a challenge drug in ill versus unaffected subjects. Neuroendocrine, autonomic, and subjective responses to the administration of **yohimbine** (an α_2-adrenergic antagonist), for example, were used to estimate the sensitivity of central α_2-adrenergic receptors in depression and anxiety disorders. However, such tests cannot provide mechanistic insights into the functioning of neurons in the brain and thus have not yielded robust pathophysiologic data.

A significant obstacle to interpreting the significance of drug-induced changes in neurotransmitter turnover and receptor sensitivity in rat brainstems from the fact that most related research has involved the use of normal laboratory rats. The brain of a depressed human being is unlikely to respond to a drug treatment in the same way that the brain of an unaffected human or laboratory rat might. Indeed, antidepressants administered to humans without depression produce no discernible responses other than typical side effects. Thus we do not know whether regulation of monoamine turnover or receptors in the rat correlates with responses to antidepressants in depressed patients. If neurotransmitter or receptor regulation were the actual mechanism by which antidepressants produce their therapeutic effects, the predicted regulation would be expected to occur in depressed patients who respond to drug treatment, but not in nonresponders. Our ability

to investigate this question most likely must await improvements in imaging technologies.

Regulation of neurotransmitter systems   Historically, antidepressant-induced adaptations were identified in the monoamine systems themselves. This research will be illustrated relatively briefly because it does not, by itself, explain the therapeutic actions of the drugs. Among the most consistently observed effects of long-term antidepressant administration in animals was the down-regulation of postsynaptic β-adrenergic receptors. Many antidepressant drugs and repeated ECT produce this effect in the cerebral cortex and other regions of rat brain. Down-regulation of β-adrenergic receptors can be viewed as a homeostatic response to the immediate actions of antidepressant drugs 14–8 . Accordingly, short-term increases in synaptic levels of norepinephrine produced by antidepressants may prompt homeostatic mechanisms to decrease β-adrenergic receptor levels over time and thereby restore noradrenergic signal transduction within the postsynaptic neuron to baseline levels.

As was typical of these early theories, there were also limitations to the hypothesis that β-adrenergic receptor down-regulation mediates antidepressant effects. Some clinically effective antidepressants, such as **bupropion**, do not down-regulate β-adrenergic receptors in rat brain. Furthermore, some compounds that modify β-adrenergic receptors exert effects that are inconsistent with a direct correlation between down-regulation of β-adrenergic receptors and mood elevation. **Thyroid hormone** can be helpful as an adjunct therapy for depression despite the fact that it augments rather than diminishes β-adrenergic receptor function; **propranolol,** a β-adrenergic receptor antagonist, is not an antidepressant and indeed can exacerbate depression in a small percentage of vulnerable individuals; and **yohimbine,** an α_2-adrenergic antagonist, that facilitates down-regulation of β-adrenergic receptors in response to tricyclic drugs does not augment the clinical efficacy of these compounds.

Other adaptations in noradrenergic systems have been reported in response to long-term treatment with antidepressants. Some evidence, both preclinical and clinical, suggests that tricyclics and certain other antidepressants down-regulate α_2-adrenergic receptors, possibly as a homeostatic response to drug-induced increases in synaptic levels of norepinephrine. Because α_2-adrenergic receptors primarily function as inhibitory autoreceptors on presynaptic noradrenergic nerve terminals (Chapter 6), down-regulation of these receptors would reduce this negative feedback and increase norepinephrine release. Many antidepressant treatments

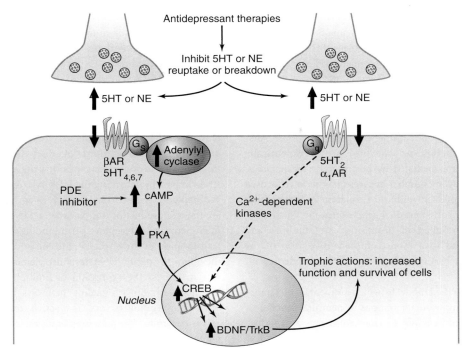

14-8 **Long-term adaptations to antidepressant treatment.** Antidepressants acutely increase levels of serotonin (5HT) and norepinephrine (NE) by inhibiting the reuptake or breakdown of these monoamines. Such increases activate several 5HT and NE receptors, including those coupled to cAMP and Ca^{2+} pathways. (G_x refers to a variety of G proteins that can influence Ca^{2+} pathways.) Long-term antidepressant administration decreases the function and expression of certain 5HT and NE receptors, such as β-AR and $5HT_2$. In contrast, the cAMP pathway is up-regulated in the hippocampus and frontal cortex by long-term treatment, resulting in increased levels of adenylyl cyclase and cAMP-dependent protein kinase A (PKA), as well as increased expression and function of the transcription factor CREB. The observation that the cAMP cascade is enhanced after long-term antidepressant treatment indicates that the functional output of 5HT and NE may be up-regulated, even though levels of certain 5HT and NE receptors are down-regulated. Brain-derived neurotrophic factor (BDNF) and TrkB represent two of many potential targets of CREB. Antidepressant-induced up-regulation of BDNF and TrkB may influence the function and survival of vulnerable hippocampal and cortical neurons (see **14-9**).

decrease levels of tyrosine hydroxylase in the LC, and in turn decrease the capacity of noradrenergic neurons to synthesize norepinephrine. However, the involvement of these antidepressant-induced adaptations in drug efficacy remains uncertain: down-regulation of α_2- and β-adrenergic receptors and of tyrosine hydroxylase would produce opposing effects on noradrenergic signal transduction, such that it is not clear whether the postsynaptic neuron is exposed to more or less norepinephrine-induced signaling compared with such signaling before drug administration, if indeed a change occurs at all. Similar uncertainties complicate the interpretation of other drug-induced changes in

neurotransmitter receptors. Overall, it seems more likely that down-regulation of these proteins are expected homeostatic responses to increased synaptic norepinephrine rather than critical mechanisms of antidepressant action.

Multiple changes in serotonergic neurotransmission in the brain also occur in response to long-term antidepressant treatment. Ligand-binding assays have indicated that many antidepressant drugs down-regulate $5HT_{2A}$ receptors. Like the down-regulation of adrenergic receptors, down-regulation of $5HT_{2A}$ receptors can be viewed as a homeostatic response to increased synaptic levels of serotonin. However, a direct correlation between $5HT_{2A}$ receptor down-regulation and the clinical effects of antidepressants must be questioned because repeated ECT up-regulates $5HT_{2A}$ receptors, and some drugs that down-regulate $5HT_{2A}$ receptors do not have antidepressant effects.

Regulation of intracellular messenger pathways and gene expression The adaptations in monoamines and monoamine receptors previously discussed, whether or not they are therapeutically relevant, are mediated by postreceptor mechanisms. Thus a growing number of investigations have focused on antidepressant-induced regulation of intracellular messengers and neuronal gene expression. Such studies have resulted in promising early findings and should lead to a more comprehensive view of the effects on brain function exerted by antidepressant drugs.

A simplified model by which antidepressants might induce long-term adaptations in neuronal function is represented in 14–8. Current antidepressants induce initial changes in the brain by increasing synaptic levels of monoamine neurotransmitters. Initial changes in monoamine function lead to many relevant and many irrelevant perturbations of intracellular signaling (Chapter 4). These changes produce alterations in gene expression and protein translation that accrue with continued drug administration. Changes in transcription and translation result in altered levels of specific neuronal proteins, which subsequently underlie long-term changes in the functional properties of target neurons. Unfortunately, despite a large catalogue of antidepressant-induced changes, the critical proteins involved in the therapeutic response remain unknown.

If intracellular signaling proteins are indeed targets of long-term administration of antidepressant agents, drugs that directly target such proteins might serve as novel antidepressants. Potential candidates for such agents include **phosphodiesterase inhibitors**. Several reports have indicated that long-term antidepressant treatment up-regulates the functioning of the cAMP pathway in the hippocampus and cerebral cortex. One consequence of this up-regulation is activation of the transcription factor, CREB (cAMP response element binding protein; Chapter 4). This has led to the proposal that increased activity of the cAMP-CREB pathway may contribute to the clinical efficacy of these treatments. Consistent with this possibility is the clinical observation that **rolipram**, a type-4 phosphodiesterase inhibitor that increases cAMP levels by decreasing its degradation (Chapter 4), may reduce the symptoms of depression. Unfortunately, rolipram is poorly tolerated by humans because of its many side effects, in particular, nausea and vomiting; however, the recent cloning of numerous subtypes of type-4 phosphodiesterase and the demonstration of their region-specific expression in brain (Chapter 4) offer promise for the development of more selective agents that may effectively relieve depression with fewer side effects.

Neurotrophic hypothesis of depression and antidepressant treatment As discussed earlier in this chapter, the brain reacts to both acute and chronic stress in part by activating the HPA axis. As described in Chapter 4, glucocorticoids, such as cortisol, which are the end product of this pathway, act by binding to their cytoplasmic receptors. Such binding induces the translocation of these receptors to the nucleus, where they bind to specific DNA response elements to activate or repress the expression of multiple genes, or interfere with other signaling pathways by binding other transcription factors. The activity of the HPA axis is controlled by numerous brain regions, including the amygdala, which exerts an excitatory influence on hypothalamic CRF–containing neurons in the PVN, and the hippocampus, which exerts an inhibitory influence (see 14–6). Glucocorticoids, by potently affecting the activity of hippocampal neurons, can provide powerful feedback to the HPA axis. Under normal physiologic circumstances, glucocorticoids appear to enhance hippocampal inhibition of HPA activity. However, sustained elevation of glucocorticoids, which occurs in response to prolonged and severe stress, suppresses hippocampal neurogenesis and may damage hippocampal neurons 14–9, thus reducing inhibitory control that the hippocampus exerts on the HPA axis, further increasing the levels of circulating glucocorticoids and resulting in additional damage to the hippocampus.

Stress may damage hippocampal neurons by several additional means. The sustained glutamatergic activation of hippocampal neurons that occurs in response to stress is potentially capable of triggering excitotoxic mechanisms of neuronal injury (Chapters 17 and 19), although this has not been proven to occur in major depression. Stress also has been shown to reduce the expression of brain-derived neurotrophic factor (BDNF; Chapter 8) in vulnerable hippocampal neurons, a mechanism by which stress may suppress neurogenesis and otherwise impair the functioning of these neurons.

In contrast, long-term administration of most antidepressants increases BDNF expression in the hippocampus. Antidepressant administration also prevents the down-regulation of BDNF that occurs in response

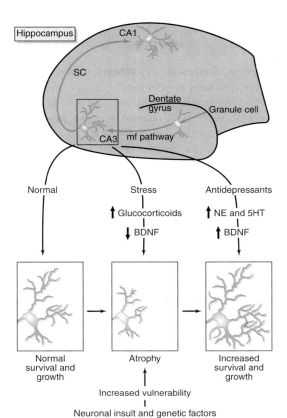

Normal

Stress
↑ Glucocorticoids
↓ BDNF

Antidepressants
↑ NE and 5HT
↑ BDNF

Normal
survival and
growth

Atrophy

Increased
survival and
growth

Increased vulnerability

Neuronal insult and genetic factors

14-9 **Model of the neurotrophic hypothesis of antidepressant treatments and stress-related disorders.** The major cell types in the hippocampus and the effects of stress and antidepressant treatments on CA3 pyramidal cells are shown. The three major subfields of the hippocampus—CA3 and CA1 pyramidal cells and dentate gyrus granule cells—are connected by the mossy fiber (mf) and Schaffer collateral (SC) pathways. Chronic stress decreases the expression of brain-derived neurotrophic factor (BDNF) in the hippocampus, which in turn may contribute to the atrophy of CA3 neurons and their increased vulnerability to a variety of neuronal insults. Chronic elevation of glucocorticoid levels is also known to decrease the survival of these neurons. In contrast, antidepressant treatments increase the expression of BDNF, as well as that of TrkB, and prevent the down-regulation of BDNF elicited by stress. Such activity may increase the dendritic arborizations and survival of the neurons, or help repair or protect the neurons from further damage.

to stress; indeed, antidepressant treatments can enhance the dendritic sprouting of certain hippocampal neurons, in contrast to the effects of stress. These effects, and the activity of antidepressants in certain behavioral models, are not observed in BDNF knockout mice. These findings are consistent with the hypothesis that antidepressants work in part by up-regulating BDNF in hippocampus and by thereby repairing stress-induced damage to hippocampal neurons and protecting vulnerable neurons from further damage (see **14-9**). Such findings could explain why responses to antidepressants are delayed: antidepressant efficacy may require sufficient time for levels of BDNF to gradually increase and exert their neurotrophic effects. Accordingly, other agents that promote BDNF function may prove to be clinically effective antidepressants. However, it is important to emphasize that this scheme remains hypothetical in human depression. As just one example, BDNF seems to be pro-depressant in other neural circuits, such as the nucleus accumbens.

An extension of the neurotrophic hypothesis of depression is the hypothesis that hippocampal neurogenesis is the required "slow step" in the action of antidepressants. In adult mammals, new neurons are born and incorporated into working neural circuits in two discrete brain areas, the subventricular zone in close proximity to the striatum, and the subgranular zone of the hippocampal dentate gyrus. In rodents, primates, and perhaps in humans, neurons arise from progenitor cells in the subgranular zone and migrate into the granule cell layer of the dentate gyrus. The function of these new hippocampal neurons is unclear, but they have properties distinct from older neurons, perhaps exhibiting enhanced plasticity. Stress and glucocorticoids inhibit, and a wide variety of antidepressant drugs, exercise, and enriched environments activate hippocampal neurogenesis.

Early experiments show that blocking neurogenesis interferes with the action of some antidepressants in behavioral paradigms that require chronic drug administration. It is still premature to conclude that neurogenesis plays a role in the therapeutic actions of antidepressants for several reasons. First, the methods used to inhibit neurogenesis might also damage existing neurons and thus block antidepressant action for other reasons. Second, both the neurotrophic hypothesis and the neurogenesis hypothesis require a more robust explanation of how the hippocampus might play a central role in depression than now exists. The ability of the hippocampus to suppress CRF secretion may not be adequate to explain how this structure can play a key role in antidepressant action. Despite these caveats, these hypotheses have generated considerable excitement; along with the **DBS** experiments described above, they constitute significant new avenues for research into therapies for depression.

Recent work with NMDA receptor antagonists
Recent novel findings have sparked interest in neuro-biologic systems that were previously unexplored in relation to depression. A dramatic example is the observation that sub-anesthetic doses of intravenously infused **ketamine** (a noncompetitive NMDA receptor antagonist whose actions are similar to those of **phencyclidine**; Chapter 5) produce a rapid but transient antidepressant effect in treatment-resistant depression. These striking effects suggest that depressive symptoms can be improved by altering glutamate signaling. Ketamine's antidepressant properties have been recapitulated in animal tests of antidepressant action such as the forced swim test, where the ability of ketamine to reduce immobility requires intact AMPA glutamate receptor signaling and is associated with increased levels of hippocampal BDNF protein. These clinical and preclinical findings have prompted investigation of the mechanisms underlying ketamine's apparent antidepressant activity and ways in which this ketamine action can be exploited as a new treatment for depression.

Lithium and Other Mood-Stabilizing Drugs

Lithium is effective in the treatment of acute mania and is used prophylactically to prevent the recurrence of manic and depressive episodes in individuals with bipolar disorder. Lithium is also used in combination with antidepressant medications to augment clinical responses in unipolar depression. As with antidepressants, the clinical effects of lithium require long-term administration. The powerful clinical effects of lithium are striking when considering its molecular simplicity: the lightest solid element in the periodic table, lithium circulates as a monovalent cation.

It is believed that lithium's therapeutic benefits are due to its effects on postreceptor intracellular signaling proteins. Long-term lithium administration has been shown to alter: (1) the coupling of some neurotransmitter receptors to G proteins, (2) the expression of $G_{\alpha i}$ and subtypes of adenylyl cyclase, (3) the modification of G proteins by ADP-ribosylation, and (4) cAMP-dependent and Ca^{2+}-dependent protein phosphorylation in specific brain regions. However, despite these numerous actions, it has been hypothesized that lithium's beneficial effects in the treatment of manic-depressive illness are related to its effects on the phosphatidylinositol or Wnt signaling pathways. A major obstacle to testing these hypotheses has been the lack of a convincing animal model of bipolar disorder.

Inositol depletion hypothesis Although this hypothesis is not new, its validity has yet to be determined. Many neurotransmitter receptors, including α_1-adrenergic, $5HT_2$-serotonergic, and muscarinic cholinergic receptors, are linked to the enzyme phospholipase C by means of the G protein Gq. Phospholipase C hydrolyzes phosphatidylinositol bisphosphate (PIP_2), a membrane phospholipid, to yield two second messengers: diacylglycerol and inositol triphosphate (IP_3). Diacylglycerol activates protein kinase C, and IP_3 binds its receptor on the endoplasmic reticulum to release intracellular Ca^{2+}. These pathways are described in detail in Chapter 4.

Phosphatidylinositol is synthesized from free inositol and a lipid moiety. Most cells can obtain free inositol directly from plasma, but neurons cannot because inositol does not cross the blood–brain barrier. Consequently, neurons must either recycle inositol by dephosphorylating inositol phosphates after they are generated from the hydrolysis of phosphatidylinositols, or synthesize it de novo from glucose-6-phosphate, a product of glycolysis. At therapeutic concentrations (0.5–1 mM), lithium inhibits several inositol phosphatases, most significantly inositol monophosphatase (IMPase). Such inhibition blocks the ability of neurons to generate free inositol from recycled inositol phosphates or glucose-6-phosphate (see **4–7** in Chapter 4). Consequently, lithium-exposed neurons have a diminished ability to resynthesize PIP_2 after it is hydrolyzed in response to neurotransmitter receptor activation. It has been hypothesized that when firing rates of neurons are abnormally high, lithium-treated neurons are depleted of PIP_2, and neurotransmission dependent on this second messenger system is dampened.

This hypothesis is intriguing because it suggests that the effects of lithium may be evident only in cells with abnormally high firing rates and that lithium may be capable of treating both manic and depressive states because of its effects on multiple neurotransmitter systems. However, the story is more complex. Chronic inhibition of inositol phosphatases may lead to a build-up of active inositol phosphates, including IP_3, and thus may facilitate rather than dampen the actions of neurotransmitters on this pathway. Indeed, whether long-term lithium administration dampens or facilitates phosphatidylinositol-dependent signal transduction in the brain is not clear. Moreover, the critical cells in the brain that are targets of lithium's therapeutic action remain unknown, and it is unclear which of the many phosphatidylinositol-dependent neurotransmitter systems must be dampened (or facilitated) to produce lithium's effects. More importantly, this hypothesis does not explain why several weeks must elapse before lithium exhibits a therapeutic effect.

Regulation of the Wnt pathway and glycogen synthase kinase 3β In addition to the antimanic properties previously discussed, several teratogenic effects have been attributed to the use of lithium. Studies have revealed, for example, that lithium has teratogenic effects on embryos of *Xenopus laevis*, an African clawed toad, that lead to dorsalization of the embryo (ie, the production of two spines). Initially it was speculated that lithium's inhibition of IMPase was responsible not only for mood stabilization, as previously discussed, but also for lithium's dramatic developmental effects. However, an important series of investigations led to the discovery that the teratogenic effects of lithium are instead related to its inhibition of glycogen synthase kinase 3β (GSK-3β). Highly selective bisphosphonate blockers of IMPase do not produce teratogenic effects in Xenopus, and lithium is capable of altering cell fate in mutants of the yeast

---

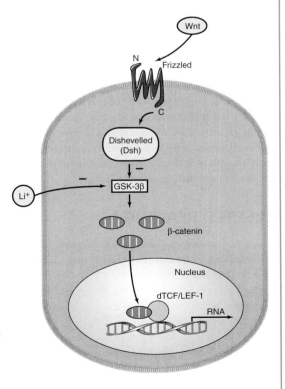

14–5 **Wnt Signaling Pathway**

Wnt genes encode a large family of secreted proteins that regulate cell proliferation and differentiation in species as divergent as nematodes, flies, frogs, and humans. In mammals, Wnt genes have been implicated in brain development. The initial gene discovery in mammals was of Int-1, a gene that became activated to produce tumors when the mouse mammary tumor virus integrated next to it in the mouse genome. Int-1 was found to be the mouse version of Wingless (Wg), a developmental control gene first discovered in *Drosophila*. The contraction of Int-1 with Wg resulted in the term Wnt, of which many members are now known.

Wnt ligands bind to receptor molecules of the Frizzled family to initiate a signal transduction cascade involving a cytosolic protein Dishevelled (Dsh). It is of interest that Dsh knockout mice are defective in social behavior and grooming, and have subtle neurologic abnormalities reminiscent of those seen in **schizophrenia** (Chapter 16). Wnt signaling through Frizzled and Dsh inhibits the serine–threonine kinase known as glycogen synthase kinase 3β (GSK3β) (see figure).

GSK3β is believed to inhibit the function of a transcriptional regulatory protein, β-catenin: phosphorylation of β-catenin triggers its degradation. By inhibiting GSK3β activity, Wnt signaling (and **lithium** which directly inhibits GSK3β) leads to stabilization of β-catenin, which in turn translocates to the nucleus, where it interacts with the transcription factor dTCF/LEF-1 to activate expression of Wnt-responsive genes. Current research is aimed at identifying Wnt-responsive genes that may contribute to lithium's clinical effects. GSK-3β is also implicated in **Alzheimer disease;** indeed, the kinase may be partly responsible for the hyperphosphorylation of tau (a microtubule-associated protein), which is believed to be a cause of neurofibrillary tangles (Chapter 17).

Dictyostelium discoideum that lack phospholipase C and thus cannot generate inositol triphosphate.

The GSK3β pathway is a negative regulator of the Wnt signaling pathway **14–5**, whose inhibition reproduces the teratogenic effects of lithium in several species. Because inhibition of GSK3β occurs at lithium concentrations similar to those used therapeutically, questions have been raised as to whether the antimanic properties of lithium may be mediated at least partly by the inhibition of this enzyme. Selective inhibitors of GSK3β must be generated before this hypothesis can be tested in humans.

Actions of other antimanic agents   Other mood stabilizers are increasingly used as substitutes for lithium in the treatment of mania. Strikingly, most of these drugs initially were developed for use as anticonvulsants (Chapter 18). **Valproic acid**, for example, appears to act by facilitating GABAergic neurotransmission, possibly by increasing GABA release through mechanisms that thus far have been poorly described. Valproic acid has been established as an effective treatment for mania and is better tolerated than lithium by some patients. Why valproic acid reduces mania is not yet understood. It has been proposed that this agent's effectiveness is consistent with the hypothesis that mania is characterized by excessive neural activity, at least in certain circuits of the brain that have yet to be identified. Other anticonvulsants have been used to treat bipolar disorder, eg, **lamotrigine** and **carbamazepine**, but the number of well-designed clinical trials remains small. The introduction of anticonvulsants as agents for the treatment of mania represents one of the few true therapeutic advances in the treatment of psychiatric disorders during the past several decades. Despite this achievement, investigators remain frustrated in their attempts to determine how these agents exert their beneficial effects.

SELECTED READING

Bechara A, Damasio H, Damasio AR. Emotion, decision making and the orbitofrontal cortex. *Cerebral Cortex*. 2000;10:295–307.

Berridge MJ, Downes CP, Hanley MR. Neural and developmental actions of lithium: a unifying hypothesis. *Cell*. 1989;59:411–419.

Berton O, Nestler EJ. New approaches to antidepressant drug discovery: beyond monoamines. *Nature Rev Neurosci*. 2006;7:137–151.

Blendy JA. The role of CREB in depression and antidepressant treatment. *Biol Psychiatry*. 2006;59: 1144–1150.

Cryan JF, Valentino RJ, Lucki I. Assessing substrates underlying the behavioral effects of antidepressants using the modified rat forced swimming test. *Neurosci Biobehav Rev*. 2005;29:547–569.

de Kloet ER, Joels M, Holsboer F. Stress and the brain: from adaptation to disease. *Nature Rev Neurosci*. 2005;6:463–475.

Duman RS, Monteggia LM. A neurotrophic model for stress-related mood disorders. *Biol Psychiatry*. 2006;59:1116–1127.

Gordon JA, Hen R. Genetic approaches to the study of anxiety. *Annu Rev Neurosci*. 2004;27:193–222.

Gould TD, Manji HK. The Wnt signaling pathway in bipolar disorder. *Neuroscientist*. 2002;8: 497–511.

Hyman SE, Nestler EJ. Initiation and adaptation: a paradigm for understanding psychotropic drug action. *Am J Psychiatry*. 1996;153:151–162.

Korte SM, Koolhaas JM, Wingfield JC, et al. The Darwinian concept of stress: benefits of allostasis and costs of allostatic load and the trade-offs in health and disease. *Neurosci Biobehav Rev*. 2005;29:3–38.

Krishnan V, Han MH, Graham DL, et al. Molecular adaptations underlying susceptibility and resistance to social defeat in brain reward regions. *Cell*. 2007;131:391–404.

Krystal JH, Staley J, Mason G, et al. Gamma-aminobutyric acid type A receptors and alcoholism: intoxication, dependence, vulnerability, and treatment. *Arch Gen Psychiatry*. 2006;63:957–968.

LeDoux JE. Emotion circuits in the brain. *Annu Rev Neurosci*. 2000;23:155–184.

Liotti M, Mayberg HS, Brannan SK, et al. Differential limbic—cortical correlates of sadness and anxiety in healthy subjects: implications for affective disorders. *Biol Psychiatry*. 2000;48:30–42.

Low K, Crestani F, Keist R, et al. Molecular and neuronal substrate for the selective attenuation of anxiety. *Science*. 2000;290:131–134.

Manji HK, Drevets WC, Charney DS. The cellular neurobiology of depression. *Nature Med*. 2001;7: 541–547.

Maren S. Neurobiology of Pavlovian fear conditioning. *Annu Rev Neurosci*. 2001;24:897–931.

Mayberg HS. Positron emission tomography imaging in depression: a neural systems perspective. *Neuroimaging Clin N Am*. 2003;13:805–815.

Mayberg HS, Lozano AM, Voon V, et al. Deep brain stimulation for treatment-resistant depression. *Neuron*. 2005;45(5):651–660.

McGaugh JL. The amygdala modulates the consolidation of memories of emotionally arousing experiences. *Annu Rev Neurosci*. 2004;27:1–28.

Nestler EJ, Carlezon WA., Jr. The mesolimbic dopamine reward circuit in depression. *Biol Psychiatry*. 2006;59:1151–1159.

Olson RW, Hanchar HJ, Meera P, et al. $GABA_A$ receptor subtypes: the "one glass of wine" receptors. *Alcohol*. 2007;41:201–209.

Ressler KJ, Nemeroff CB. Role of serotonergic and noradrenergic systems in the pathophysiology of depression and anxiety disorders. *Depress Anxiety*. 2000;12(Suppl 1):2–19.

Ron D. Signaling cascades regulating NMDA receptor sensitivity to ethanol. *Neuroscientist*. 2004;10:325–336.

Rudolph U, Mohler H. Analysis of $GABA_A$ receptor function and dissection of the pharmacology of benzodiazepines and general anesthetics through mouse genetics. *Annu Rev Pharmacol Toxicol*. 2004;44:475–479.

Rudolph U, Mohler H. GABA-based therapeutic approaches: $GABA_A$ receptor subtype functions. *Curr Opin Pharmacol*. 2006;6:18–23.

Sahay A, Hen R. Adult hippocampal neurogenesis in depression. *Nature Neurosci*. 2007;10:1110–1115.

Sanacora G, Zarate CA, Krystal JH, et al. Targeting the glutamatergic system to develop novel, improved therapeutics for mood disorders. *Nature Rev Drug Discov*. 2008;7:426–437.

Shin LM, Orr SP, Carson MA, et al. Regional cerebral blood flow in the amygdala and medial prefrontal cortex during traumatic imagery in male and female Vietnam veterans with PTSD. *Arch Gen Psychiatry*. 2004;61:168–176.

Strange BA, Dolan RJ. Beta-adrenergic modulation of emotional memory-evoked human amygdala and hippocampal responses. *Proc Natl Acad Sci USA*. 2004;101(31):11454–11458

Thome J, Sakai N, Shin KH, et al. cAMP response element-mediated gene transcription is upregulated by chronic antidepressant treatment. *J Neurosci*. 2000;20:4030–4036.

Zarate CA Jr, Singh JB, Carlson PJ, et al. A randomized trial of an N-methyl-D-aspartate antagonist in treatment-resistant major depression. *Arch Gen Psychiatry*. 2006;63:856–864.

CHAPTER 15

Reinforcement and Addictive Disorders

- The defining feature of addiction is compulsive, out-of-control drug use, despite negative consequences.

- Addictive drugs induce pleasurable states or relief from distress, thus motivating repeated drug use.

- Drugs of abuse are both rewarding and reinforcing. Rewards are stimuli that the brain interprets as intrinsically positive, and reinforcing stimuli are those that increase the probability that behaviors paired with them will be repeated.

- The brain reward circuitry targeted by addictive drugs, which normally responds to natural reinforcers such as food, water, and sex, includes the dopaminergic projections from the ventral tegmental area (VTA) of the midbrain to the nucleus accumbens (NAc) and other forebrain structures.

- Repeated use of addictive drugs produces multiple unwanted changes in the brain that may lead to tolerance, sensitization, dependence, and addiction.

- Dependence is an adaptive state that develops in response to repeated drug administration; when unmasked by cessation of drug use, this adapted state may lead to withdrawal symptoms.

- Tolerance refers to the diminished effect of a drug after repeated administration at the same dose, or to the need for an increase in dose to produce the same effect; sensitization describes the opposite response to repeated drug administration.

- Cocaine and amphetamines produce their psychoactive effects by potentiating monoaminergic transmission through actions on the dopamine transporter, together with actions on the serotonin and norepinephrine transporters.

- The reinforcing effects of opiate drugs result from their binding to endogenous opioid receptors, most importantly μ opioid receptors in both the VTA and NAc.

- The immediate effects of ethanol are believed to result primarily from facilitation of $GABA_A$ receptors and inhibition of NMDA glutamate receptors. At higher doses, ethanol inhibits the functioning of most voltage-gated ion channels as well.

- The effects of nicotine are caused by its activation of nicotinic acetylcholine (nACh) receptors; its reinforcing effects may depend on nACh receptors located on VTA dopamine neurons.

- Delta-9-tetrahydrocannabinol, the active psychotropic ingredient in marijuana, exerts its primary pharmacologic effects by binding to a G protein-coupled receptor in the brain known as the CB_1 receptor.

- The psychotomimetic drugs of abuse, phencyclidine (angel dust, PCP) and ketamine, bind specific sites in the channel of the NMDA glutamate receptor, where they act as noncompetitive NMDA antagonists.

Drug addiction is a progressive and often fatal behavioral syndrome characterized by compulsive drug seeking and consumption despite serious negative consequences. The drug-centered existence of addicts can cost them their jobs, personal relationships, financial standing, happiness, and, in some cases, their lives. Drug-addicted individuals often appear to have lost the ability to make choices that promote their own happiness and survival. Many drug addicts who seek treatment report that they realize the destructive nature of their addiction but are *unable* to alter their addictive behavior.

In laboratory settings in which social and environmental variables are controlled, normal animals with access to addictive drugs typically engage in self-administration of these substances. Such behavior indicates that addiction is the result of a conserved neurobiologic substrate in animal and human brains that is vulnerable to regulation by addictive drugs. The actions of such drugs on this neural substrate tend to promote continued drug-taking behavior in a way that becomes increasingly involuntary. In both animals and humans, roughly 50% of the risk for addiction is genetic, but the specific genes that comprise that risk remain unknown.

Understanding the biologic determinants of addiction and the biologic factors responsible for individual vulnerability to addiction will aid in the development of truly effective treatment and prevention strategies. Thus it is important to determine (1) the neurochemical and anatomic basis, and naturally intended function, of reward circuitry in the healthy brain, and (2) the changes in this circuitry produced by addictive drugs that cause the addicted brain to be fundamentally different from a drug-free brain.

BRAIN REWARD PATHWAYS

Addictive drugs are both *rewarding* and *reinforcing*. A reward is a stimulus that the brain interprets as intrinsically positive or as something to be approached. A reinforcing stimulus is one that increases the probability that behaviors paired with it will be repeated. Not all reinforcers are rewarding; for example, a negative or punishing stimulus might reinforce avoidance behaviors.

Drug-induced pleasurable states are important motivators of initial drug use. Drug actions that produce these states also produce associated, but ultimately undesirable, changes in brain reward circuitry that promote future drug use. Another form of positive reinforcement involves the alleviation of unpleasant symptoms—either from preexisting states or caused by drug withdrawal—by means of drug use. Conditioned reinforcement, which occurs when previously neutral stimuli become associated with the pleasurable effects of drugs, is yet another type of positive reinforcement. All of these mechanisms contribute to repetitive drug taking that, in vulnerable individuals, may result in an addicted state.

The reinforcing effects of drugs can be demonstrated in animals, where rodents and nonhuman primates readily self-administer certain drugs by pressing a lever or placing their noses in an aperture. In this *self-administration* paradigm, the amount of work (number of lever presses or nose pokes) an animal does to gain access to a given amount of drug indicates the strength of reinforcement induced by the drug. The strength with which different drugs reinforce behavior in animals correlates well with their tendency to reinforce drug-seeking behavior in humans. **Cocaine**, for example, is highly reinforcing when injected intravenously. Laboratory animals readily self-administer this drug, and some of them will give up survival necessities, such as food and water, or work excessively, even to the point of death, in order to gain access to cocaine. Such evidence of the power of cocaine's reinforcing properties helps to explain its addictiveness in humans. In general, drugs that are less addictive in humans (such as **marijuana**) are not as likely to be self-administered by animals, and drugs that are not addictive in humans are not reinforcing in or self-administered by animals. **Nicotine** appears to represent an exception to this rule; although it does not strongly reinforce drug-seeking behavior in animals, it produces strong addiction in some humans.

Another paradigm used to investigate drug reward in animals is known as *conditioned place preference*, where animals learn to associate a particular environment with passive drug exposure. For example, a rodent will learn to spend more time on the side of a box where it was previously given cocaine. This paradigm reflects the strong cue-conditioned effects of addictive drugs and provides an indirect measure of drug reward. In the *conditioned reinforcement* paradigm, animals learn to associate a neutral cue, such as light, with a natural reinforcer, such as water. With sufficient training, the neutral cue becomes a conditioned reinforcer, namely, something the animals will work (lever press, nose poke) to obtain. Addictive drugs dramatically potentiate the degree to which animals will work for conditioned reinforcers.

The neural substrates that underlie the perception of reward and the phenomenon of positive reinforcement are a set of interconnected forebrain structures called brain reward pathways **15-1** ; these include the

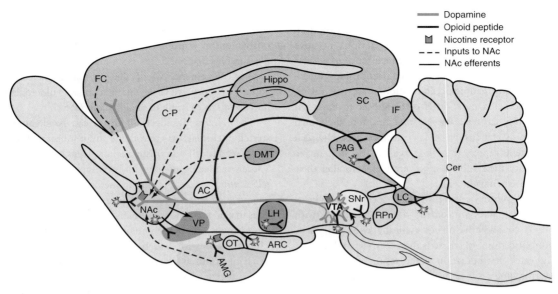

15–1 **Neural reward circuits for various drugs (cocaine, amphetamines, opiates, nicotine, and ethanol) in a sagittal section of rat brain.** A limbic–extrapyramidal motor interface is apparent. Dashed lines indicate limbic glutamatergic afferent inputs to the nucleus accumbens (NAc). Purple lines represent efferent signals from the NAc believed to be involved in drug reward. Bold blue lines indicate projections of the mesocorticolimbic dopamine system, which are believed to be critical substrates for drug reward. This dopamine system originates in the ventral tegmental area (VTA) and projects to the NAc, olfactory tubercle, ventral striatal domains of the caudate–putamen (C–P), and amygdala (AMG). Brown lines indicate opioid peptide-containing neurons, which comprise systems that may be involved in opiate, ethanol, and possibly nicotine reward; these systems include local enkephalinergic circuits (*short segments*) and the hypothalamic β-endorphin circuit (*long segment*). Gold areas indicate the approximate distribution of GABA$_A$ receptor complexes that may mediate sedative/hypnotic (ethanol) reward. Green solid structures indicate nicotinic acetylcholine receptors, which are located on dopaminergic, opioid peptidergic, and glutamatergic neurons. AC, anterior commissure; ARC, arcuate nucleus; Cer, cerebellum; DMT, dorsomedial thalamus; FC, frontal cortex; Hippo, hippocampus; IF, inferior colliculus; LC, locus coeruleus; LH, lateral hypothalamus; OT, olfactory tract; PAG, periaqueductal gray; RPn, raphe pontis nucleus; SC, superior colliculus; SNr, substantia nigra pars reticulata; VP, ventral pallidum. (Adapted with permission from Koob GF, Nestler EJ. In: Salloway S, Malloy P, Cummings JL, eds. *The Neuropsychiatry of Limbic and Subcortical Disorders.* Washington, DC: American Psychiatric Press; 1997: 179.)

nucleus accumbens (NAc; the major component of the ventral striatum), the basal forebrain (components of which have been termed the extended amygdala, as discussed later in this chapter), hippocampus, hypothalamus, and frontal regions of cerebral cortex. These structures receive rich dopaminergic innervation from the ventral tegmental area (VTA) of the midbrain. Addictive drugs are rewarding and reinforcing because they act in brain reward pathways to enhance either dopamine release or the effects of dopamine in the NAc or related structures, or because they produce effects similar to dopamine.

Roughly 50 years ago, animals were shown to press a lever to electrically stimulate discrete brain regions,

which provided the first direct evidence for specific neural substrates in the brain that are capable of mediating reinforcement. Although such *intracranial self-stimulation* of several brain structures is reinforcing, stimulation of the medial forebrain bundle and closely associated areas results in the strongest reinforcement of paired behavior. Addictive drugs and reinforcing electrical brain stimulation activate the same brain reward circuitry, as suggested by the synergistic effect that addictive drugs have on brain stimulation reward (BSR) thresholds; in the presence of drugs, less stimulation is needed to produce a particular response. Virtually all addictive drugs enhance BSR. Reinforcement produced by stimulation of the medial forebrain bundle appears to be caused primarily by activation of axons of VTA dopamine neurons coursing toward the NAc and other forebrain reward structures **15-1**. There also appear to be dopamine-independent mechanisms of the reinforcing effects of medial forebrain bundle self-stimulation. The nature of these mechanisms is unknown, although certain hypothalamic peptides have been speculated to be involved.

A Comparison Between Addictive Drugs and Natural Reinforcers

The brain reward circuitry that is targeted by addictive drugs normally mediates the pleasure and strengthening of behaviors associated with natural reinforcers, such as food, water, and sexual contact. Dopamine neurons in the VTA are activated by food and water, and dopamine release in the NAc is stimulated by the presence of natural reinforcers, such as food, water, or a sexual partner. Thus drugs tap into neural networks that apparently evolved to reinforce behaviors that are necessary for survival and reproduction. These systems can be viewed as complementary to survival networks in the brain that mediate learning about dangerous and harmful stimuli (Chapter 14).

Sensory cues produced by natural reinforcers activate reward pathways under normal circumstances, whereas addictive drugs directly activate the same neural circuitry by chemical means **15-1**, bypassing the need for evolutionarily useful behaviors. Hence, the powerful control over behavior exerted by addictive drugs may stem from the brain's inability to distinguish between the activation of reward circuitry by drugs and natural activation of the same circuitry by useful behaviors. Any activity, whether related to drug-taking or survival, that activates this circuitry is regarded as one that should be repeated. Moreover, chemical activation of reward circuitry by addictive drugs can be much more powerful than activation triggered by natural reinforcers. Exposure to addictive chemicals not only produces extreme euphoric states that may initially motivate drug use, but also causes equally extreme adaptations in reinforcement mechanisms and motivated behavior that eventually lead to compulsive use. Accordingly, the evolutionary design of human and animal brains that has helped to promote our survival also has made us vulnerable to addiction.

Repeated exposure to an addictive drug induces profound cellular and molecular changes within neurons of the brain reward circuitry, which in turn are believed to cause the alterations in reinforcement mechanisms that contribute to addiction. Drug-induced adaptations reflect both homeostatic compensations for excessive stimulation by drugs and alterations in multiple memory systems in the brain that serve to sustain addiction over long periods of time. These adaptations gradually alter normal control of motivated behavior, and eventually produce the compulsive and increasingly involuntary drug-seeking behavior that characterizes addiction. Thus compared with the normal brain, the addicted brain programs behavior in a fundamentally different way that can be long lasting and perhaps even permanent.

Pharmacological Consequences of Long-Term Drug Exposure

Familiar pharmacologic terms such as tolerance, dependence, and sensitization are useful in describing some of the time-dependent processes that underlie addiction. *Tolerance* refers to the diminishing effect of a drug after repeated administration at the same dose, or to the need for an increase in dose to produce the same effect. Tolerance may develop to some of the effects of a drug but not to others; for example, tolerance frequently develops to the analgesic, euphoric, and respiratory depressant effects of **opiates**, but not to the pupillary constriction produced by these drugs. *Pharmacokinetic* tolerance is caused by increased drug metabolism or clearance, whereas *pharmacodynamic* tolerance is a result of adaptations in the neural elements that respond to drugs initially. Pharmacodynamic tolerance is the more important mechanism in terms of its contribution to behavior, including addiction. *Sensitization,* also referred to as reverse tolerance, occurs when repeated administration of the same drug dose elicits escalating effects. *Dependence* is defined as an adaptive state that develops in response to repeated drug administration, and is unmasked during *withdrawal,* which occurs when drug-taking stops. Dependence resulting from long-term drug use may have both a somatic component, manifested by physical symptoms, and an emotional–motivational component, manifested by dysphoria and anhedonic symptoms, that occur when a drug is discontinued. While physical dependence and withdrawal occur with some drugs of abuse (**opiates, ethanol**), these phenomena are not useful in the diagnosis of an addiction because they do not occur with other drugs of abuse (**cocaine, amphetamine**) and can occur with many drugs that are not abused (**propranolol, clonidine**).

The official diagnosis of drug addiction by the *Diagnostic and Statistical Manual of Mental Disorders* (2000), which makes distinctions between **drug use**, **abuse**, and **substance dependence**, is flawed. First, diagnosis of drug use versus abuse can be arbitrary

15-1 **Examples of Acute Pharmacologic Actions of Drugs of Abuse**

Drug	Action
Opiates	Agonist at μ, δ, and κ opioid receptors[1]
Cocaine	Inhibits monoamine reuptake transporters
Amphetamine	Stimulates monoamine release[2]
Ethanol	Facilitates GABA$_A$ receptor function and inhibits NMDA glutamate receptor function[3]
Nicotine	Agonist at nicotinic acetylcholine receptors
Cannabinoids	Agonist at cannabinoid (CB$_1$ and CB$_2$) receptors[4]
Hallucinogens	Partial agonist at 5HT$_{2A}$ serotonin receptors
Phencyclidine (PCP)	Antagonist at NMDA glutamate receptors
Inhalants	Unknown

[1]μ and δ receptors mediate the reinforcing actions of opiates.
[2]Amphetamine produces this effect via actions at monoamine transporters. (see **15-3**)
[3]It is not known whether ethanol produces these effects by direct binding to these targets or by indirect mechanisms.
[4]CB$_1$ receptors mediate the reinforcing actions of cannabinoids.

and reflect cultural norms, not medical phenomena. Second, the term substance dependence implies that dependence is the primary pharmacologic phenomenon underlying addiction, which is likely not true, as tolerance, sensitization, and learning and memory also play central roles. It is ironic and unfortunate that the Manual avoids use of the term addiction, which provides the best description of the clinical syndrome.

INITIAL ACTIONS OF DRUGS OF ABUSE AND NATURAL REINFORCERS

Psychostimulants

Cocaine, amphetamines, and **methamphetamine** are the major psychostimulants of abuse. The related drug **methylphenidate** is also abused, although it is far less potent. These drugs elicit similar initial subjective effects **15-2**; differences generally reflect the route of administration and other pharmacokinetic factors. Such agents also have important therapeutic uses; cocaine, for example, is used as a **local anesthetic** (Chapter 2), and amphetamines and methylphenidate are used in low doses to treat **attention deficit hyperactivity disorder** and in higher doses to treat **narcolepsy** (Chapter 12). Despite their clinical uses, these drugs are strongly reinforcing, and their long-term use at high doses is linked with potential addiction, especially when they are rapidly administered or when high-potency forms are given.

15-2 **Acute Effects of Psychostimulants and Withdrawal Symptoms**

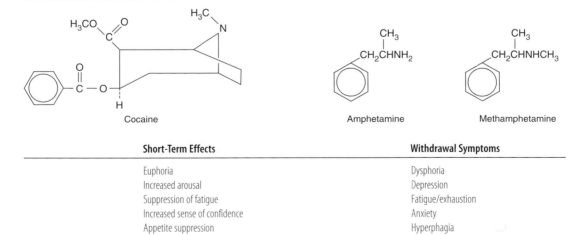

Short-Term Effects	Withdrawal Symptoms
Euphoria	Dysphoria
Increased arousal	Depression
Suppression of fatigue	Fatigue/exhaustion
Increased sense of confidence	Anxiety
Appetite suppression	Hyperphagia

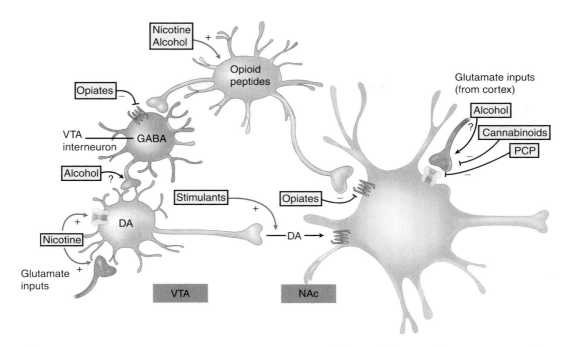

15-2 **Highly simplified scheme of converging acute actions of drugs of abuse on the VTA-NAc.** Stimulants directly increase dopaminergic transmission in the NAc. Opiates do the same indirectly: they inhibit GABAergic interneurons in the VTA, which disinhibits VTA dopamine neurons. Opiates also directly act on opioid receptors on NAc neurons, and opioid receptors, like D$_2$ dopamine receptors, signal via G$_i$, hence the two mechanisms converge within NAc neurons. The actions of the other drugs remain more conjectural. Nicotine activates VTA dopamine neurons directly via stimulation of nicotinic cholinergic receptors on those neurons, and indirectly via stimulation of its receptors on glutamatergic nerve terminals that innervate the dopamine cells. Ethanol, by promoting GABA$_A$ receptor function, may inhibit GABAergic terminals in VTA and hence disinhibit VTA dopamine neurons. It may similarly inhibit glutamatergic terminals that innervate NAc neurons. Cannabinoid mechanisms involve activation of CB$_1$ receptors (which, like D$_2$ and opioid receptors, are G$_i$ linked) on glutamatergic and GABAergic nerve terminals in the NAc and possibly on NAc neurons themselves. PCP may act by inhibiting postsynaptic NMDA glutamate receptors in the NAc. Finally, evidence suggests that nicotine and ethanol may activate endogenous opioid pathways, and that these and other drugs of abuse (eg, opiates) may activate endogenous cannabinoid pathways (not shown).

Cocaine and amphetamines produce their psychoactive effects by potentiating monoaminergic transmission **15-2** through actions on dopamine, serotonin, and norepinephrine transporters, although the precise mechanisms underlying this potentiation vary **15-3**. These proteins normally transport synaptically released neurotransmitter back into the presynaptic nerve terminal and thereby terminate transmitter action (Chapter 6). Actions at the dopamine transporter are the most important for the reinforcing effects of these drugs; for example, mice with a null mutation in the dopamine transporter (DAT) gene are much less sensitive than normal mice to the behavioral effects of cocaine or amphetamines.

The reinforcing effects of cocaine and amphetamines require an intact mesolimbic dopamine system. Systemic administration of dopamine antagonists, or of the dopamine synthesis inhibitor α-**methylparatyrosine (AMPT)**, decreases self-administration; in contrast, antagonists of various adrenergic or serotonergic receptors have little effect on such behavior. Selective antagonists for multiple dopamine receptor subtypes (D$_1$, D$_2$, and D$_3$) are effective in decreasing the reinforcing actions of cocaine. Dopamine levels are increased in the NAc during self-administration of amphetamine or cocaine, as mentioned previously, and blockade of dopaminergic transmission in the NAc—for example, in response to intra-NAc injections

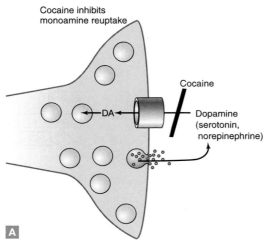

A

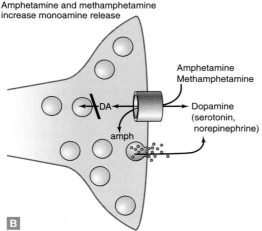

B

15-3 **Mechanism of action of cocaine and amphetamine on monoamine nerve terminals. A.** Cocaine potentiates the actions of monoamines at the synapse by inhibiting monoamine transporter proteins, which normally carry previously released transmitter back into the nerve terminal. **B.** Amphetamine serves as a substrate for monoamine transporter proteins and is transported into the nerve terminal. In the nerve terminal, amphetamine disrupts the vesicular storage of monoamine transmitters, which leads to an increase in their extravesicular levels; consequently, these transmitters are pumped out of the nerve terminal by a reverse action of the transporters.

of dopamine receptor antagonists or of the toxin **6-hydroxydopamine** (Chapter 6)—dramatically reduces drug reinforcement. The predominant effect of dopamine in the NAc is the inhibition of γ-aminobutyric acid (GABA)ergic medium spiny projection neurons;

however, why inhibition of these neurons contributes to drug reinforcement remains unknown.

Methamphetamine is an amphetamine derivative whose pharmacologic effects are very similar to those of amphetamine, but is longer acting due to pharmacokinetic considerations. Methamphetamine is easily synthesized from over-the-counter products (eg, the α-adrenergic agonist, **pseudoephedrine**), and this has led to its increasing use as an abused drug. Unlike cocaine and amphetamine, methamphetamine is directly toxic to midbrain dopamine neurons.

Opiates

The opiates and their synthetic analogs are the most effective analgesic agents known (Chapter 11), yet they are widely abused because of their effects on brain reward circuitry **15-3**. **Morphine** and **heroin**, along with a host of prescription opiates (eg, **oxycontin**), are among the most commonly abused opiates. Abuse of these drugs may be driven by a variety of factors, including their reinforcing effects, their ability to relieve both preexisting dysphoria and unpleasant symptoms related to drug withdrawal, and the intense craving they produce after long-term use. Physical dependence on opiates can occur independently of addiction; for example, patients with cancer pain may become physically dependent on these drugs but do not compulsively abuse them. Termination of opiate use is accompanied by emotional–motivational symptoms as well as somatic withdrawal symptoms **15-3**.

Immediate effects of opiate drugs result from their binding to endogenous opioid receptors. As discussed in Chapter 7, the three types of opioid receptors—μ, δ, and κ—are distinguished by their pharmacologic profiles and anatomic distributions. These receptors belong to the G protein-coupled receptor superfamily and exhibit significant homology, particularly in transmembrane and intracellular regions. Opioid receptors couple with $G_{i/o}$ proteins to inhibit adenylyl cyclase, to activate inwardly rectifying K^+ channels, and to inhibit voltage-gated Ca^{2+} channels. They typically mediate inhibitory responses that involve a reduction in excitability and cell firing, and inhibition of neurotransmitter release. Examples of neural and behavioral actions mediated by μ, δ, and κ opioid receptors are listed in **15-4**.

Opiates activate brain reward circuitry via two main mechanisms: (1) disinhibition of the VTA, which results in dopamine release in the NAc, and (2) dopamine-independent activity in the NAc. For example, reinforcing effects of intravenous heroin can be partly attenuated by administration of an opioid

15-3   **Acute Effects of Opiates and Withdrawal Symptoms**

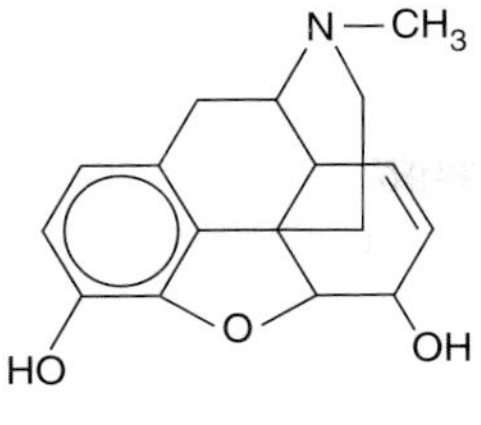

Morphine

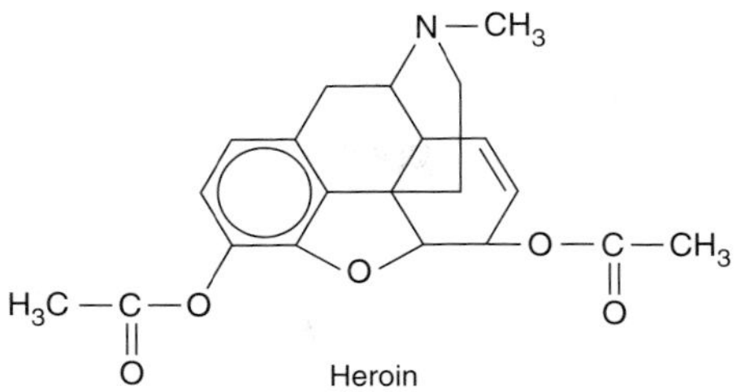

Heroin

Short-Term Effects	Withdrawal Symptoms
Analgesia	Increased pain sensitivity
Euphoria	Dysphoria; irritability
Sedation	Restlessness; insomnia
Constipation	Diarrhea
Respiratory depression	Hyperventilation

receptor antagonist directly into the VTA or by lesions of VTA dopaminergic neurons. Opiate activation of such neurons results from opiate inhibition of the GABAergic interneurons in the VTA that normally inhibit principal dopamine neurons **15-2**.

Opiates also produce reinforcement through direct dopamine-independent actions on μ, and perhaps δ, receptors expressed in NAc neurons. These receptors are normally targets of the enkephalinergic (and possibly endorphinergic) neurons that innervate this brain region. Animals will work to self-administer morphine directly into the NAc, even in the presence of dopamine receptor blockade or **6-hydroxydopamine**

lesions of dopaminergic terminals in this region of the brain. Within the NAc, opiates directly inhibit some of the same populations of medium spiny projection neurons that are inhibited by dopamine. Thus opioid and dopaminergic systems appear to converge on a common efferent reward pathway in the NAc **15-2**.

In contrast to μ and δ opioid receptor subtypes, κ opioid receptor activation is not reinforcing; indeed, it is aversive. Activation of κ receptors decreases dopamine release in the NAc; thus the mesolimbic dopamine system may mediate aversive effects of opiates as well as their reinforcing properties. See Chapter 11 for a discussion of the use of κ opioid

15-4   **Receptor Subtypes Implicated in Actions of Opiates**

	Receptor Subtype	Effect of Agonists	Effect of Antagonists
Analgesia	μ, δ, κ	Analgesia	No effect[1]
Respiratory function	μ	Respiratory depression	No effect[2]
Gastrointestinal tract function	μ, δ	Decreased motility	No effect
Sedation	μ, κ	Sedation	No effect
Reward function	μ, δ	Reinforcement	Possibly mild aversion
	κ	Aversion	Unknown

[1]Can block stress-induced analgesia.
[2]Can reverse respiratory depression caused by μ receptor agonist.

agonists (eg, **benzomorphan analgesics**) in the treatment of pain. Tonic activation of the different opioid receptors in the reward circuitry by endogenous opioid peptides may modulate responses to natural reinforcers and influence an individual's motivational state.

Ethanol

Ethanol is a CNS depressant that shares some behavioral effects with sedative–hypnotic drugs such as barbiturates and benzodiazepines (**15-5**; Chapters 5, 12, and 14). In humans it is clearly reinforcing and addictive, as evidenced by its widespread compulsive use. Ethanol reinforcement can be demonstrated in animals as well. The many serious health problems associated with long-term ethanol use, such as **gastritis**, **cirrhosis**, and **malnutrition**, most likely are related to the extremely large amounts of ethanol that are necessary for its psychoactive effects (as much as 100 mM in tolerant users), and also to the ability of this small molecule to interact with numerous physiologic systems.

Despite the high concentrations required for its psychoactive effects, ethanol exerts specific actions on the brain. The initial effects of ethanol result primarily from facilitation of GABA$_A$ receptors and inhibition of NMDA glutamate receptors. At higher doses, ethanol also inhibits the functioning of most ligand- and voltage-gated ion channels. It is not known whether ethanol selectively affects these channels via direct low affinity binding or via nonspecific disruption of plasma membranes which then selectively influences these highly complex, multimeric, transmembrane proteins.

Ethanol allosterically regulates the GABA$_A$ receptor to enhance GABA-activated Cl$^-$ flux. The anxiolytic and sedative effects of ethanol, as well as those of **barbiturates** and **benzodiazepines**, result from enhancement of GABAergic function. Facilitation of GABA$_A$ receptor function is also believed to contribute to the reinforcing effects of these drugs. Not all GABA$_A$ receptors are ethanol sensitive. As mentioned in

Chapters 5 and 14, GABA$_A$ receptor complexes comprise combinations of five distinct subunit families. The regional distribution and relative abundance of these subunit combinations vary, and thus may explain differences in the sensitivity of GABA$_A$ receptors to ethanol in different brain regions.

Ethanol also acts as an NMDA antagonist by allosterically inhibiting the passage of glutamate-activated Na$^+$ and Ca^{2+} currents through the NMDA receptor. The sensitivity of NMDA receptors to ethanol, like that of GABA$_A$ receptors, may depend on receptor subunit composition. Other NMDA antagonists, such as **phencyclidine** and **ketamine,** produce profound cognitive deficits and psychotic symptoms; thus the dissociative and psychotomimetic effects of ethanol (at higher doses) may be mediated by means of such antagonism. Because other NMDA antagonists are reinforcing, some of ethanol's addicting properties also are likely mediated by this mechanism.

The cellular mechanisms through which ethanol influences reinforcement systems is not yet known but evidence suggests the involvement of several neurotransmitter systems (see **15-2**). The reinforcing effects of ethanol are partly explained by its ability to activate mesolimbic dopamine circuitry, although it is not known whether this effect is mediated at the level of the VTA or NAc. It also is not known whether this activation of dopamine systems is caused primarily by facilitation of GABA$_A$ receptors or inhibition of NMDA receptors, or both. Ethanol reinforcement also is mediated in part by ethanol-induced release of endogenous opioid peptides within the mesolimbic dopamine system, although whether the VTA or NAc is the predominant site of such action is not yet known. Accordingly, the opioid receptor antagonist **naltrexone** reduces ethanol self-administration in animals and is used with modest effect to treat alcoholism in humans. Ethanol affects many other neurotransmitter systems in the brain, which may also contribute to its behavioral actions.

Nicotine

Nicotine is the main psychoactive ingredient of tobacco and is responsible for the stimulant effects, reinforcement, dependence, and addiction that result from tobacco use **15-6**. Cigarette smoking rapidly delivers pulses of nicotine into the bloodstream. Nicotine differs from cocaine and opiates in that it is powerfully reinforcing in the absence of subjective euphoria. The high incidence of **carcinogenicity** associated with long-term tobacco use is related to compounds other than nicotine that are either contained in tobacco or generated by its combustion.

15-5 **Acute Effects of Ethanol and Withdrawal Symptoms**

CH$_3$-CH$_2$-OH
Ethanol

Short-Term Effects	Withdrawal Symptoms
Loss of inhibition	Irritability; tremor
Anxiolysis	Anxiety
Sedation	Sleep disturbance
Decreased motor coordination	Seizures

15-6   Acute Effects of Nicotine and Withdrawal Symptoms

Nicotine

Short-Term Effects	Withdrawal Symptoms
Increased alertness	Difficulty concentrating
Mild euphoria	Dysphoria; irritability
Muscle relaxation	Restlessness; anxiety
Nausea	Increased appetite
Increased psychomotor activity	Hyperventilation

The initial effects of nicotine are caused by its activation of nicotinic acetylcholine (nACh) receptors. nACh receptors are ligand-gated cation channels (Chapters 6 and 9); in the CNS, they are located postsynaptically and also on presynaptic terminals, where they facilitate transmitter release. The reinforcing effects of nicotine, like those of other addictive drugs, depend on an intact mesolimbic dopamine system. nACh receptors located on VTA dopamine neurons are implicated in nicotine reinforcement. Systemic nicotine self-administration is disrupted when antagonists are administered directly into the VTA but not when they are administered into the NAc; moreover, nicotine is rewarding when injected directly into the VTA.

Receptors composed of $\alpha_4\beta_2$ subunits are the most important for these actions, as knockout of either receptor abolishes nicotine reward. nACh receptors on VTA dopamine neurons are normally activated by cholinergic innervation from the laterodorsal tegmental nucleus or the pedunculopontine nucleus (Chapters 6 and 12). In addition, nicotine may stimulate dopamine release in the NAc through actions on presynaptic nACh receptors located on dopamine terminals within the NAc. Nicotine self-administration also can be blocked by opioid receptor antagonists such as **naltrexone**. These findings indicate the involvement of endogenous opioid systems in the reinforcing effects of nicotine, and raise the possibility that such antagonists may be of use in the treatment of nicotine addiction.

Cannabinoids

Delta-9-tetrahydrocannabinol (THC) is one of several cannabinoid compounds contained in **marijuana,** and is primarily responsible for the psychoactive effects of cannabis preparations **15-7**. Although the addictive potential of THC has been a matter of debate, there is no question that it can be addicting, since there are many compulsive users of marijuana. Withdrawal symptoms typically do not occur with termination of long-term marijuana use, because of the persistence of accumulated THC in the tissues of long-term users. However, cannabinoid dependence can be demonstrated experimentally with the use of cannabinoid receptor antagonists, which precipitate profound withdrawal symptoms that are both physical and emotional–motivational.

15-7   Acute Effects of Cannabinoids and Withdrawal Symptoms

Delta-9-tetrahydrocannabinol   Anandamide [1]

Short-Term Effects	Withdrawal Symptoms
Euphoria	Irritability
Disinhibition	Restlessness
Cognitive deficits	Sleep disturbance
Increased hunger	Nausea
Altered sensory perception	

[1] Arachidonyl ethanolamide (for the structure of arachidonic acid, see Chapter 4).

THC exerts its primary pharmacologic effects by binding to a G protein-coupled receptor in the brain known as the CB_1 receptor—a misnomer because cannabinoids are not natural ligands for this receptor. Rather, endogenous ligands for this receptor are arachadonic acid derivatives termed *anandamide* and *2-arachidonyl glycerol (2-AG)*. THC selectively induces dopamine release in the shell of the NAc via CB_1 receptors, although the mechanism remains obscure. The best defined action of cannabinoids in NAc is induction of a unique form of long-term depression (LTD), which is mediated via activation of CB_1 receptors on glutamatergic nerve terminals leading to inhibition of glutamate release (Chapters 5 and 8). The pharmacology and psychoactive effects of cannabinoids are summarized in **15-7**. Interestingly, release of endogenous cannabinoids has been demonstrated after administration of several drugs of abuse, which has stimulated interest in the potential utility of CB_1 antagonists (eg, **rimonabant**) in the treatment of drug addiction. Such antagonists are also being considered for the treatment of **obesity** (Chapter 10).

Phencyclidine

Phencyclidine (**PCP** or **angel dust**) and **ketamine** (also known as **special K**) are structurally related drugs **15-4** that are classified as **dissociative anesthetics**. These drugs are distinguished from other psychotomimetic agents, such as hallucinogens, by their distinct spectrum of pharmacologic effects, including their reinforcing properties and risks related to compulsive abuse (Chapter 16).

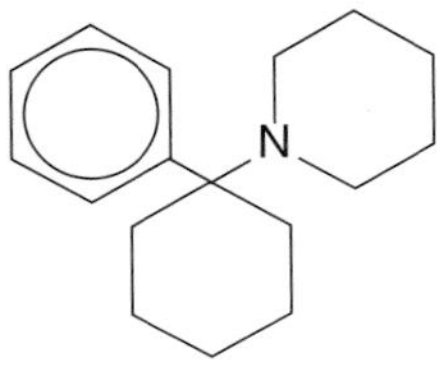

PCP

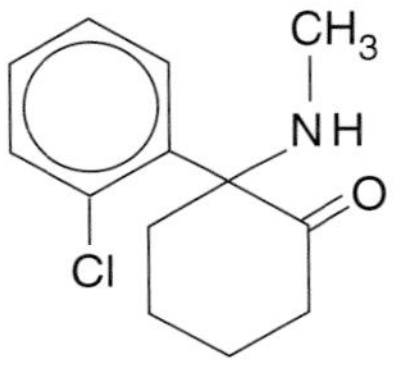

Ketamine

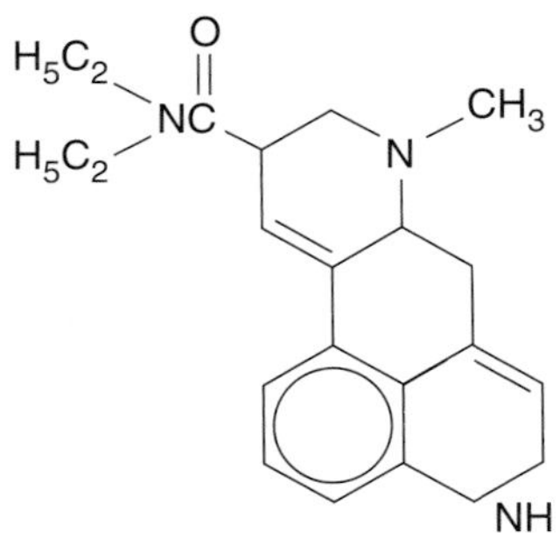

LSD

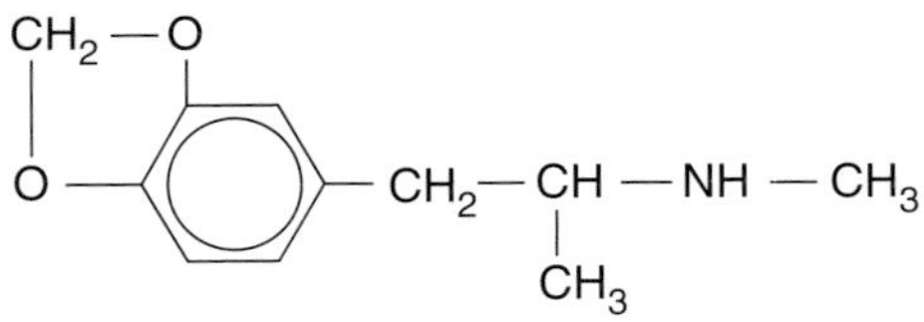

MDMA

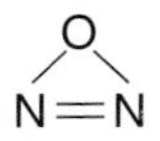

Nitrous oxide

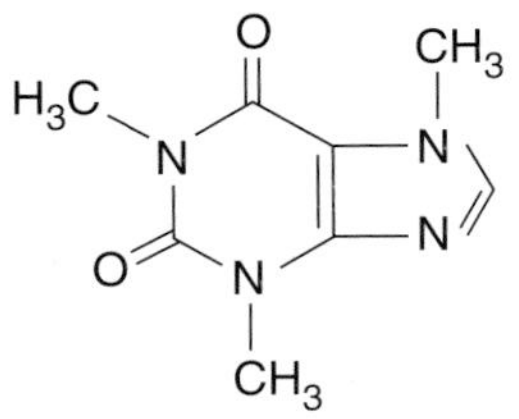

Caffeine

15-4 Chemical structures of some miscellaneous drugs that are self-administered for psychotropic effects.

The reinforcing properties of PCP and ketamine are mediated by the binding of these drugs to specific sites in the channel of the NMDA glutamate receptor, where they act as noncompetitive antagonists. PCP is self-administered directly into the NAc, where its reinforcing effects are believed to result from the blockade of excitatory glutamatergic input to the same medium spiny NAc neurons inhibited by opioids and dopamine (see 15–2).

Other Drugs of Abuse

Several other classes of drugs are categorized as drugs of abuse 15–4 but rarely produce compulsive use. These include **psychedelic** agents, such as **lysergic acid diethylamide (LSD)**, which are used for their ability to produce perceptual distortions at low and moderate doses. The use of these drugs is associated with the rapid development of tolerance and the absence of positive reinforcement (Chapter 6). Partial agonist effects at $5HT_{2A}$ receptors are implicated in the psychedelic actions of LSD and related hallucinogens.

3,4-Methylenedioxymethamphetamine (**MDMA**), commonly called **ecstasy,** is an amphetamine derivative. It produces a combination of psychostimulant-like and weak LSD-like effects at low doses. Unlike LSD, MDMA is reinforcing—most likely because of its interactions with dopamine systems—and accordingly is subject to compulsive abuse. The weak psychedelic effects of MDMA appear to result from its amphetamine-like actions on the serotonin reuptake transporter, by means of which it causes transporter-dependent serotonin efflux. MDMA has been proven to produce lesions of serotonin neurons in animals and humans.

A variety of volatile chemicals are abused as **inhalants** because of their ability to produce rapid and brief intoxication, which generally consists of some degree of euphoria and light-headedness. Abused inhalants include commercial products that are readily obtained by minors and that consist of diverse chemical classes—for example, aerosol products, formaldehydes, household solvents, adhesives, gasoline, and **nitrous oxide**. Their pharmacologic effects and toxicity vary, depending on their constituent chemicals; however, their mechanisms of action remain obscure. Compulsive use of inhalants can be severe.

Caffeine and related methylxanthines (eg, **theophylline,** and **theobromine**) stimulate the CNS, produce increased alertness, improve psychomotor performance, and decrease fatigue. Long-term caffeine use can lead to mild physical dependence. A withdrawal syndrome characterized by drowsiness, irritability, and headache typically lasts no longer than a day.

True compulsive use of caffeine has not been documented. The main mechanism responsible for the pharmacologic effects of these methylxanthines is competitive antagonism of G protein-coupled adenosine A_1 and A_{2A} receptors (Chapter 8).

Role of Reward Circuitry in "Natural Addictions"

As previously indicated, the neural circuitry activated by reinforcing brain stimulation and by addictive drugs is part of an endogenous reward mechanism that motivates individuals to pursue natural reinforcers such as food and sex. Can compulsive eating, shopping, gambling, and sex—so-called "natural addictions"—be related to abnormal regulation of endogenous reward mechanisms in certain individuals? Just as addictive drugs can powerfully activate reward pathways and consequently modify motivated behavior, it is possible that these pleasurable behaviors may excessively activate reward-reinforcement mechanisms in susceptible individuals. As with drugs, such activation may result in profound alterations in motivation that promote the repetition of initially rewarding behavior, despite the impact of negative consequences associated with the resulting compulsion. Indeed, addictions to both drugs and behavioral rewards may arise from similar dysregulation of the mesolimbic dopamine system. While speculative, such a view is supported by brain imaging studies in humans.

Dopaminergic Neurons and Reward-Dependent Learning

How does increased dopaminergic transmission in the NAc, elicited by natural reinforcers, drugs, or rewarding brain stimulation, strengthen the motivated behavior produced by these stimuli? Dopamine's precise role in reinforcement has been recently reevaluated. Instead of simply mediating subjective pleasure, dopamine may affect motivation and attention to salient stimuli, including rewarding stimuli. Several experimental findings suggest that the pleasure associated with food does not necessarily depend on dopamine; rather, it appears to be more affected by drugs that influence opioid and GABA systems. Dopaminergic lesions of the NAc and caudate nucleus, as well as dopamine receptor antagonists can alter the *motivation* to eat, but do not affect the hedonic value assigned to taste. If motivational drive is described in terms of *wanting,* and hedonic evaluation in terms of *liking,* it appears that wanting can be dissociated from liking and that dopamine may influence these phenomena differently. Differences between wanting and liking are confirmed in reports by human addicts, who state that their desire for drugs (wanting) increases with continued use even when pleasure (liking) decreases because of tolerance. Moreover, during withdrawal the desire for drugs can be more strongly associated with dysphoria than with pleasure.

The involvement of dopaminergic neurons in the regulation of attention and motivation is suggested by electrophysiologic studies of dopaminergic neurons in the midbrain of the monkey. These neurons respond robustly to reward-predicting stimuli as well as to unexpected—but not expected—rewards. Thus they appear to signal not a reward per se but salient events that warrant attention. Therefore, it is predictors of reward and *unexpected* rewarding stimuli that elicit significant responses in dopaminergic neurons of the midbrain; indeed, these neurons respond less to rewards that have become predictable based on previous experience. When predicted rewards fail to occur, dopaminergic neurons signal this deviation from expected events by a decrease in activity at the time the reward was predicted to have occurred. Based on such findings, it appears that these neurons can signal positive and negative outcomes in relation to predicted rewards. It has been suggested that the dopamine signal may constitute a mechanism of learning relevant to rewards. Dopaminergic innervation of the prefrontal cortex has been strongly associated with regulation of executive functions such as working memory (Chapter 13), a finding that further demonstrates the potent effects of dopamine—and of drugs that affect dopaminergic transmission—on attention and planning.

Extended Reward Circuitry

Dopaminergic neurons of the midbrain are believed to function in reward and reinforcement as part of a neural circuit at the interface between limbic emotional–motivational information and extrapyramidal regulation of motor behavior. The major components of this circuit and the critical substrates for drug reward are represented in **15-1**. A macrostructure postulated to integrate many of the functions of this circuit is described by some investigators as the *extended amygdala*. The extended amygdala is said to comprise several basal forebrain structures that share similar morphology, immunocytochemical features, and connectivity and that are well suited to mediating aspects of reward function; these include the *bed nucleus of the stria terminalis*, the *central medial amygdala*, the shell of the NAc, and the *sublenticular substantia innominata*.

The NAc and VTA are central components of the circuitry underlying reward and memory of reward. As

previously mentioned, the activity of dopaminergic neurons in the VTA appears to be linked to reward prediction. The NAc is involved in learning associated with reinforcement and the modulation of motoric responses to stimuli that satisfy internal homeostatic needs. The shell of the NAc appears to be particularly important to initial drug actions within reward circuitry; addictive drugs appear to have a greater effect on dopamine release in the shell than in the core of the NAc.

As mentioned earlier, the GABAergic medium spiny neurons of the NAc are believed to be a critical component of the postulated limbic–extrapyramidal interface involved in reward and reinforcement. As they do in the dorsal striatum (Chapter 13), these neurons integrate glutamatergic inputs from the cerebral cortex with dopamine inputs from the midbrain. In contrast to activity in the dorsal striatum, however, cortical inputs to the NAc arise from frontal association cortex (rather than from motor cortex and other areas) and dopamine inputs originate in the VTA (rather than in the substantia nigra). In both the NAc and dorsal striatum, the interactions between dopamine and glutamate may underlie learning and presumably involve plasticity at synapses formed between cortical pyramidal neurons and neurons of the NAc and dorsal striatum. The actions of addictive drugs in these circuits may underlie the acquisition of learned drug-seeking behaviors, in accord with dopamine's postulated involvement in the prediction of reward in animals.

Of the two main subtypes of GABAergic medium spiny neurons in the NAc (Chapter 17), the type that forms the striatopallidal pathway may be most strongly linked to reward-related behaviors. These neurons, which coexpress enkephalin and, to some extent, D_2 receptors, project from the NAc to the ventral pallidum. This pathway appears to be activated by rewarding stimulation of the VTA, and lesions of this pathway reduce cocaine and opiate reinforcement. Activation of the pathway also powerfully stimulates cocaine-seeking behavior, as described later in this chapter. However, it is important to emphasize that the other major subpopulation of GABAergic medium spiny neurons is also important in the regulation of reinforcement and motivation. These neurons project directly to the VTA and coexpress dynorphin, substance P, and predominantly D_1 receptors. A major goal of current research is to more clearly define the role of these two major cell types in reward behavior.

The amygdala regulates an individual's orientation to and memory of emotionally salient stimuli. Projections between the NAc and the amygdala are believed to be important to the formation of stimulus–reward associations. Neurons in the amygdala fire in response to food-related stimuli. Lesions of the amygdala disrupt the ability of experimental animals to remember the pairing of a stimulus with a reward (without disrupting recognition of the stimulus) and can lessen the response to a conditioned reinforcer previously paired with a natural reward. The central nucleus of the amygdala also has been implicated in aversive aspects of drug withdrawal, as described in a subsequent section of this chapter, and is associated with fear, as discussed in Chapter 14.

In addition to the amygdala, other memory circuits in the brain are affected by drugs of abuse. The *hippocampus* is likely involved in mediating the powerful associations between drug use and environmental cues. Regions of *prefrontal cortex*, as mentioned earlier, are critical for executive function. Such cortical regions provide control over impulses for destructive behavior, and their impairment, demonstrated in animals and humans after chronic drug exposure, appears to be an important mediator of the loss of control over drug intake which is central to addiction.

Finally, several peptide systems of the hypothalamus (eg, melanocortins, orexins, melanin-concentrating hormone) have been implicated recently in the actions of drugs of abuse on the brain. These systems, which normally function as an interplay between wanting and physiologically needing food (Chapter 10), may be corrupted by drugs of abuse and contribute to addictive syndromes.

MOLECULAR AND CELLULAR MECHANISMS OF ADDICTION

The loss of control over drug use that characterizes addiction develops progressively as a consequence of time-dependent, drug-induced processes in the brain, which eventually usurp normal volitional control of motivated behavior. Tolerance, dependence, and sensitization are time-dependent adaptive processes induced in neurons as a result of repeated drug exposure; when induced by drugs within reinforcement systems, such processes become critical components of addiction. These adaptations can be viewed as examples of drug-induced neural plasticity and may consist of experience-dependent changes in several molecular and cellular processes, including the regulation of receptors, ion channels, intracellular signaling proteins, and gene expression. Multiple neural circuits may undergo adaptive changes in response to a single drug; the functional consequences of the changes in each circuit are related to (1) the nature of the adaptations, and

(2) the normal function of the neurons that undergo adaptations.

A current challenge in addiction research is to determine how each adaptation contributes to long-term aspects of the addictive process, and to ascertain the cellular and molecular actions of drugs that lead to such adaptations. The sections that follow summarize some of the adaptive processes induced in neurons by long-term drug administration, many of which may underlie the alterations in reinforcement systems that cause addiction.

Adaptations Implicated in Emotional–Motivational Tolerance and Dependence

An emotional and motivational component of drug tolerance and dependence is indicated by escalation of drug intake (tolerance) and by withdrawal symptoms such as anhedonia, depression, anxiety, and negative motivational states (dependence). The fact that these symptoms can be characterized as antithetical to the initial effects of addictive drugs suggests that they may result from counteradaptations to prolonged drug exposure. Moreover, just as the reinforcing effects of addictive drugs are believed to be related to actions on brain reward circuitry, emotional and motivational aspects of tolerance and dependence associated with the long-term use of these drugs may be related to drug-induced adaptations in the same circuitry.

Indeed, work over the past decade has established that the VTA and NAc are implicated not only in the immediate reinforcing effects of addictive drugs but also in the emotional and motivational aspects of tolerance and dependence induced by long-term exposure to these drugs. Reduced VTA activity and enhanced NAc activity are associated with reduced sensitivity of an individual to the rewarding effects of the drugs and with the dysphoria associated with drug withdrawal. Thus these regions of the brain may be sites for common drug-induced adaptations related to the time-dependent changes in drug reinforcement that underlie emotional–motivational tolerance and dependence.

Up-regulation of the cAMP pathway   One of the best established molecular mechanisms of drug tolerance and dependence is up-regulation of the cAMP signaling pathway, which was first demonstrated for **opiates**. According to this scheme, depicted in **15–5**, opiates, via the activation of opioid receptors and their coupling to $G_{i/o}$, acutely inhibit the cAMP pathway. In the face of continued opiate exposure, many cells adapt

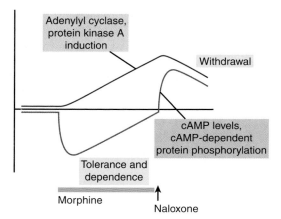

15-5 **Up-regulation of the cAMP pathway as a mechanism of opiate tolerance and dependence.** Opiates acutely inhibit the functional activity of the cAMP pathway (eg, as indicated by cellular levels of cAMP or cAMP-dependent protein phosphorylation). With continued opiate exposure, functional activity of the cAMP pathway gradually recovers and increases far above control levels upon removal of the opiate (eg, by administration of the opioid receptor antagonist, naloxone). These changes in the functional state of the cAMP pathway are mediated via the induction of adenylyl cyclase and protein kinase A (PKA) in response to chronic opiate administration. Induction of these enzymes accounts for the gradual recovery in the functional activity of the cAMP pathway seen during chronic opiate exposure (tolerance and dependence) and for the activation of the cAMP pathway seen upon removal of the opiate (withdrawal). (From Nestler EJ. Historical review: Molecular and cellular mechanisms of opiate and cocaine addiction. *Trends Pharmacol Sci.* 2004;25:210–218.)

to this inhibition by up-regulating levels of adenylyl cyclase (the enzyme that catalyzes the synthesis of cAMP) and of protein kinase A (the major effector for cAMP) (Chapter 4). Up-regulation of these enzymes compensates for opiate inhibition of the cAMP pathway and restores activity of the pathway to normal levels. This can be viewed as tolerance. When the opiate is removed, the up-regulated cAMP pathway is unopposed and causes abnormally high cAMP actions. This can be viewed as dependence and withdrawal. Such up-regulation of the cAMP pathway has been demonstrated in numerous regions of the central and peripheral nervous systems, where it has been shown to mediate diverse aspects of opiate tolerance and dependence, depending on the function subserved by these regions. For example, in the VTA and NAc, cAMP

pathway up-regulation mediates tolerance and dependence to the rewarding effects of opiates, while in the locus ceruleus (LC), a brainstem noradrenergic nucleus, cAMP pathway up-regulation causes physical dependence and withdrawal. Research over the past decade has provided detailed information concerning the molecular mechanisms by which opiates up-regulate the cAMP pathway in the LC, mechanisms which appear to also operate in other brain regions **15-1**.

Interestingly, up-regulation of the cAMP pathway in the NAc is a common adaptation to long-term exposure to several types of addictive drugs, including **opiates, cocaine, amphetamine** and **ethanol**, but it is not a feature associated with the use of nonaddictive drugs. Experimental activation of the cAMP pathway reduces the sensitivity of an animal to the rewarding effects of each of these drugs, consistent with the hypothesis that this adaptation represents a mechanism of emotional–motivational tolerance and dependence. This supports the existence of a set of common or shared molecular mechanisms of drug addiction mediated via the VTA-NAc circuit **15-6**.

Regulation of CREB The involvement of CREB in emotional and motivational aspects of dependence might be expected based on our knowledge of drug-induced up-regulation of the cAMP pathway in the NAc. Long-term opiate or psychostimulant treatment increases CREB function in the NAc, and this adaptation, like up-regulation of the cAMP pathway, functions as a mechanism of emotional-motivational tolerance and dependence and a mediator of aversive emotional symptoms during drug withdrawal. Consistent with this view are the recent findings that CREB increases the excitability of NAc neurons, which has been related directly to reduced drug sensitivity. One gene through which CREB produces this effect is that encoding pro-dynorphin. Dynorphin normally acts to decrease dopamine release in the NAc through an action on κ opioid receptors located on presynaptic dopaminergic nerve terminals in this region. This finding raises the possibility, supported by animal research, that **κ opioid antagonists** may be useful in the treatment of drug withdrawal states. A major goal of current research is to identify other CREB-regulated genes and define their influence on drug tolerance and dependence.

Regulation of GABAergic and glutamatergic transmission Changes in ion channel function and altered expression of $GABA_A$ and NMDA receptor subunits are the adaptations most often cited in connection with behavioral consequences of long-term **ethanol** exposure. Long-term use of ethanol decreases benzodiazepine- and ethanol-induced enhancement

15–1 **Molecular Mechanisms of Opiate Dependence: Studies of the Locus Ceruleus**

The locus ceruleus (LC), located in the dorsal pons, is the major noradrenergic nucleus of the brain and is important for the regulation of attentional states and autonomic nervous system activity (Chapters 6, 9, and 13). The LC also has been implicated in the autonomic and stress-like effects of opiate withdrawal. The activity of LC neurons is inhibited by opiates, but continued exposure to these drugs results in tolerance and dependence: depressed firing rates gradually return to normal and the administration of an opioid receptor antagonist causes a dramatic increase in firing rates above normal levels. The excitation of LC neurons during opiate withdrawal is necessary and sufficient to produce many of the signs and symptoms of physical withdrawal.

Up-regulation of the cAMP signaling pathway in LC neurons contributes to these opiate-induced changes in excitability (see figure). On acute exposure, opiates inhibit LC neurons primarily by increasing the conductance of an inwardly rectifying K^+ channel via direct coupling with $G_{i/o}$, and also by decreasing a Na^+-dependent inward current via coupling with $G_{i/o}$ and the consequent inhibition of adenylyl cyclase. Reduced levels of cAMP decrease protein kinase A (PKA) activity and the phosphorylation of the responsible channel or pump, which has not yet been identified. Inhibition of the cAMP pathway also decreases the phosphorylation of numerous other proteins and thereby affects many additional processes in the neuron.

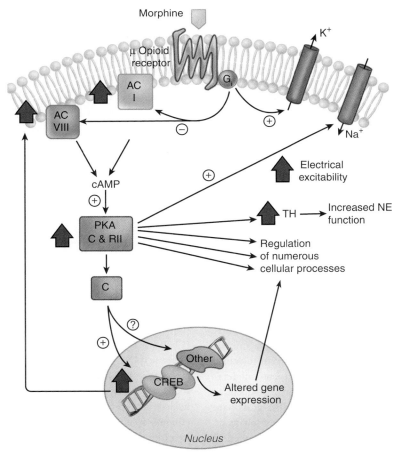

(Figure adapted with permission from Nestler EJ, Aghajanian EK. Molecular and cellular basis of addiction. *Science.* 1997;278:58.)

For example, it reduces the phosphorylation state of the transcription factor, CREB, which may initiate some of the longer-term changes in LC function. It also reduces the phosphorylation and activity of tyrosine hydroxylase (TH), the rate-limiting enzyme in norepinephrine synthesis. Upward bold arrows summarize the effects of prolonged exposure to morphine in the LC. Such long-term exposure increases levels of types I and VIII adenylyl cyclase, PKA catalytic (C) and regulatory type II (RII) subunits, and several phosphoproteins, including CREB and TH. These changes contribute to the altered phenotype of the drug-addicted state. For example, the intrinsic excitability of LC neurons is increased by enhanced activity of the cAMP pathway and Na^+-dependent inward current, which contribute to the tolerance, dependence, and withdrawal exhibited by these neurons. Up-regulation of type VIII adenylyl cyclase and of TH is mediated by CREB, whereas up-regulation of type I adenylyl cyclase and of the PKA subunits appears to occur through CREB-independent mechanisms.

of $GABA_A$-mediated responses; such findings suggest that ethanol produces a change in the $GABA_A$ receptor. The nature of this change has remained elusive, despite intensive investigation. It has been hypothesized that long-term ethanol exposure alters the expression or activity of specific $GABA_A$ receptor subunits in discrete brain regions. Regardless of the underlying mechanism, ethanol-induced decreases in $GABA_A$ receptor sensitivity are believed to contribute to ethanol tolerance, and also may mediate some aspects of physical dependence on ethanol. However, whether these changes contribute to aversive symptoms that occur during ethanol withdrawal remains unknown.

The NMDA receptor complex also undergoes adaptive changes in response to long-term ethanol exposure which appear to contribute significantly to physical dependence. Long-term use of ethanol has been reported to increase the number of binding sites for NMDA receptor ligands and also the magnitude of NMDA-mediated Ca^{2+} fluxes in certain brain regions. Increases in protein and mRNA for specific NMDA receptor subunits may mediate some of these ethanol-induced changes. Increased NMDA receptor function parallels the time course for seizure susceptibility in animals during ethanol withdrawal; this phenomenon may also explain the reduction in withdrawal signs that occurs after the administration of NMDA antagonists.

Beyond ethanol, the development of opiate tolerance and dependence has been reported to depend on glutamatergic transmission. Coadministration of competitive or noncompetitive **antagonists of NMDA glutamate receptors** can block both tolerance to the analgesic effects of opiates and the development of physical dependence on **opiates**; moreover, by implication they are proposed to block emotional–motivational dependence as well. The effects of NMDA antagonists on opiate tolerance may involve nitric oxide because the inhibition of nitric oxide production—for example, by pharmacologic inhibition of nitric oxide synthase (Chapter 4)—blocks the development of tolerance. Interactions between NMDA antagonists and opiates most likely are quite complex, and the coadministration of these agents may lead to complications. Thus, NMDA antagonists themselves are addictive and, like other addictive drugs, have powerful stimulant and reinforcing effects of their own. Consequently, long-term coadministration of an NMDA antagonist with an opiate may potentiate the addictiveness of both drugs, regardless of effects on tolerance and dependence per se. Functional interactions between dopaminergic and glutamatergic transmission in striatal and cortical regions of the brain have received a great deal of attention, and related findings should help to explain how NMDA antagonists modify responses to opiates and other addictive drugs. (See Mechanisms of Sensitization in this chapter for further discussion of the glutamate system in mechanisms of addiction.)

Drug regulation of CRF Drug regulation of corticotropin-releasing factor (CRF) is a neuropeptide that is expressed in neurons of the hypothalamus, central nucleus of the amygdala, and other brain regions (Chapter 7). It plays an important role in stress responses and has been implicated in anxiety states (Chapters 10 and 14). Moreover, recent studies have implicated CRF systems in the mediation of many of the anxiogenic and aversive aspects of drug withdrawal. Increased release of CRF, particularly in the central nucleus of the amygdala, occurs during withdrawal from **ethanol**, **opiates**, **cocaine**, **nicotine**, and **cannabinoids**. Accordingly, CRF antagonists have successfully reversed the aversive effects of cocaine, ethanol, and opiate withdrawal in laboratory animals, a finding that has led to the current evaluation of these compounds as agents for use in the treatment of drug withdrawal states.

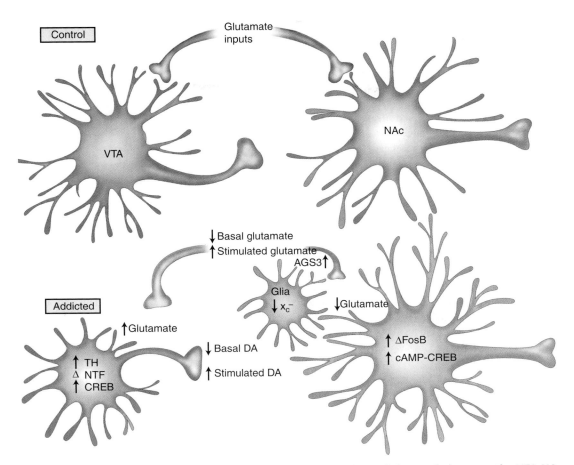

15–6 **Highly simplified scheme of some common, chronic actions of drugs of abuse on the VTA-NAc circuit**. The top panel (Control) shows a VTA neuron innervating an NAc neuron, and glutamatergic inputs to the VTA and NAc neurons, under normal conditions. After chronic drug administration, several adaptations occur. In the VTA, drug exposure induces tyrosine hydroxylase (TH) and increases AMPA glutamatergic responses (Glut), possibly via induction of GluR1 and altered trafficking of AMPA receptors. As well, VTA dopamine neurons decrease in size. In the NAc, all drugs of abuse induce the transcription factor ΔFosB, which may then mediate some of the shared aspects of addiction via regulation of numerous target genes. Several, but not all, drugs of abuse also induce CREB activity in this region, which may be mediated via up-regulation of the cAMP pathway. Several additional changes have been found for stimulant exposure. Stimulants decrease AMPA glutamatergic responses in NAc neurons, possibly mediated via induction of GluR2 or repression of several postsynaptic density proteins (eg, PSD95, Homer-1). These changes in postsynaptic glutamate responses are associated with complex changes in glutamatergic innervation of the NAc, including reduced glutamatergic transmission at baseline and in response to normal rewards, but enhanced transmission in response to cocaine and associated cues, effects mediated in part via up-regulation of AGS3 (activator of G protein signaling) in cortical neurons and down-regulation of the cystine-glutamate transporter (system x_c^-) in glia. Stimulants and nicotine also induce dendritic outgrowth of NAc neurons, although opiates are reported to produce the opposite action. The net effect of this complex dysregulation in glutamate function and synaptic structure is not yet known.

Regulation of receptor signaling One mechanism of opiate tolerance that has received a great deal of attention is the functional uncoupling of opioid receptors from their G proteins. Such uncoupling may involve phosphorylation-mediated changes in affinities of the receptors or in their G proteins that may decrease their functional interaction. Such phosphorylation may be mediated by cAMP- or Ca^{2+}-dependent protein kinases or by G protein receptor kinases (GRKs), all of which are known to be regulated by opiate exposure. As explained in Chapter 4, GRKs phosphorylate agonist-bound forms of G protein-coupled receptors, including opioid receptors, and can contribute to receptor internalization and desensitization. The efficacy of opioid receptor transduction also might be reduced by drug-induced alterations in levels of relevant G proteins. Long-term exposure to certain drugs of abuse decreases the expression of $G_{\alpha i}$ and $G_{\alpha o}$ subunits in specific brain regions, including the VTA and NAc. The $G_{i/o}$ family of G proteins represents the primary coupling mechanisms for opioid, D_2-like dopamine, and CB_1 receptors and may represent an important common substrate for drug-induced alterations in signal transduction in these receptor systems. Indeed, tolerance to D_2 receptor stimulation has been related to escalating drug intake in animals, and similar down-regulation of D_2 receptors in the NAc has been reported in human addicts.

Tolerance also may be mediated by a host of other proteins that modulate receptor–G protein interactions. RGS proteins (regulators of G protein signaling), for example, control the functioning of G protein α subunits by regulating the GTPase activity intrinsic to such subunits (Chapter 4). **Opiate**-induced increases in levels of these proteins in specific brain regions might be expected to contribute to a state of tolerance. Such mechanisms are currently undergoing investigation.

Tolerance to **nicotine** is believed to involve yet another receptor-mediated mechanism. Long-term exposure to nicotine increases the number of nACh receptors in most brain regions. This change most likely reflects the stabilization of receptor subunits because no related change in mRNA expression has been detected. Despite this increase in receptor number, most studies indicate that exposure to nicotine decreases the functional responsiveness of the receptors. Thus it appears that tolerance is related to a desensitization of nACh receptors caused by the persistent presence of nicotine (Chapter 9).

Regulation of VTA neuronal morphology Long-term exposure to **opiates** decreases the size of VTA dopamine neurons. No effect is seen on GABA VTA neurons nor on dopamine neurons in the nearby substantia nigra. Recent research has demonstrated that this effect of opiates is mediated by down-regulation of a growth factor–controlled signal transduction pathway. Specifically, chronic opiate exposure decreases activity of the IRS-PI3K (phosphatidylinositol-3-kinase)-Akt cascade (Chapter 4), which has been shown to be a potent regulator of neuronal size in several systems. This

decreased size of VTA dopamine neurons has been related directly to decreased sensitivity to the rewarding effects of opiate drugs and therefore appears to represent a mechanism of drug tolerance. Infusion of BDNF directly into the VTA prevents this reduction in VTA neuronal size and sensitizes animals to the rewarding effects of drugs of abuse. These findings have suggested novel avenues toward the development of new treatments for drug addiction.

Drug Craving and Relapse of Addiction

Drug-taking behavior associated with addiction is sustained by (1) the reinforcement produced by drug exposure, and (2) the motivation to alleviate withdrawal-related distress. However, symptoms of both physical and emotional–motivational dependence subside relatively rapidly after drug use is terminated and may not account for the high incidence of relapse among users of addictive drugs, particularly after signs of withdrawal have long subsided. Drug craving, which can be defined as the desire to reexperience the effects of a psychoactive substance, has been hypothesized to motivate drug seeking during the development of addiction, and also to trigger relapse in response to stress or conditioned stimuli even after years of abstinence. Accordingly, it has been hypothesized that withdrawal-related distress may reflect the presence of homeostatic adaptations in mesolimbic reward circuits that reverse over weeks or months, whereas late relapse may reflect relatively permanent synaptic remodeling in the same regions of the brain or in different regions. This hypothesis is discussed in greater detail in the section that follows.

These longer-term features of drug addiction can be quantified in relapse models, where animals show reinstatement of previously learned drug-seeking behaviors after a period of abstinence. In animals, as in humans, exposure to a drug of abuse, to stimuli associated with that drug, or to stress can potently reactivate drug-seeking behavior. Such animal models have enabled the identification of some neurobiologic mechanisms underlying relapse, some of which are depicted in **15–7**. Not surprisingly, several drugs of abuse induce relapse by activating the mesolimbic dopamine system, an effect mediated primarily via the activation of D_2 dopamine receptors, a finding that supports the close relationship between mechanisms relevant to relapse and those related to drug reinforcement.

Stimulation of drug-seeking behavior by drug-associated stimuli and stress is believed to be mediated by dopamine-dependent and dopamine-independent

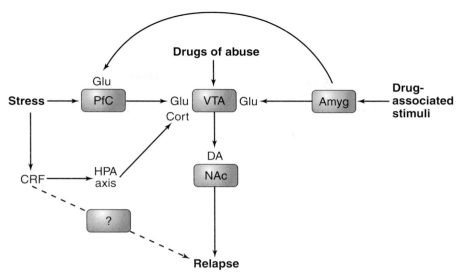

15-7 **Primary pathways through which stress, drugs of abuse, and drug-associated stimuli are hypothe-sized to trigger relapse of drug-seeking behavior.** Stress and drug-associated stimuli activate excitatory gluta-mate (Glu) projections to the VTA from the prefrontal cortex (PfC) and amygdala (Amyg), respectively. Drugs of abuse stimulate dopamine (DA) release from dopaminergic neurons of the VTA that project to the nucleus accum-bens (NAc). Projections from the amygdala to the prefrontal cortex represent a secondary pathway through which drug-associated stimuli may access dopaminergic neurons of the VTA. Stress-induced relapse may involve corticotropin-releasing factor (CRF) and the hypothalamic–pituitary–adrenal (HPA) axis, and subsequently, the acti-vation of VTA dopaminergic neurons by means of cortisol (Cort) secretion. Although dopamine release in the NAc may be the common neurochemical event by which all three stimuli trigger relapse, stress and CRF also may act on unknown brain regions by means of dopamine-independent mechanisms to cause a return to drug-seeking behavior. (From Self DW, Nestler EJ. Relapse to drug seeking: Neural and molecular mechanisms. *Drug Alcohol Depend.* 1998;51:49.)

mechanisms. The mechanisms that depend on dopamine are becoming increasingly well understood (see **15-7**). Drug-associated stimuli are believed to activate circuits of the amygdala, which are implicated in memories of emotionally salient events. The amyg-dala, in turn, is believed to activate dopaminergic neu-rons of the VTA directly, by means of glutamatergic or CRF inputs and, indirectly, through the prefrontal cor-tex. Stress is believed to activate the mesolimbic dopamine system through effects on the prefrontal cor-tex, amygdala, and hypothalamic–pituitary–adrenal (HPA) axis (Chapter 10). The effect of stress-induced activation of the HPA axis may be mediated by CRF or by increased levels of circulating glucocorticoids.

Although mechanisms of sensitization have been most closely associated with mechanisms of relapse, we still have a relatively rudimentary understanding of the molecular and cellular changes in the VTA-NAc and of other parts of the reward circuitry that mediate relapse to drugs, drug-associated cues, and stress. This remains one of the most important areas of drug abuse research.

Sensitization of Neural Processes May Underlie Drug Craving

Drug craving can intensify with repeated drug use and can persist during prolonged periods of drug absti-nence. Unlike the homeostatic types of adaptations that are believed to underlie tolerance and dependence, the intensification of drug craving is hypothesized to involve adaptations that augment rather than counter-act drug reinforcement. It is proposed that sensitization of neural processes related to drug craving, or to envi-ronmental stimuli associated with drugs (known as cues), leads to the progressive increase in drug-seeking behavior that characterizes addiction. Such sensitization appears to increase the attractiveness of drug taking and that of drug-associated stimuli.

Sensitization of some drug-responsive systems has been demonstrated in rodents after repeated exposure to addictive drugs and drug-associated stimuli. Well-characterized behavioral sensitization, involving an increase in locomotor activity and the development of stereotyped movements, has been observed after repeated intermittent administration of virtually all drugs of abuse. Moreover, cross-sensitization to many of these agents occurs and is consistent with the involvement of common neurobiologic mechanisms (see 15-6).

Because the precise molecular and cellular mechanisms underlying drug-seeking behavior are unknown, it is difficult to demonstrate the extent to which sensitization contributes to an increase in this behavior. However, the desire for a drug is clearly different from the initial rewarding aspect of drug action; indeed, addiction continues in many cases after drugs have lost some of their associated euphoria as a result of tolerance or illness (eg, alcoholic gastritis, lung cancer, AIDS).

Mechanisms of Sensitization

The reinforcing effects of addictive drugs are subject to sensitization. Repeated systemic or intra-VTA administration of psychostimulants, opiates, or ethanol, among others, causes a progressive enhancement of their reinforcing actions. Sensitization resulting from such administration requires persistent activation of the mesolimbic dopamine system. Because activation of this system is implicated in initial drug reinforcement, the sensitization observed with repeated drug administration might be mediated by changes in the mesolimbic dopamine system that enhance its responsiveness to subsequent drug exposure.

Adaptations in the VTA   Effects of drugs on the VTA are essential for the *induction* of behavioral sensitization. **Morphine** or **amphetamine** injected locally into the VTA can enhance drug-induced behavioral responses, and intra-VTA injections of dopamine antagonists can block the ability of systemic amphetamine to produce sensitization. In contrast, drugs injected locally into the NAc are ineffective in producing sensitization of behavioral responses. Induction of behavioral sensitization in the VTA may involve D_2 autoreceptor subsensitivity. The receptors themselves do not appear to be down-regulated, but levels of G proteins that transduce the D_2 signal ($G_{\alpha i}$ and $G_{\alpha o}$ subunits) are decreased transiently in the VTA after long-term drug treatment. Experimental inactivation of these G proteins with **pertussis toxin** (Chapter 4) can cause behavioral sensitization to subsequently administered cocaine.

Drug treatment also produces adaptations in the VTA's glutamate system that may be relevant to the sensitization of drug responses. Short- or long-term administration of any of several drugs of abuse induces a long-term potentiation (LTP)-like effect at excitatory synapses on VTA dopamine neurons by increasing AMPA glutamate responses. This may be mediated initially by increased trafficking of AMPA receptor subunits to the synapse and, in more chronic situations, by induction of subunit expression. Experimental overexpression of AMPA receptor subunits in VTA neurons has been shown to sensitize animals to locomotor-activating and reinforcing effects of drugs of abuse, which further suggests that changes in VTA AMPA receptors contribute to sensitization.

Dopaminergic and glutamatergic adaptations in the NAc and frontal cortex   Enhanced drug-induced dopamine levels in the NAc, a measure of enhanced mesolimbic dopamine activity, can persist for weeks in association with behavioral sensitization after long-term **psychostimulant** or **opiate** treatment. The molecular mechanism that underlies such facilitation of dopamine release is unknown but may be related to the adaptations in dopaminergic cell bodies (eg, up-regulation of AMPA receptor function) outlined in this chapter.

Sensitization to psychostimulants is associated with an LTD-like effect at excitatory synapses in the NAc. This effect is manifested by reduced responses to AMPA glutamate receptor stimulation. The LTD-like actions of psychostimulants may be mediated by increased trafficking of AMPA receptor subunits away from the synaptic membrane as well as by altered expression of particular AMPA subunits. Psychostimulant sensitization is also associated with reductions in the activity of voltage-gated Na^+ and Ca^{2+} channels, which may be caused by altered expression or phosphorylation of channel subunits. These findings underscore the association between reinforcement and reduced excitability of NAc medium spiny neurons, and indicate that long-term reductions in such excitability may contribute to sensitization.

Recent research has also begun to identify molecular alterations in glutamatergic neurons in frontal cortex as important mechanisms of drug sensitization. Some of these changes are depicted in 15-6 and suggest fundamentally new strategies for treatment development of addictive disorders.

Induction of ΔFosB in the NAc   In contrast to all other members of the Fos family of transcription factors, which are induced rapidly and transiently in response to various perturbations, ΔFosB is induced only slightly by initial stimuli. However, with repeated stimulation, ΔFosB accumulates in neurons because of its unusual stability (see 4-27 in Chapter 4). This phenomenon occurs within the NAc and certain other brain areas with many classes of addictive drugs, including **cocaine, amphetamines, opiates, nicotine,**

ethanol, **cannabinoids**, and **PCP**. Recent studies involving the selective expression of ΔFosB in the NAc of adult mice has provided direct evidence that induction of ΔFosB in this region causes sensitized behavioral responses to drugs of abuse. This is yet another example of common adaptations to drugs of abuse which contribute to shared aspects of addiction (see **15–6**).

Work is now underway to identify the target genes through which ΔFosB mediates sensitization. One apparent target is the AMPA glutamate receptor subunit GluR2; its induction could partly mediate the LTD-like responses induced by drugs in the NAc, since GluR2-containing AMPA receptors carry less current than AMPA receptors without these subunits (Chapter 5). Another target is Cdk5 (cyclin-dependent kinase-5), whose induction may contribute to the sprouting of dendritic spines on NAc neurons, as will be discussed in the next section. Many additional targets for ΔFosB have been identified. Importantly, research has suggested that >25% of all of the genes regulated by long-term cocaine use in the NAc may be mediated via induction of ΔFosB. An interesting question raised by these studies is whether antagonists of ΔFosB might be useful in the treatment of addictive disorders.

Induction of dendritic spines on NAc neurons
Chronic exposure to certain drugs of abuse has been shown to cause long-lasting increases in the length and degree of branching of dendrites, and in the density of dendritic spines, in neurons of the NAc and prefrontal cortex. These morphological changes have been documented for several stimulant drugs of abuse, including **cocaine**, **amphetamine**, and **nicotine**, and are proposed to underlie the sensitized behavioral responses to drugs and their associated cues. Moreover, there is early evidence that induction of ΔFosB, via its induction of Cdk5 and other target genes, is partly responsible for these morphological changes. It is surprising, however, that **morphine** causes the opposite changes in the morphology of NAc neurons, despite the fact that it too causes ΔFosB induction and behavioral sensitization. The induction of dendritic spines by stimulants also has not been reconciled with the LTD-like effects of these drugs in the NAc. Thus, further work is needed to better understand the molecular basis of these morphological changes in NAc and prefrontal cortical neurons and to understand their functional consequences.

TREATMENT OF ADDICTION

The primary goals of addiction treatment are the facilitation of abstinence and the prevention of relapse. Such goals have proven difficult to attain in the treatment of many forms of addiction; indeed, maintenance on long-acting **opiates** has been accepted as an alternative to abstinence for many opiate-addicted individuals. Pharmacologic treatment often is used to reduce withdrawal symptoms, but thus far has not been effective in preventing relapse. The potential for relapse lasts longer than withdrawal symptoms and involves complex mechanisms that include associative learning. Yet it remains a theoretical possibility that medications that block the reinforcing effects of drugs or drug-induced plasticity might reduce drug craving and the likelihood of relapse **15–7**. Such medications might prove to be effective if they can act without producing potent reinforcing or anhedonic effects by themselves, and if they can exert their beneficial effects without interfering with the body's responsiveness to natural rewards. Unfortunately, with the exception of **naltrexone**, which is only partly efficacious in the treatment of alcoholism, no reward-reducing drug treatment (eg, agonists or antagonists of κ opioid receptors, CB_1 receptors, CRF_1 receptors) has yet been established for clinical use.

Psychostimulants

Pharmacologic treatment for psychostimulant addiction is generally unsatisfactory. As previously discussed, cessation of cocaine use and the use of other psychostimulants in dependent individuals does not produce a physical withdrawal syndrome but may produce dysphoria, anhedonia, and an intense desire to reinitiate drug use. In rodents, withdrawal from these drugs is characterized by a greater threshold for brain stimulation reward, which may represent a model of anhedonia. It has been hypothesized that these symptoms result from the decreased responsiveness of the mesolimbic dopamine system that is characteristic of withdrawal from psychostimulants; accordingly it has been postulated that dopamine agonists might ameliorate such symptoms and that these agents might be clinically useful as long as they are not themselves highly reinforcing.

Unfortunately, dopamine D_2 agonists such as **bromocriptine** and the weak dopamine indirect agonist **amantadine** have been unimpressive clinically. Dopamine D_1 agonists, which have shown some promise in animal models, have not yet been adequately tested in clinical trials.

Several classes of **antidepressant** medications (Chapter 14) have been used to ameliorate dysphoric mood and other depression-like symptoms but have not proven to be especially effective. Likewise, several other serotonin-based drugs, including $5HT_{1A}$ or

$5HT_{2A/2C}$ agonists, or $5HT_3$ antagonists, have proven to be ineffective as well.

Attempts have been made to immunize animals to cocaine, and thereby decrease the bioavailability of subsequently administered drug. Such **immunotherapy** remains controversial for drugs such as cocaine that already have an extremely short half-life; it also would be selective for one type of drug, such as cocaine, and would not work for a replacement drug such as amphetamine. A related approach is to develop a medication that binds to the cocaine-binding site on the dopamine transporter and thereby blocks the binding of cocaine, without affecting transporter function. Currently, **cognitive–behavioral therapies** are the most successful treatment available for preventing the relapse of psychostimulant use.

Opiates

Treatment of opiate addiction is twofold. The first and most straightforward step involves the detoxification of an addicted patient, which is undertaken with an effort to minimize physical withdrawal symptoms. The second, and far more difficult, step involves the treatment of emotional–motivational symptoms of withdrawal and efforts that enable the patient to maintain abstinence. One type of detoxification involves the substitution of a safer drug. For example, a long-acting opiate agonist, such as **methadone,** may be substituted for heroin, which has a much shorter half-life 15–8; subsequently the methadone may be slowly tapered. An alternative approach involves the use of an α_2-adrenergic receptor agonist, such as **clonidine,** which acts in part on autoreceptors of neurons in the LC to counteract the rebound hyperactivity implicated in physical withdrawal syndromes (see 15–1). Clonidine permits a relatively comfortable and rapid withdrawal from methadone and other opiates. Its use also is compatible with the administration of an opioid receptor antagonist, such as **naltrexone,** in rapid detoxification protocols. In the absence of clonidine, naltrexone precipitates a very severe and intolerable withdrawal syndrome.

A long-acting opiate antagonist, naltrexone has been used not only for detoxification but also to prevent relapse in detoxified opiate users. Morning use of naltrexone blocks the euphoria that accompanies heroin or other opiates and thereby makes drug relapse less likely. Over time this treatment also may help extinguish the association of drug-taking behaviors with reinforcement. However, the clinical use of naltrexone is limited because it is associated with low rates of compliance, apparently due to the fact that naltrexone induces dysphoria.

Many opiate addicts cannot achieve abstinence. For these individuals, pharmacologic treatment involves maintenance on a long-acting oral opiate, such as levo-α-acetylmethadol (**LAAM**) or **methadone** 15–8. Such treatment has several advantages. It suppresses craving and drug-seeking behavior, and limits intravenous drug use and associated risks of **hepatitis** and **AIDS.** Moreover, by smoothing out the peaks and valleys that often characterize **heroin** use, and blocking the urge to seek heroin during the day, this treatment facilitates rehabilitation and increases an individual's ability to sustain employment and stabilize social relationships. Methadone and LAAM are generally administered in the context of highly structured psychosocial interventions. An alternative agent is **buprenorphine** 15–8, a partial μ opioid receptor agonist. This drug, which has only mild reinforcing effects by itself, blocks the effects of heroin by binding to the μ receptor. However, unlike naltrexone, buprenorphine does not produce dysphoria. **Suboxone,** a fixed ratio combination of buprenorphine and naloxone, looks promising in the long-term treatment of opiate addiction in early clinical experience.

Ethanol

Detoxification from ethanol typically involves the administration of benzodiazepines such as **chlordiazepoxide,** which exhibit cross-dependence with ethanol at $GABA_A$ receptors (Chapters 5 and 14). A dose that will prevent the physical symptoms associated with withdrawal from ethanol, including tachycardia, hypertension, tremor, agitation, and seizures, is given and is slowly tapered. Benzodiazepines are used because they are less reinforcing than ethanol among alcoholics. Moreover, the tapered use of a benzodiazepine with a long half-life makes the emergence of withdrawal symptoms less likely than direct withdrawal from ethanol.

Disulfiram, while approved for the treatment of alcoholism, is not widely used. It irreversibly inhibits *aldehyde dehydrogenase*, and thereby leads to the buildup of the toxic compound acetaldehyde after ethanol consumption. The ethanol–disulfiram reaction is characterized by flushing, dizziness, nausea, and vomiting. The rationale for disulfiram use is that it devalues ethanol consumption by associating ethanol use with a strongly aversive experience. Yet clinical trial data do not support the use of disulfiram in most cases; although the drug may decrease total drinking days for some individuals, it is not effective in preventing a return to heavy drinking. In addition, the ethanol–disulfiram reaction may produce serious morbidity, including severe hypotension. Some clinicians believe that disulfiram may be useful in selected,

15-8 **Chemical structures of some clinically useful opioid receptor agonists and antagonists.** (See Chapter 11 for structures of opiate agonists used in the treatment of pain.)

highly motivated patients. Disulfiram has more recently been suggested for **cocaine** addiction, given its weak activity as a dopamine β-hydroxylase inhibitor, but definitive evidence for its efficacy remains to be obtained.

Two other medications are approved in the United States for the treatment of alcoholism in conjunction with psychosocial interventions; however, neither is widely used due to relatively modest efficacy. As mentioned earlier, part of ethanol's rewarding effects are

mediated via activation of endogenous opioid pathways, which suggests the potential utility of **naltrexone** in the treatment of alcoholism. While naltrexone has been shown to reduce ethanol reward and risk of relapse in numerous clinical trials, its effects are modest in most patients. **Acamprosate** is a homotaurine derivative that has some structural similarities to GABA but has no appreciable effect at GABA receptors. It weakly modulates NMDA receptor function in rodents, with facilitation of the receptors in some brain regions, and antagonistic effects in other regions. Unfortunately, acamprosate is not adequately effective for most alcoholics.

Nicotine

Nicotine addiction is currently treated with substitution therapy, that is, with nicotine itself in safer preparations than tobacco (eg, patches, chewing gum). Several antidepressants (in particular, **bupropion**) are effective in some individuals. Recent research has focused on the development of selective antagonists or partial agonists at the $\alpha_4\beta_2$ nAChR for the treatment of nicotine addiction. One such drug, **varenicline**, has recently been approved in the United States, but its efficacy remains unproven.

SELECTED READING

Crabbe JC, Phillips TJ, Harris RA, et al. Alcohol-related genes: contributions from studies with genetically engineered mice. *Addiction Biol.* 2006;11:195–269.

Everitt BJ, Robbins TW. Neural systems of reinforcement for drug addiction: from actions to habits to compulsion. *Nature Neurosci.* 2005;8:1481–1489.

Howlett AC, Breivogel CS, Childers SR, et al. Cannabinoid physiology and pharmacology. 30 years of progress. *Neuropharmacology.* 2004;47 (Suppl 1): 345–358.

Hyman SE, Malenka RC, Nestler EJ. Neural mechanisms of addiction: the role of reward-related learning and memory. *Annu Rev Neurosci.* 2006;29: 565–598.

Kalivas PW, Hu XT. Exciting inhibition in psychostimulant addiction. *Trends Neurosci.* 2006;29:610–616.

Kauer JA, Malenka RC. Synaptic plasticity and addiction. *Nature Rev Neurosci.*2007; 8:844–858.

Koob GF, Ahmed SH, Boutrel B, et al. Neurobiological mechanisms in the transition from drug use to drug dependence. *Neurosci Biobehav Rev.* 2004;27: 739–749.

Koob GF, LeMoal M. *Neurobiology of Addiction.* Academic Press, New York; 2006.

Kreek MJ, Bart G, Lilly C, et al. Pharmacogenetics and human molecular genetics of opiate and cocaine addictions and their treatments. *Pharmacol Rev.* 2005;57:1–26.

Luscher C, Ungless MA. The mechanistic classification of addictive drugs. *PLoS Med.* 2006;3:e437.

Nestler EJ. Is there a common molecular pathway for addiction? *Nature Neurosci.* 2005;8:1445–1449.

Nestler EJ. Molecular basis of long-term plasticity underlying addiction. *Nature Rev Neurosci.* 2001;2: 119–128.

Olson RW, Hanchar HJ, Meera P, et al. GABA$_A$ receptor subtypes: the "one glass of wine" receptors. *Alcohol.* 2007;41:201–209.

Robinson TE, Kolb B. Structural plasticity associated with exposure to drugs of abuse. *Neuropharmacology.* 2004;47(Suppl 1):33–46.

Self DW. Regulation of drug-taking and -seeking behaviors by neuroadaptations in the mesolimbic dopamine system. *Neuropharmacology.* 2004;47 (Suppl 1):242–255.

Schultz W. Behavioral theories and the neurophysiology of reward. *Annu Rev Psychol.* 2006;57:87–115.

Shaham Y, Shalev U, Lu L, et al. The reinstatement model of drug relapse: history, methodology and major findings. *Psychopharmacology.* 2003;168:3–20.

Thomas MJ, Malenka RC. Synaptic plasticity in the mesolimbic dopamine system. *Phil Trans Royal Soc London B: Biol Sci.* 2003;358:815–819.

Volkow ND, Li TK. Drug addiction: the neurobiology of behaviour gone awry. *Nature Rev Neurosci.* 2004;5:963–970.

Wise RA. Dopamine, learning and motivation. *Nature Rev Neurosci.* 2004;5:483–494.

Wolf ME, Sun X, Mangiavacchi S, et al. Psychomotor stimulants and neuronal plasticity. *Neuropharmacology.* 2004;47(Suppl 1):61–79.

CHAPTER 16

Schizophrenia and Other Psychoses

- Schizophrenia is characterized by positive ("psychotic") symptoms such as hallucinations and delusions, negative symptoms such as amotivation and social withdrawal, and cognitive deficits such as poor working memory.

- The risk of schizophrenia is highly influenced by genes. Nongenetic factors, such as environmental factors, also appear to be important, although they remain poorly defined.

- Relatives of individuals with schizophrenia may have symptoms such as suspiciousness, social isolation, eccentric beliefs, and cognitive deficits—but not psychotic symptoms. This condition is currently classified as schizotypal personality disorder.

- Schizophrenia is characterized by loss of gray matter in frontal and temporal regions of the cerebral cortex. Unaffected first-degree relatives may have similar, but milder gray matter thinning.

- The mainstay of treatment for schizophrenia are the antipsychotic drugs. These drugs are also efficacious in the treatment of acute mania, schizoaffective disorders, and psychosis associated with depression or drug intoxication,

hence their designation as antipsychotic—not antischizophrenic—drugs.

- The main benefit of antipsychotic drugs is in treatment of positive symptoms. They have more modest efficacy in treating negative symptoms and lack significant benefits for the cognitive symptoms of schizophrenia and related disorders.

- The therapeutic action of all available antipsychotic drugs depends on their ability to antagonize D_2 dopamine receptors. This action can also cause significant motor side effects termed extrapyramidal symptoms. Newer (ie, second-generation) antipsychotic drugs partly mitigate these side effects due to weaker antagonism of D_2 receptors and by possessing other receptor binding properties (eg, $5HT_{2A}$ receptor antagonism) but have other significant side effects.

- All current antipsychotic drugs exert their full therapeutic actions over weeks, suggesting that, like lithium and antidepressants, slowly developing adaptations (in this case to initial D_2 dopamine receptor blockade) are required for their antipsychotic effects.

PSYCHOSIS

Psychotic symptoms are disturbing and often dramatic psychological phenomena in which an individual appears to have lost touch with reality. *Hallucinations* are perceptions disconnected from external stimuli; individuals may report hearing voices that others cannot hear or seeing things that others cannot see. *Illusions* that can be considered psychotic symptoms are not optical problems or common misperceptions, but rather severely distorted perceptions or misinterpretations of stimuli, for example, seeing an object as pulsating that others see as still. *Delusions* are fixed, false beliefs that are not shared by others in an individual's culture. Examples include bizarre delusions such as the belief that the fillings in one's teeth are radio transmitters receiving messages from outer space, or paranoid delusions such as a fixed, false belief that one is being spied on or persecuted. *Ideas of reference* are beliefs that ordinary objects, such as license plates, contain specific messages for the person. These are called *delusions of reference* when the person holding these beliefs is unable to question them. Some patients describe *thought insertion or deletion*, the belief that some outside agency has removed or added thoughts to their brain.

Schizophrenia is the best known disorder in which individuals have psychotic symptoms, but it is by no means the only such disorder. Psychotic symptoms can occur in **mood disorders**; they are common in full episodes of **mania** and occur also in the most severe cases of **depression** (Chapter 14). When they occur in mood disorders, psychotic symptoms are generally congruent with the person's elevated or depressed mood. Thus, during a manic episode, a person may have the delusion that he or she is a prophet or deity or is endowed with supernatural powers. During depression with psychotic features, patients may hear voices hectoring them or describing them as worthless or may have delusions that they are rotting from the inside and emitting an intolerable odor. In these cases, the psychotic symptoms remit when the underlying mood disorder responds to treatment. Symptoms of mania or depression can also occur in cases in which chronic schizophrenia-like symptoms predominate; these patients are often said to have **schizoaffective disorder,** although evidence from family and genetic studies suggests that this is a highly heterogeneous grouping. There are also several nonaffective psychotic disorders that lack the course or full symptoms of schizophrenia. Individuals may develop acute and transient schizophrenia-like syndromes followed by full recovery. This is referred to as **schizophreniform disorder.** Other individuals may harbor chronic delusions without other symptoms of schizophrenia such as hallucinations or cognitive symptoms (**delusional disorder**). As well, psychotic symptoms may occur as a result of **drugs of abuse**, toxins, or metabolic derangements (Chapters 10 and 15). Delusions and hallucinations may occur in neurodegenerative disorders such as **Alzheimer disease** or **Huntington disease.** For example, as patients with Alzheimer disease begin to lose track of possessions, they may develop the delusion that their house is being frequented by burglars and robbed.

SCHIZOPHRENIA

The symptoms of schizophrenia form three major clusters: positive, negative, and cognitive symptoms. The term *positive symptoms* signifies mental phenomena that are absent in healthy individuals and refers to psychotic symptoms such as hallucinations and delusions. In schizophrenia, hallucinations are more commonly auditory than in other sensory modalities, often taking the form of sounds or voices. Patients may hear voices carrying on a conversation, which may be about the sufferer; the voices can be derogatory or can issue commands. Delusions are often bizarre or paranoid. Patients also typically exhibit some form of thought disorder such as those described in the preceding section.

The term *negative symptoms* is used to describe loss or significant impairment of normal psychological functions such as loss of motivation (amotivation), social interaction (asociality), blunting of affect, or impoverishment of the content of thought and speech. The cognitive symptoms of schizophrenia include deficits in executive function, including impairment of working memory, the ability to hold information "on line" that can be used to guide thought or behavior (Chapter 13). Deficits in episodic memory may occur as well.

Schizophrenia most often manifests in late teen years or in the early 20s (although earlier and later onsets may occur). Typically, there is a period of prodromal symptoms in which the person begins to have difficulties at school or work, becomes socially isolated, and often increasingly eccentric. Some individuals become intermittently belligerent, while others develop negative symptoms. The diagnosis is generally made with the appearance of psychotic symptoms, which may arrive acutely and dramatically, often leading to hospitalization **16–1**. The course of schizophrenia is chronic, with periods of milder residual symptoms punctuated by relapses of florid psychosis. With treatment, individuals often have a good recovery from their first psychotic episode,

16-1   Schizophrenia: A Case History

Martin is a 35-year-old man who is currently homeless and living in shelters or on the street. His childhood was unremarkable until high school, when he began to withdraw from his peers. He tended to eat and play by himself at school and spent much of his time reading science fiction. In college, Martin developed a preoccupation with mysticism and religion, often writing lengthy but confusing manifestos that described his beliefs. His parents became concerned at the end of his sophomore year when final exams were approaching, and he seemed to become more and more preoccupied with his theories which he believed were sure to revolutionize society. Finally, Martin broke off contact with his parents, believing that they had been recruited into a conspiracy to prevent him from developing his philosophy. During his junior year, Martin's behavior continued to change. He began to wear large hats because he believed that people could hear his thoughts and were trying to steal them. When he heard news stories about overseas civil disturbances or wars he believed that they were being waged between forces trying to help him and others who were trying to stop him. One night, as Martin was putting aluminum foil around his dorm room to prevent people from using electrical devices to steal his ideas, he began to hear two voices discussing his work and his philosophy. Their discussion confirmed his fear that his ideas had been stolen. He became more and more frightened and angry as the voices began to ridicule his ideas, until finally he fled his apartment. On the street he saw a policeman he believed was sent to kidnap him. Martin attacked the policeman in what he believed was self-defense.

Martin was brought to a psychiatric hospital where he was given **antipsychotic** medication and additional short-term treatment with a **benzodiazepine** (Chapter 14) to calm him until the antipsychotic drug could begin to work. With treatment, his auditory hallucinations and paranoid delusions subsided over the course of a few weeks, but he remained adamant that he did not want to see his parents. Soon after he was released from the hospital, Martin stopped taking his medications because they made him feel tired and gain weight. He attempted to continue his studies but within six months dropped out of school because of the return of paranoid delusions about people stealing his ideas and because he was having great difficulty keeping up with his assignments. For the next 6 years, he tried to work at a series of jobs but was unable to keep any of them because of unexplained absences and frequent clashes with his bosses and coworkers. During these years he was hospitalized involuntarily six times and given many different first- and second-generation antipsychotic drugs. Each time he was given an antipsychotic medication there was an initial reduction in his paranoia and auditory hallucinations. He rarely continued to take these drugs for more than a few months, however, because of the side effects he experienced or because the hallucinations began to return despite medication.

At one point Martin reconciled with his parents and lived with them for several years, but they became increasingly frustrated with his resistance to taking his medications followed by frightening outbursts and hospitalization. Because discussions about this issue caused considerable tension, Martin would occasionally become very angry and disappear to live with his one remaining friend or on the street for weeks at a time. He began drinking **alcohol** and using **marijuana** and **cocaine**, because he was bored and because these substances would help him ignore the voices that frequently bothered him. Eventually, when he was 29, Martin had a major fight with his parents over his illicit drug use and he moved out of their house, never to return.

During the past 6 years Martin has been living in shelters and on the street. He receives medication from a local public health clinic. Although he continues to take such medication inconsistently, he takes it more frequently because he has come to recognize that it helps him stay out of the hospital. He knows some of the other people at the shelters he visits, but in general people make him uncomfortable and he keeps to himself. His parents occasionally send him money but he talks to them only about once a year. Although he still thinks of his philosophy occasionally, it makes less sense to him than it used to. Mostly he spends time alone, making small talismans out of wire and glass to help him feel safe.

but such episodes recur, and functioning between episodes tends to deteriorate. **Antipsychotic drugs** not only treat acute episodes of psychosis, but also clearly extend the period between relapses. Unfortunately, the existing drugs do not abolish relapses; moreover, the side effect burden of antipsychotic drugs contributes to their discontinuation by patients. The cognitive symptoms respond poorly to current medications and tend to be unremitting. Overall, individuals with schizophrenia lose functional capacities until they reach a plateau well below their best prior level of functioning.

Epidemiology and Genetics of Schizophrenia and Related Disorders

It has long been thought that schizophrenia affects 1% of the population worldwide and attacks men and women in equal numbers. Indeed, it is difficult to accurately identify individuals with psychotic symptoms in surveys in general (nonclinical) populations. Individuals with active or prior psychosis may be homeless, deny access to surveyors, or hide their symptoms if questioned. Examination of clinical populations fails to detect individuals who have never been treated, because they either actively avoid medical attention or lack access to services. Despite such challenges, recent epidemiologic surveys have called into question longstanding beliefs about the prevalence of schizophrenia. Like virtually every other chronic disease with complex genetic and environmental risk factors, schizophrenia does not have uniform prevalence, but exhibits significant variations in different populations with a global mean somewhere between 0.5% and 1.0%. There is also emerging evidence that males are at higher risk for schizophrenia than females (approximately 1.4 to 1) and tend to have earlier onset of the illness. The lifetime prevalence of psychosis of all causes may be between 3% and 4% of the population.

Genetic and Nongenetic Risk Factors for Schizophrenia

Schizophrenia has long been observed to run in families, but not to exhibit typical Mendelian patterns of dominant or recessive transmission. Nonetheless, twin and adoption studies demonstrate that the familiality of schizophrenia results predominantly from shared genes. Monozygotic twin pairs, whose DNA sequences are 100% identical, have a concordance for schizophrenia of nearly 50%. In contrast, dizygotic twin pairs, whose DNA sequences, on average, exhibit 50% identity, have a concordance for schizophrenia of 15%. Overall, the more DNA sequences one shares with a person who has schizophrenia, the higher one's risk **16–1**.

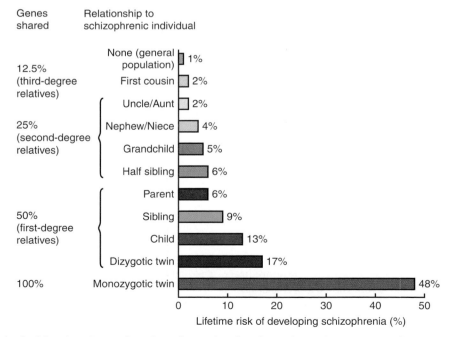

16–1 Risk of schizophrenia as a function of genetic relatedness. (From Gottesman 1991)

Despite their power to detect genetic influences, twin studies do not fully separate genetic from environmental influences. An alternative strategy to demonstrate a role for genes is to study people with schizophrenia who were adopted early in life. Such studies have demonstrated that adoptees resemble their biologic rather than their adoptive families with respect to schizophrenia. However, as for all common psychiatric disorders, genes do not act alone. For a co-twin in a monozygotic twin pair, there is a 50- to 100-fold increase in risk of schizophrenia (over the population base rate of 0.5%–1%) if the other member of the pair has schizophrenia. However, 50% of pairs are discordant (ie, the other twin does not develop schizophrenia), underscoring an important role for nongenetic factors.

Interestingly, the risk of schizophrenia is nearly twice as high for a member of a dizygotic twin pair with a schizophrenic co-twin (17%) as for a nontwin sibling (9%) despite both sharing approximately 50% of DNA sequences. The leading hypothesis to explain this variance is *epigenetic* modification of the genome by such processes as methylation of DNA or covalent modification of the histone proteins that are the major constituent of chromatin (Chapter 4). Such modifications, which partly result from environmental signals and which are partly stochastic, produce persistent changes in gene expression that could strongly influence brain development. Since twins share a uterine environment at the same time, they are thought more likely to have shared epigenetic modifications of their DNA than nontwin siblings or other first-degree relatives.

Adoption, twin, and family studies also find that blood relatives of schizophrenic probands, who do not have psychotic symptoms, nevertheless may exhibit some degree of social isolation, suspiciousness, eccentric beliefs, or magical thinking. This constellation of symptoms is described as *schizotypy*, and is classified in current diagnostic nomenclatures as **schizotypal personality disorder**. Whether or not schizotypal symptoms are present to a significant degree, nonschizophrenic monozygotic twins and unaffected siblings of individuals with schizophrenia tend to exhibit cognitive impairments and neuroanatomic abnormalities similar to but milder than those observed in their schizophrenic relatives. These considerations further underscore the heritability of schizophrenia and the likely existence of a spectrum of schizophrenia-like syndromes.

A deeper understanding of these observations, as well as insights into the pathophysiology of schizophrenia and other psychotic disorders, will benefit enormously from the identification of genes that confer risk. Gene identification should identify molecular pathways involved in disease pathogenesis and may also provide clues for treatment development. As for other common, heterogeneous, and genetically complex disorders (such as diabetes mellitus, inflammatory bowel disease, mood disorders, and autism), the search has proved challenging. Genetically complex disorders result from the interaction of multiple genes of small effect and nongenetic factors. Moreover, different constellations of risk genes may act in different families. While disorders such as diabetes mellitus type II and inflammatory bowel disease are also heterogeneous and genetically complex, there are objective medical tests that draw boundaries around core phenotypes. Thus, the use of advanced genomic technologies to study very large numbers of affected individuals has yielded the first replicated disease risk genes for these disorders.

In contrast, schizophrenia and other psychiatric disorders lack objective measures that can limit heterogeneity for genetic study. Accordingly, while several interesting candidate genes have been identified, none is yet certain **16-1**. One candidate, Disrupted in Schizophrenia (DISC1), was found in a Scottish family with a balanced chromosomal translocation that interrupted the gene. The DISC1 story speaks directly to the challenges of phenotype in psychiatric disorders. First, it is not yet certain that DISC1 causes schizophrenia in this family: rather, disruption of DISC1 may be an epiphenomenon. However, even assuming a causal role for DISC1 in this family, it is unclear what symptoms a DISC1 mutation might produce. Some family members with the mutation have schizophrenia-like symptoms, but others have a syndrome that is more akin to depression with psychotic features.

Another putative schizophrenia risk gene, neuregulin 1 (NRG1), was discovered by positional (linkage) methods in an Icelandic population and replicated in a Scottish population. In one study, levels of erbB-3, one

16-1 **Schizophrenia Candidate Genes**

Protein	Gene Name
Disrupted in schizophrenia	DISC1
Dysbindin (dystrobrevin binding protein 1)	DTNBP1
Neuregulin 1	NRG1
D amino acid oxidase activator	DAOA
Catechol-O-methyl transferase	COMT
Regulator of G-protein signaling 4	RGS4

of the receptors for neuregulin 1, were found to be 42% decreased in the prefrontal cortex of affected individuals studied at autopsy compared to unaffected controls. NRG1 is an interesting candidate because, among its many other functions in the nervous system, it regulates neuronal migration, a process that may be aberrant in schizophrenia, and also regulates the expression of the NMDA glutamate receptor, also implicated in schizophrenia-like behaviors. Despite this promising evidence, based on the most rigorous current statistical genetic methods, NRG1 cannot be said with certainty to confer risk of schizophrenia.

Potential environmental risk factors that have been identified in epidemiologic studies include urban birth, increasing paternal age, and intrauterine exposure to viral infection, among several others. Maternal starvation during pregnancy has been identified as a risk factor for schizophrenia based on famine in the Netherlands following World War II and in China. It has been hypothesized that lack of critical nutritional factors may result in de novo germ line mutations that could contribute to schizophrenia and other disorders. However, it must be emphasized that, to date, causal evidence is lacking for any particular environmental factor. It is likely that genetic factors must be found before environmental factors, which specifically influence that genetic potential, can be identified with certainty.

Pathophysiology of Schizophrenia

Cognitive deficits in schizophrenia Individuals with schizophrenia have preservation of basic sensori-motor skills and associative abilities, but tasks that require symbolic or verbal representation may be impaired. Individuals with schizophrenia also have difficulty integrating novel stimuli with older memories or concepts, and tend to treat familiar associations as though they were unusual and new situations as if they occurred in the recent past. The disorganization of speech and loosening of associations that characterize schizophrenia may stem from an inability to keep recent thoughts or words in mind.

These and other difficulties reflect deficits in *working memory,* the short-term, capacity-limited ability to hold information online (Chapter 13). Working memory, sometimes described as "scratch pad" memory, involves the ability to represent information, manipulate it, and order it, thus permitting a person to exert "cognitive control" over thoughts, emotions, and behavior. Without an ability to hold goals, plans, and relevant information in mind, it is difficult to complete a task, suppress automatic responses to familiar stimuli, and overcome distractions. As a result, deficits

in working memory would interfere with the ability of a person to complete complex tasks at school or work. It is believed that impairments in working memory is a major contributor to disability in schizophrenia.

In the lab, people with schizophrenia have difficulty with working memory tasks. In one task, for example, a visual target is presented on a screen to a human subject for 200 milliseconds, and after a delay of 5 to 30 seconds during which the target is absent, a distraction is introduced to keep the image from being converted into a verbal representation. At the end of the delay period, the subject is asked to look at the original location of the target. People with schizophrenia perform poorly on such tests compared with healthy subjects. Such tasks in human subjects have their basis in physiological studies that have been performed in monkeys in which electrodes are implanted in the brain to record the activity of neurons. Monkeys may be trained, for example, in spatial working memory tasks, and then tested while recordings are being made. In such tasks, a subset of neurons in the dorsolateral prefrontal cortex actively fire, perhaps serving as the internal representation of the (now absent) target (see **13–3**). In humans, invasive recordings are not ethical, but functional neuroimaging can reveal ensembles of neurons that fire during working memory and other cognitive tasks **16–2**. Humans with strokes or injuries that affect the dorsolateral prefrontal cortex, like monkeys that have received experimental lesions in this region, perform poorly in similar paradigms.

Another task at which schizophrenic individuals perform poorly is the Wisconsin Card Sorting Test (WCST). Subjects who take this test are asked to sort a deck of cards marked with symbols that vary in number, color, and shape. As each card is dealt, the subject must match the card to a reference deck based on its color, number, or shape. The experimenter indicates whether the subject's match is correct or incorrect, and over time the subject learns the rule of sorting. After a specified number of trials, the experimenter changes the sorting rule without telling the subject, who must realize the task has changed and learn the new rule. Schizophrenic individuals perform well when learning the initial sorting rule but have difficulty recognizing and adopting a new sorting rule. Both normal and schizophrenic subjects learn to associate a card (an external stimulus) with a response (correct or incorrect) until a sorting rule, such as sort by color, is internalized and becomes rapid and automatic. Schizophrenic individuals are deficient in the working memory component of this task, and thus cannot exert cognitive control to suppress an initial associative sorting rule when it is no longer correct.

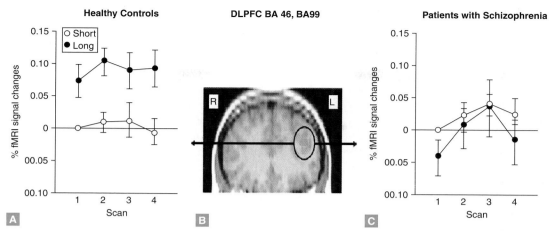

16-2 **Deficits in a working memory task correlated with impairment in recruitment of dorsolateral prefrontal cortex in schizophrenia.** Functional MRI (fMRI) was used to examine activation of dorsolateral prefrontal cortex in patients with first-episode schizophrenia who had never been given antipsychotic drugs compared with healthy controls during performance of a working memory task. Subjects were presented with a sequence of letters and instructed to respond to a particular letter (the "probe" letter) only if it immediately followed another specified letter (the "contextual cue" letter). Demands on working memory were varied by altering the delay between the cue and the probe letters. A longer delay places greater demands on working memory relative to a short delay. Panel **B** shows a deficit of activity in patients with schizophrenia compared with healthy controls in a specific region of dorsolateral prefrontal cortex (Broadman areas 46/49). Panels **A** and **C** plot the percent change in the fMRI signal for the region shown in the scan in response to the long and short delay tasks. This region of prefrontal cortex does not activate normally in the subjects with schizophrenia correlating with a deficit in performance during the long delay task that puts greater demands on working memory function. (Adapted from Barch et al. Selective deficits in prefrontal cortex function in medication-naive patients with schizophrenia. *Arch Gen Psychiatry*. 2001;58:280–288.)

Patients with schizophrenia also demonstrate deficits in cognitive control when performing the Stroop test. Cards used in this test have the name of a color written on them, but the name is printed in the ink of another color—for example, green is written in red ink **16-3**. Subjects are asked to give the name of the color in which the word is written, while suppressing the natural tendency to recite the color represented by the word. Patients with schizophrenia have difficulty performing this task because it requires keeping the rule in working memory and ignoring the stimulus of the semantic representation of the word.

Working memory depends on optimal stimulation of D_1 dopamine receptors (Chapter 13) located on pyramidal cells in the prefrontal cortex. In multiple species, including rats, monkeys, and humans, an inverted-U–shaped dose response curve has been observed, with either too little or too much D_1 dopamine receptor stimulation causing degradation of working memory. The tuning of working memory by D_1 dopamine receptor stimulation appears to depend on the cAMP pathway, as would be expected since D_1

receptors are G_s linked (Chapter 4). These findings not only have potential relevance for the development of therapies based on the D_1 dopamine receptor pathway, but may also explain why antipsychotic drugs (many of which have D_1 dopamine receptor antagonist properties) may worsen working memory performance in schizophrenic individuals beyond their already impaired baseline.

Neuroanatomic correlates of schizophrenia
Neuroanatomic studies have demonstrated differences in the brains of schizophrenic patients compared with the brains of matched controls. The most consistent finding, based on structural magnetic resonance imaging (MRI) of living patients and postmortem brain examinations, is thinning of gray matter in the prefrontal and temporal regions of the cerebral cortex **16-4** with compensatory enlargement of the third and lateral ventricles. The most severe gray matter loss occurs in the dorsolateral prefrontal cortex, the brain region required for working memory. It can therefore be hypothesized that the cognitive deficits

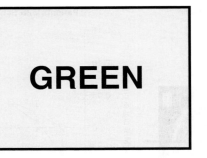

GREEN

16-3 **Example of the Stroop task.** The subject is asked to name the color in which a word is printed. When the word names objects such as "BALL" or "TABLE", reaction time is faster than when the meaning of the word is dissonant, such as "GREEN" printed in red ink. That is because the automatic (prepotent) response to read the word is stronger than to name the color. Working memory is required to hold the instructions in mind in order to exert cognitive control, ie, to suppress the prepotent response, which is to say "green," and follow the instruction and say "red." People with schizophrenia have substantially worse performance on Stroop tasks than healthy individuals.

and corresponding abnormalities in the dorsolateral prefrontal cortex observed with functional imaging **16-2** may result from regionally specific gray matter abnormalities. Abnormal functioning of the hippocampus—anterior regions of this structure, in particular—also has been reported in individuals with schizophrenia and correlates with impaired performance on various cognitive tasks.

The observed loss of volume in the frontal and temporal cortical regions, or observed aberrant functioning of hippocampus, does not appear to result from loss of cell bodies, but rather from a reduction in neuropil, which is composed of dendritic and axonal processes. Some studies have found that the loss of dendritic processes is accompanied by loss of dendritic spines and, hence, very likely loss of synapses.

Postmortem examinations of cerebral cortex and hippocampus of schizophrenic subjects have not found evidence of cell loss, gliosis, or inflammation. These findings have been interpreted to mean that schizophrenia is not a neurodegenerative disorder, but more likely a result of abnormal brain development.

The neurodevelopmental hypothesis also receives support from the typical age of onset of schizophrenia in the late teens or early adulthood. During this period, the brain undergoes its last significant period

of maturation in the context of significant developmental events such as sexual maturation, leaving the parental home, and taking up more adult responsibilities. These hormonal and developmental events are accompanied by completion of the myelination of axon fibers in frontal regions of cerebral cortex and by significant *synaptic pruning* in this and other regions. Synaptic pruning describes a process believed to maintain those synaptic connections that have been used effectively during brain development and to remove those connections that have been ineffective. Synaptic pruning may be a particularly robust process in the prefrontal cortex. Moreover, it coincides with major changes in dopaminergic neurotransmission in this brain area during late adolescence. A final piece of evidence that argues for a neurodevelopmental pathogenesis of schizophrenia are the results of a longitudinal study of individuals who have onset of schizophrenia in childhood. Individuals with these relatively rare early onsets exhibit accelerated loss of gray matter compared with healthy matched control subjects.

Neurotransmitter Systems Implicated in Psychotic Disorders or Their Treatment

Dopamine The neurotransmitter most frequently implicated in schizophrenia is dopamine, although much of the evidence is inferential, being based on the fact that all effective **antipsychotic drugs** (described below) are antagonists at D_2 dopamine receptors (Chapter 6). Psychostimulants, such as **amphetamine** and **cocaine**, and L-dopa (Chapter 6), which increase synaptic levels of dopamine, can cause delusions, most commonly paranoid delusions, ideas of reference, and auditory hallucinations. The putative involvement of dopamine in schizophrenia and other psychotic syndromes is consistent with the significant dopaminergic innervation of the prefrontal cortex and other limbic regions (Chapter 6) implicated in psychosis. Despite such evidence, the hypothesis that dopamine is a direct contributor to the pathogenesis of psychotic disorders has significant weaknesses. Antipsychotic drugs block D_2 receptors upon initial drug exposure, but specific antipsychotic effects are seen only after several days, and often weeks, of drug administration. Conversely, psychostimulants and L-dopa increase synaptic dopamine with each dose, but generally cause psychosis only after prolonged use at high doses.

It must be emphasized that neurotransmitter-related hypotheses that attempt to explain the etiology of schizophrenia are based solely on pharmacologic evidence, and thus are likely to be incomplete or

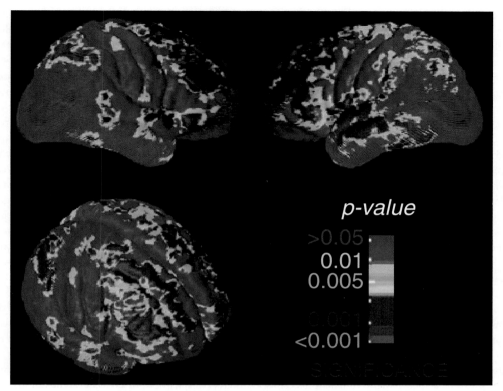

16-4 **Gray matter loss in the cerebral cortex in schizophrenia and in co-twins.** A study of monozygotic and dizygotic twin pairs discordant for schizophrenia compared with healthy matched control twins demonstrated gray matter loss in schizophrenia, and significant but milder gray matter thinning in their "unaffected" co-twins. Beyond the gray matter deficits shared with family members, the affected co-twin had more severe "disease-specific" deficits in dorsolateral prefrontal, superior temporal, and superior parietal association areas (red pseudo-color in figure), presumably reflecting the action of nongenetic factors acting against a background of genetic risk. The gray matter deficits in the schizophrenic co-twins correlated with symptom severity and cognitive dysfunction rather than with duration of illness or drug treatment. The images here show gray-matter deficits in schizophrenic monozygotic twins relative to their healthy co-twins viewed from the right, left, and right-oblique perspectives. A pseudocolor scale is superimposed on cortical surface maps. (From Cannon et al. Cortex mapping reveals region-ally specific patterns of genetic and disease-specific gray-matter deficits in twins discordant for schizophrenia. *Proc Natl Acad Sci USA.* 2002;99:3228–3233.)

misleading. Although pharmacologic manipulation of neurotransmitter systems may exacerbate or amelio-rate psychotic symptoms, aberrations in these systems do not necessarily underlie psychotic disorders.

Glutamate   Glutamate, the major excitatory neuro-transmitter in the brain, gained attention as a possible contributor to schizophrenia because of the actions of drugs that block NMDA glutamate receptors (Chapter 5). **Phencyclidine** (**PCP**) and **ketamine**, developed as **dis-sociative anesthetics**, both have significant abuse potential. Phencyclidine is known on the street as **angel dust** and ketamine as **special K**. These drugs produce a sense of depersonalization and dissociation

of subjective experience from sensory stimuli. As a result, during surgery, nociceptive signals might not be experienced as aversive. These drugs also produce dra-matic psychotic-like symptoms in a dose-dependent manner including visual and auditory hallucinations. Finally, these drugs can result in addiction (Chapter 15). As a result of its side effects and abuse potential, phen-cyclidine is no longer used therapeutically, although ketamine is still used in limited circumstances for pediatric and veterinary anesthesia.

The major actions of PCP were once believed to be mediated by the *sigma receptor*, to which the drug binds with a relatively high (200 n*M*) affinity. This receptor was originally thought to be an opioid receptor because it is bound by **benzomorphan** opiate drugs such as **pentazocine** (Chapter 11). However, it is not blocked by the nonselective opioid receptor antagonist naloxone, and it binds diverse drugs that are unrelated to opioids. The sigma receptor remains poorly understood. Subsequently, PCP, ketamine, and other dissociative anesthetics were shown to have a higher affinity for the NMDA glutamate receptor, where they function as open channel blockers (Chapter 5). This action of PCP has suggested that the glutamate system may be exploited in the treatment of schizophrenia, as discussed at the end of this chapter. Interestingly, PCP often causes profound retrograde amnesia; it has been hypothesized that this effect can be explained by the drug's interference with NMDA receptor function, which is critically important for long-term potentiation in the hippocampus and other brain regions and for certain forms of long-term memory (Chapters 5 and 13).

The mechanism by which blockade of NMDA receptors induces a psychotic state is unknown. In animal models, NMDA antagonists have been shown to increase glutamate release in prefrontal cortex, perhaps as a homeostatic response to NMDA receptor blockade, which raises the possibility that increased glutamatergic transmission at non-NMDA glutamate receptors (eg, at AMPA receptors) may be responsible for the psychotic symptoms. While this scheme remains highly conjectural, such studies with PCP and ketamine have led to the hypothesis that schizophrenia may result from an aberration in glutamatergic function, for example, decreased NMDA receptor function or increased overall glutamatergic transmission. However, it is important to point out that postulating a role for abnormal glutamatergic neurotransmission in schizophrenia is akin to proposing that the brain is involved in schizophrenia since every single neuron in the brain receives thousands of excitatory synapses that utilize glutamate as their neurotransmitter. It is, therefore, essential to further develop this hypothesis and specify which specific glutamatergic circuits malfunction in which direction to cause this devastating disorder.

Antipsychotic Drugs

Chlorpromazine and **reserpine,** the first antipsychotic drugs, were introduced in the 1950s and revolutionized the treatment of psychotic disorders and acute **mania**. Chlorpromazine ⬛16-5 was initially developed as an antihistamine intended for use as a preanesthetic. An astute surgeon observed that it was highly sedating in surgical patients, and suggested its experimental use in agitated psychiatric patients. Its effectiveness in psychotic patients, beyond the simple sedation produced by **barbiturates**, then widely used to sedate schizophrenic

and manic patients, was later demonstrated: chlorpromazine caused psychotic symptoms such as hallucinations and delusions to remit over a period of days to weeks. In fact, schizophrenic patients habituated to the sedative properties over time, making chronic use of chlorpromazine tolerable. Unfortunately, chlorpromazine produced extrapyramidal motor side effects reminiscent of **Parkinson disease** such as tremor and rigidity. It was soon recognized that both the therapeutic effects and the Parkinson-like effects were due to a shared mechanism, which ultimately turned out to be antagonism of the D_2 dopamine receptor. This resulted in the use of motor side effects such as catalepsy (rigidity of the limbs) as a screening tool for new antipsychotic drugs in laboratory animals. The term *neuroleptic,* Greek for *neuron clasping,* was applied to the first generation antipsychotic drugs and referred to the motor side effects of these medications.

Studies of chlorpromazine roughly coincided with the discovery of antipsychotic properties of the drug reserpine. Reserpine, the active component of snakeroot or *Rauwolfia serpentina,* had traditionally been used in India to treat psychiatric disorders. However, it was initially used as an antihypertensive agent in the United States (Chapter 6) until clinical trials demonstrated its effectiveness as an antipsychotic drug. Interestingly, therapeutic doses of reserpine caused motor side effects that are similar to those associated with the use of chlorpromazine. Despite very different molecular structures and different molecular targets in the brain, both compounds interfered with dopamine neurotransmission.

Early studies of antipsychotic drug action   In the mid-1950s reserpine was shown to reduce the levels of dopamine, norepinephrine, and serotonin in rat brain. (As described in Chapter 6, the molecular target of reserpine proved far more recently to be the vesicular monoamine transporter.) The reduction in dopamine was a particularly compelling finding because it explained the motor side effects of reserpine; by this time **Parkinson disease** had been attributed to the death of dopamine neurons in the substantia nigra and the resulting depletion of dopamine from the striatum (Chapter 17). Initial studies of chlorpromazine did not support involvement of dopaminergic systems in its mechanism of action because it did not have a significant effect on catecholamine levels in the brain. However, it was observed that administration of chlorpromazine or other antipsychotic drugs caused an increase in the dopamine metabolite homovanillic acid (HVA) in the striatum. This observation lead to the proposal that these antipsychotic drugs worked by blocking dopamine receptors, leading to a compensatory increase

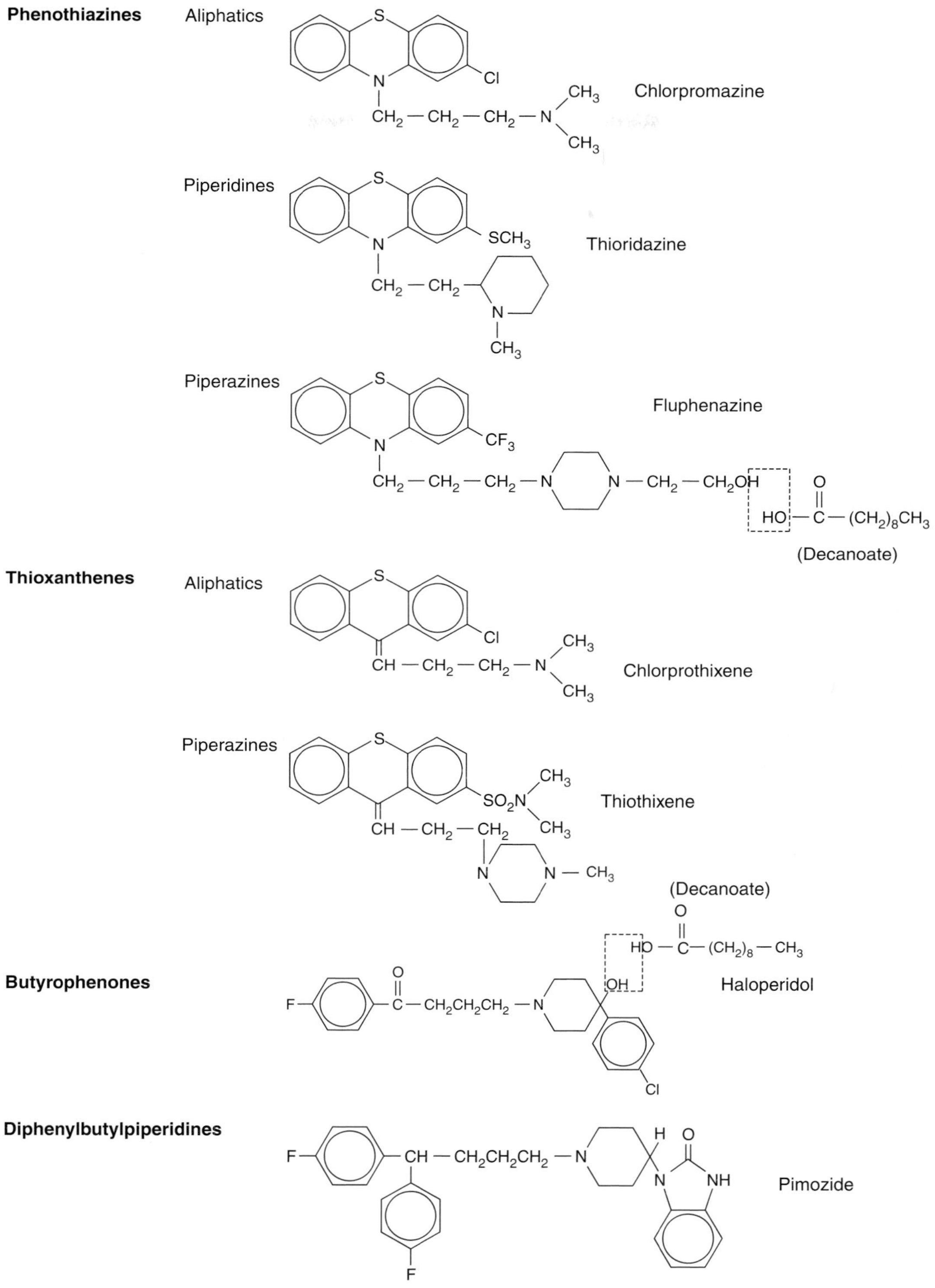

Phenothiazines Aliphatics Chlorpromazine

Piperidines Thioridazine

Piperazines Fluphenazine

(Decanoate)

Thioxanthenes Aliphatics Chlorprothixene

Piperazines Thiothixene

(Decanoate)

Butyrophenones Haloperidol

Diphenylbutylpiperidines Pimozide

16-5 Chemical structures of representative first generation antipsychotic drugs.

in dopamine release in the striatum and thereby to an increase in dopamine breakdown products such as HVA.

Effects of antipsychotic drugs on D$_2$ dopamine receptors The dopamine hypothesis of antipsychotic drug action was bolstered by studies of dopamine receptor binding and function in rat striatum. Such studies identified two major dopamine binding sites, termed D$_1$ and D$_2$. Although some older antipsychotic drugs, such as chlorpromazine, are potent antagonists of both receptor types, antagonism of the D$_2$ receptor correlates with antipsychotic efficacy 16–6 . **Haloperidol**, for example, a

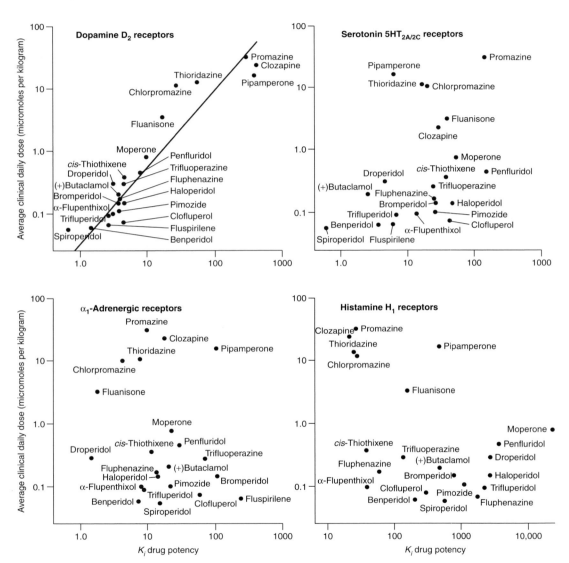

16–6 **Relationship between clinical potencies of antipsychotic medications (as measured by therapeutic dose) and their affinities for various receptors.** Each graph shows clinical potency as a function of binding to D$_2$ dopamine, 5HT$_{2A/2C}$ serotonin, α_1-adrenergic, and H$_1$ histamine receptors. Clinical potency correlates with affinity for D$_2$ dopamine receptors. In fact, dosing and D$_2$ dopamine receptor affinity were not entirely independent of each other, as receptor affinity is used to select doses to test in clinical trials. Affinity and receptor occupancy can be judged in human subjects using positron emission tomography. (From Snyder SH. *Drugs and the Brain*. New York: Scientific American Library; 1996.)

butyrophenone compound that is a highly potent antipsychotic medication, has a high affinity for the D_2 but not the D_1 receptor (see **16–5** and **16–6**). Molecular cloning studies later revealed that the D_1 binding site consists of D_1 and D_5 receptors and that the D_2 binding site consists of D_2, D_3, and D_4 receptors (Chapter 6). Although antagonism of the D_2 receptor remains most strongly associated with antipsychotic drug action, the involvement of D_3 and D_4 receptors in such activity has been considered in recent years although without much success. For example, at least 1 selective D_4 receptor antagonist failed to show efficacy in early clinical trials.

The mechanism by which antagonism of D_2 receptors produces an antipsychotic effect remains unknown. Certain complexities present themselves, however. First, antipsychotic drugs take several weeks to exert their full antipsychotic effects. Accordingly, it is probably not antagonism of D_2 receptors per se that decreases psychosis; rather, this effect is most likely explained by slowly accumulating adaptations of cells, synapses, and neural circuits to sustained blockade of D_2 receptors. Second, the effects of D_2 receptor antagonism must be understood within the context of the cells and neural circuits in which these receptors function. D_2 receptors are both presynaptic and postsynaptic (Chapter 6) and are expressed on neurons in the striatum (at high levels), in multiple subcortical forebrain limbic structures including the amygdala and hippocampus, and at lower levels in the prefrontal cortex (where D_1 dopamine receptors predominate). Pyramidal neurons in the prefrontal cortex, for example, receive glutamatergic inputs both from other cortical neurons and from thalamic neurons. These cortico-cortical and thalamocortical glutamatergic synapses are modulated by local GABAergic interneurons and by numerous afferent projections, which include dopamine projections from the ventral tegmental area as well as inputs from other monoaminergic and cholinergic neurons. A goal of current research is to delineate how dopamine, acting on D_1 family and D_2 family dopamine receptors, modifies these various synaptic inputs and pyramidal neuron excitability, and how chronic blockade of D_2 receptors alters the functioning of these circuits to reduce psychosis. Similar questions can be raised about other cells and circuits expressing D_2 receptors.

Side effects of antipsychotic drugs Although antipsychotic drugs revolutionized the treatment of schizophrenia and other psychotic disorders, serious side effects have limited their clinical use. These side effects can have significant negative medical consequences and can also be distressing, thus causing doctors and patients to change medications frequently or causing patients to stop their medications entirely. Side effects of the first generation of antipsychotic drugs resulted from both "on target" effects mediated by D_2 receptor blockade and "off target effects" mediated by actions at many other receptors **16–2**.

Side effects due to D_2 receptor antagonism include extrapyramidal motor side effects and hyperprolactinemia. Synthesis and release of prolactin by anterior pituitary lactotrophs are inhibited by dopamine released from the arcuate nucleus of the hypothalamus acting on D_2 receptors (Chapter 10). Antipsychotic drugs with high affinity for D_2 receptors can thereby cause elevated levels of prolactin resulting in galactorrhea and sexual dysfunction.

Extrapyramidal side effects can be divided into four major categories (see **17–1** and **17–3** in Chapter 17). The first consists of a syndrome that resembles **Parkinson disease**. This syndrome is characterized by rigidity, difficulty in initiating movements, mask-like facial expressions, and a resting tremor. A second type is **acute dystonia**, which is characterized by a sudden and spastic contraction of muscles—often those of the face and neck. Dystonic reactions may be dramatic and disturbing, as well as excruciatingly painful, to individuals who experience them. A third category of extrapyramidal symptoms consists of **akathisia**, characterized by a subjective sense of anxiety and intense restlessness. Such drug-induced akathisia is commonly mistaken for psychotic agitation, which may lead to mistaken decisions to increase doses of antipsychotic drugs when an opposite strategy may be indicated. The fourth category of extrapyramidal side effect is **tardive dyskinesia**, late onset involuntary abnormal choreiform movements (Chapter 17). Tardive dyskinesia occurs mainly with long-term drug exposure and is not readily reversible after cessation of drug treatment. A potentially debilitating side effect, risk of tardive dyskinesia has severely limited the use of first-generation antipsychotic drugs.

Because D_2 receptor antagonism is both the therapeutic mechanism of antipsychotic drugs and the cause of elevated prolactin levels and extrapyramidal side effects, all antipsychotic drugs have some liability for these adverse reactions. However, the risk correlates with the affinity of a drug for the D_2 dopamine receptor and the dose used. High-potency antipsychotic drugs such as haloperidol have a high affinity for D_2 dopamine receptors, and thus have a greater liability for these side effects than lower potency drugs, such as chlorpromazine. In addition, many low-potency first-generation antipsychotic drugs possess anticholinergic (antimuscarinic) properties that

16–2   Pharmacologic Properties of Classic Neuroleptics

Drug	Approximate Dose Equivalent (mg)	Sedative Effect	Hypotensive Effect	Anticholinergic Effect	Extrapyramidal Effect
Phenothiazines					
Aliphatic					
Chlorpromazine (Thorazine)	100	High	High	Medium	Low
Triflupromazine (Vesprin)	30	High	High	Medium	Medium
Piperidines					
Mesoridazine (Serentil)	50	Medium	Medium	Medium	Medium
Thioridazine (Mellaril)	95	High	High	High	Low
Piperazines					
Acetophenazine (Tindal)	15	Low	Low	Low	Medium
Fluphenazine (Prolixin, Permitil)	2	Medium	Low	Low	High
Perphenazine (Trilafon)	8	Low	Low	Low	High
Trifluoperazine (Stelazine)	5	Medium	Low	Low	High
Thioxanthenes					
Aliphatic					
Chlorprothixene (Taractan)	75	High	High	High	Low
Piperazine					
Thiothixene (Navane)	5	Low	Low	Low	High
Dibenzodiazepines					
Loxapine (Loxitane, Daxolin)	10	Medium	Medium	Medium	High
Clozapine (Clozaril)	100	High	High	High	Very low
Butyrophenones					
Droperidol (Inapsine—injection only)	1	Low	Low	Low	High
Haloperidol (Haldol)	2	Low	Low	Low	High
Indolone					
Molindone (Moban)	10	Medium	Low	Medium	High
Diphenylbutylpiperidine					
Pimozide (Orap)	1	Low	Low	Low	High

Reproduced with permission from Hyman SE, Arana GW, Rosenbaum JF. *Handbook of Psychiatric Drug Therapy*, 3rd ed. Boston: Little Brown and Co.1995.

ameliorate extrapyramidal side effects, although not hyperprolactinemia. In fact, when high-potency first-generation antipsychotic drugs are used, they are often coadministered with drugs that have antimuscarinic properties such as **benztropine** or **diphenhydramine** (Chapter 6).

Off-target effects of antipsychotic drugs include sedation, which results from the blocking H_1 histamine receptors, muscarinic cholinergic receptors, and possibly α_1-adrenergic receptors in the CNS. Hypotension results from the antagonism of α_1-adrenergic receptors. Autonomic side effects such as dry mouth, blurred vision, urinary retention, and constipation (Chapter 9) are caused by the antagonism of muscarinic cholinergic receptors. Delirium, which may occur in the elderly or in patients receiving multiple anticholinergic drugs, is most often due to blockade of muscarinic cholinergic receptors in the CNS. Even among the first-generation drugs there is a wide diversity of affinities for different neurotransmitter receptors permitting some ability to trade off side effects depending on the situation of a particular patient.

Second-generation antipsychotic drugs   The first-generation antipsychotic drugs were quite successful in their ability to treat the positive psychotic symptoms of schizophrenia and other disorders. They had significant limitations, however, because of side effects, most notably extrapyramidal symptoms, and limited efficacy.

Specifically, these drugs produced only modest benefits for negative symptoms and had no significant efficacy against cognitive symptoms. These limitations stimulated a search for better antipsychotic drugs.

The prototype for a second generation of antipsychotic drugs was an older drug with "atypical" properties, **clozapine** 16–7 . Clozapine was initially believed to be an ordinary low-potency antipsychotic drug. However, it produced far fewer extrapyramidal symptoms than expected compared with other drugs. Despite this apparent benefit, its introduction into the United States was delayed for many years because approximately 1% of patients develop agranulocytosis (a significant decrease in white blood cells), a potentially fatal side effect. Clozapine had other problematic side effects as well, among them sedation, weight gain, drooling, and a decrease in seizure threshold. However, clinical trials demonstrated that clozapine could produce significant benefit to schizophrenic patients who had failed to respond to other antipsychotic drugs, including significant improvement in negative symptoms. As a result, clozapine was approved in the United States in 1990 with a requirement for weekly white blood cell counts. It is now recognized that clozapine has a very low risk of producing extrapyramidal side effects including tardive dyskinesia. The combination of unique efficacy and diminished risk of motor side effects stimulated the development of new drugs, using some of the properties of clozapine as a prototype, while trying to avoid its liabilities.

Pharmacology of second-generation antipsychotic drugs   Detailed examination of the receptor binding properties of clozapine revealed that it has antagonist or possibly inverse agonist properties at many neurotransmitter receptors 16–8 . An important characteristic that explains its low risk of extrapyramidal side effects and lack of effect on prolactin levels appears to be its relatively low affinity for D_2 receptors. Clozapine exhibits a relatively higher affinity for the D_3 and D_4 dopamine receptors, which are expressed at low levels in the dorsal striatum but at higher levels in the ventral striatum and in the prefrontal cortex. However, the role of D_3 and D_4 receptors in antipsychotic drug action remains unclear. Many first-generation antipsychotic drugs, including haloperidol, display high affinity for the D_3 receptor. Furthermore, a selective D_4 antagonist failed to exhibit antipsychotic properties in clinical trials, as stated earlier.

Serotonergic mechanisms had once elicited interest as a possible contributor to psychotic disorders because LSD, a $5HT_{2A}$ partial agonist (Chapter 6), produces hallucinations. It was recognized, however, that the effects of LSD and related hallucinogens were quite unlike the symptoms of schizophrenia. Clozapine rekindled interest in serotonin because it is a high affinity antagonist of multiple serotonin receptors, notably including the $5HT_{2A}$ receptor. While evidence for an independent antipsychotic action of $5HT_{2A}$ receptor blockade is very weak, several lines of evidence suggest that blockade of these receptors might limit the extrapyramidal liability of antipsychotic medications. Consequently, a high ratio of $5HT_{2A}$ to D_2 receptor affinity became a design principle for many second-generation drugs. Examples include **risperidone, olanzapine** (a close chemical analog of clozapine), **quetiapine, ziprasidone, sertindole,** and **paliperidone** (an active metabolite of risperidone). **Aripiprazole,** another second-generation antipsychotic drug, is similar to the aforementioned drugs by virtue of being a high affinity antagonist at $5HT_{2A}$ receptors. However, it differs in that the other second-generation drugs are D_2 receptor antagonists or possibly inverse agonists, whereas aripiprazole is a high affinity D_2 receptor partial agonist. Its high D_2 receptor affinity means that its ratio of $5HT_{2A}$ to D_2 receptor affinity is low. Yet, as a partial agonist aripiprazole can act as an agonist or antagonist depending on the strength of endogenous dopamine neurotransmission. It would act as an agonist in low dopaminergic states and as an antagonist in hyperdopaminergic states. In practice it has low extrapyramidal liability and does not elevate prolactin.

The second-generation medications are effective antipsychotic drugs and cause fewer extrapyramidal symptoms than first-generation drugs, although they are not free of this risk. Depending on D_2 receptor affinity, these drugs vary in the actual incidence of extrapyramidal side effects; for instance, risperidone, with a higher D_2 receptor affinity, has a somewhat higher risk than olanzapine. As experience has accumulated, however, and as large-scale comparative clinical trials have been completed, these drugs have not met the high expectations with which they were introduced. While olanzapine may have somewhat greater efficacy than first-generation drugs in some circumstances, none of the second-generation drugs are as efficacious as clozapine and all appear in most cases to be no better than first-generation drugs with respect to the treatment of positive, negative, or cognitive symptoms.

The precise mechanism responsible for clozapine's unique clinical properties has therefore not yet been defined. Clozapine binds many receptors 16–8 , for example, it has relatively high affinity for the $5HT_{2C}$, $5HT_3$, and $5HT_6$ receptors as well as the $5HT_{2A}$ receptor. In addition, there is some thought that the metabolite **desmethylclozapine** may contribute to the unique

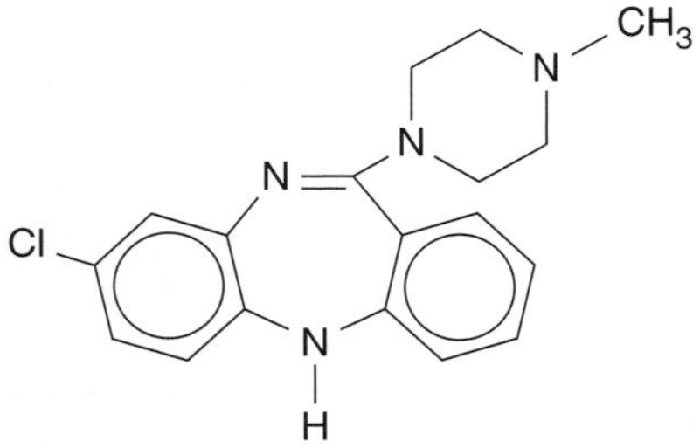

Clozapine

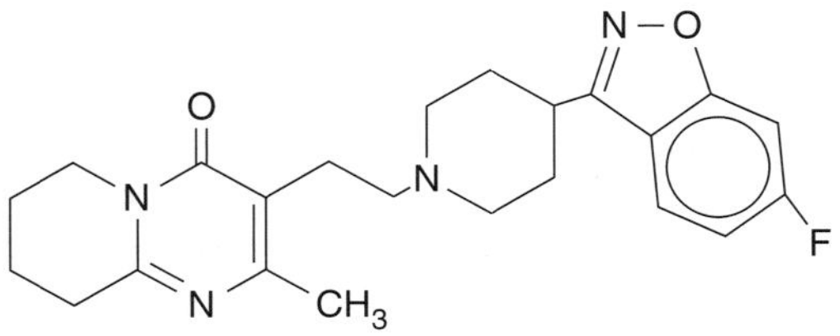

Risperidone

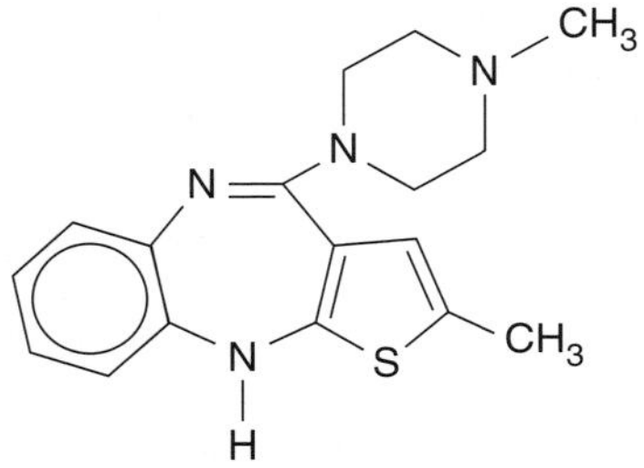

Olanzapine

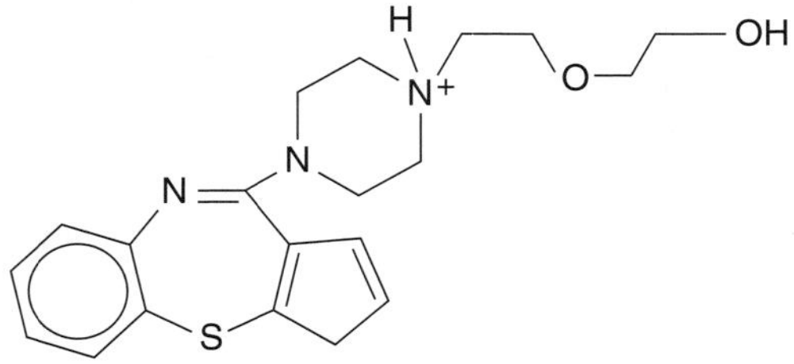

Quetiapine

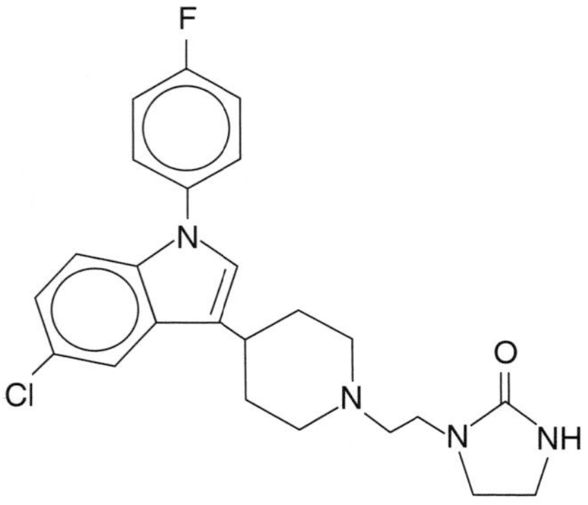

Sertindole

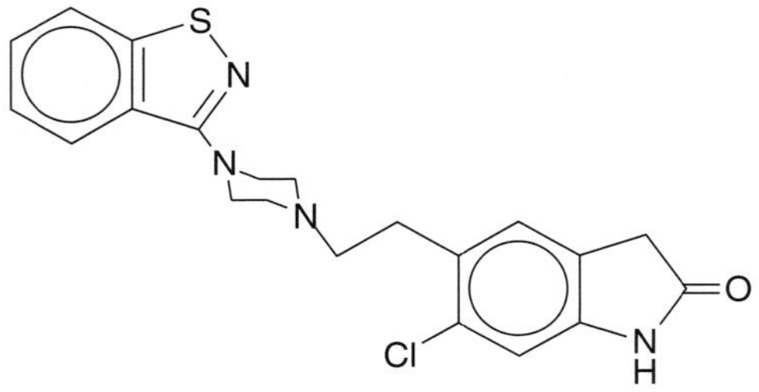

Ziprasidone

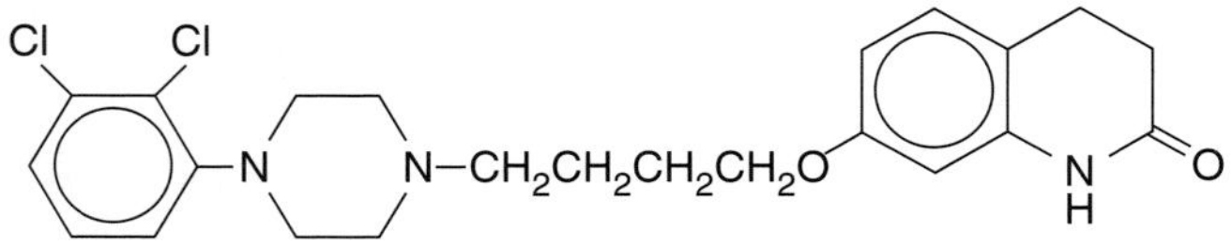

Aripiprazole

16–7 **Chemical structures of clozapine and several other second-generation antipsychotic drugs.**

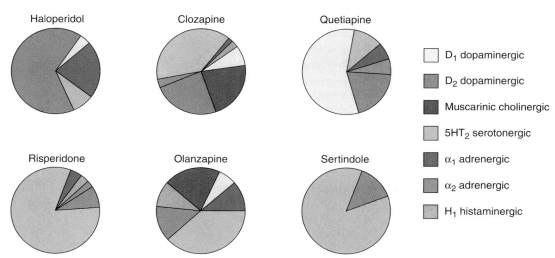

16-8 **Pie graphs comparing pharmacologic profiles of haloperidol, clozapine, and several second generation antipsychotic drugs.** (From Casey DE. The relationship of pharmacology to side effects. *J Clin Psychiatry.* 1997;58(Suppl)10:55.)

efficacy of clozapine treatment. At present, however, there is no fully convincing explanation for its greater efficacy.

While the second-generation drugs have a lower risk of extrapyramidal side effects, they bring their own side effect liability. Olanzapine and some of the other agents cause dramatic weight gain and elevate serum glucose and cholesterol. Over time this drug-induced **metabolic syndrome** would produce a high risk of **diabetes** and **cardiovascular disease**. The pharmacologic basis of the metabolic side effects of second-generation antipsychotic drugs remains unknown, although blockade of $5HT_{2C}$ receptors in melanocortin-expressing neurons of the hypothalamus is one leading hypothesis (Chapter 10).

Other strategies for treating schizophrenia As described, the NMDA glutamate receptor has been proposed as a target for antipsychotic drug action based primarily on the actions of **PCP** and like drugs. Postmortem brain studies have reported altered levels of expression of NMDA receptor subunits in the fore-brains of schizophrenics compared with normal brains. Such results offer a highly speculative possibility that hypofunction of glutamatergic neurotransmission may contribute to the pathogenesis of schizophrenia.

If indeed NMDA receptor hypofunction contributes to schizophrenia-like psychosis, it has been reasoned

that agents that augment NMDA receptor function might reverse psychotic symptoms. This hypothesis led to clinical trials involving the use of glycine to treat schizophrenia. As discussed in Chapter 5, glycine promotes NMDA receptor function by binding to a positive allosteric regulatory site on the receptor complex. **D-Cycloserine** **16-9**, a partial agonist at this glycine site, has been administered as an adjunct to antipsychotic

16-9 **Chemical structures of proposed antipsychotic drugs that act on glutamate receptors.** Note that LY2140023 is a prodrug for LY404039; it is orally absorbed and metabolized into LY404039.

drugs in clinical trials. Some small trials have reported modest benefit; others have been negative. Used as a sole agent, D-cycloserine was no better than placebo in treating negative or cognitive symptoms. The endogenous agonist for the glycine site on the NMDA receptor may be *D-Serine*, generated by *serine racemase* (Chapter 5). Accordingly, activators of this enzyme, or inhibitors of D-amino acid oxidase which metabolizes D-serine, are currently being pursued for potential use as novel antipsychotic agents.

More recently, agonists at group II metabotropic glutamate receptors (mGluRs) have been considered as possible treatments for schizophrenia. mGluR$_2$ and mGluR$_3$, which are G$_i$-linked receptors (Chapter 5), are localized at several sites at the synapse, including presynaptically on glutamatergic nerve terminals where their activation decreases glutamate release 16-10. Animal studies have documented antipsychotic-like actions of **mGluR$_{2/3}$**

agonists and one human proof of concept study has demonstrated antipsychotic effects of an mGluR$_{2/3}$ agonist 16-9 that are comparable to those of currently available medications. Importantly, this mGluR$_{2/3}$ agonist is devoid of any binding activity at dopamine or other monoamine receptors, which would suggest a fundamentally new basis of antipsychotic activity. The mechanism by which an mGluR$_{2/3}$ agonist would exert antipsychotic actions is not known, but could be related to its blockade of glutamate release in prefrontal cortex. As mentioned earlier in the chapter, animal studies have led to the speculation that psychosis may be related to *hyper*function (not *hypo*function) of overall glutamatergic transmission. While much further work is clearly needed to study the efficacy of this agent and its mechanism of action, the preclinical and early clinical studies show that this highly novel strategy deserves further investigation for the treatment of schizophrenia.

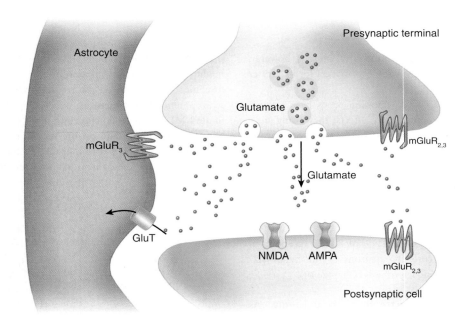

16-10 **An agonist of group II (types 2 and 3) metabotropic glutamate receptors (mGluRs) showed a therapeutic effect in schizophrenia in a clinical proof of concept (Phase II) trial.** Such mGluR$_{2/3}$ agonists act by modulating neurotransmission. As shown, the receptors (predominantly GluR$_2$) are found on presynaptic neurons where they inhibit neurotransmitter release (including that of glutamate) and postsynaptically where they modify the actions of glutamate at ionotropic glutamate receptors (ie, AMPA and NMDA receptors). Group II mGluRs (predominantly GluR$_3$) are also found on glia where they regulate expression of the glial glutamate transporter, which would further modify glutamatergic transmission. Which action mediates the putative antipsychotic activity of an mGluR$_{2/3}$ agonist is not known with certainty.

The Future

Despite the extraordinary advances in the treatment of schizophrenia and other psychotic disorders that have occurred during the second half of the past century, much work remains to be done. In particular, it will crucial to discover genes that confer risk for schizophrenia and identify environmental and perhaps epigenetic factors that modify this genetic risk. These advances will be important in gaining a much more sophisticated understanding of the etiology and pathophysiology of psychotic disorders, at the molecular, cellular, and neural circuit levels, so that rational drug treatments of greater efficacy and safety can be developed.

SELECTED READING

Arnold SE, Trojanowski JQ, Gur RE, et al. Absence of neurodegeneration and neural injury in the cerebral cortex in a sample of elderly patients with schizophrenia. *Arch Gen Psychiatry.* 1998;55: 225–232.

Barch DM, Carter CS, Braver TS, et al. Selective deficits in prefrontal cortex function in medication-naive patients with schizophrenia. *Arch Gen Psychiatry.* 2001;58:280–288.

Boos HBM, Aleman A, Cahn W, et al. Brain volumes in relative of patients with schizophrenia. A meta-analysis. *Arch Gen Psychiatry.* 2007;64:297–304.

Buchanan RW, Javitt DC, Marder SR, et al. The cognitive and negative symptoms in schizophrenia trial (CONSIST): the efficacy of glutamatergic agents for negative symptoms and cognitive impairments. *Am J Psychiatry.* 2007;164: 1593–1602.

Cannon TD, Thompson PM, van Erp TG, et al. Cortex mapping reveals regionally specific patterns of genetic and disease-specific gray-matter deficits in twins discordant for schizophrenia. *Proc Natl Acad Sci USA.* 2002;99:3228–3233.

Craddock N, O'Donovan MC, Owen MJ. The genetics of schizophrenia and bipolar disorder: dissecting psychosis. *J Med Genet.* 2005;42:193–204.

Glantz LA, Lewis DA. Decreased dendritic spine density on prefrontal cortical pyramidal neurons in schizophrenia. *Arch Gen Psychiatry.* 2000;57:65–73.

Goldman-Rakic PS. Cellular basis of working memory. *Neuron.* 1995;14:477–485.

Harrison PJ. The neuropathology of schizophrenia. A critical review of the data and their interpretation. *Brain.* 1999;122:593–624.

Kane J, Honigfeld G, Singer J, et al. Clozapine for the treatment-resistant schizophrenic. A double-blind comparison with chlorpromazine. *Arch Gen Psychiatry.* 1988;45:789–96.

Keefe RS, Bilder RM, Davis SM, et al. Neurocognitive effects of antipsychotic medications in patients with chronic schizophrenia in the CATIE Trial. *Arch Gen Psychiatry.* 2007;64: 633–647.

Kety SS, Rosenthal D, Wender PH, et al. The types and prevalence of mental illness in the biological and adoptive families of adopted schizophrenics. *J Psychiatry Res.* 1968;6:345–362.

Kishi T, Elmquist JK. Body weight is regulated by the brain: a link between feeding and emotion. *Mol Psychiatry.* 2005;10:132–146.

Laursen TM, Labouriau R, Licht RW, et al. Family history of psychiatric illness as a risk factor for schizoaffective disorder. *Arch Gen Psychiatry.* 2005;62: 841–848.

Leonard BE. Sigma receptors and sigma ligands: background to a pharmacological enigma. *Pharmacopsychiatry.* 2004;37 Suppl 3:S166–S170.

Lewis DA, Levitt P. Schizophrenia as a disorder of neurodevelopment. *Annu Rev Neurosci.* 2002;25: 409–432.

Lieberman JA, Stroup TS, McEvoy JP, et al. Effectiveness of antipsychotic drugs in patients with chronic schizophrenia. *N Engl J Med.* 2005;353: 1209–1223.

Mamo D, Graff A, Mizrahi R, et al. Differential effects of aripiprazole on D(2), 5HT(2), and 5HT(1A) receptor occupancy in patients with schizophrenia: a triple tracer PET study. *Am J Psychiatry.* 2007;164: 1411–1417.

Meyer-Lindenberg A, Weinberger DR. Intermediate phenotypes and genetic mechanisms of psychiatric disorders. *Nature Rev Neuroscience.* 2006;7: 818–827

Moghaddam B. Targeting metabotropic glutamate receptors for treatment of the cognitive symptoms of schizophrenia. *Psychopharmacology.* 2004;174: 39–44.

Owen MJ, Craddock N, Jablensky A. The genetic deconstruction of psychosis. *Schizophr Bull.* 2007;33:905–911.

Patil ST, Zhang L, Martenyi F, et al. Activation of mGlu2/3 receptors as a new approach to treat schizophrenia: a randomized Phase 2 clinical trial. *Nat Med.* 2007;13:1102–1107.

Perala J, Suvisaari J, Saarni SI, et al. Lifetime prevalence of psychotic and bipolar I disorders in a general population. *Arch Gen Psychiatry.* 2007;64: 19–28.

Ross CA, Margolis RL, Reading SA, et al. Neurobiology of schizophrenia. *Neuron.* 2006;52:139–153.

Siever LJ, Davis KL. The pathophysiology of schizophrenia disorders: perspectives from the spectrum. *Am J Psychiatry*. 2004;161:398–413.

Tamminga CA, Holcomb HH. Phenotype of schizophrenia: a review and formulation. *Mol Psychiatry*. 2005;10:27–39.

Thompson PM, Vidal C, Giedd JN, et al. Mapping adolescent brain change reveals dynamic wave of accelerated gray matter loss in very early-onset schizophrenia. *Proc Natl Acad Sci USA*. 2001;98:11650–11655.

Vidal CN, Rapoport JL, Hayashi KM, et al. Dynamically spreading frontal and cingulate deficits mapped in adolescents with schizophrenia. *Arch Gen Psychiatry*. 2006;63:25–34

Vijayraghavan S, Wang M, Birnbaum SG, et al. Inverted-U dopamine D_1 receptor actions on prefrontal neurons engaged in working memory. *Nature Neurosci*. 2007;10:376–384.

CHAPTER 17

Neurodegeneration

- Neurodegenerative diseases, of which Alzheimer disease and Parkinson disease are the most common, are a large and diverse group of neurologic disorders characterized by death of neurons.

- The major processes by which neurons die are necrosis and apoptosis (programmed cell death); both processes involve cascades of proteins including proteolytic enzymes of the caspase family. These mechanisms, once thought entirely distinct, appear to have significant overlap.

- Processes that can initiate cell death include mitochondrial dysfunction, excitotoxicity, oxidative stress, and abnormal protein aggregation.

- Abnormal mitochondrial function plays a key role in apoptosis and other forms of neurodegeneration.

- Excitotoxicity involves excessive activation of neurons via stimulation of glutamate receptors or other mechanisms of depolarization, which trigger biochemical cascades that lead to cell death.

- The pathologic hallmarks of Alzheimer disease, the most common cause of severe memory impairment in the elderly, are senile plaques, neurofibrillary tangles, dystrophic neurites, and neuronal loss.

- The development of Alzheimer disease may be due to the improper biochemical processing of amyloid precursor protein (APP) and the subsequent accumulation of β amyloid.

- Inherited forms of Alzheimer disease have been linked to mutations in APP or in proteins called presenilins, which regulate the processing of APP.

- Currently there is no effective treatment for Alzheimer disease, although several pharmacologic strategies for preventing the buildup of β amyloid appear promising.

- Loss of dopamine input to the basal ganglia causes the symptoms of Parkinson disease; restoration of dopamine function, for example, with the dopamine precursor L-dopa, remains the mainstay of therapy for the disease.

- Rare familial forms of Parkinson disease are caused by mutation in several genes related to protein aggregation, including α-synuclein and parkin.

- Huntington disease is caused by a mutation in the gene for huntingtin; the mutation increases the number of glutamine residues expressed in the protein, which is pathogenic.

- Amyotrophic lateral sclerosis or ALS is caused by the selective death of upper motor neurons in the cerebral cortex and/or lower motor neurons in the spinal cord.

Because the vast majority of neurons in an adult are postmitotic, the brain has limited capacity to compensate for cells lost during pathologic processes, such as neurodegeneration, stroke, and traumatic injury. As a result, enormous attention has been focused on understanding mechanisms of neuronal cell death in the hope that novel therapeutics can be developed to minimize or prevent cell loss. Cell death has typically been categorized as either programmed (*apoptotic*) or *necrotic*, although recent findings have revealed overlapping molecular pathways underlying the two. Identification of multiple forms of nonapoptotic programmed cell death has further blurred the distinction between necrosis and apoptosis. In addition, two forms of cell death appear to be unique to neurons: *excitotoxicity* and *protein aggregation*. This chapter begins with a basic overview of the molecular and cellular mechanisms of these distinct processes of neurodegeneration. The second portion of the Chapter focuses on several severe brain disorders, including **Alzheimer disease**, **frontotemporal dementia**, **Parkinson disease**, **Huntington disease,** and **amyotrophic lateral sclerosis** (**ALS**), each of which is characterized by a unique pattern and mechanism of neurodegeneration. Although disease-altering treatments for these disorders remain lacking, we will discuss new approaches to intervene therapeutically based on our evolving knowledge of the molecular mechanisms of disease pathogenesis.

NECROSIS

In response to several types of environmental insults, often termed "cellular stress," neurons activate a series of intracellular stress pathways. Examples of such cellular stresses include ischemia (lack of oxygen), UV irradiation, virus infection, free radicals, and various toxins. Intracellular pathways activated by these cellular stresses are designed to turn off nonessential cellular functions, limit the internal damage, activate repair mechanisms, and allow the cell to survive homeostatic challenges. However, when a neuron receives excessive injury, these stress response pathways are overwhelmed, resulting in depletion of energy stores and loss of membrane integrity. The resulting necrotic neurons and the organelles they contain swell until their membranes eventually burst. Necrosis is exactly what might be expected of a cell undergoing failure of active transport, membrane integrity, and osmotic stability, all of which ultimately result in disintegration. Necrosis is accompanied by the leakage of cytoplasmic and organelle contents into the extracellular space;

such leakage can be toxic to neighboring cells and can promote inflammatory processes. The molecular mechanisms underlying responses to cellular stress are becoming increasingly well understood **17-1**.

APOPTOSIS

Apoptosis, a process of programmed cell death, is essential for the survival of an organism. In the nervous system, it enables the pruning of excess neurons during development, and thereby contributes to the formation of anatomically precise and correct connections between nerve cells. However, increasing evidence indicates that apoptotic mechanisms of neuronal death also contribute to several neurodegenerative disorders and to decrements in brain function associated with aging. Consequently, considerable attention is focused on understanding the precise molecular basis of apoptosis and on developing medicinal agents that interfere with these processes. A brief overview of molecular mechanisms of apoptosis is provided in **17-1**.

Apoptotic neurons undergo a series of tightly regulated changes characterized by chromatin aggregation, exocytosis of membrane-bound cytoplasmic fragments (apoptotic bodies), and progressive loss of cell volume. Apoptosis is generally recognized as a series of steps undertaken by a doomed cell in order to prevent necrosis. In contrast to necrosis, during apoptosis potentially dangerous intracellular material is packaged into vesicles that can be safely taken up into surrounding cells by endocytosis and metabolized. Unlike necrosis, which is a passive process, cell death by apoptosis results from the execution of active and well-regulated genetic programs. In many biologic systems, inhibition of gene transcription or protein synthesis can prevent apoptosis, underscoring its active nature.

Apoptosis may result in the death of neurons only moderately affected by injury. For instance, it may affect neurons that undergo a mild or short-lived ischemic event, such as those in a peri-infarct area, which is the area between severely ischemic and normal tissue in the period immediately following a **stroke**. In cortical cell cultures treated with very high levels of N-methyl-D-aspartate (NMDA) (which activates NMDA glutamate receptors; see Chapter 5) or nitric oxide (NO) plus superoxide, neuronal death is generally observed to be necrotic; however, with lower levels of NMDA or NO–superoxide, apoptosis occurs. These findings suggest that severely damaged neurons undergo necrosis before a more controlled process of apoptosis can occur, whereas in moderately damaged

17–1 **Cell Death and Survival Pathways**

Tremendous progress has been made in understanding the dynamic balance between death signals (orange in figure) and survival signals (purple in figure) in neurons. The figure depicts just a small portion of the complex intracellular signaling pathways governing cell death and survival. There is considerable overlap between mechanisms of necrosis and apoptosis, such that many of the pathways shown in the figure contribute to both processes.

Cell death can be triggered by intracellular or extracellular pathways. The extracellular pathway involves transmembrane receptors, such as Fas (the name comes from an antibody screen), TNFα (tumor necrosis factor-α), and p75 (also called the

low affinity neurotrophin receptor; see Chapter 8). These proteins contain a conserved death domain, which recruits and activates caspases (Casp) 8 or 10 by means of death-domain adaptor proteins such as TRADD (TNF receptor-associated death domain) and FADD (Fas-associated death domain). These caspases, in turn, activate effector caspases, caspases-3, -6 and -7, which trigger cell death via the fragmentation of cell structures.

In contrast to the extracellular pathway, the intracellular pathway relies on permeabilization of the outer membrane of mitochondria by pro-death Bcl-2 family members. Proteins such as Bax (Bcl-2 associated protein X), Bak (Bcl-2 homologous

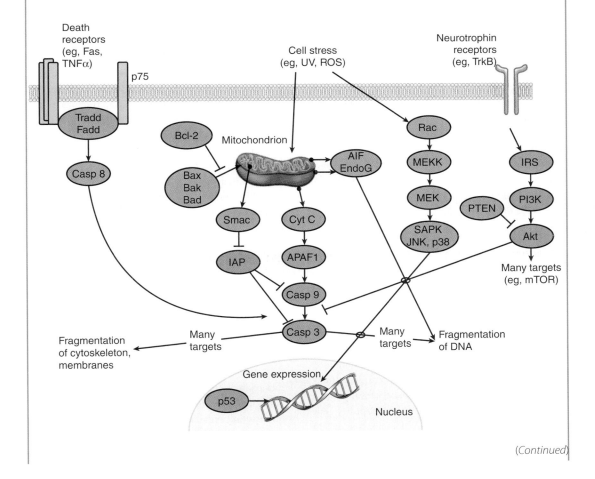

(Continued)

17–1   **Cell Death and Survival Pathways (*Continued*)**

antagonist/killer), or Bad oligomerize in the mito-chondrial membrane and permit the release of pro-death proteins such as cytochrome c (Cyt c), SMAC (second mitochondrial activator of caspases), Endo G (endonuclease G), and AIF (apoptosis inducing factor). Prosurvival Bcl-2 family members, including Bcl-2 and Bcl-Xl, interfere with Bax and inhibit mitochondrial permeabilization. Upon release from the mitochondria, cytochrome c binds to a cytoplasmic adapter protein called apoptosis-activating factor 1 (Apaf1) which allows for oligomerization and autoproteolytic activation of caspase-9. Activated caspase-9, much like caspase-8, can cleave caspases-3, -6, and -7 to initiate a self-amplifying cascade which leads to apoptosis. SMAC induces apoptosis by inhibiting the prosurvival IAPs (inhibitors of apoptosis) which inhibit caspases. Endo G and AIF promote apoptosis by translocating to the nucleus where they induce large-scale fragmentation of DNA.

Cellular stress, which can be produced by a variety of agents and environmental factors, induces deleterious effects on cells in part via activation of Jun N-terminal kinase (JNK) and p38, both types of SAP-kinase (stress-activated protein kinase). JNK and p38 are protein serine–threonine kinases that are involved in one branch of the MAP-kinase cascades (see Chapter 4 for more detailed discussion of these cascades). Activation of specific forms of MAP-kinase kinases (MEK kinases), a process that depends on the Ras-like small G protein Rac, leads to activation of a series of MEKs and ultimately to

the activation of JNK or p38. In vitro and in vivo studies have indicated that JNK and p38 are involved in both necrotic and apoptotic forms of cell death. A primary target of JNK is the activation of transcription factors c-Jun and ATF2 (activating transcription factor 2). c-Jun levels are elevated in the CNS after cellular stress, and dominant negative forms of c-Jun protect cells from certain forms of injury.

An interesting question raised by these findings is: What is the normal function of cellular stress pathways? Presumably, transient activation of JNK and p38 triggered by more mild forms of stress serves to protect the cell from long-term injury by initiating homeostatic responses. Perhaps excessive or more sustained activation of these pathways, as seen under abnormal conditions, leads to cell death. Further work is needed to better understand the normal functioning of these pathways and to assess whether their pharmacologic inhibition may be of use under certain pathophysiologic conditions.

One of the prototypical triggers for apoptosis, at least in vitro, is the withdrawal of neurotrophic factors. Neurotrophic factor receptors, such as the TrkA receptor for NGF or the IGF-I receptor for insulin-like growth factor, activate prosurvival signaling cascades; these involve the sequential activation of insulin receptor substrate (IRS), phosphatidylinositol-3-kinase (PI3K), and Akt (a serine/threonine kinase). Akt phosphorylates proapoptotic proteins such as Bad and caspase-9, inhibiting their apoptotic action.

---

neurons apoptotic processes may be initiated as a way to dispose of damaged neurons in a safer manner.

Thus, apoptosis provides a safe means of removing damaged cells, including those that are potentially cancerous. For example, the tumor suppressor *p53* is a transcription factor that activates pro-apoptotic gene expression in response to DNA damage that might lead to cell transformation (see figure in **17–1**). For this reason, as the field strives to develop inhibitors of apoptosis to limit neuronal loss in neurodegenerative disorders, caution must be exercised with respect to potentially serious side effects of inhibiting this crucial physiologic process.

Cellular Markers of Apoptosis

One of the hallmark characteristics of apoptosis involves the breakdown of double-stranded DNA into nucleosomal segments (Chapter 4). This breakdown makes it possible for apoptosis to be observed, because the resulting segments are equally spaced and can be visualized as DNA "laddering" on an electrophoretic gel. Histologically, apoptosis can be distinguished from necrosis with the use of a technique called terminal transferase-mediated dUTP-biotin nick end-labeling (*TUNEL*). This technique involves the end-labeling of DNA in tissue sections with a fluorescent marker.

Because the fragmented DNA in apoptotic cells has many free ends, TUNEL-labeled cells incorporate more of the fluorescent probe and glow brightly.

Role of Mitochondria

Mitochondria are critically involved in the regulation of apoptosis. The triggering of apoptosis is mediated by altering ratios of members of the B-cell lymphoma protein 2 (*Bcl-2*) family of proteins. Proapoptotic Bcl-2 family members promote cell death by permeabilizing the outer membrane of mitochondria and releasing numerous pro-death proteins into the cytoplasm (see figure in 17-1). These proteins cannot exert their pro-death actions when contained in the intramembrane space between the inner and outer membranes of the mitochrondria due to the actions of antiapoptotic members of the Bcl-2 family. Once in the cytoplasm, the released mitochondrial proteins promote cell death by systematically dismantling specific targets important to cell functioning. Some translocate into the nucleus and induce large-scale DNA fragmentation. Others, like cytochrome c, activate a family of proteases, termed caspases, which induce apoptosis.

Caspases

Caspases (short for cysteine aspartate proteases) cleave and inactivate prosurvival proteins and activate proapoptotic proteins in an amplifying cascade that leads to the rapid fragmentation of cell structures (see 17-1). Under basal conditions, caspases exist as inactive proenzymes until they are activated by proteolytic cleavage. After it enters the cytoplasm, cytochrome c triggers the cleavage and activation of caspase-9. Activation of caspase-9 then triggers the cleavage and activation of several other caspases including caspases-3, -6, and -7. After they are activated, caspases cleave numerous types of proteins that trigger fragmentation of DNA, cytoskeletal proteins, and other cell structures.

Potential Antiapoptotic Therapies

Researchers are now trying to determine whether interference with apoptotic processes will improve treatment outcomes, such as decreasing the area of infarction caused by **stroke**. For instance, overexpression of the antiapoptosis Bcl-2 gene, or knockout of the proapoptosis Bax gene, reduces infarction in rodent brains subjected to focal ischemic insults (see Chapter 19 for further discussion of stroke). These findings indicate that inhibition of apoptotic pathways may indeed be neuroprotective. New treatments have focused on combining apoptosis inhibition with additional agents, such as antioxidants, neuronal growth factors, ion channel blockers, or thrombolytic compounds to achieve synergistic benefits.

Caspase inhibitors offer an attractive target for pharmaceutical development in part because of the relative ease in designing a drug to inhibit the active site of a protease. Some of the most effective treatments for **HIV (human immunodeficiency virus)** are aspartyl protease inhibitors. Currently available caspase inhibitors consist of small peptides that do not readily cross the blood-brain barrier or enter cells. Major efforts are under way to develop small molecule inhibitors that might overcome such limitations. However, as stated earlier, such inhibitors must be developed with caution, given the evidence that apoptosis is important in protecting the organism from damaged and potentially cancerous cells. Under some circumstances, interference with apoptosis may worsen stroke-related damage. If neurons were to undergo necrosis instead of apoptosis, increased damage to healthy neighboring neurons might result.

BASIC MECHANISMS OF EXCITOTOXICITY

One form of cell death unique to neurons is excitotoxicity. When blood flow to brain tissue is interrupted, eg, during a stroke, conduits through which oxygen and nutrients enter cells, and potentially toxic metabolites exit, are severed. Interference with blood flow triggers many biochemical changes in the extracellular environment of the affected area of the brain. These changes lead rapidly to a large number of cellular disruptions including depletion of ATP stores, loss of ion gradients, Ca^{2+} pouring into cells through open channels, and activation of numerous second messenger systems. Many of these biochemical changes are very harmful to neurons and contribute to the neuronal death that results from prolonged ischemia. However, some of the sequelae of ischemia may have little effect on neuronal survival and some may even have neuroprotective effects, representing homeostatic responses to ischemic insult that neurons produce in self-defense. Accordingly, strategies designed to minimize infarct-related neural damage must be based on a clear understanding of how each ischemia-related process affects neuronal survival 17-1 .

Depletion of Energy Stores

Under normal conditions, the brain uses oxygen and glucose to produce adenosine triphosphate (ATP)

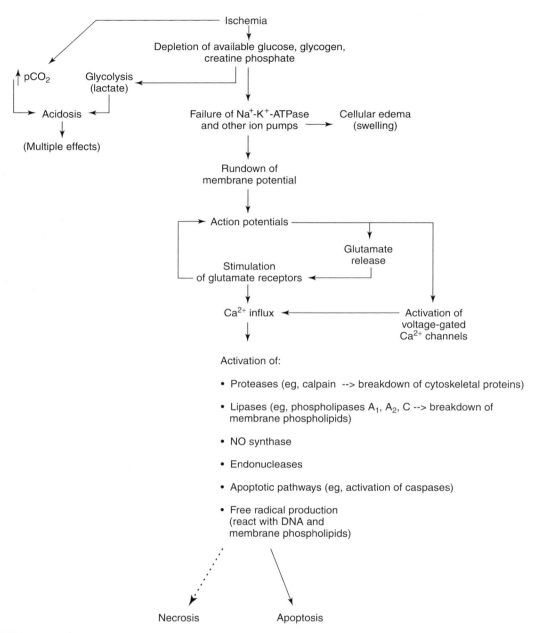

17–1 Events that lead to cell death, including apoptosis and necrosis, after ischemia.

through the processes of glycolysis and oxidative phosphorylation. Complete interruption of brain blood flow can deplete the brain's supply of oxygen within 10 seconds. In the absence of oxygen, oxidative phosphorylation ceases, and anaerobic glycolysis becomes the only source of ATP for neurons. Anaerobic glycolysis supplies less than 10% of the ATP garnered from complete oxidation of glucose and leads to the production of lactic acid. Moreover, without incoming blood to supply glucose, neurons must rely on the glycolytic processing of preexisting stores of glucose and glycogen. During ischemia, these reserves are depleted within 2 to 3 minutes. Phosphocreatine stores also are consumed during this time. Consequently, ischemia can lead to the depletion of neuronal ATP within minutes. Because the basal metabolic activity of neurons is so great, such depletion rapidly leads to serious consequences.

Failure of Ion Pumps

One of the most important consequences of the loss of available ATP is the failure of ATP-dependent ion pumps and the subsequent dissipation of the resting membrane potential of neurons. As discussed in Chapter 2, the maintenance of the resting membrane potential is ultimately dependent on Na^+-K^+-ATPase, which exports Na^+ and imports K^+ against their concentration gradients at the cost of ATP. Although very large neurons can maintain a negative resting potential for some time after the inhibition of Na^+-K^+-ATPase, small and highly branched neurons of the mammalian brain are extremely vulnerable to loss of Na^+-K^+-ATPase activity because of their very large surface area to volume ratio. Accordingly, many CNS neurons depolarize rapidly after ATP depletion.

Loss of Na^+-K^+-ATPase activity has other consequences in addition to depolarization. Many ion pumps, including the Na^+–Ca^{2+} exchanger, are dependent on the transmembrane Na^+ gradient for their activity. As this gradient declines, so does the activity of these exchange systems, which leads to further disruptions of ionic equilibrium. Moreover, many ATP-dependent ion pumps, such as ATP-dependent Ca^{2+} pumps, are disabled when neuronal energy stores are depleted.

Neuronal Depolarization and Firing

As neurons depolarize they fire more action potentials and, as such firing escalates, further depolarization occurs, causing a still further rundown of the many ionic gradients required for normal neuronal function. Increased neuronal firing and increased cellular levels of free Ca^{2+} trigger the uncontrolled release of neurotransmitters including the powerful excitatory neurotransmitter, glutamate (Chapter 5). Released glutamate can then trigger neighboring neurons to depolarize and fire action potentials, further extending the injurious chain of events.

Neural damage caused by excessive release of glutamate is potentiated by the failure of glutamate transporters. As explained in Chapter 5, these transporters, which are expressed by glial and neural cells, assist in terminating the actions of synaptically released glutamate by removing glutamate from the synaptic cleft. This reuptake process depends on ATP; thus when ATP stores in the brain become depleted in response to ischemia, the functioning of these transporters is compromised. Subsequently, higher than normal levels of glutamate accumulate in synapses and cause activation of glutamate receptors for abnormally long periods of time.

The role of glutamate in excitotoxicity has spurred the investigation of drugs that block glutamate action in situations of ischemia such as **stroke** (Chapter 19). Early studies evaluated the utility of potent NMDA receptor antagonists, such as **MK-801**. However, all of these drugs can induce cognitive distortions, dissociation, and hallucinations. Indeed, **phencyclidine** (**PCP**), also known as angel dust, is abused to produce these symptoms. Unfortunately, it has not been possible to separate the neuroprotective effects of potent NMDA antagonists from their unwanted psychotropic actions (Chapter 16). One potential intervention is **memantine**, a weaker NMDA antagonist, although the clinical efficacy of memantine is limited, and the mechanism for these modest clinical effects may be unrelated to NMDA receptor blockade, as described below under **Alzheimer disease**.

Increases in Intracellular Calcium

Under normal conditions, concentrations of cytosolic Ca^{2+} are under extremely tight regulation (Chapter 2). In a neuron at rest, these concentrations are approximately 100 nM, whereas extracellular Ca^{2+} concentrations are in the millimolar range. With extracellular Ca^{2+} approaching concentrations that are 10,000 times greater than cytosolic concentrations, there is normally a tremendous driving force for Ca^{2+} to enter the neuronal cytoplasm. The great effort that a neuron expends in maintaining a low cytosolic Ca^{2+} concentration is compromised during ischemia **17–2**. Ca^{2+} that enters the cytosol is removed by a variety of mechanisms, including the ATP-dependent Ca^{2+} pumps and Na^+–Ca^{2+} exchangers previously mentioned. Both of these pumps are ultimately ATP-dependent because ATP-dependent maintenance of the Na^+ gradient is required for the effective performance of the Na^+–Ca^{2+} exchanger; indeed, as the Na^+ gradient dissipates, it may even reverse and cause Ca^{2+} to be pumped into the cell. Depolarization also can lead to the opening of various voltage-gated Ca^{2+} channels, and glutamate release from neighboring cells can induce the entry of Ca^{2+} through NMDA and certain AMPA receptors. As a result, **Ca^{2+} channel blockers**, alone or in combination with other agents, are being studied as potential novel treatments for excitotoxicity, such as that seen during **stroke** (Chapter 19).

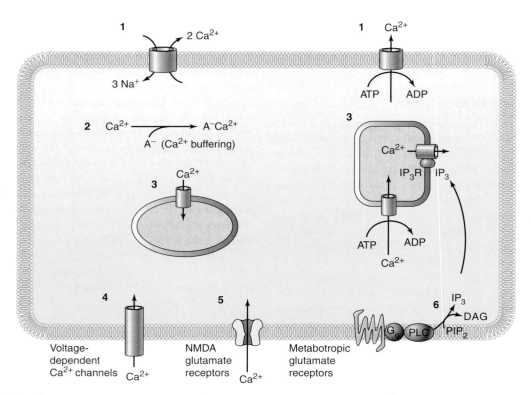

17-2 **Ca²⁺ homeostasis in neurons. 1.** Ca^{2+} is removed from the cytoplasm by Ca^{2+}–Na^+ exchangers and adenosine triphosphate (ATP)-dependent pumps. **2.** Ca^{2+} is buffered by intracellular anions (A^-). **3.** Subsequently it is sequestered in organelles, such as mitochondria and endoplasmic reticulum, in an ATP-dependent fashion. During ischemia, Ca^{2+} pumps fail because of the lack of ATP. **4.** Decreases in membrane potential lead to Ca^{2+} entry through voltage-dependent Ca^{2+} channels. Release of glutamate by neighboring cells permits Ca^{2+} entry through NMDA and other Ca^{2+}-conducting glutamate receptors **5.** and activates G_q-coupled metabotropic glutamate receptors **6.** which increase the formation of inositol triphosphate (IP_3) and the release of Ca^{2+} from internal stores. ADP, adenosine diphosphate; PLC, phospholipase C; PIP_2, phosphatidylinositol bisphosphate; IP_3R, IP_3 receptor; DAG, diacylglycerol.

Activation of Intracellular Enzymes by Ca²⁺

Increases in neuronal Ca^{2+} may be the ultimate cause of ischemia-related neuronal death. When Ca^{2+} entry is restricted in vitro, for example, through the removal of Ca^{2+} from the extracellular medium or through the blockage of certain Ca^{2+}-conducting ion channels, neurons are protected against excitotoxic damage. Moreover, neurons that express subtypes of AMPA receptors that conduct Ca^{2+} exhibit heightened vulnerability to glutamate receptor–induced toxicity. Why does a high cytosolic Ca^{2+} concentration induce neuronal death? This question remains under investigation, but there are several clues to the answer. One clue lies in the fact that Ca^{2+} functions as a signaling molecule (Chapter 4). As described in

previous chapters, many neuronal enzymes, and hence many neural processes, respond to this signal. It is possible that excessive activation of these various enzymes and processes, caused by inappropriate Ca^{2+} levels in cells, may contribute to neuronal stress and death. Identification of the key proteins involved would help drug discovery efforts to potentially intervene therapeutically.

Among the many enzymes that have been implicated in Ca^{2+}-mediated neuronal damage are *Ca²⁺-activated proteases*, particularly calpain, which can produce widespread cellular damage. Calpain cleaves cytoskeletal proteins which leads to severe cytoskeletal damage. *Phospholipases*, such as phospholipase A_2 (PLA_2), also can be activated by Ca^{2+}. PLA_2 targets membrane phospholipids and hydrolyzes the bond between the fatty acid portions and the polar head groups. When activated en masse, phospholipases may disrupt membrane integrity by changing the numbers and proportions of phospholipids in the neuronal membrane. Moreover, the resulting free fatty acids, which include arachidonic acid, are metabolized by cyclooxygenases and lipoxygenases to yield numerous biologically active products, such as prostaglandins (Chapter 4). The highly reactive $\cdot O_2^-$ radical is formed as part of these reactions.

Nitric oxide synthase (NOS), which is activated on binding to Ca^{2+}–calmodulin complexes, produces gaseous NO from arginine. As explained in Chapter 4, NO is an important messenger molecule; among its other actions, it activates guanylyl cyclase, which catalyzes the formation of cGMP. NO also can inhibit many cellular enzymes, particularly those containing iron–sulfur complexes, such as mitochondrial NADH–ubiquitone oxidoreductase and NADH–succinate oxidoreductase which are crucial to metabolism. Other reactions of the NO molecule—especially its reaction with oxygen to yield peroxynitrate—also may be important in neuronal demise because they may lead to the formation of free radicals.

Formation of Free Radicals

In vitro studies have demonstrated that excitotoxicity is frequently associated with the production of large numbers of free radicals. Free radicals are molecules with an unpaired electron in an outer shell; this unpaired electron causes the molecule to be unstable and highly reactive. Free radicals can peroxidize membrane fatty acids, and in turn can induce alterations in membrane fluidity and integrity. They also can oxidize protein sulfhydryl groups the products of which can subsequently be metabolized to yield a variety of products, including $\cdot O_2^-$. Activation of NOS by Ca^{2+} increases levels of NO, which can react with oxygen or O_2^- to yield peroxynitrate (ONOO); ONOO decomposes with the production of $\cdot OH$, a highly toxic free radical.

Regardless of the source, many experiments have shown that free radical scavengers protect against excitotoxicity in vitro. Such scavengers may effectively reduce ischemic injury only when given soon after the occurrence of an ischemic event and may be good candidates to combine with thrombolytic medications (which dissolve blood clots; see Chapter 19). Only a small number of free radical scavengers have been investigated in clinical trials of **stroke**, and none have yet been shown to be efficacious.

Acidosis

Interruption of blood supply to the brain leads to both increased CO_2 tension—due to decreased CO_2 removal—and increased lactate accumulation caused by forced glycolysis in the absence of aerobic respiration. These two events result in acidosis. Ischemia-related acidosis can be severe; indeed, pH values in an ischemic region often approach 6.0. Acidosis affects cellular function in multiple ways, including the promotion of free radical formation; inhibition of the Na^+–Ca^{2+} exchanger; decomposition of nicotinamide–adenine dinucleotide (NAD), which is essential for oxidative phosphorylation; and inhibition of neurotransmitter reuptake.

Despite our knowledge of these effects, the significance of acidosis to the ultimate death or survival of ischemic neurons is unclear. In fact, acidosis may have certain neuroprotective functions. Neurons exposed to high levels of glutamate in vitro undergo injury at a neutral pH; however, much of this damage is avoided when such experiments are performed at an acidic pH of 6.6. Although many plausible explanations for the protective effect of acidosis exist, one of the most likely involves the pH sensitivity of the Ca^{2+}-conducting NMDA receptor. At acidic pH, NMDA currents are drastically reduced, which may in turn significantly reduce Ca^{2+} accumulation in challenged neurons.

PROTEIN AGGREGATION–INDUCED CELL DEATH

Despite widely divergent etiologies, many neurodegenerative diseases are charactized by the inappropriate accumulation of protein aggregates. The protein aggregates can occur either intracellularly in diseases such as **Parkinson disease**, **Huntington disease**, neurofibrillary tangles in **Alzheimer disease, familial amyotrophic lateral sclerosis,** and **spinocerebellar ataxia type 1**, or extracellularly as in the β-amyloid plaques of Alzheimer disease. Although precise mechanisms have yet to be determined, these protein aggregates have been shown to interfere with a wide variety of intracellular processes which could be deleterious to the functioning of the cell.

Proteasomal Mechanisms

The proteasome endopeptidase complex has been likened to an intracellular "trash can." When a protein is no longer necessary for cellular functioning, it is targeted for destruction by polyubiquitination, the enzymatic addition of small proteins called *ubiquitin* by enzymes called ubiquitin ligases **17–3**. Once a protein has been tagged with four or more ubiquitins, it is transported to the proteasome, unfolded, and cleaved into short peptides, which can then be further degraded into amino acids by cytosolic peptidases.

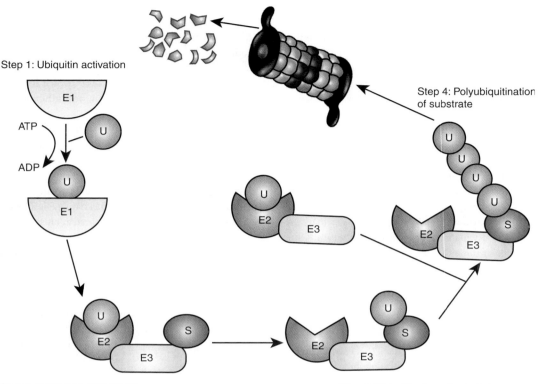

Step 5: Proteolysis of substrate in proteasome

Step 1: Ubiquitin activation

Step 4: Polyubiquitination of substrate

Step 2: Formation of U:E2:E3 complex with substrate

Step 3: Ubiquitination of substrate

17-3 **Ubiquitin-dependent degradation of proteins by the proteasome.** E1 ligases activate ubiquitin (U) (Step 1), and the activated ubiquitin is transferred to E2 ligases which recruit E3 ligases bound to specific substrate proteins (S) (Step 2). This leads to ubiquitination of the substrate on specific lysine residues (Step 3). The process is repeated as the substrate is polyubiquitinated (Step 4). The polyubiquitinated protein is then digested in the proteasome complex.

As will be seen below, several neurodegenerative disorders (eg, **Huntington disease,** several **spinocerebellar ataxias**) are characterized by the genetic expansion of a chain of glutamine residues within a particular protein. These proteins can undergo polyubiquitination, but are unable to be processed by the proteasome due to inefficient cleavage between glutamine residues. Another example for proteasome involvement in neurodegeneration comes from identification of one particular ubiquitin ligase, parkin, as a gene involved in **Parkinson disease.** Loss of function in the parkin gene decreases the ability to add ubiquitin to certain proteins, the identity of which remain unknown. Diminished proteasome activity, either by accumulation of uncleavable aggregates (as with polyglutamine diseases) or genetic loss of function of

ubiquitinating enzymes (as with parkin mutations), results in a buildup of unwanted and potentially toxic proteins within the cell. Intensive research efforts are now aimed to identify the mechanism by which protein aggregates lead to neuronal death and to develop novel methods to intervene to limit such mechanisms of neurodegeneration.

Endoplasmic Reticulum Stress and the Unfolded Protein Response

The most dramatic example of the medical consequences of protein folding is provided by **Prion diseases**, where a particular conformational state of prion protein becomes the etiologic agent in profound neurodegenerative disorders, including **Creutzfeld-Jakob** disease, **kuru**, and **spongiform encephalopathies**, among others. More recently, the misfolding of many additional proteins has been implicated in the pathogenesis of several other neurologic disorders.

The endoplasmic reticulum (ER), an intracellular system of membranes (Chapter 2), has unique mechanisms for managing protein aggregates. Unfolded or misfolded proteins are recognized and bound by the ER chaperone protein called BiP for binding protein. BiP normally binds to and inhibits three signal transduction proteins within the ER membrane: PERK, ATF6 (activating transcription factor-6), and IRE1 (inositol-requiring endoribonuclease). However, when all available BiP is completely bound by misfolded proteins, these signaling proteins are released and activate a process termed the "unfolded protein response," which functions to help the cell adapt to the increased load of misfolded protein. PERK reduces the ER protein load by phosphorylating eIF2α (elongation initiating factor-2α), a protein required for protein translation. Free ATF6 is processed into an active transcription factor, which is translocated to the nucleus where it activates the transcription of proteins involved in protein folding. Finally, once IRE1 is released from BiP, it processes a transcription factor called XBP1 (X-box binding protein 1) which upregulates expression of proteins involved in protein degradation and in the transport of proteins from the ER to the cytosol.

In neurodegenerative diseases associated with intracellular protein aggregates, it is possible that these normal homeostatic mechanisms for handling misfolded proteins are overwhelmed, enabling the proteins to aggregate and damage the cells in other ways. There is also evidence that chronic activation of the unfolded protein response may be injurious itself, for example, by inducing apoptosis through a mitochondrial pathway dependent on proapoptotic Bcl-2 family members (see 17-1).

Autophagy

Autophagy refers to a cellular method for clearing items too large for proteasome degradation, such as damaged organelles or large protein aggregates. In this process the target is engulfed by an autophagosome which then fuses to a lysosome to allow for degradation of the target by lysosomal enzymes. In addition to eliminating large structures, autophagy is used by the cell to free amino acids for synthesis of critical proteins during periods of protein starvation. While this process is initially adaptive for the cell, excessive activation of autophagy can lead to a nonapoptotic form

of programmed cell death through inappropriate degradation of proteins and organelles. Abnormal autophagy has been implicated in **Parkinson disease** (see below). Importantly, pharmacologic inhibition of apoptotic caspases has been shown in some systems to induce autophagy, indicating that redundant pathways may exist to kill severely damaged cells. Therefore, multiple pathways may need to be targeted medicinally to prevent neuron loss in the context of a chronic neurodegenerative disorder.

Potential Therapies for Protein Aggregation

Several strategies to treat abnormal, pathogenic protein aggregation are currently in development. Most approaches involve the use of drugs that prevent protein aggregation in cultured cells or in mouse models of neurodegeneration. Promising medications in this class include **cystamine**, **geldanamycin**, and **minocycline**, which are now in early clinical trials. Cystamine forms disulfide bonds with and inhibits several enzymes, including certain caspases. Geldanamycin activates heat shock protein-90, an important chaperone, which, by binding to toxic proteins, may protect cells from proapoptotic signals. Although the molecular mechanism of action of minocycline is unknown, the drug has been shown to inhibit microglial activation in vitro and in vivo.

Another potential therapy currently under study in **Huntington disease** is **rapamycin** which can induce autophagy and potentially speed the clearance of toxic aggregates. Rapamycin acts by inhibiting mTor (mammalian target of rapamycin), a protein downstream of several neurotrophic factor signaling pathways, including Akt (see figure in 17-1 ; see also Chapter 8), which exerts powerful control over protein synthesis. Because of their central role in apoptosis, medications that stabilize mitochondrial function, such as **coenzyme Q10** and **creatine**, are of great interest. Both compounds are antioxidants.

Recent work has implicated the generation of toxic peptides from protein aggregates in the pathogenesis of neurodegeneration. Mice carrying mutant huntingtin (the cause of **Huntington disease**; see below) or mutant β-amyloid precursor protein (the cause of certain familial cases of **Alzheimer disease**; see below) exhibit increased cell death. When the caspase recognition sites in the mutant proteins are altered to prevent their cleavage by caspases, neurons become resistant to cell death in these mouse models. These findings suggest that release of toxic peptides by proteolytic cleavage of protein aggregates may be important for the progression of certain neurodegenerative diseases. The findings further substantiate the potential utility of **caspase inhibitors** in the treatment of these illnesses.

ALZHEIMER DISEASE AND RELATED DEMENTIAS

Alzheimer disease has become a major public health problem as human life span has been extended by modern medicine. Alzheimer disease is characterized by a gradual decline in cognitive function over a period of years. Although the disease processes begin earlier, symptoms are generally noticed later in life. Among individuals older than 65 years of age, 6% to 8% have Alzheimer disease; among persons aged 85 and older, the prevalence of Alzheimer disease is approximately 30%. Rare monogenic forms of the disease may begin in midlife.

Among the earliest symptoms of Alzheimer disease is memory impairment. As Alzheimer disease advances, the ability to learn new information is increasingly compromised. Access to distant memories, which is relatively intact in the initial stages of the disease, begins to diminish. As cognitive impairment progresses, patients may become lost while walking or driving, and become increasingly unable to perform tasks such as preparing meals, taking regular medications, or managing finances. As cognition declines, patients may experience depression and irritability and later delusions and hallucinations. Patients also may become aggressive, even toward their caretakers. The end-stage of Alzheimer disease is generally characterized by a complete loss of independence. The disease exacts an enormous toll from not only affected individuals but also the friends and family members who care for them and society at large.

As the number and percentage of elderly persons increase steadily, the prevalence of Alzheimer disease almost certainly will rise. It is estimated that by the year 2040, there will be 11 million people in the United States and 80 million people worldwide with Alzheimer disease. Thus, there is an enormous need to develop effective medications to slow or halt the disease process.

Pathology

Even cursory inspection reveals that the brain of a patient with mid- to late-stage Alzheimer disease is noticeably different from that of a normal person of the same age. The diseased brain appears shrunken compared with the normal brain, and has wider gyri, larger ventricles, and less overall mass. However, the pathologic hallmarks of Alzheimer disease and clues as to its etiology can be observed only at the microscopic level.

In addition to loss of neurons and synapses, these hallmarks include the presence of various abnormal protein deposits. *Senile plaques* are dense, extracellular deposits that are composed primarily of the 39- to 43-amino-acid amyloid β peptide (Aβ), the biochemistry of which is discussed later in this chapter. Two types of senile plaques—diffuse plaques and neuritic plaques—have been identified. *Diffuse plaques* are extracellular deposits of Aβ; most of these are formed by the 40-amino-acid form of the peptide (A$β_{40}$). Neuritic plaques also consist of extracellular masses of Aβ, but are distinguished from diffuse plaques by the presence of dystrophic dendrites and glia. Intracellular accumulations of abnormally phosphorylated helical filaments known as *neurofibrillary* tangles also are hallmarks of Alzheimer disease. The major constituent of the tangles is the microtubule-associated protein tau, a protein present in normal brain tissue that becomes abnormally phosphorylated in Alzheimer disease.

For reasons that currently are unclear, tangle formation and neuron loss tend to develop preferentially in the hippocampus and medial temporal neocortex, and plaques form first in the frontal, parietal, and other association cortices. Cholinergic nuclei such as the nucleus basalis (Chapter 6) are highly impaired while primary sensory cortices and subcortical brain regions tend to be spared. This pattern correlates with early onset memory impairment (declarative memory is dependent on the medial temporal lobe) and progressive cognitive decline (Chapter 13).

The significance of the defining pathologic features of Alzheimer disease has been the topic of intense research. Among the most important questions that investigators have attempted to answer are those related to causality. Are plaques and tangles toxic to neurons? Or are they coping mechanisms that the cell uses to detoxify other, more toxic forms of Aβ and tau? While answers to these questions are still unclear, there is increasing evidence that small, soluble oligomers of Aβ (ranging from dimers to dodecamers and larger species) are particularly pathogenic and may be a major mediator of Alzheimer disease.

Genetics

Two primary risk factors for Alzheimer disease have long been recognized: advanced age and genetics. Common forms of Alzheimer disease begin later in life and appear to be genetically complex. There are, however, inherited forms in which symptoms appear in middle age and follow autosomal dominant inheritance patterns. More than 100 different mutations in three known genes (amyloid precursor protein, presenilin-1, and presenilin-2) can each cause early-onset, familial Alzheimer disease, with some differences in age of onset and rate of progression.

In late onset forms, the disease does not occur in a Mendelian inheritance pattern. Nonetheless, family studies have revealed that between 25% and 50% of relatives of patients with Alzheimer disease eventually are afflicted with the disease themselves, compared with approximately 10% among control groups. The apolipoprotein E (apoE) gene is the most important known genetic factor that modifies the risk for Alzheimer disease and the age at which the disease emerges. Other genetic loci are still being investigated, and environmental factors are probably also important in determining whether or not an individual will develop the disease.

Role of APP and Aβ

The first major genetic advance in the study of Alzheimer disease occurred with the discovery of a linkage in some families with the region of chromosome 21 that codes for *amyloid precursor protein (APP)*, whose products include Aβ peptides. Duplication of the APP locus, which increases APP gene dose, also causes early-onset Alzheimer disease. Further evidence consistent with a role for APP in Alzheimer disease is that patients with **Down syndrome (Trisomy 21)** and thus an extra copy of the APP gene generally develop early-onset Alzheimer disease.

The cellular functions of APP and its metabolites in healthy individuals include regulating synaptic transmission, axonal transport, gene expression, and neuronal growth. APP is a transmembrane protein that is expressed in many tissues, including the brain. It has multiple splice variants, the longest of which (APP770) contains 770 amino acid residues. It has a short half-life and is metabolized rapidly by proteases by means of two pathways, designated α and β. The β pathway, which leads to the production of Aβ 17-4, involves cleavage of APP by β-secretase between

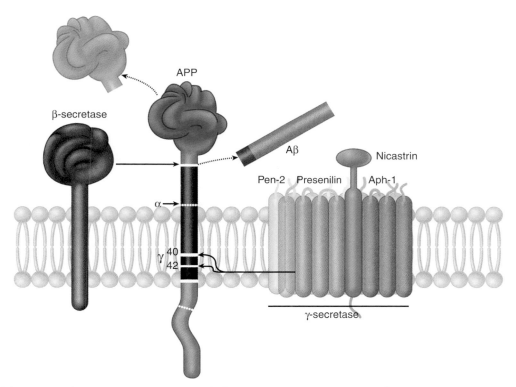

17-4 **Diagram of APP and the production of Aβ.** The APP ectodomain is shed by β-secretase cleavage. The multiprotein γ-secretase complex then cleaves APP to generate either Aβ40 or Aβ42. This complex consists of presenilin, Pen-2 (presenilin enhancer-2), nicastrin, and Aph-1 (anterior pharynx defective-1, named for its role in Notch signaling). α-Secretase cleavage prevents formation of Aβ. (From Roberson ED, Mucke L. 100 years and counting: prospects for defeating Alzheimer's disease. *Science.* 2006;314:781–784.)

residues 671 and 672, and subsequent cleavage by γ-secretase near residue 712. The location of the second cleavage is not precise. When it occurs at residues 712–713, a 40-amino-acid protein termed $A\beta_{40}$ is produced. When it occurs after residue 714, the resultant product is $A\beta_{42}$, which is more toxic and more prone to aggregate than $A\beta_{40}$. The α pathway involves cleavage by α-secretase between APP residues 687 and 688, which are located within the Aβ domain. Thus cleavage of APP by means of the α pathway precludes the generation of Aβ peptides. A product of the α pathway

is the p3 peptide, whose physiologic function is largely unknown.

Several different mutations of the APP gene have been determined to lead to early-onset Alzheimer disease **17-5**. The biochemical effects of these mutations on APP processing have been studied extensively. Some of these mutations, particularly the Swedish mutation near the β-secretase cleavage site, lead to increased production of Aβ, including both $A\beta_{40}$ and $A\beta_{42}$. Other mutations, especially those near the γ-secretase site, selectively increase the production of

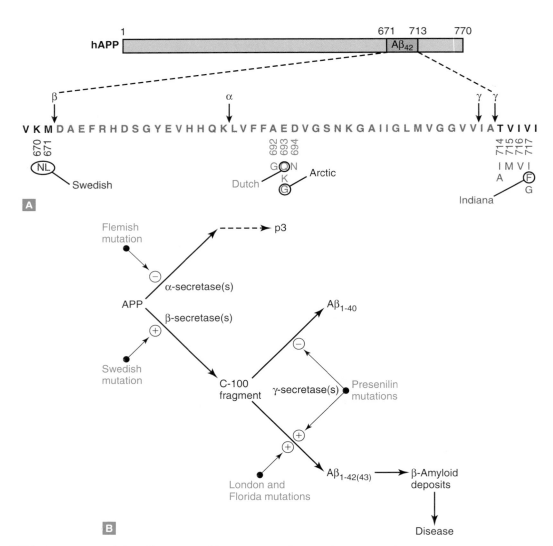

17-5 **A. Diagram of the Aβ portion of human APP (hAPP)** shows sites of genetic mutations and sites of cleavage by β-, α-, and γ-secretases. **B.** Initial steps in the cascade leading from APP to Aβ. (Adapted with permission from Hardy J. Amyloid, the presenilins, and Alzheimer disease. *Trends Neurosci.* 1997;20:154.)

$A\beta_{42}$. A third group of mutations changes the sequence of $A\beta$ and its aggregation properties. The mutations cause Alzheimer disease and **cerebral amyloid angiopathy,** a condition in which amyloid deposition in blood vessel walls leads to frequent intracerebral hemorrhages. Together with the known neurotoxic effects of $A\beta$, these genetic observations have led to the "amyloid hypothesis" that Alzheimer disease is caused by excessive $A\beta$, particularly $A\beta_{42}$, which ultimately leads to neural damage.

How does $A\beta_{42}$ harm neurons? Aggregation seems to be a key step. $A\beta$ can aggregate into small oligomers that remain soluble, and also into large, insoluble filaments that form plaques. Both types of $A\beta$ aggregates are toxic to neurons. Amyloid plaques can damage nearby neurites, potentially interfering with proper signaling. $A\beta$ oligomers appear to be even more toxic, and data from animal models indicate that they can disrupt learning and memory in the absence of plaques. $A\beta$ oligomers, for example, block long-term potentiation and other forms of synaptic plasticity. $A\beta$ binds to many different cellular proteins and it is not yet known which is the primary effector of its toxic effects. Other factors may also contribute to $A\beta$-induced neuronal injury. Microglial activation and inflammatory responses help clear $A\beta$ aggregates, but release of cytokines and other mediators may disrupt normal neuronal function. $A\beta$-initiated neurotoxic and inflammatory processes may in addition cause the generation of free radicals, which are also damaging to neurons, as outlined earlier in this chapter.

Role of Presenilins

Shortly after mutations in APP were linked to the inheritance of early-onset Alzheimer disease, germline mutations in two other genes, *presenilin 1* (PS1) and *presenilin 2* (PS2), were also found to cause Alzheimer disease. Mutations in PS1 account for the majority of autosomal dominant cases of early-onset Alzheimer disease. PS1 and PS2 are integral membrane proteins that are widely expressed and have multiple functions.

Presenilin is the catalytically active component of the γ-secretase complex, which is formed along with other proteins including Nicastrin, Aph-1, and Pen-2 **17-4**. γ-Secretase mediates intramembranous proteolytic cleavage of type I membrane proteins with small ectodomains. One substrate is APP, after its ectodomain has been shed by β-secretase; γ-secretase cleavage of this APP carboxy-terminal fragment yields $A\beta$. Mutations in PS1 seem to increase its tendency to generate $A\beta_{42}$, relative to $A\beta_{40}$. In this way, the resulting increase in toxic $A\beta_{42}$ production is similar to the effect of APP mutations near the γ-secretase cleavage site. This effect is believed to be a major mechanism through which presenilin mutations cause Alzheimer disease. Thus, inhibiting γ-secretase may be an ideal therapeutic strategy for Alzheimer disease, but the situation is complicated by the fact that γ-secretase also cleaves many other protein besides APP (see below).

Presenilins have functions other than their role in the γ-secretase complex that may contribute to Alzheimer disease. For example, presenilins play important roles in calcium homeostasis by regulating loading of endoplasmic reticulum calcium stores. This function does not depend on γ-secretase activity, but is disrupted by disease-causing PS1 mutations. The degree to which loss of these normal functions—versus gain of toxic $A\beta_{42}$-producing γ-secretase activity—mediates the effects of presenilin mutations remains to be determined.

Role of ApoE

Apolipoprotein E (apoE) is a 34-kDa protein that plays an important role in cholesterol transport, uptake, and redistribution. The three common alleles of apoE (ε2, ε3, and ε4) are inherited in a codominant fashion. The inheritance of each copy of the ε4 allele tends to increase the risk and decrease the age of onset of Alzheimer disease **17-6**. Conversely, each ε2 allele results in lower risk and increased age of onset in most populations studied to date. Thus ε4 conveys higher risk while ε2 is protective, relative to the most common ε3 allele. Based on these observations, it has been proposed that in the general population the apoE gene is an important modifier of the risk for common (nonfamilial) forms of Alzheimer disease; in fact, apoE4 may account for 30% to 50% of the genetic risk of developing the disease in some populations.

How might a lipoprotein have such a profound influence on the risk of developing Alzheimer disease? One strong possibility is through effects on $A\beta$ deposition and plaque formation. Three principal lines of evidence support the hypothesis that apoE promotes amyloidogenesis. First, unlike wildtype mice, mice that lack the gene for apoE are protected against amyloid deposition. Second, in vitro experiments have demonstrated that apoE, especially apoE4 (the protein product of ε4), can enhance the ability of $A\beta$ to form fibrils. Third, transgenic mice that overexpress various forms of $A\beta$ develop more plaques when they also overexpress apoE4.

Although its effect on amyloid deposition is probably the most well-studied role of apoE in Alzheimer disease, there are other mechanisms that may contribute.

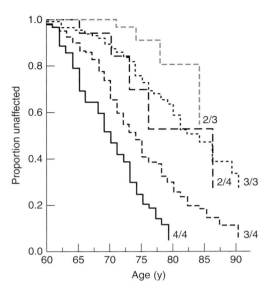

17-6 **Probability of remaining unaffected by Alzheimer disease as a function of ApoE genotype.** Note that an increased incidence and decreased age of onset of the disease occurs among individuals with two copies of ApoE$_4$, whereas those with even one copy of ApoE$_2$ are relatively protected. The numbers on the curves designate alleles. (Adapted with permission from Strittmatter WJ, Roses AD. Apolipoprotein E and Alzheimer disease. *Annu Rev Neurosci.* 1996;19:53.)

ApoE4 may increase Aβ production, apart from its effect on Aβ aggregation. ApoE also binds to tau and is found in tangles, and apoE4 stimulates tau phosphorylation more than other apoE isoforms. ApoE is normally made and secreted by astrocytes, but is produced by neurons after injury. Neuronal apoE may aid in neuronal repair, but apoE4 in neurons can be proteolytically cleaved, which renders a toxic truncated form of the protein. Finally, the ε4 allele is also associated with a higher risk of cerebrovascular disease, which probably interacts with the pathogenic processes underlying Alzheimer disease.

Role of Tau

The microtubule-associated protein tau is involved in several neurodegenerative diseases. Some, including **frontotemporal dementia** (discussed later), can be caused by tau gene mutations and are termed *primary tauopathies*. Alzheimer disease is a *secondary tauopathy*; tau mutations apparently do not cause disease, but tau protein nonetheless accumulates and plays an important pathogenic role.

The tau gene on chromosome 17 is very complex and alternatively spliced to generate six different isoforms **17-7**. Three of the isoforms contain three microtubule-binding domains (3R tau), while the other three have four such domains (4R tau). Tau is expressed primarily in neurons and at lower levels in glia. Tau is involved in neurite outgrowth and regulates axonal transport, yet tau knockout mice have no dramatic defects.

Interest in tau has focused on neurofibrillary tangles, which are composed primarily of aberrantly phosphorylated tau. Several kinases are thought to contribute to tau hyperphosphorylation, including Cdk5 (cyclin-dependent kinase 5) and GSK3β (glycogen synthase kinase 3β) (Chapter 4). The amount of tangle pathology is highly correlated with the degree of neuronal loss and the severity of cognitive impairment in Alzheimer disease patients. This suggests that pathologic aggregation of tau may be a final pathway leading to neurodegeneration in Alzheimer disease. There is abundant evidence that Aβ can stimulate modification and aggregation of tau. Aβ activates many of the kinases that phosphorylate tau, and also increases pathologic tau cleavage. Mouse models expressing high levels of both Aβ and human tau develop plaques and tangles, and treatments aimed at Aβ reverse some aspects of the tau pathology. Thus, one model for Alzheimer pathogenesis postulates that Aβ triggers downstream changes in tau, leading to tangle formation and neuronal death, thereby causing cognitive impairment.

While many aspects of this model have been validated, other mechanisms undoubtedly also contribute. For example, animal models indicate that, much like soluble oligomers of Aβ, soluble forms of tau contribute to neuronal dysfunction and cognitive deficits, even apart from any role in tangle formation and cell death. Other important questions about tau's role in Alzheimer disease remain, such as which phosphorylation sites are most important in the disease and the extent to which various tau posttranslational modifications contribute to pathogenesis.

Treatment

Because Alzheimer disease is so disabling and yet so common, intense research efforts in the pharmaceutical industry and in academic settings have been devoted to developing agents that will prevent or retard the disease process. Currently used agents focus on symptomatic improvement only and include drugs that increase cholinergic neurotransmission or block glutamate receptors. Still in development are several strategies aimed at altering the disease processes themselves, such as regulating Aβ or tau.

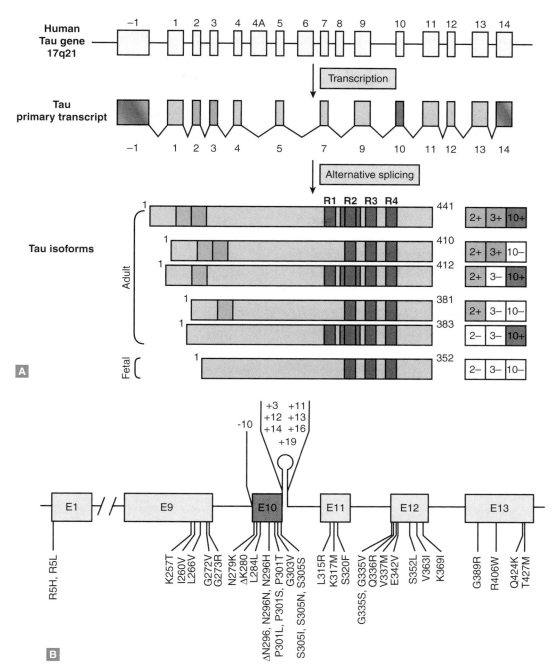

17-7 **Structure of the tau gene and isoforms, and their pathogenic mutations. A.** The tau gene (top) is transcribed into a primary RNA (middle) that is alternatively spliced and translated to produce six mRNA and protein isoforms. The isoforms contain either zero (0N), one (1N), or two (2N) amino-terminal inserts, and either three (3R) or four (4R) carboxy-terminal microtubule-binding domains. (Adapted with permission from Buée L, Bussière T, Buée-Scherrer V, et al. Tau protein isoforms, phosphorylation and role in neurodegenerative disorders. *Brain Res Rev.* 2000;33:95–130.) **B.** Summary of mutations in the tau gene that are causative of rare familial forms of frontotemporal dementia or related neurodegenerative disorders. (Figure borrowed with permission from Michel Goedert, Medical Research Council, Cambridge, UK).

Cholinergic agents Because cholinergic neurons of the nucleus basalis are prominently affected in Alzheimer disease, and because cholinergic activity regulates memory processing, enhancement of cholinergic functioning was one of the earliest treatment goals. The initial attempts to increase cholinergic functioning involved administration of the acetylcholine precursors, **choline** and **lecithin**. Although the analogous strategy has proven effective for **Parkinson disease**—L-dopa, a precursor of dopamine, improves symptoms of the illness (see below)—multiple studies have established that cholinergic precursors are not effective in the treatment of Alzheimer disease.

Subsequent efforts met with partial success by inhibiting the cholinesterase activity that clears acetylcholine from the synaptic cleft (see Chapter 6 for a general discussion of cholinergic systems). Four cholinesterase inhibitors are currently approved for the treatment of Alzheimer disease in the United States: **tacrine, donepezil, galantamine,** and **rivastigmine** 17–8 . These agents do not reverse the course of the disease, nor are they dramatically effective at restoring cognitive function, but in some patients they can temporarily delay the inevitable symptomatic deterioration.

In addition, cholinergic neurotransmitter receptors are potential targets of medicinal agents, as both α_7

nicotinic and M_1 muscarinic receptors modulate the pathogenic effects of APP/Aβ. The α_7 receptor is highly enriched in hippocampus, and several α_7 selective nicotinic receptor agonists are in early clinical trials as cognitive enhancers in Alzheimer disease.

Other cholinergic treatment strategies include targeting the nerve growth factor signaling pathway, which provides trophic support for cholinergic neurons. However, as discussed in Chapter 8, it is challenging to deliver growth factors directly into the brain and to design small molecules that activate endogenous growth factor signaling pathways, and there is no evidence to date that this approach will work clinically.

NMDA receptor antagonists In addition to the cholinesterase inhibitors, the other approved treatment for Alzheimer disease is **memantine**. Memantine is a low affinity antagonist of the NMDA glutamate receptor, which is integrally involved in synaptic plasticity (Chapter 13) but also mediates excitotoxic injury as discussed earlier. Because its effects are voltage dependent, it has been proposed that memantine preferentially inhibits excessive NMDA receptor activation associated with excitotoxicity, without blocking the receptor's function under most normal conditions. However, this speculation is counter to our knowledge of NMDA receptor function in brain and the use of memantine to treat the cognitive symptoms of Alzheimer disease: one would predict that NMDA agonists might improve cognitive function, while NMDA antagonists might reduce longer-term excitotoxicity. Hence the use of an NMDA antagonist for symptomatic improvement, not as a disease-altering agent, does not make sense. It is, of course, quite possible that memantine's modest clinical effects are mediated via alternative mechanisms not yet identified.

Tacrine

Donepezil

Galantamine   Rivastigmine

17–8 **Structures of clinically used cholinesterase inhibitors.**

Anti-inflammatory agents and antioxidants The buildup of Aβ into plaques causes some local microglial and astrocytic activation, with concomitant release of cytokines and acute-phase proteins. Thus, inflammatory processes are implicated in the neurodegeneration that is characteristic of Alzheimer disease. Consistent with this suspicion, retrospective epidemiologic studies suggest that patients taking **nonsteroidal anti-inflammatory drugs** (**NSAIDs**), eg, **ibuprofen**, on a regular basis—for example, for arthritis—have a reduced risk of developing Alzheimer disease. Unfortunately, prospective trials have failed to support the efficacy of several different NSAIDs. It is likely that inflammation can in some ways be beneficial, perhaps by contributing to plaque clearance, and that anti-inflammatory therapies will need to be specifically targeted to the harmful aspects of these processes.

A related treatment strategy involves the use of antioxidants and free-radical scavengers. Activated microglia secrete hydrogen peroxide, superoxides, and hydroxyl radicals; these are useful in combating foreign cells or organisms but can damage neurons. It is therefore possible that antioxidants and free-radical scavengers may serve a protective function in Alzheimer disease and in other neurodegenerative disorders. **Vitamin E (α-tocopherol)** has been extensively studied. While early studies suggested that it might slow progression, larger studies have been disappointing. Combined with reports of increased all-cause mortality in patients on high-dose vitamin E, it is no longer recommended for patients with Alzheimer disease.

Disease-altering strategies **Targeting Aβ** Much of the current excitement in Alzheimer disease treatment surrounds strategies for counteracting the effects of Aβ. Several different compounds, including **cyclohexanehexols** and **tramiprosate**, are able to block aggregation of Aβ into oligomers or fibrillar plaques. These agents reduce plaques and improve cognitive deficits in mice and are advancing to clinical trials in Alzheimer disease patients.

Immune-based approaches to stimulate Aβ clearance are also under clinical investigation. Vaccination with Aβ plus adjuvant was highly effective in mouse models, profoundly reducing amyloid plaque load and improving cognitive performance. However, a clinical trial in patients was terminated early because a subset of patients developed encephalitis related to the immune reaction. Because the trial still gave hints of benefit in at least some patients, second-generation approaches using different immunologic strategies are under investigation.

Considerable effort is devoted to inhibiting Aβ production by blocking β- or γ-secretase. Challenges in the chemical synthesis of β-secretase inhibitors (termed **BASE inhibitors**) have slowed their development; it has not yet been possible to generate selective, blood-brain barrier–permeable inhibitors that show good oral bioavailability. While BASE inhibitors remain a highly favored treatment strategy by the pharmaceutical industry, they are unfortunately still in preclinical stages of development. In addition, there is recent evidence that β-secretase may regulate myelin thickness, raising questions about possible side effects of any new drugs.

It has proven easier to block γ-secretase, but concerns over side effects related to substrate specificity have been the limiting issue. Besides APP, γ-secretase cleaves many other type I transmembrane proteins with small extracellular domains. One of the most important is *Notch*, a signaling molecule with critical roles in differentiation and development. Notch cleavage by γ-secretase releases the Notch intracellular domain (NICD), which acts in the nucleus to regulate gene expression. Presumably through inhibition of Notch cleavage, **γ-secretase inhibitors** have demonstrated adverse effects on lymphoid and gastrointestinal tissues, which have large populations of rapidly dividing cells. Attempts to create γ-secretase inhibitors that are more selective for APP are underway. A related approach is to develop modulators of γ-secretase rather than direct inhibitors of the enzyme's catalytic activity. Certain drugs, such as **R-flurbiprofen**, alter the exact site of γ-secretase-mediated cleavage. These compounds cause γ-secretase to produce more $A\beta_{40}$ and less $A\beta_{42}$, essentially the reverse effect of presenilin mutations, and thus may lessen Alzheimer disease pathogenesis.

Additional approaches to reducing Aβ levels are being considered. As mentioned, α-secretase cleavage of APP initiates a nonamyloidogenic pathway by cleaving within the Aβ sequence, so increasing α-secretase activity should reduce Aβ levels. In addition, many endogenous peptidases that serve to degrade Aβ have been identified, including **neprilysin** and **insulin-degrading enzyme**. Activating either α-secretase or one of these peptidases may be effective in lowering Aβ levels and treating Alzheimer disease.

Other disease-altering strategies Pharmaceutical approaches to directly target tau or apoE are not as advanced as approaches toward Aβ. Compared to Aβ, it is less clear how to pharmacologically reduce levels of these "normal" proteins, or indeed if that would be effective. Rather, attempts are focused on identifying specific conformations, posttranslational modifications, or intermolecular interactions that might be pathogenic and could be targeted to treat the disease. For example, because tau phosphorylation is such a hallmark of Alzheimer disease, inhibitors of the several protein kinases that are known to phosphorylate tau (eg, Cdk5, GSK3β) are being investigated, but the multiple roles of these protein kinases raise significant challenges for developing drugs that are safe. Inhibitors of tau aggregation are also under development.

Frontotemporal Dementia

The frontotemporal dementias (FTDs) are a group of related neurodegenerative disorders that are distinguished in several ways from Alzheimer disease, perhaps foremost because of their heterogeneity, both clinically and pathologically.

Clinical syndromes Whereas the signature cognitive deficit in Alzheimer disease is memory impairment, FTD patients classically have preserved memory, but severe problems in other cognitive domains. Several different syndromes can be diagnosed, depending on which symptoms occur earliest or are most severe. Patients with classical FTD withdraw from their friends and families and lack normal emotional responses, such as empathy when a loved one is injured. They often develop unusual compulsions, personality changes, altered food preferences, and disinhibited behaviors, and lack insight into their own illnesses. Patients with *semantic dementia* show some of these behavioral abnormalities, but are affected primarily by a loss of semantic knowledge, or information about what things are. This leads to problems in naming objects that are shown to them, and eventually with being able to describe anything about the item. Other patients show problems primarily in language expression and are diagnosed with *progressive aphasia*. Finally, some patients present primarily with parkinsonism and other motor symptoms and are diagnosed with *progressive supranuclear palsy* or *corticobasal degeneration* (see **Parkinson disease** below). Patients who present with one of these syndromes often go on to develop one or more of the others as their disease worsens.

FTD tends to occur in somewhat younger patients than Alzheimer disease, with an average age of onset in the late 50s. In fact, among patients under 65, FTD is as common as Alzheimer disease.

Pathology   The neuropathology of FTD syndromes is also more heterogeneous than that of Alzheimer disease. Amyloid plaques are not observed, and Aβ is not believed to play a prominent role in causing these diseases. About half of patients show some type of tau-positive inclusions, although usually not the classic neurofibrillary tangles seen in Alzheimer disease. Often, the tau pathology occurs in glial cells or takes the form of spherical neuronal inclusions termed *Pick bodies*. (FTDs were originally referred to as **Pick disease**.) The other half of patients do not have tau-positive inclusions, but most have inclusions composed of some ubiquitinated protein. For years, the identify of this protein was unknown, but it has now been identified as TDP-43 (TAR DNA-binding protein of 43 kD). TDP-43 is a nuclear protein, the exact role of which in neuropathogenesis remains to be determined.

Genetics   Mutations in the tau gene are one cause of FTD. Because these cases often have parkinsonism and the tau gene is on chromosome 17, these cases are often referred to as **FTDP-17**. Many different tau mutations have been described, most of which are around the microtubule-binding domains of the protein **17-7**. Many mutations seem to increase the

proportion of 4R tau, while others seem to favor tau aggregation. Current research is aimed at understanding precise molecular mechanisms through which tau mutations cause FTD.

The other major genetic cause of FTD is mutation in the *progranulin* gene. Progranulin is a secreted growth factor, and the many different mutations that have been described lead to a destabilization of the mRNA and resulting haploinsufficiency of progranulin. The leading hypothesis is that a resulting loss of progranulin's trophic effects contributes to neurodegeneration.

Less common genetic forms of FTD are caused by mutations in valosin-containing protein (VCP) or charged multivesicular body protein 2B (CHMP2B), both of which have roles in protein handling.

Treatment   There are no approved drugs for FTD. Cholinesterase inhibitors used for Alzheimer disease are not effective, although **memantine** may be. Serotonergic systems seem to be strongly affected by FTD, and selective serotonin reuptake inhibitors are currently the most commonly used treatment for the illness.

Other Causes of Dementia

Vascular disease is a major cause of cognitive impairment in the elderly. Both large infarctions and chronic ischemia due to changes in small vessels, as occurs with long-standing hypertension, can lead to dementia. These cases are termed **vascular dementia** or **multi-infarct dementia**. They are usually diagnosed based on a combination of stepwise (as opposed to steadily progressive) decline, the presence of cardiovascular risk factors, and neuroimaging evidence of vascular disease. The primary form of treatment is prevention (see Chapter 19 on stroke).

Dementia with Lewy bodies may clinically resemble Alzheimer disease. Distinguishing features include parkinsonism, frequent and severe fluctuations, and the occurrence of visual hallucinations. Pathologically, Lewy bodies containing α-synuclein, identical to those seen in Parkinson disease, are found throughout the neocortex. Treatment is similar to that for Alzheimer disease.

PARKINSON DISEASE

Parkinson disease is characterized by tremor at rest, bradykinesia, and cogwheel rigidity. The characteristic resting tremor is typified by a pill-rolling motion at a frequency of 3 to 5 Hz. Bradykinesia refers to a slowness of movements—in particular, a difficulty in initiating movements—which interferes with the performance of daily tasks. Rigidity and impaired reflexes are partly responsible for the parkinsonian gait, which is traditionally described as festinating, or characterized by short rapid steps. Patients with Parkinson disease also may experience micrography, or small handwriting; weight loss; and alterations in autonomic function; masked facies, or a blank facial expression caused by less frequent eye blinking, and bradykinesia of the facial muscles also are common among affected individuals. Clinical definitions of abnormal movements are given in **17-1**.

Pathophysiology

Parkinson disease is caused by the death of dopamine neurons in the substantia nigra pars compacta, with consequent dopamine depletion in the caudate nucleus and putamen. Pathologic manifestations include degenerative changes, such as neuronal deterioration and depigmentation in the substantia nigra, and the appearance of intracellular inclusions called *Lewy bodies* in dopamine neurons. Death of dopaminergic neurons in the VTA and that of other monoaminergic neurons (eg, noradrenergic and serotonergic neurons in the brainstem) also may occur on a much smaller scale.

The functional effects of the loss of dopamine in patients with Parkinson disease can be understood, to some degree, based on our knowledge of striatal circuits (see **17-9** and **17-10**; see also Chapter 13). Normally, dopamine exerts an inhibitory influence on GABAergic projection neurons of the striatum. Consequently, the loss of dopamine causes increased activity among these neurons, and in turn causes increased inhibitory output from the basal ganglia to the thalamus (see **17-9**). Increased activity among striatal GABAergic neurons decreases the activity of GABAergic neurons in the globus pallidus. These events lead to increased activity among glutamatergic neurons in the subthalamic nucleus, which in turn leads to increased activity among GABAergic neurons of the substantia nigra pars reticulata. Such activity causes increased inhibition of the thalamic ventral tier nuclei. Because these nuclei are responsible for the activation of cortical areas involved in the initiation of movements, the ultimate effect of dopamine deficiency is paucity of movement.

Healthy individuals possess a large reserve of nigrostriatal dopaminergic neurons; consequently, overt parkinsonian symptoms do not occur until approximately 80% of these neurons have been lost. Compensatory responses in remaining neurons, such as the up-regulation of tyrosine hydroxylase (Chapter 6), enable these cells to make more dopamine. The

17-1 Types of Abnormal Movements Associated With Movement Disorders

Type of Movement	Description
Akathisia	Subjective feeling of inner restlessness that is relieved by stereotypic and complex movements (eg, squirming, crossing/uncrossing legs, rocking and pacing)
Asterixis	Periods of sudden cessation of muscle contraction, most easily observed when patient's arms are extended in front; considered a form of myoclonus
Athetosis	Sinuous, slow, writhing or wormlike movements involving the extremities, trunk, and neck
Ballismus	Wild flinging, flailing movements of the arm and leg that represent proximal choreiform movements; often unilateral (hemiballismus)
Bradykinesia	Movements that are slow or of diminished frequency or amplitude
Catalepsy	Maintenance of abnormal positions; passive movement of limbs, often characterized by waxy flexibility
Chorea	Rapid irregular muscle jerks that occur involuntarily and unpredictably in alternating parts of the body in a continuous and nonpurposeful pattern; disappear during sleep
Dyskinesia	Any excessive movement
Dystonia	Twisting movements sustained for variable periods of time
Freezing	Brief episodes during which a motor act is temporarily blocked or halted; most often affect walking
Myokymia	Quivering or rippling of muscle
Rigidity	Increased muscle tone during passive motion in all directions (ie, affects flexors and extensors equally)
Tachykinesia	Movements of speech that are characterized by continuous acceleration or loss of amplitude
Tics	Sudden, quick, coordinated, repetitive movements or sounds that are voluntarily suppressible for short periods; diminish during voluntary activity and disappear during sleep
Tremor	Regular, rhythmic, oscillatory movements that may be present at rest or during action

functional reserve provided by these adaptations causes most cases of Parkinson disease to be characterized by a slow, progressive loss of function. Rapidly evolving lesions, such as those produced by

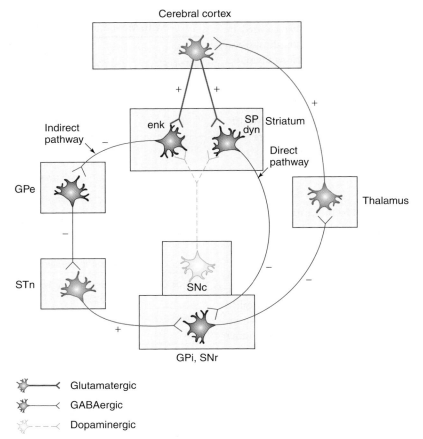

17-9 **Simplified representation of neural circuitry in the basal ganglia.** Glutamatergic neurons from the cortex innervate two major types of GABAergic medium spiny neurons in the striatum. One type, which coexpresses the neuropeptides dynorphin (dyn) and substance P (SP), projects directly to the globus pallidus pars interna (GPi) and substantia nigra pars reticulata (SNr). These "direct projecting" neurons also predominantly express D_1 dopamine receptors. The other type of GABAergic neuron, which coexpresses enkephalin (enk), projects indirectly to the GPi and SNr by means of the globus pallidus pars externa (GPe) and subthalamus nucleus (STn). These "indirect projecting" neurons predominantly express D_2 dopamine receptors. The functioning of the direct and indirect pathways remains incompletely understood. However, cortical activation of direct-projecting striatal neurons is thought to promote motor activity by inhibiting the GPi and SNr which thereby disinhibits the thalamus, while cortical activation of indirect-projecting striatal neurons is thought to inhibit motor activity by inhibiting the GPe's inhibition of the STn and thereby activating the thalamus. Dopaminergic neurons in the substantia nigra pars compacta (SNc) modulate these striatal outputs. The activity of these dopamine neurons is controlled by GABAergic projections from the striatum and by GABAergic neurons in the SNr (not shown). The major output neurons of the basal ganglia are GABAergic neurons in the GPi and SNr, which project to the thalamus and to the brainstem (not shown).

neurotoxins, can produce parkinsonian symptoms in response to the loss of many fewer dopaminergic neurons. Interestingly, a very slow, progressive loss of dopamine neurons occurs—even in the absence of Parkinson disease—in normal individuals throughout adult life.

Genetic Factors

Increasing evidence suggests that there may be a genetic contribution to the etiology of common forms of Parkinson disease, but the exact nature of this contribution remains unclear. In most cases, the disease

Normal

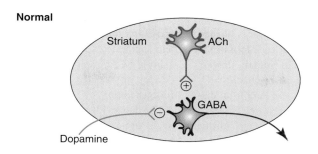

Parkinson disease

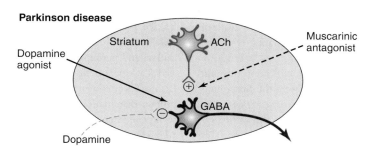

Huntington disease

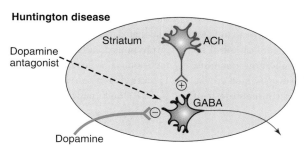

17–10 **Dopamine-acetylcholine (Ach) interactions in the striatum.** According to a simplified scheme, the net activity of striatal GABAergic projection neurons is determined by the relative activity of inhibitory dopaminergic input (mediated by D_1 and D_2 receptors) and of excitatory cholinergic input (mediated by muscarinic receptors). In individuals with Parkinson disease, the degeneration of dopaminergic neurons leads to increased excitation of GABAergic projection neurons and to motor symptoms associated with parkinsonism. Such symptoms can be reduced by L-dopa, which partially restores the inhibitory influence of dopamine, or by muscarinic cholinergic antagonists. Huntington disease is characterized by the degeneration of the GABAergic projection neurons, which leads to motor symptoms such as choreoathetoid dyskinesias. GABAergic function in affected individuals can be partially restored by dopamine receptor antagonists; theoretically, GABAergic function also should be restored by muscarinic cholinergic agonists, but the use of these agents has not resulted in clinical improvement.

appears to be sporadic; that is, it occurs in individuals who do not have a family history of the disease. However, this pattern of disease may reflect genetic susceptibility that only gives rise to illness when certain environmental factors, such as exposure to dopaminergic neurotoxins, are also present.

In addition to the sporadic, common forms of Parkinson disease, there are rare familial forms that are characterized by Mendelian transmission. Several genes responsible for such transmission have been identified by genetic linkage analysis and several more genes are likely to be identified from families known to have Mendelian patterns of inherited Parkinson disease without mutations in the several genes already identified **17-2**. The normal cellular functions of the proteins encoded by these genes remain largely unknown and the pathophysiologic mechanisms by which mutations in these genes cause Parkinson disease remain the subject of intense research. Current leading hypotheses for the causative mechanisms include protein aggregation or disruption of protein degradation, mitochondrial dysfunction, and oxidative stress. Another major unanswered question is why mutations in proteins widely expressed throughout the brain and in other tissues cause selective death of dopamine neurons in the substantia nigra.

Evidence for protein aggregation as a causative mechanism emerged upon the identification of point mutations in α-*synuclein*, which were the first mutations linked to familial Parkinson disease. α-Synuclein is a major component of Lewy bodies, the pathognomonic inclusions of sporadic Parkinson disease. This suggested that α-synuclein aggregation may cause sporadic Parkinson disease and that α-synuclein point mutations linked to familial Parkinson disease increase the propensity of α-synuclein to form intracellular aggregates that may be toxic and may also lead to Lewy body formation. The subsequent identification of α-synuclein gene duplication and triplication mutations linked to familial Parkinson disease reinforced the hypothesis that increased cellular concentrations of even wild-type α-synuclein may cause disease by increasing the rate of formation of α-synuclein protein aggregates. Consistent with this idea, transgenic animals overexpressing wild-type or mutant α-synuclein develop intracellular α-synuclein inclusions and neurodegeneration.

Further evidence supporting protein aggregation or disruption of protein degradation as a pathogenic mechanism comes from the linkage of familial Parkinson disease to loss-of-function mutations in a novel E3 ubiquitin ligase named *parkin*. As stated in an earlier section of this chapter, ubiquitin ligases are critical for protein degradation via the proteasome (see **17-3**). It is thought that one or more proteins accumulate and perhaps aggregate in the absence of normal Parkin function, thus leading to cell death. Lysosomes are the other major cellular mechanism for protein degradation. Recessively inherited mutations in a gene encoding a putative lysosomal membrane ATPase of unknown function, ATP13A2, have also been linked to familial Parkinson disease.

The first evidence that mitochondrial dysfunction may cause Parkinson disease came not from genetics but from the discovery of a severe form of parkinsonism that developed in a group of young adults after intravenous use of a preparation of **meperidine**, a synthetic opiate, which contained the harmful by-product 1-methyl-4-phenyl-1,2,3,6-tetrahydropyridine (**MPTP**). Such patients exhibited rapid and extensive

17-2 Genetic Causes of Parkinson Disease

Gene	Chromosome	Age of Onset	Effect of Mutations
PINK1 (PARK6)	1	20–40 years	Recessive loss of function
DJ-1 (PARK7)	1	20–40 years	Recessive loss of function
UCHL1 (PARK5)	4	Late onset	Associated with susceptibility to sporadic cases
SNCA (PARK1,4)	4	20–65 years	Dominant gain of function
PARK2	6	20–40 years	Recessive loss of function
LRRK2 (Dardarin)	12	Late onset	Dominant gain of function

PINK1, PTEN-induced kinase 1; UCHL1, ubiquitin C-terminal hydrolase L1; SNCA, α-synuclein; PARK2, parkin (a ubiquitin E3 ligase); LRRK2, leucine-rich repeat kinase 2.

loss of dopamine neurons, resulting in severe parkinsonism. Investigators have since learned that MPTP is converted within the brain to its active metabolite MPP+, which selectively accumulates in dopaminergic neurons via the dopamine transporter and is directly neurotoxic by inhibiting mitochondrial respiration (Chapter 6). MPTP, and another selective dopaminergic toxin, **6-hydroxydopamine**, are used to induce Parkinson-like syndromes in animals. Mitochondrial respiration defects also occur in sporadic Parkinson disease and in patients bearing parkin mutations.

Direct genetic evidence of mitochondrial dysfunction as a cause of Parkinson disease comes from the linkage of loss-of-function mutations in the *PINK1* (PTEN-induced kinase 1) gene to recessively inherited Parkinson disease. PINK1 is a kinase that localizes to mitochondria, and is induced by PTEN, a dual function lipid and protein phosphatase upstream of the Akt cell survival pathway mentioned earlier (see **17-1**). Although the precise function of PINK1 remains unknown, it may be important for preventing cell death through regulation of mitochondrial function.

Another kinase of unknown function with mutations linked to familial Parkinson disease, *LRRK2* (leucine-rich repeat kinase 2; also called Dardarin), partially localizes to mitochondria. Although LRRK2 mutations were initially believed to be rare, the G2019S point mutation in LRRK2 has been reported in 30% to 40% of familial Parkinson disease patients of Ashkenazi Jewish or North African Arab origin. LRRK2 polymorphisms may also be a significant risk factor for Parkinson disease in the Asian population.

Oxidative stress has long been hypothesized to be a cause of sporadic Parkinson disease because dopamine itself readily reacts to form chemical species that can cause oxidative damage to cells. Age is the greatest risk factor for Parkinson disease, which implicates cumulative oxidative damage to cells. *DJ-1* is a protein, first identified as a product of an oncogene, believed to protect cells from oxidative stress. Loss-of-function mutations in DJ-1 have been linked to parkinsonism. Mice deficient in DJ-1 are hypersensitive to MPTP and oxidative stress.

Environmental Factors

Prior to the identification of genes with mutations linked to familial Parkinson disease, it was commonly thought that Parkinson disease was strictly caused by environmental factors. This belief was reinforced by the discovery in the early 1980s that MPTP exposure can cause a severe and rapid-onset form of parkinsonism.

The possibility that environmental neurotoxins may cause sporadic cases of Parkinson disease—albeit with less dramatic effects than MPTP—has been further supported by epidemiologic evidence, not always verified, that the disease may be more common in people who reside in rural areas, drink well water, and have regular exposure to herbicides and pesticides. Potential disease-causing toxins have been identified. The pesticide **rotenone** can reproduce features of Parkinson disease in animal models. In Guam a very high incidence of Parkinson disease and other neurodegenerative syndromes, such as **ALS** and **dementia,** has been explained by reliance on the **cycad plant** as a dietary staple; it is believed that the seeds of this plant contain one or more neurotoxins that kill dopaminergic and other neurons. **Heavy metal** poisoning, particularly from exposure to Mn^{2+} or Al^-, also has been associated with Parkinson disease. Moreover, a high incidence of the disease has been noted after certain viral epidemics; thus a viral contribution to the disease is conceivable. However, specific toxins and viruses that cause common forms of Parkinson disease have yet to be identified with certainty.

Epidemiologic studies suggest that inflammation may be involved in sporadic Parkinson disease, because users of **NSAIDs** are less likely to have Parkinson disease. Smoking and increased caffeine intake are also associated with reduced risk of Parkinson disease. The putative protective mechanisms of caffeine and smoking remain speculative and it cannot be excluded that patients with Parkinson disease are less prone to **caffeine** or **nicotine** addiction, especially given the well-established role of dopamine in reward and addiction. Nicotine has been reported to protect against neurodegeneration in the striatum but not in the substantia nigra of animals treated with MPTP. By contrast, caffeine and other antagonists of adenosine A_{2A} receptors, which are highly enriched in striatum, have been reported to protect against nigral cell loss as well as depletion of dopamine in striatum of animals treated with MPTP. Targeted disruption of the A_{2A} receptor gene also confers protection from MPTP toxicity in mice.

Drug-Induced Parkinsonism and Dyskinesias

As described in Chapter 6, **antipsychotic drugs** that potently block D_2 dopamine receptors can cause a reversible parkinsonian-like syndrome. Drug-induced parkinsonism is most common among elderly patients, presumably because they have a smaller reserve of dopamine neurons. Symptoms develop within days to months after use of the offending drug commences **17-3** and disappear over weeks or months after cessation of the drug.

17-3   **Extrapyramidal Side Effects of Antipsychotic Drugs**

Side Effect	Features	Period of Maximal Risk	Treatment
Acute dystonia	Spasms of muscles in tongue, face, neck, and back	First 5 days of treatment	Antiparkinsonian agents
Akathisia	Motor restlessness	5–60 days after treatment begins	Reduction of dose or change to different drug; antiparkinsonian agents, benzodiazepines, or propranolol may help
Parkinsonism	Bradykinesia, rigidity, variable tremor, mask-like facies, shuffling gait	5–30 days after treatment begins	Antiparkinsonian agents
Neuroleptic malignant syndrome	Catatonia, stupor, fever, unstable blood pressure, myoglobinemia; can be fatal	Weeks after treatment begins; can persist for days after neuroleptic is discontinued	Immediate discontinuation of neuroleptic; dantrolene or bromocriptine may help; antiparkinsonian agents not effective
Tardive dyskinesia	Oral-facial dyskinesia; widespread choreoathetosis or dystonia	After months or years of treatment; is exacerbated by withdrawal	Prevention is crucial; treatment is unsatisfactory

Parkinsonian-like symptoms caused by typical antipsychotic medications are among a large number of so-called extrapyramidal side effects produced by these drugs **17-3**. The most dramatic such effect produced in rodents is *catalepsy*, a waxy-like rigidity of the extremities. Such side effects are caused by the D_2 dopamine receptor antagonist properties of these agents. Blockade of these receptors produces functional effects that mimic those of increased activity of GABAergic projection neurons, such as occurs with the loss of dopaminergic neurons **17-10**.

The fact that antipsychotic drugs reduce psychosis, presumably through D_2 antagonism in the mesocorticolimbic dopamine system, and cause extrapyramidal side effects, presumably through D_2 antagonism in the nigrostriatal dopamine system, has provided clinicians with a dilemma. Agents that tend to reduce psychosis also tend to increase the severity of motoric side effects, and agents that reduce motoric side effects likewise tend to aggravate psychosis. A similar dilemma is encountered in the treatment of Parkinson disease: although L-**dopa** is effective in replacing lost dopamine, it can cause dyskinetic side effects and psychotic symptoms after prolonged use. Likewise, agents that are used to reduce the dyskinetic side effects associated with L-dopa tend to increase the severity of parkinsonian symptoms. As discussed in Chapter 16,

the introduction of newer antipsychotic medications has helped to reduce some of these complications.

Tardive dyskinesia   Antagonism of D_2 receptors has been implicated in a particularly severe extrapyramidal side effect of traditional antipsychotic medications known as tardive dyskinesia (TD). TD is unlike other extrapyramidal side effects in that it requires prolonged exposure to the offending drug; indeed, the longer the exposure, the greater the likelihood of developing this syndrome. Moreover, unlike other extrapyramidal side effects, it can persist for long periods, even for a lifetime, after the precipitating medication has been discontinued. TD involves excessive, abnormal movements, particularly choreoathetoid movements that are reminiscent of **Huntington disease**. These abnormal movements, which predominate in the head and neck and typically involve the mouth and tongue, can be debilitating. TD must be distinguished from withdrawal dyskinesias that occur in many individuals after the cessation of antipsychotic treatment and gradually subside over weeks or months.

The Huntington disease–like features of TD symptoms have led to the proposal that TD represents a state of supersensitivity to dopamine in the striatum that develops as an adaptation to persistent D_2 receptor antagonism. Indeed, one treatment for TD symptoms involves raising the dose of the precipitating D_2 antagonist, a practice that is not ultimately beneficial because it leads to a vicious cycle of TD symptoms followed by increasing doses of medication, which in turn cause a worsening of TD symptoms. Despite a great deal of research, the drug-induced changes in the striatum or elsewhere in the brain that cause TD are not yet known. Fortunately, the incidence of TD has decreased dramatically with the introduction of second-generation antipsychotic agents and with the use of lower doses of first-generation antipsychotic drugs (Chapter 16).

Treatment of Parkinson Disease

The treatment of Parkinson disease currently consists of the administration of medications that enhance dopaminergic function in the basal ganglia. As described in Chapter 6, oral administration of L-**dopa** is the most effective symptomatic treatment available for Parkinson disease **17–10**. L-dopa is transported across the blood-brain barrier and is converted to dopamine within remaining dopaminergic nerve terminals and, perhaps, by other monoaminergic terminals that can transport L-dopa via their plasma membrane transporters.

L-dopa efficiently restores neurologic function, particularly during the early stages of Parkinson disease. Yet systemically administered L-dopa cannot possibly replicate dopaminergic innervation of the striatum, either spatially or temporally. Moreover, the efficacy of L-dopa decreases after several years and, as previously mentioned, side effects in addition to dyskinesias begin to appear, including visual hallucinations and other psychotic symptoms, sleep disturbances, and confusion. A late complication of L-dopa therapy, referred to as the *on–off* phenomenon, involves abrupt and transient fluctuations in the severity of parkinsonism at different intervals of the day; such fluctuations are unrelated to drug dosage. To minimize this phenomenon, individuals often restrict their use of L-dopa to times of the day when therapeutic relief is required.

Peripheral side effects caused by the conversion of L-dopa into dopamine by aromatic amino acid decarboxylase expressed in liver and other peripheral tissues may include severe hypotension and nausea. Such problems with L-dopa have been controlled by aromatic amino acid decarboxylase inhibitors such as **carbidopa** and **benserazide** **17–11**. When administered with L-dopa, such agents, which cannot cross the blood-brain barrier, inhibit peripheral aromatic amino acid decarboxylase and reduce the peripheral conversion of L-dopa into dopamine. Such actions reduce the peripheral side

effects of L-dopa and enable the drug to be administered in much smaller doses. L-dopa and carbidopa are available in a fixed-ratio preparation called **Sinemet**. **Entacapone,** an inhibitor of catechol-*O*-methyltransferase (COMT), is also used in conjunction with L-dopa in the treatment of Parkinson disease. Because L-dopa is metabolized peripherally by COMT (Chapter 6) as well as by aromatic amino acid decarboxylase, entacapone can prolong the efficacy of a dose of L-dopa.

Dopamine agonists, which theoretically should be effective during later stages of Parkinson disease, mimic endogenous dopamine by directly stimulating dopamine receptors and, unlike L-dopa, do not require enzymatic transformation. Many dopamine agonists also are not metabolized by L-dopa oxidative pathways and thus do not produce the potentially toxic metabolites of this agent. **Bromocriptine** is an ergot derivative that directly stimulates dopamine D_2-like receptors. It is less effective than L-dopa in providing symptom relief, but produces less dyskinesia and less of the on–off phenomenon, possibly because of its direct receptor activation. Like bromocriptine, **pergolide** is an ergot derivative and dopamine receptor agonist, but it acts on both D_1-like and D_2-like receptors. These medications are used most commonly as an adjunct to L-dopa and, by reducing the amount of L-dopa needed, can decrease the long-term complications of L-dopa therapy. The development of more selective D_1 and D_2 receptor agonists remains a goal of the pharmaceutical industry.

Muscarinic cholinergic antagonists are helpful in alleviating tremor and rigidity but are generally less effective than dopaminergic drugs. However, they are the mainstay of treatment for parkinsonism induced by D_2 antagonists because dopaminergic therapy increases the severity of associated psychiatric symptoms. The mechanism by which muscarinic anticholinergic agents reduce parkinsonism can be understood based on the actions represented in **17–10**. Normally, cholinergic interneurons provide an excitatory influence on striatal medium spiny neurons; consequently, the loss of dopaminergic inhibition of these medium spiny neurons can be compensated for by a decrease in cholinergic excitation. Muscarinic antagonists commonly used to treat parkinsonism include **benztropine, trihexyphenidyl,** and **diphenhydramine** **17–11**.

Amantadine, introduced originally as an anti-influenza medication, has more recently proven to be useful in the treatment of Parkinson disease. It may be given alone or in combination with anticholinergic medications and is believed to potentiate the release of

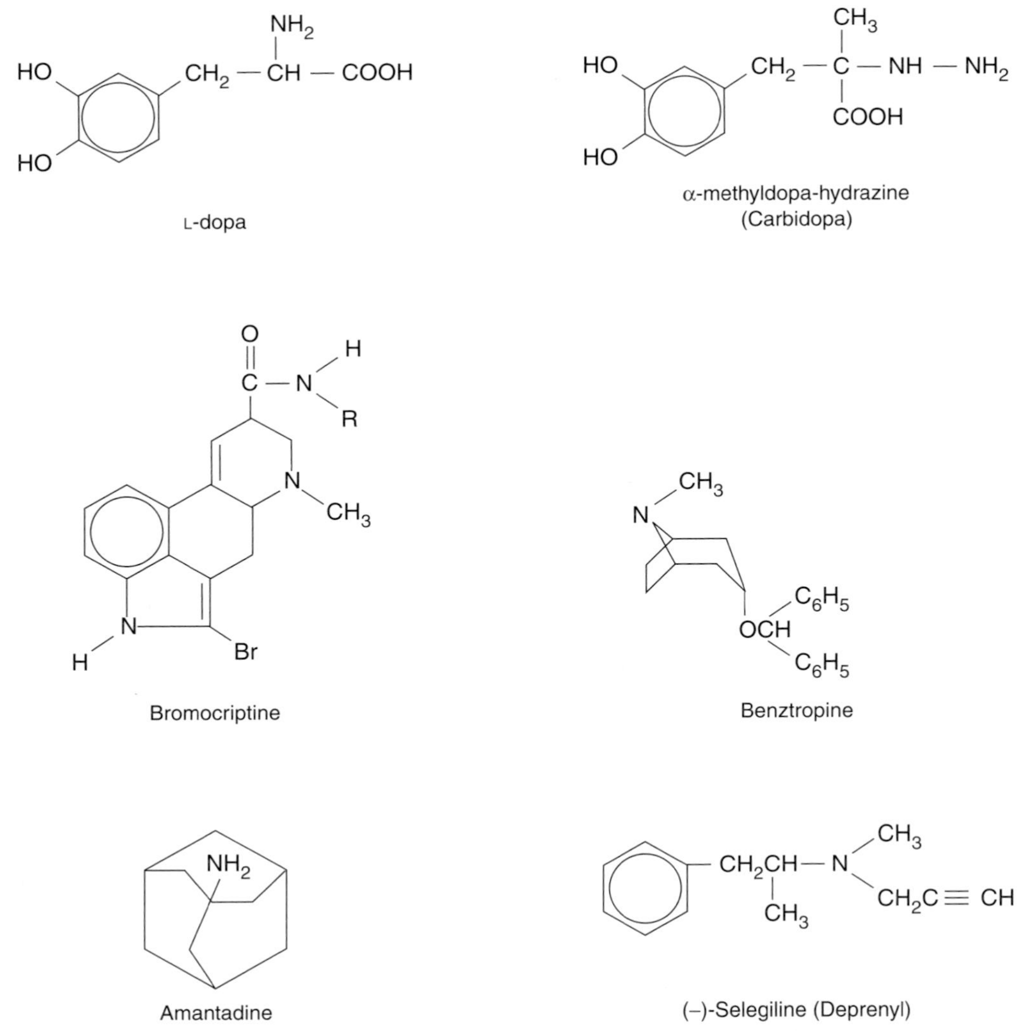

L-dopa

α-methyldopa-hydrazine
(Carbidopa)

Bromocriptine

Benztropine

Amantadine

(−)-Selegiline (Deprenyl)

17–11 Chemical structures of drugs commonly used in the treatment of Parkinson disease.

dopamine. It appears to exert this effect by acting as a weak antagonist at *N*-methyl-D-aspartate (NMDA) glutamate receptors, although precisely how this action leads to enhanced dopamine release is not yet known. Amantadine improves all of the clinical features of parkinsonism, and associated side effects are uncommon. However, the benefits of this drug are relatively modest and short lived.

Selegiline (**deprenyl**) is a selective inhibitor of monoamine oxidase B (MAOB) (Chapter 6). It was introduced into clinical use because MAOB converts MPTP into its active neurotoxic form, MPP+. It was hypothesized that the progression of idiopathic Parkinson disease may involve neurotoxins that act

like MPTP but are as yet unidentified; accordingly, it was speculated that selegiline might retard the progression of Parkinson disease. Large multicenter studies indicate that although selegiline may offer benefits during early stages of the illness, its efficacy wanes as the disease progresses. In addition, selegiline may not provide a neuroprotective effect but may simply increase dopamine levels by inhibiting monoamine oxidase.

Rasagiline is a newer FDA-approved selective inhibitor of MAOB that shows both symptomatic benefit and potentially neuroprotective properties perhaps by antioxidant or antiapoptotic effects. In initial large-scale clinical trials, new Parkinson patients receiving rasagiline for 12 months showed less functional decline compared to a control group receiving placebo for the first 6 months and rasagiline for the remaining six months. Confirmation of these promising effects is needed.

The antioxidants, **coenzyme Q10** and **creatine**, mentioned earlier in the chapter, are also undergoing clinical trials for Parkinson disease. Coenzyme Q10 is a component of the mitochondrial respiratory chain that is neuroprotective in animal and cell models of dopamine neurotoxicity. A phase II trial in Parkinson patients suggested that high doses of coenzyme Q10 may slow the progression of motor symptoms. Further studies are in progress. Like coenzyme Q10, dietary creatine supplementation is thought to promote mitochondrial function which is likely deficient in Parkinson disease. A clinical trial is being conducted with creatine combined with minocycline which is hypothesized to inhibit apoptosis and inflammation.

Drugs that act at various types of adenosine receptors, in particular, A_1 or A_{2A} **antagonists**, are currently under evaluation for use in the treatment of Parkinson disease. These compounds may act by means of interactions at dopaminergic synapses in the striatum, as previously discussed. (See Chapter 8 for further discussion of adenosine systems in brain.)

New approaches to treatment Because patients treated pharmacologically soon become refractory to L-dopa and related therapies, other treatment strategies have been explored. Excess output from the subthalamic nucleus is postulated to play a critical role in the pathophysiology of Parkinson disease (see 17–9). Surgical lesions of this nucleus, or of the internal segment of the globus pallidus (called a **pallidotomy**) have reduced major motor disturbances such as akinesia, rigidity, and tremor. However, because such treatment involves an irreversible lesion, it is reserved for the most severe and medication-refractory cases. More recently, **deep brain stimulation** with a stimulating electrode in the subthalamic nucleus has shown promise as a reversible alternative to placing a lesion. At appropriate stimulation frequencies, the subthalamic nucleus is inactivated and symptoms are relieved, at least temporarily.

Cell transplantation, for example, the administration of fetal mesencephalic dopaminergic neurons–or **stem cells** programmed to differentiate into dopaminergic neurons–into the striatum, remains an area of interest for the treatment of Parkinson disease. This approach is based on the expectation that such cells will proliferate, establish synaptic connections, and synthesize and release dopamine in the striatum.

Indeed, Parkinson disease would appear to be particularly well-suited, compared to other neurologic or psychiatric disorders, for cell transplantation or stem cell therapies, given the fact that it involves the loss of a highly localized cell population in the adult brain. Yet, clinical trials with fetal dopaminergic neurons have been highly disappointing. Further, while the use of stem cells, which has not yet been evaluated in humans, offers some promise, it also remains very speculative; a tremendous amount of progress will be needed to (1) deliver programmed stem cells into the substantia nigra, and (2) prompt those cells to form synaptic connections in the adult brain which normally form early in development.

Gene therapy refers to the transfer of a therapeutic gene into a target tissue and the maintenance of its function for a sufficient length of time. Gene therapy for neurologic disorders can be achieved when genes are delivered into the brain either by transplantation of genetically modified cells or by direct injection of genes (eg, by means of viral vectors) into the striatum. Several strategies for **viral-mediated gene transfer** are under active investigation. Early studies focused on delivering the tyrosine hydroxylase gene to striatal neurons as a way to increase local dopamine synthesis. More recent efforts have focused on the delivery of various types of neurotrophic factors into the substantia nigra or striatum, either by viral gene transfer or by direct delivery of the growth factor into the brain. **BDNF** (brain-derived neurotrophic factor), **GDNF** (glial cell line–derived neurotrophic factor), and **nurturin** have received the most attention given their ability to promote the survival of dopamine neurons in animal models. Still other approaches have involved delivering genes that encode proteins that alter the functional activity of neurons, eg, in the subthalamic nucleus, as a way to correct the abnormal circuitry seen in Parkinson disease. All of these approaches remain at the earliest stages of development, although trials in humans are underway.

HUNTINGTON DISEASE

Huntington disease is an autosomal dominant disorder caused by a mutation of the *huntingtin* gene on the short arm of chromosome 4. The clinical manifestations of the disease typically begin in midlife, with a mean age of onset of 40 years. Initially, the symptoms are subtle and include minor coordination problems, jerky eye movements, and occasional movements of the fingers, limbs, or trunk. Such symptoms may be accompanied by depression, psychotic symptoms, irritability, impulsiveness, and cognitive changes. Deterioration leads to progressive dementia, emotional lability and personality changes, and choreiform movements. Progressive cognitive decline causes disruption of memory and difficulty with complicated tasks; in addition, mood swings, depression, and apathy become more pronounced. During late stages of the disorder choreiform movements regress and dystonia and rigidity are typical symptoms.

In approximately 10% of cases of Huntington disease, symptoms occur before age 20. Individuals with juvenile-onset disease exhibit a more rapidly progressive course and are more likely to experience dystonia with seizures and cerebellar ataxia than chorea. As discussed in the next section, genetic factors are an important determinant of early onset of disease.

Pathophysiology

Huntington disease is associated with degenerative changes that are most apparent in the caudate nucleus and putamen. Such destruction is selective and is restricted to populations of GABAergic medium spiny projection neurons, particularly those that form the previously described indirect pathway and project to the globus pallidus (see **17-9**). Neuronal loss also occurs in the thalamus and cerebral cortex. Striatal cholinergic interneurons, as well as midbrain dopaminergic neurons, are largely unaffected. Indeed, choreiform activity is believed to result from excessive activity of preserved nigrostriatal dopaminergic neurons in conjunction with decreased activity of striatal GABAergic neurons (see **17-9** and **17-10**). However, the connection between a loss of GABAergic output from the striatum and choreiform movements is not yet understood.

Genetics and Pathogenesis

Huntington disease is a Mendelian dominant genetic disorder; individuals who inherit only one mutated copy of the gene do not differ clinically from individuals who possess two defective copies. The molecular basis of Huntington disease is an expansion of a trinucleotide repeat sequence $(CAG)_n$ within the coding region of the huntingtin gene, which was first identified in a linkage study of a large lineage with the disease. In normal individuals, the repeated CAG triplet encodes an average of 5 to 30 copies of the amino acid glutamine within the huntingtin protein. Huntington disease results from an expansion of these triplet repeats that yields 37 to 86 or more glutamines. Such expansion of nucleotide repeats is common to several inherited neuropsychiatric diseases **17-4**. Longer

17-4 Examples of Diseases Caused by Trinucleotide Repeats

Disease	Repeat
Fragile X	$(GGC)_n$ on *FMR1* gene promoter
Myotonic dystrophy	$(CTG)_n$ on myotonin protein kinase gene
Spinobulbar muscular atrophy	$(CAG)_n$ on coding sequence of the androgen receptor gene
Huntington disease	$(CAG)_n$ on huntingtin gene
Spinocerebellar ataxia 1	$(CAG)_n$ on ataxin-1 gene

FMR1, Fragile X mental retardation gene.

repeats in individuals with Huntington disease are associated with an earlier age of onset and, in some cases, with more severe symptoms. Moreover, repeat lengths are unstable and tend to increase from one generation to the next through transmission from both sexes. This expansion most likely occurs during gametogenesis and is believed to be characterized by average increases of 0.4 and 9 repeat units in female and male transmissions, respectively. Such changes result in the clinical phenomenon of *anticipation*—an earlier age of onset or an increase in the severity of disease across successive generations. As expected, individuals with juvenile onset of Huntington disease have the largest number of glutamine repeats in huntingtin.

Although the age of onset of Huntington disease is most dependent on repeat length, it also is influenced by modifying genes and environmental factors. Accordingly, two individuals with the same number of repeats can exhibit very different courses of the disease when they are members of different families. There is great interest in identifying genetic and environmental factors that lead to such modifications because such knowledge might improve management or prevention of the disease and shed light on its pathogenesis. The expanded repeats in huntingtin can be detected in gene carriers by a simple polymerase chain reaction (PCR)-based assay. Consequently, family members can be tested before they are symptomatic to determine whether they carry the defective gene, and the gene also can be detected in fetuses through prenatal testing.

The mechanism underlying Huntington disease represents a classic example of a gain-of-function mutation. The disease is caused by a single copy of a mutant gene that leads to a new biologic effect, rather than a simple increase or decrease in the normal effect of the gene. The new function of mutant huntingtin remains incompletely understood. However, according to an emerging hypothesis, the longer the glutamine repeat is, the more likely the huntingtin protein is to accumulate within vulnerable neurons as intranuclear inclusion bodies, which are seen in the striatum of patients with Huntington disease. Such inclusion bodies lead to disruptions in critical cellular functions, including RNA processing, and eventually cause cell death. It has been hypothesized that the gain of function in mutant huntingtin is the neural toxicity of the expanded polyglutamine domain of the mutant protein. Consistent with this theory are recent findings from mice that overexpress a mutant huntingtin gene; these animals exhibit nuclear inclusion bodies and morphologic changes in vulnerable neurons—early signs of apoptosis that parallel the patterns of cell death associated with Huntington disease. Such mice represent models that can be used to develop new therapies. Interestingly, the huntingtin gene is widely expressed throughout the brain and most other organs; therefore, why mutant huntingtin leads to a relatively selective pathologic process within striatal GABAergic neurons remains a mystery.

The normal function of huntingtin is also something of a mystery. Knockout mice that lack huntingtin die early during embryonic development, exhibiting features of apoptotic cell death. Such findings indicate that huntingtin plays a critical role in many cell types, yet investigators have yet to uncover clues to its function.

Treatment of Huntington Disease

Unfortunately, no specific treatment is available for Huntington disease. The drugs most commonly used for controlling associated dyskinesias are dopamine receptor antagonists, including first generation antipsychotic agents such as **haloperidol** and **chlorpromazine**. These drugs are effective because the blockade of dopamine action relieves dopamine's inhibitory influence on dying GABAergic neurons, thereby increasing net GABAergic output from the striatum (see 17–10). The use of antipsychotic drugs also has the beneficial effect of reducing psychosis in patients who experience such symptoms. Other pharmacologic treatment of Huntington disease targets specific symptoms, such as depression and impulsive behavior, for which **antidepressants** and **propranolol** have been used, respectively. However, the therapeutic efficacy of the latter agent, a β-adrenergic antagonist, is limited.

The interactions represented in 17–10 suggest that drugs that increase GABAergic or cholinergic function in the striatum should ameliorate the symptoms of Huntington disease. However, attempts to alleviate chorea and other dyskinesias with drugs that exert such effects have not yielded consistent clinical responses.

Lessons From Huntington Disease

Experience with Huntington disease has raised several points that are essential to remember as we strive to identify the causes of other neuropsychiatric disorders. First, the gene that causes Huntington disease was previously unknown; its discovery illustrates the power of "reverse genetics"—that is, approaches to finding a disease-related gene that can proceed without prior knowledge of the disease's pathophysiology. Second, the discovery of a disease-related gene provides essential tools for investigating pathogenesis. Indeed, classic approaches to understanding disease pathophysiology did not succeed in explaining Huntington disease. Classic neuropharmacologic approaches would have been based on the assumption that GABAergic and dopaminergic mechanisms were central to the disease. Yet the culprit is a protein that is expressed throughout the body, is not even enriched in the striatum, and is not directly involved in neurotransmission.

Third, the path that leads from the identification of a disease-related gene to definitive treatment can be long and arduous. Many years after identification of the gene, little is known about the normal product of the gene and we are just beginning to understand how the mutant product generates disease. Definitive treatment of Huntington disease and preventive measures await our ability to discover and exploit such information.

Finally, it should be emphasized that Huntington disease is caused by a single genetic mutation and characterized by a straightforward diagnosis, uncomplicated familial transmission, and definitive pathologic findings. The process of determining the mechanisms that underlie other neuropsychiatric disorders and of developing pathophysiologically based treatments for the disorders, particularly those that represent heterogeneous, genetically complex syndromes, is likely to be far more challenging.

AMYOTROPHIC LATERAL SCLEROSIS

Also known as **Lou Gehrig disease** in the United States, amyotrophic lateral sclerosis or ALS is a motor neuron disease that generally occurs in individuals between 30 and 60 years of age. It is characterized by the degeneration of upper and lower motor neurons in both the corticospinal and corticobulbar tracts 17–12. The distribution of resulting deficits in movement can

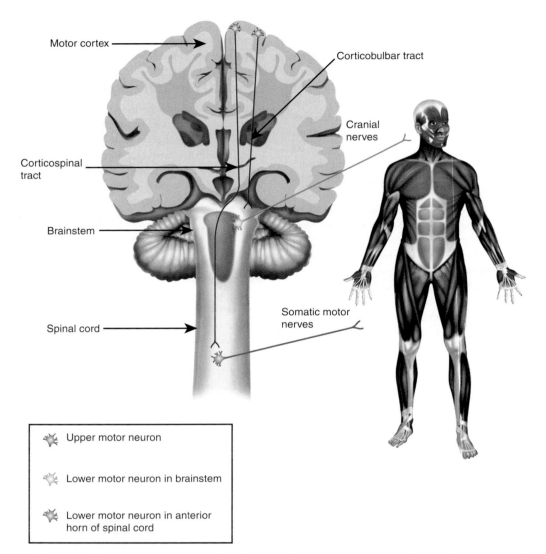

Motor cortex

Corticobulbar tract

Cranial nerves

Corticospinal tract

Brainstem

Somatic motor nerves

Spinal cord

✦ Upper motor neuron

✦ Lower motor neuron in brainstem

✦ Lower motor neuron in anterior horn of spinal cord

17–12 **Upper and lower motor neurons that die in ALS.** Corticobulbar and corticopinal tracts, arising from upper motor neurons in the cerebral cortex, innervate lower motor neurons in the brainstem and spinal cord, respectively. Brainstem motor neurons innervate the muscles of the head and neck via cranial nerves. Spinal motor neurons innervate the rest of the body's skeletal muscle via motor nerves.

be traced to predominant involvement of either the limbs or cranial nerves, and the predominant involvement of either upper or lower motor neurons, and can be used to distinguish the clinical variations of this disorder. In approximately 20% of patients, for example, the disease is limited to weakness of the bulbar muscles; bulbar involvement is characterized by difficulty in swallowing, chewing, coughing, breathing, and speaking. ALS is progressive and typically results in a fatal outcome within three to five years. Patients

with bulbar involvement generally are given a poorer prognosis because of breathing and swallowing difficulties and associated aspiration and pulmonary infections. Motor neuron disease in children, such as **Werdnig-Hoffmann disease** (infantile spinal muscular atrophy), typically presents early in life and is characterized by impaired swallowing or sucking and muscle wasting of the limbs.

Most cases of ALS are sporadic; only 10% to 20% are characterized by familial transmission. In approximately

20% of familial cases (a very small percentage of all cases), the disease is caused by mutations in the gene for the enzyme *Cu/Zn superoxide dismutase* (*SOD*), which is involved in removing reactive oxygen species from cells. Accordingly it was believed that mutations in SOD lead to a loss of its function, which in turn increases oxidative stress on cells. However, further investigation indicates a more complicated situation, because knock-out mice that lack SOD do not develop signs of ALS, some disease-causing mutations in the protein do not result in reduced enzyme activity, and transgenic mice that overexpress such disease-causing mutant forms of SOD exhibit a loss of motor neurons.

Currently it is believed that mutant forms of SOD cause familial ALS by a toxic gain of function likely involving protein aggregation; such mutant proteins cause the development of inclusions in the cytoplasm and cellular processes that in turn cause damage to cells. Details regarding this process remain controversial; for example, some researchers argue that these inclusions initially form in astrocytes of the spinal cord, reducing their ability to transport glutamate and thereby interfering with the termination of synaptic glutamate signals (Chapter 5). Such interference might result in excitotoxicity. Others argue that inclusions initially form in motor neurons and thereby directly disrupt aspects of neuronal function; such disruption most likely would not depend on excitotoxicity.

Other aspects of ALS remain puzzling. Because the expression of SOD is ubiquitous, researchers have yet to determine why the mutation of its gene results in the selective degeneration of upper and lower motor neurons, and why this degeneration occurs relatively late in life, in a relatively synchronized fashion. Also, very little is known about the molecular pathogenesis of familial ALS as well as of the much larger number of sporadic cases of the illness.

Until recently, treatment of ALS has been symptomatic. There are no treatments that halt motor neuron loss; however, the one medication currently approved by the Food and Drug Administration for the treatment of ALS, **riluzole**, has been shown to prolong survival by approximately three months. Riluzole is believed to exert ameliorative effects by decreasing synaptic levels of glutamate, although it has several other actions as well (eg, inhibiting SK (small K^+) channels). Such activity is consistent with the hypothesis that ALS may be caused by glutamate-mediated excitotoxicity. Other treatments that have shown some ability to increase survival time in ALS animal models, such as the anti-inflammatory agent **minocycline**, have yet to show significant benefit in human clinical trials. There is hope that multidrug combinations will prove to be more effective.

SELECTED READING

Ascherio A, Chen H, Weisskopf MG, et al. Pesticide exposure and risk for Parkinson's disease. *Ann Neurol.* 2006;60:197–203.

Blennow K, de Leon MJ, Zetterberg H. Alzheimer's disease. *Lancet.* 2006;368:387–403.

Bonuccelli U, Del Dotto P. New pharmacologic horizons in the treatment of Parkinson disease. *Neurology.* 2006;67:S30–S38.

Bredesen DE, Rao RV, Mehlen P. Cell death in the nervous system. *Nature.* 2006;443:796–802.

Carri MT, Grignaschi G, Bendotti C. Targets in ALS: designing multidrug therapies. *Trends Pharmacol Sci.* 2006;27:267–273.

Citron M. Strategies for disease modification in Alzheimer's disease. *Nature Rev Neurosci.* 2004;5: 677–685.

Cuervo AM, Stefanis L, Fredenburg R, et al. Impaired degradation of mutant alpha-synuclein by chaperone-mediated autophagy. *Science.* 2004;305: 1292–1295.

Dawson TM, Dawson VL. Molecular pathways of neurodegeneration in Parkinson's disease. *Science.* 2003;302:819–822.

Dawson VL, Dawson TM. Mining for survival genes. *Biochem Soc Trans.* 2006;34:1307–1309.

DeArmond SJ, Prusiner SB. Perspectives on prion biology, prion disease pathogenesis, and pharmacologic approaches to treatment. *Clin Lab Med.* 2003;23:1–41.

de Lau LM, Breteler MM. Epidemiology of Parkinson's disease. *Lancet Neurol.* 2006;5:525–535.

Farrer MJ. Genetics of Parkinson disease: paradigm shifts and future prospects. *Nature Rev Genet.* 2006;7:306–318.

Feigin A, Kaplitt MG, Tang C, et al. Modulation of metabolic brain networks after subthalamic gene therapy for Parkinson disease. *Proc Natl Acad Sci USA.* 2007;104:19559–19564.

Gatchel JR, Zoghbi HY. Diseases of unstable repeat expansion: mechanisms and common principles. *Nature Rev Genet.* 2005;6:743–755.

Graham RK, Deng Y, Slow EJ, et al. Cleavage at the caspase-6 site is required for neuronal dysfunction and degeneration due to mutant huntingtin. *Cell.* 2006;125:1179–1191.

Graybiel AM. The basal ganglia: learning new tricks and loving it. *Curr Opin Neurobiol.* 2005;15: 638–644.

Krantic S, Mechawar N, Reix S, et al. Molecular basis of programmed cell death involved in neurodegeneration. *Trends Neurosci.* 2005;28:670–676.

Lansbury PT, Lashuel HA. A century-old debate on protein aggregation and neurodegeneration enters the clinic. *Nature.* 2006;442:774–779.

Lee VM, Trojanowski JQ. Mechanisms of Parkinson's disease linked to pathological alpha-synuclein: new targets for drug discovery. *Neuron.* 2006;52: 33–38.

Lin MT, Beal MF. Mitochondrial dysfunction and oxidative stress in neurodegenerative diseases. *Nature.* 2006;443:787–795.

Lleó A, Greenberg SM, Growdon JH. Current pharmacotherapy for Alzheimer's disease. *Annu Rev Med.* 2006;57:513–533.

Mahley RW, Weisgraber KH, Huang Y. Apolipoprotein E4: a causative factor and therapeutic target in neuropathology, including Alzheimer's disease. *Proc Natl Acad Sci USA.* 2006;103:5644–5651.

May BC, Govaerts C, Cohen FE. Developing therapeutics for the diseases of protein misfolding. *Neurology.* 2006;66(Suppl 1):S118–S122.

McLaurin J, Kierstead ME, Brown ME, et al. Cyclohexanehexol inhibitors of Aβ aggregation prevent and reverse Alzheimer phenotype in a mouse model. *Nature Med.* 2006;12:801–808.

Neumann M, Sampathu DM, Kwong LK, et al. Ubiquitinated TDP-43 in frontotemporal lobar degeneration and amyotrophic lateral sclerosis. *Science.* 2006;314:130–133.

Orr HT, Zoghbi HY. Trinucleotide repeat disorders. *Annu Rev Neurosci.* 2007;30:575–621.

Roberson ED. Frontotemporal dementia. *Curr Neurol Neurosci Rep.* 2006;6:481–489.

Roberson ED, Mucke L. 100 years and counting: prospects for defeating Alzheimer's disease. *Science.* 2006;314:781–784.

Rubinsztein DC. The roles of intracellular protein-degradation pathways in neurodegeneration. *Nature.* 2006;433:780–786.

Shults CW. Therapeutic role of coenzyme Q10 in Parkinson's disease. *Pharmacol Ther.* 2005;107: 120–130.

Stoothoff WH, Johnson GV. Tau phosphorylation: physiological and pathological consequences. *Biochim Biophys Acta.* 2005;1739:280–297.

Tanzi R, Bertram L. Twenty years of the Alzheimer's disease amyloid hypothesis: a genetic perspective. *Cell.* 2005;120:545–555.

Walsh DM, Selkoe DJ. Deciphering the molecular basis of memory failure in Alzheimer's disease. *Neuron.* 2004;44:181–193.

Wichmann T, Delong MR. Deep brain stimulation for neurologic and neuropsychiatric disorders. *Neuron.* 2006;52:197–204.

Wolfe MS. The γ-secretase complex: membrane-embedded proteolytic ensemble. *Biochemistry.* 2006;45:7931–7939.

CHAPTER 18

Seizure Disorders

KEY CONCEPTS

- A seizure is caused by the abnormal synchronous firing of large ensembles of neurons. Epilepsy refers to any neurologic disorder that is characterized by recurrent seizures.

- Seizures can be classified as focal, which indicates that the initial abnormal firing is limited to a specific area in one hemisphere, or generalized, which indicates that a large population of neurons in both hemispheres is involved.

- Seizures occur because of a change in the brain's delicate balance of excitatory and inhibitory synaptic processes. This change can be caused by any number of different brain insults, including tumors, strokes, and head injury as well as developmental abnormalities.

- Many forms of epilepsy have a genetic component, although the inheritance of epilepsy is rarely simple.

- Most anticonvulsants work by modifying the function of sodium or calcium channels or by enhancing GABA-mediated inhibitory synaptic transmission.

This chapter is devoted to seizure-related disorders such as **epilepsy.** Seizures are characterized by uncontrolled firing of sets of neurons in the brain and can have devastating consequences. Seizure disorders are common: they affect approximately 2.5 million individuals in the United States, many of whom are children. Fortunately, the treatment of seizures has steadily improved with the introduction of safer and more effective anticonvulsant agents.

SEIZURES AND EPILEPSY

A seizure is a paroxysmal derangement of cerebral function caused by excessive and generally synchronized activity of a group of neurons. Seizure activity can occur in many different regions of the brain, and its physical manifestations vary according to the region in which it occurs. Thus, the term *seizure* may refer to a 3-second lapse of consciousness that is barely noticeable to the affected individual or to witnesses of the event. The same term also applies to a "grand mal" tonic–clonic seizure that causes an individual to contract all muscles of the body followed by a jerking of his or her entire body so violent that the ensuing muscle damage and electrolyte abnormalities can prove fatal.

Approximately one individual in 20 experiences a seizure at some point during his or her lifetime. In most cases a seizure can be traced to a specific insult, such as **head trauma**, **high fever**, or **alcohol withdrawal**. Approximately one individual in 200 can be described as **epileptic,** or as having a propensity for recurring seizures. Inherited vulnerabilities, focal brain injury, or chronic illness can produce lower seizure thresholds in epileptic individuals, who generally require medication to control their seizures.

Because there are many varieties of seizures, there are many types of epilepsy. Patients who visit epilepsy clinics exhibit a wide diversity of symptoms, from grand mal tonic-clonic seizures to seizures that consist of lapses of consciousness and odd behavior such as lip smacking. Patients also vary in terms of seizure control, ranging from those who are receiving successful therapy and have not had a seizure for years to those who have difficulty maintaining employment because of recurrent seizures resistant to treatment with multiple drugs. Accordingly, the impact of seizures on quality of life varies. Some epileptic patients are inconvenienced only by their need for daily medication, whereas others can be nearly incapacitated by their condition. The effectiveness of treatment also can be highly variable. Some types of epilepsy, including juvenile absence epilepsy, are eminently treatable; other types, especially those related to gross developmental disorders, cannot be adequately treated. Moreover, some patients readily tolerate pharmacotherapy, while others experience distressing side effects such as fatigue, forgetfulness, and medical complications.

The treatment of seizures, along with our understanding of their biologic basis, has undergone slow, steady progress during the last few decades. Newer anticonvulsant drugs, such as **levetiracetam,** are improving seizure control and reducing side effects for many patients. The genetic factors that underlie seizure vulnerability are increasingly well understood, and the physiology of certain types of seizures is slowly being elucidated. Moreover, the molecular events that contribute to epileptogenesis in previously healthy neuronal tissue are beginning to be discovered. Although epilepsy remains a serious disorder for many, effective treatment continues to be developed.

GENERATION OF A SEIZURE

In a normal, conscious state, the net neuronal activity recorded by an *electroencephalogram* (EEG) reveals few waves and no large shifts in polarity (Chapter 12). Such activity does not indicate that the brain is quiet; rather it indicates that neuronal activity is asynchronous. To maintain balance, posture, and fine motor control, for example, some cortical motor neurons may fire action potentials while others are hyperpolarized.

At the onset of a seizure, the EEG reveals characteristic changes **18–1**. Events that may include dramatic upward and downward shifts of polarity begin to appear. Such events indicate that a large number of neurons are firing and repolarizing in synchrony; the summation of their activity produces a noticeable effect on the EEG recording. This type of synchrony can be accompanied by abnormalities in movement, sensation, or consciousness. If synchronous firing occurs in cortical motor neurons, for example, twitching and jerking of affected body parts may replace the fine gradations of muscle activity needed to maintain balance, posture, and smooth, controlled motion. When synchrony occurs in other brain regions, the result may be strange sensations, such as the perception of a particular odor, confusion, or the loss of consciousness.

What causes this change from normal neuronal activity to abnormal synchronized firing of large ensembles of neurons? Many factors can set the stage for a seizure. Abnormal synchronized activity often arises from a particular area in the brain, referred to as a *seizure focus.* Brain imaging and electroencephalography can be used to identify seizure foci, which may

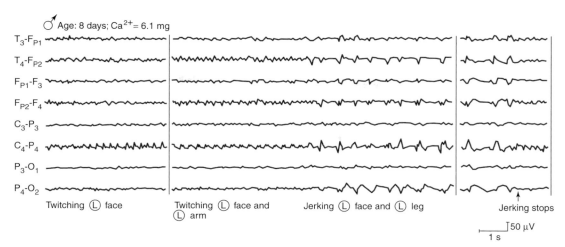

18-1 **Scalp-recorded right hemisphere seizure in a neonate with hypercalcemia.** Note that the onset of large shifts in potential correspond to the progression of the seizure. L, left. (Adapted with permission from Wyllie E. *The Treatment of Epilepsy: Principles and Practice,* 2nd ed. Baltimore: Williams & Wilkins; 1997.)

be associated with areas of neuronal maldevelopment, degeneration, or a structural abnormality such as a tumor **18-2**. A decrease in the overall level of inhibitory transmission in the brain also can precipitate a seizure. Such decreases can occur after the administration of γ-aminobutyric acid (GABA) antagonists, or during withdrawal from repeated exposure to GABA agonists such as **alcohol** or **benzodiazepines**. Moreover, events that do not cause seizures in most people, such as hyperventilation or

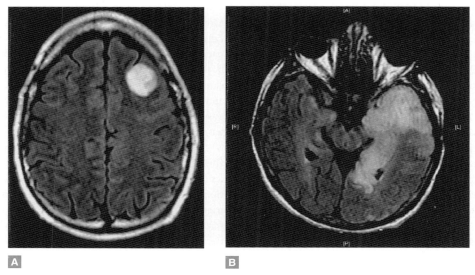

18-2 **MRI scans of patients with brain lesions causing seizures. A.** The patient is a 26-year-old man who presented with complex partial seizures and was found to have a left frontal oligodendroglioma. **B.** Patient with HSV encephalitis showing signal change throughout the left medial temporal lobe, extending to the temporal tip. (Images courtesy of Steven Feske, MD.)

flashing lights, may precipitate seizures in vulnerable individuals.

Although the exact chain of events that trigger individual seizures may be poorly understood, the tendency of neurons to fire in synchrony is related to their extensive interconnectedness. Neurons in different regions of the brain, as well as those within single regions, often have extensive reciprocal connections with one another; for example, glutamatergic neurons in the thalamus project to glutamatergic neurons in the cortex, which in turn project to the thalamus. After they emerge, waves of activity can become self-sustaining and can even propagate from one region of the brain to another.

CLASSIFICATION OF SEIZURES

Seizures can be broadly categorized as *focal* (partial) or *generalized*. As their name suggests, focal seizures are characterized by clinical and electroencephalographic changes that indicate an initial activation of neurons in a relatively small, discrete region of the brain, whereas generalized seizures are characterized by involvement of both hemispheres and widespread neuronal activation. These two broad classifications comprise dozens of subtypes of seizures that have distinct clinical manifestations and involve particular brain regions (see Selected Readings).

Seizure classification aids in the selection of optimal treatment regimens. However, one individual can undergo multiple seizures of varying types; indeed, a single seizure event can involve more than one type of seizure. Focal seizures, for example, commonly evolve into a generalized seizure as activity spreads from the seizure focus to other areas of the brain. The identification of seizure type and progression also helps to determine an optimal treatment regimen 18–1 .

As previously mentioned, the clinical manifestations of *focal seizures* reflect the region of brain in which they occur; for example, a focal seizure in sensory cortex may produce an odd sensory experience, such as a noxious smell or a clicking sound. Other types of focal seizures include aphasic/phonatory, somatosensory, and adversive seizures. *Aphasic/phonatory*

18–1   Rasmussen Encephalitis: An Autoimmune Disorder?

During the early 1990s, experimenters attempting to generate antibodies to the external portion of GluR3, an AMPA glutamate receptor subunit (Chapter 5), noticed that two of the three rabbits they had immunized with GluR3 protein developed recurrent seizures. The brains of these two rabbits exhibited pathology similar to that seen in **Rasmussen encephalitis,** a rare syndrome characterized by seizures, progressive dysfunction, and inflammatory histopathology that typically is confined to a single cerebral hemisphere. The onset of this syndrome usually occurs between 2 and 10 years of age and is followed by progressive atrophy and dysfunction of the affected cerebral hemisphere.

Historically, treatment of Rasmussen encephalitis has been frustratingly ineffective, ultimately necessitating a hemispherectomy—literally removing the affected half of the brain. The pathogenesis of this syndrome had not been determined, and typical anticonvulsant drugs provide little benefit. However, because of the serendipitous finding regarding GluR3, investigators currently believe that the ultimate cause of Rasmussen encephalitis is an autoimmune response to this protein. Serum from individuals with Rasmussen displays immunoreactivity against GluR3, unlike serum from control subjects. Moreover, plasma exchange reduces seizure frequency and increases cognitive function in many patients. Although GluR3 autoimmunity appears to be the cause of Rasmussen encephalitis, how the disease starts and progresses, why circulating GluR3 antibodies are produced, and how antibodies slip past the blood-brain barrier after they are generated has yet to be established.

Some GluR3 antibodies are capable of activating GluR3-containing AMPA receptors; these antibodies can therefore generate seizures by direct activation of glutamate receptors. After a seizure is triggered, a damaging cycle may ensue, involving seizure-induced disruption of the blood–brain barrier, increased entry of GluR3 antibodies, recurring seizures, and further neural injury. Regardless of the exact mechanism of progression, the discovery of the autoimmune basis of Rasmussen encephalitis has advanced the treatment of this once baffling condition.

seizures result in a sudden inability to speak, write, or read. Related seizure foci often are found in the temporal, inferior frontal, or inferior parietal cortex. *Somatosensory seizures* cause paresthesias often referred to as pins and needles, or hot or cold sensations, with corresponding seizure foci often found in somatosensory cortex. *Adversive seizures* result in sudden movements of the head and eyes to the contralateral side of the seizure focus, and related foci often are found in the frontal lobe or precentral gyrus.

Focal motor seizures are characterized by clonic twitching of the contralateral muscles consequent to a localized epileptic discharge from the motor cortex. The muscles involved depend on the affected area of the brain. The motor activity can be moderate (inconspicuous twitching) or extreme (massive jerking of the affected muscles). Focal motor seizures can spread from the focus to neighboring areas of motor cortex. For example, the seizure may spread from one twitching area of the body to the next until the entire half of the body shows clonic activity. Focal motor seizures also may progress into full-blown generalized tonic-clonic (grand mal) attacks.

Complex partial seizures are focal seizures characterized by an impairment of consciousness and can arise from virtually any area of cortex that subserves a complex function such as speech, emotion, or memory. These seizures can produce a variety of effects, including auditory or visual hallucinations, feelings of familiarity (déjà vu) or strangeness (jamais vu), or automatisms such as lip smacking or chewing motions. Although complex partial seizures involve impaired consciousness, the affected individual often continues to interact with the environment, in ways that are sometimes bizarre `18-2`.

The behaviors and experiences that occur during a complex partial seizure are usually initiated in higher-level association cortices, which may explain why resulting behaviors are complex, including automatisms, rather than gross, for example, tonic–clonic movements of an appendage. The involvement of high-level auditory and visual association cortices most likely explains the occurrence of hallucinations during some complex partial seizures. The temporal lobe is a particularly common focus for complex partial seizures. **Temporal lobe epilepsy** is often associated with complex partial seizures involving aphasia and sensations of jamais vu or déjà vu. The hippocampus, which is critical for learning and memory (Chapter 13), is believed to be the source of many temporal lobe epilepsies which in some cases are associated with atrophy of the hippocampus and reorganization of dentate granule cell axons.

Generalized seizures are those that involve multiple, bilateral areas of the brain. The exact cause of most generalized seizures is unknown. Although a focal seizure can spread or generalize, there are many instances in which the entire cortex seems to give rise to seizure activity all at once. Many generalized seizures are associated with developmental disorders.

Tonic seizures are characterized by an extension of the extremities and a rigid stretching of the body.

`18-2` Complex Partial Seizures

Complex partial seizures can be amazingly intricate, as illustrated by a patient, Mary. At the beginning of her seizure, Mary suddenly began to raise and lower the tilting top of her desk in class. When the teacher asked her to stop, Mary looked at the teacher blankly and began to fumble with the buttons on her sweater. When the teacher walked toward Mary to find out what was wrong, Mary put out her arms as though to ward off the teacher. Mary subsequently stood up and wandered aimlessly around the classroom. After a few minutes she stopped, looked around as though puzzled, returned to her desk, put her head down, and fell asleep. Mary had little memory of what had happened except for an awareness that she had behaved strangely; she was embarrassed by the episode and was reluctant to return to school.

After examining Mary, her doctor was convinced that she had experienced many other such lapses. An EEG revealed frequent sharp-wave discharges from Mary's right temporal lobe. After she adopted a regimen that included regular use of **carbamazepine,** Mary stopped experiencing seizures. The details of Mary's complex partial seizure disorder explain why such symptoms are sometimes misconstrued as conduct problems. (Gumnit RJ. *The Epilepsy Handbook: The Practical Management of Seizures.* New York: Raven Press; 1995.)

These attacks are common in children with **Lennox–Gastaut syndrome**. This syndrome is characterized by a slow spike-and-wave complex on EEG recordings, impaired cognitive function, and multiple types of seizure, including atonic drop attacks. Lennox–Gastaut syndrome typically becomes evident between 1 and 10 years of age, and often is refractory to anticonvulsant medications. The cause of this syndrome remains unknown; however, it has been associated with **brain malformations**, **hypoxic–ischemic brain injury**, **encephalitis**, **meningitis**, and **tuberous sclerosis**. A heritable susceptibility also may be a factor in the acquisition of this syndrome: a family history of epilepsy is evident in 3% to 27% of cases.

Atonic seizures are accompanied by a sudden loss of muscle tone, which is sometimes preceded by a myoclonic jerk; if standing, the affected individual typically falls to the ground. These attacks generally last only a few seconds, and do not involve a loss of consciousness. A patient generally recovers immediately after an atonic seizure; however, a risk of injury is present during the fall, and many affected individuals must wear protective gear such as helmets to prevent fall-related injuries. *Clonic seizures* involve repetitive muscle twitching; such attacks can last as long as 1 minute. *Myoclonic seizures* are rapid involuntary muscle contractions; the term *myoclonic* is used to denote a single twitch event, which is distinct from repetitive, or clonic, twitching.

Generalized tonic-clonic (grand mal) seizures are associated with immediate profound coma and orderly sequences of motor activity. This activity comprises distinct tonic phases (arms in semiflexion and legs extended) that are followed by a clonic phase (full-body spasms with intermittent relaxations). EEGs exhibit massive fast spiking during the tonic phase and bursts of polyspikes interrupted by slow waves during the clonic phase. Such seizures are frequently preceded by focal seizures.

Generalized absence seizures, or *petit mal seizures*, are characterized by a brief lapse of consciousness (approximately 10 seconds or less) accompanied by an EEG recording of a spike-and-wave discharge of approximately 3 Hz 18-3 . The earliest clinical description of a generalized absence seizure appeared in 1705 in a report by a French physician: "At the approach of an attack the patient would sit down in a chair, eyes open, and would remain there immobile and would not afterward remember falling into this state. If she had begun to talk and the attack interrupted her, she took it up again at precisely the point at which she stopped and she believed she had talked continuously." Although this description gives the essence of an absence seizure, additional phenomena such as mild atonia, automatisms,

and mild tonic or clonic components may occur in some patients. The 3-Hz spike-and-wave pattern that accompanies an absence seizure reflects a widespread phase-locked oscillation between excitation (spike) and inhibition (wave) in mutually connected thalamocortical neuronal networks.

The activity of a group of neurons in the nucleus reticularis thalami (NRT) is particularly important for determining the behavior of thalamocortical networks and therefore the occurrence of absence seizures. GABAergic neurons of the NRT project densely to one another and to almost all thalamic relay nuclei. They also receive excitatory, glutamatergic inputs from the collaterals of both thalamocortical axons and corticothalamic axons 18-4 . During periods of reduced conscious awareness, NRT neurons exhibit firing in rhythmic bursts, whereas during alert wakefulness, they exhibit tonic single-spike firing. The cellular event that is responsible for the rhythmic burst firing mode of NRT neurons is the low-threshold (T-type) Ca^{2+} spike (Chapter 2). What causes this type of rhythmic firing during absence seizures is unclear but the role of T-type channels elegantly explains the actions of **ethosuximide**, the drug of choice in the treatment of absence seizures. At clinically relevant concentrations, ethosuximide diminishes T-channel currents in NRT neurons; it is believed that this action quells the 3-Hz spike-and-wave activity that characterizes the absence seizure. Interestingly, absence seizures are among the few types of seizure that are actually made worse by the administration of GABA agonists. Drugs that promote GABAergic transmission such as **vigabatrin** may enhance the ability of NRT neurons to adopt rhythmic firing mode by enhancing their hyperpolarization, which leads to greater activation of T-channels when the cells are subsequently depolarized.

WHAT CAUSES EPILEPSY?

Had epilepsy never existed, it would have been discovered eight times over the past year by those intent on knocking out mouse genes one at a time.

Noebels, 1996

The many different causes of epilepsy are too numerous to list. Many knockout mice experience spontaneous seizures, and the various forms of human epilepsy that appear to have a genetic basis have been traced to many different genes. Moreover, as previously mentioned, epilepsy frequently occurs after brain trauma or infection.

Why is the brain predisposed to seizure activity? Because neurons are so extensively and often reciprocally

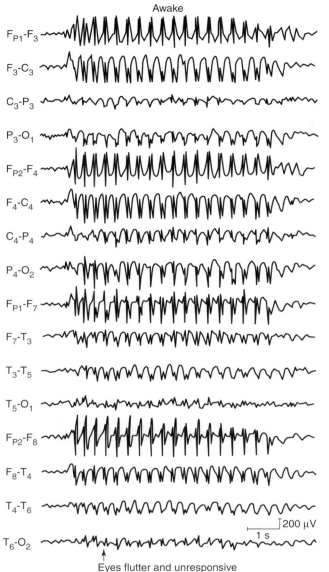

18-3 **Absence seizure recorded in a 7-year-old girl.** The 3-Hz spike-and-wave activity occurs simultaneously across the entire cortex. Less than one second after the beginning of this activity, the girl becomes unresponsive. *Inset*: expansion of the 3-Hz spike and wave. (From Wyllie E. *The Treatment of Epilepsy: Principles and Practice*, 2nd ed. Baltimore: Williams & Wilkins; 1997.)

interconnected, it appears that any excitatory activity can propagate and perpetuate itself across a brain or brain circuit. In healthy individuals, inhibitory circuitry generally limits the degree to which any neural activity is propagated, either spatially or temporally. As a result, any condition that upsets the delicate balance between excitation and inhibition is likely to cause a seizure. The sections that follow discuss a few of the many different ways such imbalance can occur.

Genetic Influences

More than 20 strains of knockout mice exhibit spontaneous seizures, as do several strains of mice in which

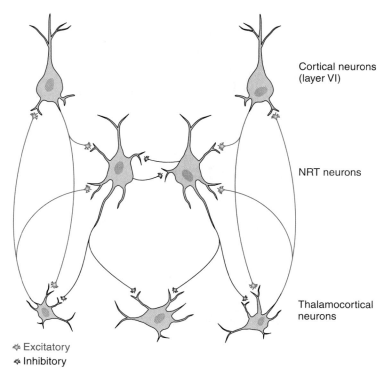

Cortical neurons
(layer VI)

NRT neurons

Thalamocortical
neurons

✧ Excitatory
✦ Inhibitory

18–4   **Thalamocortical circuitry believed to be involved in absence seizures.** Note that nucleus reticularis thalami (NRT) neurons are excited by both cortical and thalamic inputs and inhibited by one another. The NRT also provides inhibitory input to the thalamus.

particular proteins have been overexpressed **18-1**. Spontaneous seizures are seen, for example, in mice that lack the genes for ion channels, such as the delayed rectifier K^+ channel mKv1.1; for neurotransmitter receptors, such as GluR2 and serotonin $5HT_{2c}$; for enzymes, such as Ca^{2+}/calmodulin kinase II; and for transcription factors. That such a wide variety of gene products can influence seizure susceptibility is not surprising. Ion channels and neurotransmitter receptors influence the excitability of neurons directly; enzymes, which modify neurotransmitter receptors and ion channels, influence neuronal excitability in many ways; DNA-binding proteins influence the repertoire of proteins expressed by neurons, which might in turn affect excitability. These proteins might also influence epileptogenesis in a more complex manner; for example, they might alter developmental processes so that abnormal neural circuits are produced.

Many cases of human epilepsy appear to have a genetic component, although the inheritance of epilepsy is rarely simple (Mendelian). Numerous human epilepsy syndromes have been mapped to specific chromosomes and, in a few cases, the specific genes have been identified. These types of epilepsy are listed in **18-2**. All known epilepsy-causing mutations in humans affect channels or receptors, and represent deficits that would be expected to directly affect neuronal excitability.

Neuronal Death, Neurogenesis, and Sprouting: Keys to Epileptogenesis?

In addition to the large number of genetic abnormalities that can lead to epilepsy, trauma, such as a blow to the head, can cause epilepsy in humans as well as in experimental animals. Seizure-inducing trauma is generally associated with discrete anatomic changes, which have been most intensively studied in the hippocampus, a particularly epileptogenic area of the brain. In animal models, seizure-inducing trauma is associated with selective loss of inhibitory interneurons of the dentate hilus, and also with an increase in the number of excitatory dentate granule cell axons (mossy fibers). Loss of hilar cells and sprouting of mossy fibers are also a

18-1 Examples of Mouse Genes Linked to an Epileptic Phenotype

Gene	Protein	Age of Onset	Postnatal Lethality
Spontaneous seizures			
Deletions			
5HT$_{2C}$	Serotonin receptor	<5 weeks	+
Synapsin I, II	Synaptic vesicle proteins	>2 months	−
CaMKIIα	Ca^{2+}/calmodulin protein kinase		−
TNAP	Nonspecific alkaline phosphatase	2 weeks	+
Centromere BP-B	Brain-specific DNA binding protein	3–4 months	−
mKv1.1	K$^+$ channel	2 weeks	+
Weaver	G protein–gated inward rectifier (GIRK2)	Adult	+
GluR2	Q/R site editing of glutamate receptor subunit	2 weeks	+
Overexpression			
GAP–43	Neural growth-associated protein	>4 weeks	−
Pip	Myelin protected protein	<4 weeks	+
No seizures, but decreased threshold for epileptogenesis			
Tyn	Tyrosine kinase receptor		−
tPA	Tissue plasminogen activator		−
BDNF (−/+)	Brain–derived neurotrophic factor		−

Reproduced with permission from Noebels JL. *Neuron.* 1996; 16:241.

prominent aspect of the pathologic changes observed in human temporal lobe epilepsy.

These observations raise several questions. The loss of hilar inhibitory interneurons is consistent with the imbalance of excitation and inhibition that might be expected to lead to seizures. However, why do hilar interneurons die in greater numbers than excitatory neurons? Moreover, what mechanisms underlie the increased number of mossy fibers, and what are the consequences of this sprouting? An increase in mossy fibers may result from the sprouting of existing dentate granule cells or it may be related to an increase in the total number of these cells. Indeed, the generation of new dentate granule cells, neurogenesis, which occurs at low levels during adulthood, has been found to increase after trauma, as well as after seizures.

The ultimate effects of the increase in mossy fiber density are uncertain. It is possible that mossy fiber sprouting contributes to epileptogenesis by increasing excitatory input to hippocampal circuits. Alternatively, mossy fibers may selectively synapse onto remaining hilar interneurons in an attempt to return the overall level of inhibition to normal. Mossy fiber proliferation may be manipulated by means of pharmacologic and molecular interventions. The NMDA glutamate receptor antagonist **MK-801** retards seizure development and mossy fiber sprouting, as does elimination of the gene for the transcription factor c-Fos. Neurotrophic factors most likely play a role in mossy fiber proliferation, and research into the effects of neurotrophins such as brain-derived neurotrophic factor (BDNF) (Chapter 8) on mossy fiber sprouting has begun to yield interesting results. If mossy fiber sprouting is proven to contribute directly to the development of seizures, these findings might be exploited to inhibit epileptogenesis.

TREATMENT OF EPILEPSY

Along with advances in our understanding of the etiologies of seizure disorders, there has been slow but steady progress in the development of new and safer anticonvulsants. Nevertheless, most individuals with recurrent seizures continue to be treated with anticonvulsant drugs that have been available for many years **18-5**.

Almost all anticonvulsants work by directly modifying neural excitability through alterations either in ion channels or in the availability of amino acid neurotransmitters. The key to seizure prevention is

18-2 Molecular Genetics of Idiopathic Epilepsies

Epilepsy Syndrome	Linkage	Gene
Epilepsies with simple inheritance		
Benign familial neonatal convulsions	20q	KCNQ2[2]
	8q	KCNQ3[2]
Benign familial infantile convulsions	19q	?
	16	?
Autosomal dominant nocturnal frontal lobe epilepsy	20q	CHRNA4[3]
	15q[1]	?
Familial partial epilepsy with auditory features	10q	?
Familial partial epilepsy with variable foci	2q[1]	?
Epilepsies with complex inheritance		
Juvenile myoclonic epilepsy	6p	?
	15q[1]	?
Idiopathic generalized epilepsy, unspecified	8q[1]	?
Idiopathic generalized epilepsy, unspecified	3p[1]	?
Persisting absence with later myoclonic epilepsy	1p[1]	?
Persisting absence with tonic–clonic seizures	8q[1]	?
Generalized epilepsy with febrile seizures	2q[1]	?
	19q	SCN1B[4]
Benign rolandic epilepsy	15q[1]	?
Febrile seizures	8q[1]	?
	19p[1]	?

[1]Single report to date so linkage should be regarded as tentative.
[2]KCNQ2 and KCNQ3 are novel neuronal potassium channel genes.
[3]CHRNA4 is the gene for the alpha-4 subunit of the neuronal nicotinic acetylcholine receptor.
[4]SCN1B is the gene for the beta-1 sodium channel subunit.
? Unknown.
Reproduced with permission from Berkovic SF, Scheffer IE. *Curr Opin Neurol.* 1999; 12:177–182.

interference of rapid, synchronized firing of neurons. The ideal anticonvulsant drug must prevent the excessive, synchronized discharges that occur during a seizure without impeding normal neuronal function. Most anticonvulsants can be divided into three general categories according to their mechanisms of action: agents that act on Na$^+$ channels, those that affect GABAergic transmission, and those that act on Ca^{2+} channels.

Drugs that selectively stabilize the inactive state of Na$^+$ channels decrease a nerve's ability to fire rapid bursts of action potentials (Chapter 2). Drugs that enhance inhibitory GABAergic transmission are able to increase GABA availability or to enhance the effect of GABA on GABA receptors. The activities of drugs that inhibit Ca^{2+} channels were discussed earlier in this chapter; inhibitors of T-type Ca^{2+} channels are especially effective against generalized absence seizures.

Although most anticonvulsant drugs have at least one of these mechanisms of action, many appear to affect other aspects of neurotransmission. Some anticonvulsant drugs, for example, are believed to reduce glutamatergic neurotransmission by altering glutamate metabolism or by blocking glutamate receptors directly.

Drugs That Enhance Na$^+$ Channel Inactivation

Phenytoin, carbamazepine, oxcarbazepine, lamotrigine, topiramate, and **felbamate** all enhance Na$^+$ channel inactivation, although some of these substances produce additional effects that may contribute to their anticonvulsant activity. Because these drugs bind to and stabilize Na$^+$ channels that are inactivated, their binding is dependent on the opening of Na$^+$ channels, which leads to the inactivated state. Stabilization of the inactivated state of the voltage-gated Na$^+$ channel has the ultimate effect of reducing sustained high-frequency firing of action potentials **18-6**.

18-5 Chemical structures of commonly used anticonvulsants.

Drugs with this mechanism act specifically on rapidly firing neurons, and the ability of neurons to fire one or a few action potentials is little affected.

Valproate is another use-dependent Na^+ channel blocker, although it is weaker in this regard than drugs such as phenytoin and carbamazepine. However, valproate exerts other effects as well. Not only is it a Ca^{2+} channel blocker, but, based on the results of many studies, it also may be able to increase levels of GABA in the brain, albeit via as yet unknown mechanisms.

Interestingly, several of these anticonvulsant agents, particularly valproate and lamotrigine, are used clinically in the treatment of **bipolar disorder.**

The mechanism by which these drugs exert such mood-stabilizing effects is a matter of considerable debate (Chapter 14).

Drugs That Enhance Inhibitory GABAergic Transmission

Benzodiazepines and **barbiturates** bind to distinct sites on the $GABA_A$ receptor and increase the receptor's affinity for GABA, thereby increasing its chloride conductance (**18-7** ; see Chapter 5). These agents, such as **phenobarbital,** are not as frequently prescribed for epilepsy as they once were. They often produce unwanted sedative effects in patients, who may complain of tiredness, forgetfulness, and confusion. Moreover, patients are subject to rapid tolerance to the anticonvulsant effects of benzodiazepines with repeated administration. However, several newer anticonvulsants with different mechanisms of action may be more effective and better tolerated.

Vigabatrin, a relatively new anticonvulsant medication approved for use outside of the United States, is a synthetic structural analogue of GABA that acts as a specific inhibitor of GABA transaminase, an enzyme critical to the breakdown of GABA in the nerve terminal (Chapter 5). As might be expected, patients who take vigabatrin have increased levels of GABA in their cerebrospinal fluid. This is consistent with the model that vigabatrin may exert its anticonvulsant action by increasing the overall availability of GABA.

Tiagabine is an inhibitor of the plasma membrane GABA transporter that removes released GABA from the synaptic space and returns it to the nerve terminal for recycling or catabolism (Chapter 5). By inhibiting the GABA transporter, tiagabine most likely acts to increase the time that GABA remains in the synaptic cleft after its release. In hippocampal CA1 cells, tiagabine increases the duration of inhibitory postsynaptic currents—an action that is consistent with its ability to produce a prolonged effect of GABA at inhibitory synapses.

Gabapentin and the related drug **pregabalin** are GABA analogues; however, they have not been proven to bind to the GABA receptor or affect GABA metabolism or reuptake. Nonetheless, gabapentin increases total GABA concentrations in human cerebrospinal fluid. It has been suggested that gabapentin increases GABA availability by stimulating the release of nonvesicular pools of GABA. It also may stimulate GABA synthesis. However, these actions remain speculative.

Zonisamide is a relatively new anticonvulsant used for the treatment of partial seizures. The exact mechanism of action is unknown, but it may bind to GABA

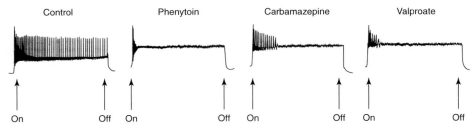

18-6 **Effects of three anticonvulsant drugs on sustained high-frequency firing of action potentials.** In control neurons, a depolarizing pulse leads to repetitive firing of action potentials. In the presence of phenytoin, carbamazepine, or valproate, the number of action potentials is drastically reduced. (Adapted with permission from Katzung BG. *Basic and Clinical Pharmacology*, 7th ed. Originally published by Appleton and Lange. Copyright © 1998 by The McGraw-Hill Companies, Inc.)

receptors, similar to the actions of benzodiazepines, as well as inhibit GABA reuptake.

Levetiracetam is a member of a family of cyclic derivatives of GABA (eg, **piracetam**) that were originally promoted as so-called **nootropic** agents to enhance cognitive function. While this effect of the drugs is weak at best, levetiracetam was approved recently for the treatment of several forms of epilepsy, and early experience with the drug is promising. The mechanism of action of levetiracetam is unknown; it is proposed to bind to a

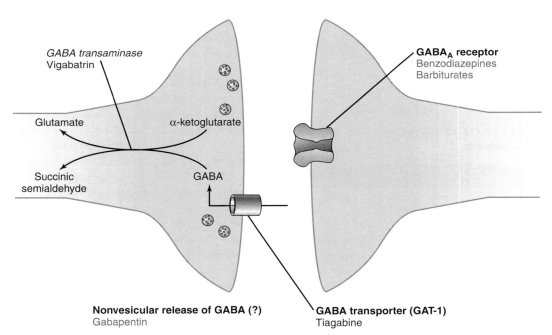

18-7 **Actions of various anticonvulsant drugs that act at γ-aminobutyric acid (GABA) synapses.** Vigabatrin inhibits GABA transaminase, and in turn prevents the breakdown of GABA. Tiagabine inhibits GABA reuptake. Benzodiazepines and barbiturates enhance the function of GABA$_A$ receptors. Gabapentin's mechanism of action remains unknown; however, it may promote the nonvesicular release of GABA from synaptic terminals.

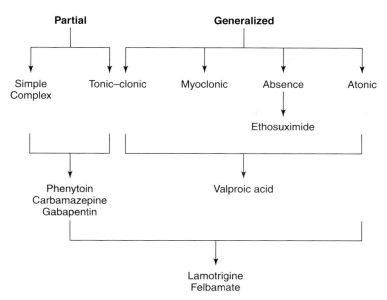

18-8 **Specificity of anticonvulsant drugs in the treatment of partial and generalized seizures.**

synaptic vesicle protein SV2A, whose role in exocytosis is poorly defined.

Rhyme and Reason: Determining the Appropriate Drug

Clinical trials and experience, rather than an understanding of the pathophysiology of epilepsy and the mechanisms of action of anticonvulsant medications, have provided the best guidelines for determining the medication that is most effective in controlling each type of seizure. Valproate, for example, is effective in controlling primary generalized epilepsy of the absence, myoclonic, or tonic–clonic type, and is less effective in the treatment of partial seizures, for which phenytoin and carbamazepine are the drugs of choice. As previously mentioned, the T-channel blocker ethosuximide is most useful in treating generalized absence seizures; this finding is consistent with what is known about the processes that underlie this type of seizure.

In general, agents that are effective in controlling partial seizures appear to produce relatively effective use-dependent Na^+ channel blockade compared with drugs that are most useful for treating generalized seizures. Conversely, drugs effective in controlling generalized seizures tend to be better Ca^{2+} channel blockers **18-8**.

We look forward to a day when the pathophysiology underlying a particular seizure disorder will more accurately guide the use of drugs with specific mechanisms of action and greater tolerability.

SELECTED READING

Adams SM, Knowles PD. Evaluation of a first seizure. *Am Fam Physician.* 2007;75:1342–1347.

Andrews PI, McNamara JO. Rasmussen's encephalitis: an autoimmune disorder? *Curr Opin Neurobiol.* 1996;6:673–678.

Borgeois BF. Chronic management of seizures in the syndromes of idiopathic generalized epilepsy. *Epilepsia.* 2003;44(Suppl 2):27–32.

Chang BS, Lowenstein DH. Epilepsy. *New Engl J Med.* 2003;349:1257–1266.

Manning JP, Richards DA, Bowery NG. Pharmacology of absence epilepsy. *Trends Pharmacol Sci.* 2003;24: 542-549.

Marsh ED, Brooks-Kayal AR, Porter BE. Surgeries and anti-epileptic drugs: does exposure alter normal brain development? *Epilepsia* 2006;47:1999–2010.

McNamara JO, Huang Yz, Leonard AS. Molecular signaling mechanism underlying epileptogenesis. *Science STKE.* 2006;re12.

Meldrum BS, Rogawski MA. Molecular targets for epilepsy drug development. *Neurotherapy.* 2007;4:18–61.

Moshe SL. Mechanisms of action of anticonvulsant agents. *Neurology.* 2000;55(Suppl):S32–S40.

Murdoch D. Mechanisms of status epilepticus: an evidence-based review. *Curr Opin Neurol.* 2007;20: 213–216.

Noebels JL. The biology of epilepsy genes. *Annu Rev Neurosci.* 2003;26:599–625.

Rogawski MA, Loscher W. The neurobiology of antiepileptic drugs. *Nature Rev Neurosci.* 2004;5: 553–564.

Steinlein OK. Genetic mechanisms that underlie epilepsy. *Nature Rev Neurosci.* 2004;5:400–408.

Tsuchida TN, Barkovich AJ, Bollen AW, et al. Childhood status epilepticus and exitotoxic neuronal injury. *Pediatr Neurol.* 2007;36:253–257.

CHAPTER 19

Stroke and Migraine

- Stroke occurs when blood flow to the brain is disrupted and the areas of brain deprived of oxygen die. This can be caused by obstruction or hemorrhage of blood vessels.

- Loss of oxygenation causes death of neurons through complex processes, which include excitotoxicity–mediated by excessive release of glutamate from damaged neurons, and subsequent increases in intracellular calcium levels and overactivation of calcium-dependent enzymes.

- Loss of oxygenation also causes neuronal death through the formation of free radicals and through genetically programmed cell death, called apoptosis.

- Despite increased understanding of the biochemical processes underlying neuronal death, the best therapy for stroke remains rapidly restoring the brain's blood supply and preventing the formation of clots and emboli.

- This includes the use of anticoagulants such as aspirin, heparin, and warfarin, as well as thrombolytic agents such as tissue plasminogen activator (tPA).

- Migraine headaches are believed to result from waves of inhibitory neuronal activity called "cortical spreading depression" that stimulate trigeminal nerve endings innervating the brain's vasculature. This causes release of proinflammatory substances into and around the vessels, resulting in vasodilation and pain.

- Treatment regimes for migraine headaches typically employ both prophylactic and abortive strategies.

- The mainstay in abortive treatment are the triptan drugs, such as sumatriptan.

STROKE

Vertebrate neurons are exquisitely specialized for the functions they perform. As explained in previous chapters, a single neuron may receive information from and relay information to thousands of other neurons; consequently, the nervous system is capable of remarkably complex functions. Moreover, the brisk flux of ions across neural membranes permits extremely rapid interneuronal signaling. However, this specialization comes at a cost. A tremendous amount of energy is required to maintain ionic gradients across the membranes of the approximately 100 billion neurons that comprise the human brain. Although the brain represents only 2% of the body's total mass, it uses approximately 20% of the body's oxygen supply, and blood flow to the brain accounts for about 15% of total cardiac output. Ischemia, or insufficient blood supply, results in oxygen and glucose deprivation and in the buildup of potentially toxic metabolites such as lactic acid and CO_2. Interruption of blood flow to the brain can lead to complete loss of consciousness within 10 seconds, the approximate amount of time required to consume the oxygen contained in the brain.

Stroke occurs upon disruption of blood flow to brain tissue caused by obstruction or hemorrhage. The exquisite vulnerability of neurons to energy deprivation caused by stroke results in vast medical, economic, and personal costs. In the United States alone, roughly 550,000 strokes occur each year. Approximately 150,000 of these strokes are fatal, which makes stroke the third leading cause of death in the United States. Survivors of stroke often are beset by serious long-term disabilities, including paralysis and disruption of higher cognitive functions such as speech. Individuals with such disabilities may be unable to resume work and other daily activities, and often require extensive long-term care by healthcare professionals or friends and family.

The term stroke, also referred to as **cerebrovascular accident (CVA),** broadly refers to neurologic symptoms and signs that result when blood flow to brain tissue is interrupted. The two primary types of stroke are occlusive and hemorrhagic. An *occlusive* stroke is caused by the blockage of a blood vessel **19–1**. Vascular occlusion, which generally restricts blood flow to a discrete area of the brain, results in neurologic deficits and in a loss of functions controlled by the affected region. Occlusive strokes typically are caused by embolic, atherosclerotic, or thrombotic occlusion of cerebral vessels **19–2**.

A *hemorrhagic* stroke is caused by bleeding from a vessel. Intracranial bleeding can occur in the intraparenchymal, epidural, subdural, or subarachnoid

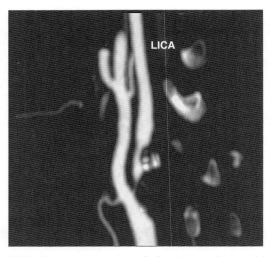

19–1 **Critical stenosis of the internal carotid artery (ICA) at the bifurcation of the common carotid artery into the internal and external carotids.** In addition to the 99% stenosis of the ICA, note the ulcerated atherosclerotic plaque.

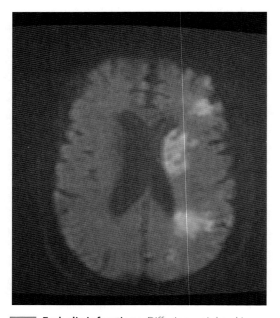

19–2 **Embolic infarctions.** Diffusion weighted imaging MRI revealing embolic infarcts (white) within the left middle cerebral artery (MCA) territory. Such emboli may have arisen from blood clots in the heart (cardioembolic) or from clots or atheromatous plaque from an artery such as the carotid (artery-to-artery emboli).

spaces. Intraparenchymal hemorrhage may be caused by acute elevations in blood pressure or by a variety of disorders that weaken blood vessels. Chronic hypertension is the most common predisposing factor, but coagulation disorders, brain tumors that promote the development of fragile blood vessels, and the use of **cocaine** or **amphetamines**—both of which cause rapid elevation of blood pressure—are among the risk factors for intraparenchymal hemorrhages. Intraparenchymal hemorrhaging can lead to the formation of blood clots (hematomas) in the cerebrum, cerebellum, or brainstem, which in turn may limit the blood supply to nearby brain regions and exacerbate the injurious effects of a stroke.

Epidural, subdural, and subarachnoid bleeding often results from head trauma or the rupture of an aneurysm. In addition to the damage caused by the loss of blood supply to affected areas of the brain, hemorrhages can cause damage by increasing intracranial pressure which further compromises neuronal health. Moreover, through mechanisms that are not completely understood, subarachnoid hemorrhage can cause reactive vasospasm of cerebral surface vessels, which in turn can lead to a further reduction in blood supply.

Mechanisms of Neuronal Injury During Stroke

When neurons are deprived of the nourishment they require, they quickly become unable to maintain their resting membrane potentials and, as they depolarize, they fire action potentials. Their firing triggers the release of neurotransmitters, in particular, glutamate, which in turn promotes depolarization of neighboring neurons. Such activity sets the stage for a destructive cycle of neuronal activation, neurotransmitter release, and further activation. Prolonged periods of neuronal activation can lead to the disruption of ionic gradients, massive Ca^{2+} influx, cellular swelling, activation of cellular proteases and lipases, mitochondrial damage, generation of free radicals, and eventually widespread neuronal death. Ischemia of only a few minutes' duration can result in permanent brain damage. The basic biochemical mechanisms responsible for these processes of neuronal injury and death, broadly termed *necrosis* or *apoptosis* (or programmed cell death), are described in detail in Chapter 17.

Treatment of Stroke

Despite our growing knowledge of the mechanisms that underlie ischemic neuronal death, our ability to treat stroke remains limited. Among the treatment strategies currently available, the best are geared toward prevention through the maintenance of cardiovascular health,

restoration of blood supply, and the slowing of metabolism with hypothermia. Although none of these therapies has capitalized on the sophisticated studies of the biochemical events underlying neuronal cell death, efforts to prevent stroke nevertheless have been successful. The incidence of stroke has been reduced markedly by primary preventive measures aimed at controlling hypertension, hypercholesterolemia, diabetes, and tobacco use. HMG-CoA reductase inhibitors, known as the **statin** class of cholesterol-lowering agents, appear to confer additional benefit in stroke prevention beyond cholesterol control, as treatment with statins in individuals with normal cholesterol levels significantly reduces the incidence of future stroke. Prophylactic use of drugs that inhibit platelet function, such as **aspirin, clopidogrel,** or **dipyridamole,** have proven to be effective in reducing the risk of occlusive stroke at the cost of slightly increasing the risk of hemorrhagic stroke.

One reason that stroke prevention is so important is that current stroke therapies are pitted against an unforgiving opponent: *time*. By the time an individual becomes aware of the occurrence of a stroke, travels to a hospital, and is diagnosed, hours often have elapsed. Even in current clinical trials, several hours usually elapse between the onset of stroke and the administration of treatment. As previously emphasized, serious neural damage can occur within minutes of an ischemic event. Barring round-the-clock observation of all individuals at risk for stroke, the effectiveness of treatment in humans is unlikely to approach that of laboratory animals because researchers in the laboratory have the luxury of administering therapy during or immediately after an ischemic insult.

The Peri-Infarct Area: An Important Treatment Target

Many of the approaches to treatment discussed in the sections that follow involve actions that occur primarily in the peri-infarct area, the "penumbra," and serve to salvage at-risk neurons that would otherwise be destined to die within hours or days after a stroke. The peri-infarct area constitutes compromised but potentially salvageable tissue between the severely ischemic core and adequately perfused brain tissue. Although potentially salvageable, the peri-infarct area is quite vulnerable because it is subject to high levels of excitotoxic neurotransmitters and free radicals, waves of cellular depolarization, and inflammatory processes (Chapter 17).

Restoring Blood Supply

After an occlusive stroke, blood supply can be restored with anticoagulants and thrombolytic agents, which dissolve the clots that impede the normal flow of blood. Thrombolytic agents have been found to improve the outcome of this type of stroke in clinical trials. However, these agents must be used with great caution because they increase the risk of hemorrhage. Consequently, the presence of hemorrhagic stroke must be ruled out, by use of computerized tomography (CT) scans or other brain imaging modalities before anticoagulant and thrombolytic agents are used. Even occlusive strokes are accompanied by a small but real risk of hemorrhagic transformation.

Thrombolytics   Urokinase, streptokinase, prourokinase, desmoplase, reteplase, and tissue plasminogen activator (tPA) are proteins that promote the conversion of the proenzyme plasminogen into plasmin, an enzyme that degrades fibrin, a key structural protein in most blood clots 19-3 ; 19-1 . Currently, **tPA** is the only

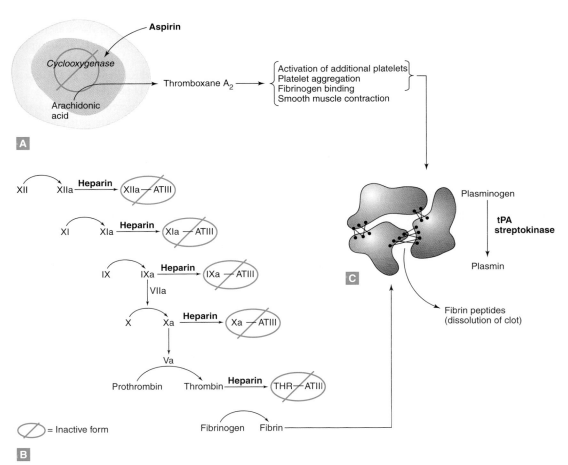

19-3 **Mechanisms of action of anticoagulants and thrombolytics. A.** Platelets are activated by molecules exposed during tissue injury. Aspirin inhibits cyclooxygenase, which catalyzes the formation of thromboxane A_2, a key intermediary in the clotting process. **B.** During the clotting cascade, a chain of precursor proteins activate one another, a process that results in amplification of the signal. Heparin catalyzes the binding of antithrombin III (ATIII) to several of the activated clotting proteins denoted by roman numerals; the antithrombin-bound clotting factors are inactive. **C.** Thrombolytics such as tissue plasminogen activator (tPA) and streptokinase catalyze the conversion of the inactive precursor plasminogen to the active enzyme plasmin, which catalyzes the breakdown of fibrin polymers. Fibrin is a key component of the clot; it is produced from its precursor fibrinogen through catalysis by thrombin, a major product of the clotting cascade.

19-1 Treatment of Stroke

Category	Name	Action/Type of Agent	Clinical Efficacy
Anticoagulation and thrombolysis	Aspirin	Inhibits synthesis of thromboxane A_2, inhibiting platelet aggregation	Modest
	Heparin	Activates antithrombin III, which inhibits clotting factor proteases	Modest
			Being tested
	Nadroparin	Heparin-like anticoagulants	Being tested
	Orgaron		
	tPA	Converts plasminogen to plasmin, which cleaves thrombin	Modest
	Urokinase		Being tested
	Streptokinase		None
Glutamate receptor blockade	Aptiganel	NMDA receptor channel blocker	None
	Dextrorphan		None
	Dextromethorphan		None
	Magnesium		Being tested
	NPS 1506		Being tested
	Remacemide		Minimal
	ACEA 1021 (licostinel)	NMDA glycine-site antagonist	None
	GV 150526		Being tested
	Eliprodil	NMDA polyamine-site antagonist	None
	YM872	AMPA receptor antagonist	Being tested
	ZK-200775 (MPQX)		None
Voltage-gated Ca^{2+} channel blockers	Nimodipine	Reduces Ca^{2+} influx	None
	Lifarizine		?
	Flunarizine		None
Na^+ channel blockers	Lubeluzole	Reduces excitability and glutamate release	?
	Riluzol		?
	Phenytoin		None
Voltage-dependent K^+-channel agonist	BMS-204352	Reduces Ca^{2+} influx	Being tested
Enhancement of inhibitory neurotransmission	Clormethiazole[1]	GABA receptor agonist	Being tested
Free radical scavengers/ antioxidants	Pergorgotein	Reduces free-radical-mediated injury	?
	Tirilazad		None
	Ebselen		Minimal
Neural repair	Citicoline	Phospholipid precursor	?
	Trofermin	bFGF receptor agonist	Minimal

[1]Clormethiazole enhances the action of GABA at $GABA_A$ receptors, although its exact mechanism of action is unknown.

None—either a clinical trial of the drug was completed and no efficacy was found or the clinical trial had to be stopped because of adverse side effects.

?—either no data on clinical efficacy are available or the clinical data are preliminary.

tPA, tissue plasminogen activator.

thrombolytic substance approved for intravenous use in the United States. Clinical trials demonstrate that intravenously delivered tPA reduces the disability of patients with acute ischemic stroke who were treated within the first 3 hours of the onset of symptoms. Although administration of intravenous tPA in the emergency room setting within 3 hours of symptom onset is now standard of care in the United States, only 3% to 5% of stroke patients actually receive tPA because of the difficulty of administering it within 3 hours of the acute event.

Even when intravenous tPA is successfully administered in time, the affected vessel does not always open or open completely. At academic centers, intravenous therapy is increasingly followed by interventional procedures, where a catheter is guided from a peripheral artery (usually the femoral artery in the groin) to the affected cerebral artery. The clot is then treated with a combination of mechanical clot disruption or direct instillation of a thrombolytic agent into the clot itself. Because a smaller dose of the thrombolytic agent is used when given at the site of the clot itself, as compared to systemic (intravenous) administration, intra-arterial therapy is in some ways safer and can be performed up to six hours after symptom onset. In cases of basilar artery thrombosis, when the brainstem is at risk and the matter of opening the artery is literally life and death, intra-arterial therapy will sometimes be given up to 24 hours after symptom onset. **Prourokinase, urokinase, reteplase,** and **desmoplase** are additional thrombolytics that are used in intra-arterial therapy.

Anticoagulants Heparin is a heterogeneous mixture of sulfated mucopolysaccharides. It is found in mast cells and in the extracellular matrix of most tissues. It has a molecular mass of 750 to 1000 kDa and is composed of long polymers of glycosaminoglycan chains that are attached to a core protein **19-4**. Because of its structure, heparin is not effective after oral administration and must be given parenterally. It inhibits clot formation by enhancing the activity of antithrombin III, a protein that forms equimolar complexes with the

19-4 Chemical structures of representative antiplatelet and anticoagulant drugs.

various proteases activated during the clot formation process (see 19-3). By binding directly to antithrombin III, heparin causes a conformational change in the protein that enhances its binding to the clotting factor proteases. Because heparin works by inhibiting the formation of clots, rather than by degrading existing clots, its use typically is considered a preventive measure against the recurrence of stroke. Patients treated with heparin for 1 to 2 weeks after an initial episode of stroke show a significant improvement in their condition compared with patients who receive a placebo. However, this improvement in overall outcome may not persist long after the treatment period.

As discussed in Chapters 4 and 11, **aspirin** 19-4 inhibits cyclooxygenase, which in platelets catalyzes the conversion of arachidonic acid to thromboxane A_2, among other products. Thromboxane A_2 is a critical intermediate in the recruitment of platelets necessary for the clotting cascade. Aspirin administered to patients during hospital admission for stroke produces a small but significant net benefit: its use prevents death or disability in approximately 13 per 1000 affected individuals compared with placebo. Other cyclooxygenase inhibitors, including some nonsteroidal anti-inflammatory drugs (**NSAIDs**) (Chapter 11), may have similar activity. **Clopidogrel** is another antiplatelet agent in current use. It acts by inhibiting the binding of fibrinogen to activated platelets through interactions with glycoproteins on platelet membranes.

Dipyridamole, used for similar purposes clinically, inhibits clot formation and causes vasodilation, although it is not known which of its many actions (eg, phosphodiesterase, adenosine reuptake, or adenosine deaminase inhibition) is responsible for the drug's clinical effects.

Patients at risk for cardioembolic strokes, such as those with atrial fibrillation, severe congestive heart failure, or a mechanical heart valve, conditions that predispose patients to form intracardiac clots, often are treated with **warfarin** (see 19-4). Warfarin is a synthetic derivative of a related compound in sweet clover, which was found in the early 20th century to promote bleeding. Warfarin acts as a **vitamin K** antagonist. Vitamin K is a required cofactor for the enzymes that activate several clotting factors, including II, VII, IX, and X. Warfarin prevents the reduction of oxidized vitamin K into its active form. Warfarin and related compounds are the most potent oral anticoagulants known; indeed, they are so potent that severe hemorrhage is a significant side effect of their use. (This effect, at high doses, is exploited in warfarin's use as a rat poison.) Patients who take warfarin must have regular blood tests to ensure that their bleeding times are within safe boundaries.

Aspirin, warfarin, and other oral anticoagulants are used not only to treat stroke but also to prevent **transient ischemic attacks** (**TIAs**), which are brief periods of brain ischemia that resolve without a lasting neurologic deficit (ie, without appreciable neuronal death). These attacks are believed to be caused by transient occlusions of the cerebral vasculature. The symptoms of TIAs are similar to those of stroke, except that they resolve within minutes to hours of onset.

Minimizing Ca^{2+} Influx Into Cells

Because Ca^{2+} appears to be critically involved in promoting the biochemical processes that lead to neuronal destruction, the reduction of Ca^{2+} influx might be considered a promising strategy in the treatment of stroke. However, the effectiveness of drugs that reduce the influx of Ca^{2+} into neurons (see 19-1) has yet to be demonstrated in clinical trials. Inhibitors of voltage-dependent Ca^{2+} channels (Chapter 2) such as **nimodipine,** an L-type Ca^{2+} channel blocker that penetrates the brain, and **flunarizine,** a T-type Ca^{2+} channel blocker, have been investigated as potential therapies for stroke but thus far have not been shown to improve the functional outcome of patients after ischemic stroke. **NMDA receptor antagonists** exhibit a robust protective effect on neurons in culture but have not proven to be effective in humans. Even if they were effective, many of these antagonists have **phencyclidine**-like adverse effects, such as psychosis and dissociation (Chapter 16), which severely limit the dose that can be used. **Magnesium** blocks the NMDA receptor, and a current trial of intravenous magnesium sulfate given within 2 hours of symptom onset is underway. Because of the relative safety of magnesium and the narrow time window defined by the study, the trial design allows intravenous magnesium to be given by paramedics in the field, prior to arrival and evaluation in the emergency room. Antagonists of voltage-dependent Na^+ channels, such as **phenytoin,** which can be very effective in the treatment of seizure disorders, have failed to improve clinical outcomes of stroke. Likewise, drugs that promote GABAergic function in brain have been considered for stroke, but efficacy of this mechanism too has not yet been demonstrated in humans.

Reducing Free Radical Damage and Cell Death Pathways

There is evidence that the increased generation of free radicals in ischemic brain tissue may contribute to neuronal injury and death 19-5 (Chapter 17). Free radical scavengers are agents that are oxidized by oxygen-reactive species without deleterious effects to the cell

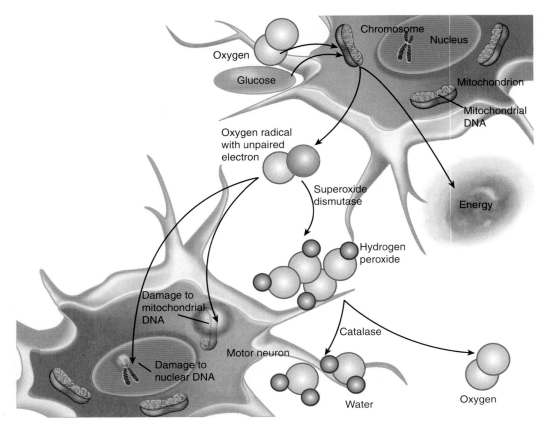

19-5 **Free-radical damage to subcellular structures.** Reactive oxygen species (ROS) and radicals are generated as a result of metabolic processes. These free radicals have at least one unpaired electron which renders them chemically unstable and highly reactive with other molecules in the body. Mitochondrial DNA (miDNA) is located near the inner mitochondrial membrane and lacks advanced DNA repair mechanisms; this makes miDNA particularly susceptible to damage from ROS. Cells respond to oxidative damage by neutralizing free radicals through antioxidant enzymes such as superoxide dismutase (SOD) and catalase. Eventually damage accumulates due to the inability of cells to repair damage as quickly as it arises.

and thus might be expected to have positive effects in stroke. **Tirilazad,** a nonglucocorticoid steroid that inhibits lipid peroxidation, has been shown to reduce infarct area in animals treated within 10 minutes of complete focal ischemia. However, tirilazad has no effect on functional outcome when administered to humans approximately 4 hours after stroke. **Ebselen,** another free radical scavenger, was reported to produce a very modest reduction in damaged tissue when given 6 to 12 hours after acute occlusion of the middle cerebral artery in one clinical study. **Disufenon,** a free radical trapping agent, showed modest initial promise in one trial in terms of functional outcome at 90 days, but those results were not replicated in a subsequent trial. Thus, currently there are no accepted stroke therapies based on blocking free radical damage.

Knowledge of the biochemical basis of necrotic and apoptotic mechanisms of neuronal death has suggested many additional potential approaches to the treatment of stroke. Indeed, genetic manipulation of numerous cell death or survival proteins in rodents has been shown to alter the brain's vulnerability to a stroke. However, none of these strategies has to date been validated in clinical trials. Among the promising strategies under investigation in animal models is the use of **caspase inhibitors;** caspases (short for cysteine aspartate proteases) are enzymes that promote apoptosis and necrosis (Chapter 17).

Another potential strategy is the use of agonists of PPARγ (peroxisome proliferators activated receptor-γ). PPARγ is a member of the nuclear receptor superfamily, which also includes the receptors for steroid hormones, vitamin D, and retinoic acid (Chapter 4). PPARγ, and its PPARα and PPARδ isoforms, heterodimerize with the retinoid X receptor to form an active transcription factor complex that regulates many genes involved in intermediary metabolism. While the endogenous ligands for PPARγ remain uncertain, synthetic agonists exert beneficial clinical effects: the thiazolidinediones, **pioglitazone** and **rosiglitazone,** are effective antidiabetic agents and act by increasing the sensitivity of peripheral tissues to insulin. A recent study showed that diabetics treated with these agents exhibited a lower incidence of stroke. This is consistent with the ability of the drugs to reduce brain injury in animal models of ischemia possibly by inhibiting excitotoxicity and apoptosis. Further research is now required to understand the molecular mechanisms by which activation of PPARγ, which is expressed in neurons and microglia, exerts these protective effects and determine whether PPARγ agonists are useful in the treatment or prevention of stroke.

Still another experimental approach involves inhibitors of nitric oxide synthesis, based on the animal literature that the generation of nitric oxide during ischemia, mediated by excessive glutamatergic transmission and intracellular Ca^{2+} levels, may contribute to neuronal injury perhaps via free radical formation. However, other studies of nitric oxide in stroke suggest that it might be protective, highlighting some of the complexities of translating findings from animal models to the clinical situation 19–1 .

Strategies with Pleotropic Agents

Several neuroprotective strategies act at multiple levels in the cascade of postischemic damage. **Statins,** mentioned earlier as agents that play a key role in preventing strokes from occurring, appear to also confer benefit on stroke recovery in several animal and human studies. Effects of statins include improving endothelial function, reducing inflammation, and increasing cerebral blood flow. In animal models, statins reduce infarct size and improve functional recovery. These benefits of statins are bearing out in clinical studies as well. It will be interesting in future research to understand the mechanisms underlying these diverse, palliative effects of the statins.

Another broad spectrum strategy is **hypothermia.** Controlled hypothermia confers benefit in cases of global ischemia after cardiac arrest, and so interest has been sparked as to its effect in cases of focal ischemia or stroke. Several studies have demonstrated neuroprotective effects of hypothermia in animal models of stroke. The clinical utility in human stroke is a matter

still under investigation, with mixed results in initial clinical trials.

Promoting Neural Recovery

Another approach to stroke therapy is to promote the self-repair of damaged neurons or the growth of healthy neurons to help compensate for the loss of neurons destroyed during an ischemic attack. Two general strategies can be used to this end. A nutritive strategy involves ensuring that neurons have the molecules they need for repair and growth, and a signaling strategy involves providing the chemical signals that instruct neurons to grow. The first strategy has been attempted with administration of the phospholipid precursor **citicoline,** for which a small beneficial effect on outcome has been claimed, as measured by functional recovery and examination of mental status. Citicoline is a key intermediate in the biosynthesis of phosphatidylcholine, an important component of the neural cell membrane.

Neurotrophic factors such as basic fibroblast growth factor (bFGF; Chapter 8) also are being considered for restorative therapy. In animal stroke models, bFGF reduces infarct volume when given shortly after the onset of focal ischemia. Although bFGF did not reduce infarct size when given 24 hours after experimentally induced stroke, it did improve outcome as measured by behavioral tests. This neurotrophic factor and others have yet to be assessed in human clinical trials.

Despite all of the advances in our understanding of neural injury related to stroke, the best-established way to ensure long-term recovery of function is through rehabilitation. Research involving laboratory animals has provided insight into how rehabilitation might work at the neurobiologic level 19–2 . The results of such research raise the possibility that neurobiologic mechanisms underlying the inherent plasticity of the brain may be exploited in the future to ensure maximal return of function after stroke.

MIGRAINE HEADACHES

Subtypes of Migraine

Migraine disorders are characterized by periodic, often unilateral, frequently pulsatile headaches. It is a common disorder, with prevalence estimated at as much as 15% of Caucasian women and 5% of Caucasian men; the incidence is lower in Asian and African populations. *Classic migraine,* also known as migraine with aura or neurologic migraine, is characterized by a disturbance

19-1 Role of Nitric Oxide in Stroke

Nitric oxide (NO) functions as an intracellular and intercellular messenger in the brain (Chapter 8). It is synthesized by the Ca²⁺-activated enzyme, nitric oxide synthase (NOS). The importance of NOS activation in neuronal injury has been tested through the use of specific **NOS inhibitors,** such as **L-nitroarginine.** Initial studies produced inconsistent results: NOS inhibitors displayed neuroprotective effects in some experiments, especially those conducted in cell culture, and produced either no effect or a detrimental effect in others. These conflicting results most likely were attributable to the multiple roles and sources of NO in the brain.

Three different isoforms of NOS exist, each of which is the product of a distinct gene. Neuronal NOS (nNOS) is expressed exclusively in neurons, endothelial NOS (eNOS) originally was identified in endothelial cells, and inducible NOS (iNOS) originally was identified in certain immune system cells. Some neurons express eNOS and iNOS in addition to nNOS. NO produced by eNOS acts as an endothelial relaxing factor: it promotes the relaxation of the smooth muscle surrounding arterioles and leads to vasodilation and increased blood flow.

Gene knockout technology has helped to elucidate the roles of these NOS isoforms in neuronal

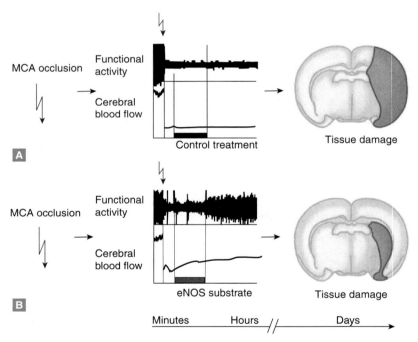

Intravenous treatment with the NOS substrate, L-arginine, promotes functional recovery in an experimental stroke model. **A.** Occlusion of the middle cerebral artery (MCA; onset indicated by red lightening) results in a profound reduction in regional cerebral blood flow (measured by laser-Doppler flowmetry; lower graph) and functional activity of the brain (measured by electrocorticogram; upper graph). Days later, a large cerebral infarct evolves in the ischemic middle cerebral artery territory (indicated in red on the coronal brain section). **B.** In comparison, intravenous infusion of the eNOS substrate L-arginine after MCA occlusion in another rat augments cerebral blood flow, improves functional activity, and reduces the area of infarct compared with control treatment. These findings suggest that augmenting NO bioavailability can promote functional recovery in the ischemic brain. (Adapted with permission from Dalkara T, Morikawa E, Panahian N, et al. Blood flow-dependent functional recovery in a rat model of focal cerebral ischemia. *Am J Physiol.* 1994;267:H678–H683.)

injury. Compared with their wild type counterparts, mice deficient in nNOS typically have smaller infarct volume (ie, amount of necrotic tissue) after an experimentally induced ischemic stroke. This finding suggests that nNOS activity may be detrimental to neuronal survival during ischemia. In contrast, mice deficient in eNOS tend to have greater than normal infarct volumes after experimentally induced stroke, which indicates that eNOS has neuroprotective activity. Most likely, eNOS exerts its beneficial effect by promoting the reperfusion of the ischemic area. This is demonstrated in the figure. Interestingly, iNOS knockout mice, like nNOS knockout mice, display diminished infarct

volume after ischemic stroke; it is speculated that a decreased inflammatory response may reduce infarct size in these mice.

The multiple effects of NO on ischemic injury provide an excellent lesson in the complexity of the brain's response to ischemia. Other events that take place during ischemia, such as Ca^{2+} entry into cells, also may have multiple and varied effects, and these actions must be carefully examined if effective therapies are to be devised. If, for example, NOS inhibition can be developed as a clinical treatment for ischemic neuronal injury, such inhibition most likely will have to be carefully targeted to nNOS or perhaps iNOS.

---

of neurologic function that precedes the headache. This disturbance can take numerous forms, most commonly visual symptoms such as seeing scintillating dots or shapes. Following the "aura," pulsatile head pain develops, which can be bilateral or hemicranial and is often accompanied by nausea and even vomiting, as well as sensitivity to light and sound (photophobia and phonophobia). The headache typically develops within 10 to 30 minutes of the aura, and then intensifies, lasting several hours to even days. In the throes of a migraine, people tend to lay down in a quiet, dark room and are frequently all but incapacitated by the headache.

Common migraine is much the same, without the preceding neurologic disturbance to serve as a warning. The ratio of classic to common migraine is about 1:5. Migraine variants also exist, including the restriction of neurologic dysfunction to one eye (ocular and ophthalmoplegic migraine), as well as neurologic dysfunction so severe as to cause dramatic motor deficits (hemiplegic migraine) or even a reversible coma (so-called basilar migraine).

Migraine tends to run in families. In classic migraine, 60% to 80% of patients have an affected family member, with somewhat lower family frequency in common migraine. Inheritance of migraine is not classically Mendelian and is thought to be polygenic in most cases. In hemiplegic migraine, however, several families have been described that display autosomal dominant inheritance. In about one-third of families with hemiplegic migraine, the responsible gene appears to be on chromosome 19 and codes for a voltage-gated P/Q-type Ca^{2+} channel (Chapter 2). This finding raises the

possibility that other forms of migraine are caused by as-of-yet undiscovered channelopathies.

In addition to genetic factors, there are clearly environmental triggers as well. Association with a long list of food triggers is well established; common agents include caffeine, red wine, and chocolate. Moreover, women find that their headache pattern is often strongly influenced by their menstrual cycle and by pregnancy, indicating hormonal influences on headache frequency and severity. Sleep deprivation and stress may also play roles.

Etiology of Migraine Headaches

The etiology of migraine headaches is an area of continued investigation and debate, with competing vascular and neurogenic hypotheses. It is agreed that activation of the trigeminovascular system—the trigeminal nerve innervation running along the intracranial and extracranial vasculature—accounts for the throbbing pain of migraine. It is also agreed that the neurologic dysfunction associated with classic migraine and variants such as hemiplegic migraine result from an electrophysiologic phenomenon called *cortical spreading depression*, waves of inhibitory activity that spread at a rate of approximately 3 millimeters per minute. Alterations in blood flow in the affected region of brain, most often in the visual cortex, have been demonstrated using functional MRI (fMRI) `19-6`. During a migraine attack, there is an initial increase and subsequent decrease in blood flow, measured during fMRI as changes in the blood oxygen level-dependent (BOLD) signal. These alterations in

19-2 Neurobiologic Basis of Rehabilitation

Stroke patients with large initial deficits often can exhibit striking improvement. The length of the recovery process (typically 1-2 years) suggests that events other than the resolution of edema and inflammation are responsible for improvement in function. In some cases, restoration of blood flow through the development of collateral circulation may contribute to the regaining of function. However, several lines of evidence indicate that neurons undergo anatomic and functional changes that significantly assist in functional improvement after a stroke. In rats, for example, increased expression of the growth cone-associated protein GAP-43 and of the synaptic vesicle protein synaptophysin have been detected near experimentally induced infarct areas. *Growth cones* are specialized endings of growing axons before they form mature synapses. Increased expression of GAP-43 also has been noted in the periphery of infarcted human brain tissue examined at autopsy. Interestingly, dendritic sprouting has been observed contralateral to cortical lesions produced by electrocauterization in rats. This finding suggests that recovery of function may occur as the corresponding, contralateral area of the brain assumes the function of its injured counterpart.

The occurrence of compensatory neural remodeling after stroke has been demonstrated experimentally. Electrophysiologic experiments have revealed a reassignment of function after ischemic infarct in squirrel monkeys: when small infarcts are produced in the area of the motor cortex that corresponds to the hand, new areas of the cortex, previously responsible for movements of the arm and shoulder, slowly gain the ability to control hand motions. This topographic reorganization of neuronal function required that the monkeys perform tasks that necessitated the use of their debilitated hand. Thus, frequent activation may stimulate the growth of remaining neuronal processes responsible for control of the hand into arm-and-shoulder territory. Alternatively, such activation may increase the potency of a small number of "hand neurons" that preexisted in the arm and shoulder space.

Similar reassignment of function likely takes place in the human brain. Positron emission tomography (PET) and magnetic resonance imaging (MRI) studies indicate that adjacent or contralateral brain regions may indeed work to compensate for damaged tissue. Verbal tasks typically cause activation of speech areas in the left hemispheres of normal subjects; however, in some recovered aphasic patients, increased activation of homologous areas in the right hemisphere have been observed. Is this an indication that the right hemisphere can undergo changes that allow compensation for the damaged left hemisphere? Unfortunately, current experiments have not conclusively answered this question. It is possible, for example, that speech centers in the right hemispheres of certain aphasics participated in verbal tasks to an unusual degree before the onset of stroke. However, in light of anatomic and physiologic data from animal models, dendritic and axonal growth and other forms of neural plasticity are mechanisms worth investigating in stroke patients. Knowledge of the molecular and cellular events that influence such rearrangement may eventually lead to techniques for aiding the recovery of stroke victims. Moreover, because shifts of function depend on the use of an affected area after stroke, it is likely that aggressive physical or speech therapy will continue to be a critical tool in promoting recovery after stroke.

---

blood flow are believed to result from vasomotor changes (vasodilation and vasoconstriction).

The relationship of cortical spreading depression to the vascular changes seen in migraine is a point of debate. The leading theory is that cortical spreading depression activates the trigeminovascular system, thereby causing the vascular changes, including vasomotor changes as well as blood-brain barrier leakiness, which result in *"neurogenic inflammation"* and pain 19-7. According to this neurogenic hypothesis, currently in favor, cortical spreading depression causes vascular changes via trigeminal nerve-mediated release of vasoactive substances. While early attention focused on substance P, current work indicates a particularly important role for calcitonin gene-related peptide (CGRP). After a migraine attack, CGRP (but not substance P) can be measured in blood from the jugular vein. A likely source is the trigeminal ganglion; in human trigeminal ganglia, more than 40% of neurons express CGRP, while about half as many express substance P. The competing

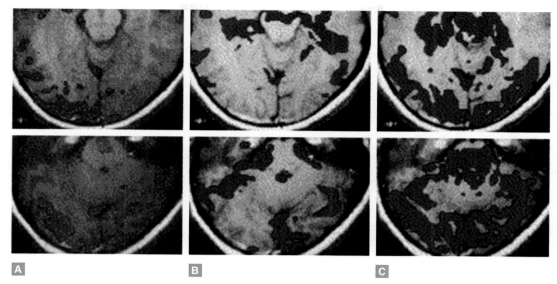

19-6 **BOLD-fMRI of the occipital cortex during a migraine attack.** A migraine attack was provoked using an alternating red-green checkerboard pattern projected to the patient in the magnet. Two adjacent axial images (upper, lower) through the occipital cortex are shown; BOLD intensities show changes from baseline. **A.** In the right occipital lobe (ie, left of image), significant decreases (blue) in BOLD signal occurred before symptom onset; these changes were observed only in patients who reported visual symptoms. **B.** Significant increases in BOLD signal (red) were observed later in the attack, especially in the left visual cortex (ie, right of the image) but also in association cortex. **C.** Still later, increased BOLD signal had spread into the left hemisphere (ie, right of the image). The increases in BOLD signal might reflect vasodilation similar to that observed during early phases of cortical spreading depression. (Modified, with permission, from Cao Y, Welch KMA, Aurora S, et al. Functional MRI-BOLD of visually triggered headache in patients with migraine. *Arch Neurol.* 1999;56:548–554; and from James MF, Smith JM, Boniface SJ, et al. Cortical spreading depression and migraine: new insights from imaging. *Trends Neurosci.* 2001;24:266–271.)

vascular hypothesis states that vasodilation and constriction, which alter blood flow and cause relative ischemia, cause the cortical spreading depression.

Environmental and genetic factors associated with migraine may function to alter the threshold for cortical spreading depression. In support of this idea, the mutation in the P/Q Ca^{2+} channel linked to familial hemiplegic migraine has been shown in a mouse model to decrease the threshold of cortical spreading depression.

Treatment of Migraine

Typical treatment of migraine headaches incorporates both prophylactic and abortive strategies **19-2**. Agents such as the nonspecific β-adrenergic antagonists **propranolol** or **timolol,** antiepileptic agents such as **topiramate** and **carbamazepine,** tricyclic antidepressants

such as **amitriptyline,** and L-type Ca^{2+} channel blockers such as **verapamil** are taken daily to decrease headache frequency. The mechanisms by which these prophylactic medications work remain obscure, although it has been proposed that they inhibit the generation of cortical spreading depression and subsequent neurogenic inflammation.

When a migraine does occur, several abortive therapies are available. Abortive agents must be taken early in the headache for maximal efficacy and are less effective if taken after a full blown migraine has developed. For mild to moderate headaches, standard analgesic agents may be effective such as **aspirin, acetaminophen,** or **NSAIDs** (Chapter 11). However, these agents are not effective in treating severe migraines. Historically, nonselective serotonin agonists such as **ergotamine** **19-8** were widely used. More recently, selective agonists

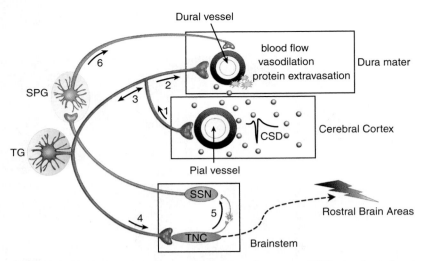

19-7 **Neurogenic hypothesis of migraine.** Cortical spreading depression (CSD) stimulates the trigeminovascular system, resulting in release of vasoactive neuropeptides (eg, calcitonin gene-related peptide, substance P, neurokinin A; gold triangles in nerve terminals) and other vasoactive molecules (eg, K^+, H^+, nitric oxide, adenosine, arachidonic acid metabolites; orange circles) into the extracellular and perivascular space and causes transient hyperemia and vasodilation in cortex, pial vessels, and dura mater. Within the perivascular space, these molecules activate or sensitize perivascular trigeminal afferents (arrow 1) and transmit impulses centrally to trigeminal ganglia (TG) and trigeminal nucleus caudalis (TNC) (arrows 3 and 4). Impulses from TNC are carried rostrally to brain structures involved in transmitting and processing pain. Dural trigeminal afferents are either directly activated or stimulated indirectly (via bifurcating axons; arrow 2) and possibly sensitized by edema (yellow stars) following the release of vasoactive neuropeptides. Activation of ipsilateral TNC, in turn, leads to stimulation of the superior salivatory nucleus (SSN; arrow 5) and parasympathetic efferents via the sphenopalatine ganglia (SPG) (arrow 6). Postganglionic parasympathetic fibers promote vasodilation and augment flow by releasing vasoactive intestinal polypeptide, nitric oxide, and acetylcholine (small blue circles in nerve terminals) into the dura mater. (From Bolay H, Reuter U, Dunn A, et al. Intrinsic brain activity triggers trigeminal meningeal afferents in a migraine model. *Nature Med.* 2002;8(2):136–142.)

19-2 **Examples of Drugs Used to Prevent Migraines[1]**

Drug	Potential Mechanism
ACE inhibitors	Enkephalinase inhibition, enhance antinociception
Anticonvulsants *Topiramate, valproate, gabapentin, lamotrigine*	Inhibit cortical spreading depression, block neurogenic inflammation, enhance antinociception
Antidepressants *TCAs, SNRIs, SSRIs*	Inhibit cortical spreading depression, enhance antinociception
β-adrenergic antagonists *Propranolol, timolol, nadolol, atenolol*	Inhibit cortical spreading depression, decrease sympathetic activity
Calcium channel antagonists *Flunarizine, verapamil*	Inhibit cortical spreading depression, block neurogenic inflammation

[1]Many of these treatments have not been validated in well-controlled clinical trials, and their use for migraine remains empirical.
TCA, tricyclic antidepressants; SNRIs, serotonin-norepinephrine reuptake inhibitors; SSRIs, selective-serotonin reuptake inhibitors.
Adapted from Silberstein SD. Preventive treatment of migraine. *Trends Pharmacol Sci.* 2006;27:410–415.

Sumatriptan

Zolmitriptan

Naratriptan

Rizatriptan

Eletriptan

Ergotamine

19-8 Chemical structures of triptan antimigraine drugs and the older medication, ergotamine.

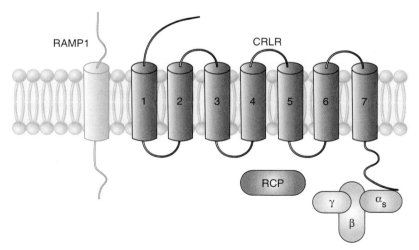

19-9 The calcitonin gene-related peptide (CGRP) receptor complex consists of a seven-transmembrane G protein-coupled calcitonin receptor-like receptor (CRLR) linked to receptor activity modifying protein 1 (**RAMP1**). RAMP1 is involved in receptor trafficking and ligand binding. CGRP-receptor component protein (RCP) is a 17-kDa intracellular protein, which is important for coupling the receptor with G proteins (G protein α, β, and γ subunits are shown).

at the $5HT_{1B/D}$ receptor, which belong to a class of agents called **triptans**, have been shown to be highly effective and have largely transformed the treatment of migraine headache and its associated neurologic and other symptoms (eg, nausea and vomiting). Several triptans are currently marketed in the United States, including **sumatriptan, zolmitriptan, naratriptan, rizatriptan,** and **eletriptan** `19-8`. $5HT_{1B/D}$ receptors are inhibitory autoreceptors on presynaptic serotonergic nerve terminals; the $5HT_{1B}$ receptor is expressed in rodents, and the $5HT_{1D}$ receptor is expressed in humans (Chapter 6). However, the mechanisms by which activation of these receptors alleviates the symptoms of migraine remain unclear. Receptor agonists are thought to act as vasoconstrictors that return dilated blood vessels to normal caliber. This may be achieved by blocking CGRP (and perhaps substance P) release from trigeminal nerve terminals, which has been observed in animal models. In human trials, **NK_1 receptor antagonists** did not relieve migraine symptoms, but in early, small trials, **CGRP receptor antagonists** show promise. The CGRP receptor is anomalous for a G protein-coupled receptor in that the typical seven-transmembrane receptor protein appears to require two additional subunits for activity `19-9`. This novel structure may assist in the development of selective CGRP receptor antagonists.

SELECTED READING

Amerenco P, Bougousslav J, Callahan A, et al. Stroke Prevention by Aggressive Reduction in Cholesterol Levels (SPARCL) investigators. High dose Atorvastatin after stroke or transient ischemia event. *N Engl J Med.* 2006;355:549–559.

Bolay H, Reuter U, Dunn A, et al. Intrinsic brain activity triggers trigeminal meningeal afferents in a migraine model. *Nature Med.* 2002;8: 136–142.

Brain SD. Poyner DR. Hill RG. CGRP receptors: a headache to study, but will antagonists prove therapeutic in migraine. *Trends Pharmacol Sci.* 2002;23: 51–53.

Chollet F, DiPiero V, Wise RJ, et al. The functional anatomy of motor recovery after stroke in humans: a study with positron emission tomography. *Ann Neurol.* 1991;29:63–71.

Coughlin SR. Thrombin signaling and protease-activated receptors. *Nature.* 2000;407:258–264.

Culman J, Zhao Y, Gohlke P, et al. PPAR-gamma: therapeutic target for ischemic stroke. *Trends Pharmacol. Sci.* 2007;28:244–249.

Dalkara T, Zervas NT, Moskowitz MA. From spreading depression to the trigeminovascular system. *Neurol Sci.* 2006;27:S86–S90.

Dawson VL, Dawson TM. Nitric oxide in neurodegeneration. *Prog Brain Res.* 1998;118:215–229.

Doods H, Arndt K, Rudolf K, et al. CGRP antagonists: unraveling the role of CGRP in migraine. *Trends Pharmacol Sci.* 2007;28:580–587.

Endres M, Laufs U, Liao JK, et al. Targeting eNOS for stroke protection. *Trends Neurosci.* 2004;27:283–289.

Green AR, Hainsworth AH, Jackson DM. GABA potentiation: a logical pharmacological approach for the treatment of acute ischemic stroke. *Neuropharmacology.* 2000;39:1483–1494.

Heart Protection Study Collaborative Group. Effects of cholesterol lowering with simvastatin on stroke and other major vascular events in 20,536 people with cerebrovascular disease and other high-risk conditions. *Lancet.* 2004;363:757–767.

James MF, Smith JM, Boniface SJ, et al. Cortical spreading depression and migraine: new insights from imaging. *Trends Neurosci.* 2001;24:266–271.

Johnston SC. Clinical practice. Transient ischemic attack. *N Engl J Med.* 2002;347:1687–1692.

Leifer D. Neuronal plasticity and recovery from stroke. *The Neuroscientist.* 1998;4:68–70.

Majerus PW, Tollefsen DM. Anticoagulant, thrombolytic, and antiplatelet drugs. In: Hardman JG, Limbird LE, eds. *Goodman and Gilman's The Pharmacological Basis of Therapeutics,* 10th ed. New York: McGraw-Hill; 2001:1519–1538.

May A, Matharu M. New insights into migraine: application of functional and structural imaging. *Curr Opin Neurol* 2007;20:306–309.

Mehdiratta M, Caplan LR. Stroke thrombolysis 2006: an update progress in cardiovascular diseases. *Prog Cardiovasc Dis.* 2007;49:430–438.

Muir KW, Tyrell P, Sattar N, et al. Inflammation and ischemic stroke. *Curr Opin Neurol.* 2007;20: 334–342.

Nudo RJ, Wise BM, SiFuentes F, et al. Neural substrates for the effects of rehabilitative training on motor recovery after ischemic infarct. *Science.* 1996;272: 1791–1794.

Patrono C, Garcia Rodriguez LA, Landolfi R, et al. Low-dose aspirin for the prevention of atherothrombosis. *N Engl J Med.* 2005;353:2373–2383.

Pietrobon D, Striessnig J. Neurobiology of migraine. *Nature Rev Neurosci.* 2003;4:386–398.

Ropper AH, Brown RH. *Adams and Victor's Principles of Neurology,* 8th ed. New York: McGraw-Hill; 2005.

Sacco RL, Chong JY, Prabhakaren S, et al. Experimental treatments for acute ischemic stroke. *Lancet.* 2007;369:331–341.

Silberstein SD. Preventive treatment of migraine. *Trends Pharmacol Sci.* 1006;27:410–415.

Suwanwela N, Koroshetz WJ. Acute ischemic stroke: overview of recent therapeutic developments. *Annu Rev Med.* 2007;58:89–106.

van der Worp HB, van Gijn J. Clinical practice. Acute ischemic stroke. *N Engl J Med.* 2007;357: 572–579.

Waeber C, Moskowitz MA Migraine as an inflammatory disorder. *Neurology.* 2005;64:S9–S15.

Warfarin Aspirin Symptomatic Intracranial Disease (WASID) Investigators. Warfarin vs aspirin for symptomatic intracranial stenosis: subgroup analysis from WASID. *Neurology.* 2006;67:1275–1278.

INDEX

Page numbers followed by *f* or *t* indicate figures or tables, respectively.